Video Contents

*Used with the permission of the American Academy of Facial Plastic and Reconstructive Surgery.

Master Techniques
in Rhinoplasty

Master Techniques in Rhinoplasty

■ **BABAK AZIZZADEH**, MD, FACS
Director
The Center for Advanced Facial Plastic Surgery;
Associate Clinical Professor
David Geffen School of Medicine at UCLA;
Attending Surgeon
Cedars-Sinai Medical Center
Beverly Hills, California

■ **MARK R. MURPHY**, MD
Director
Palm Beach Facial Plastic Surgery
Palm Beach Gardens, Florida

■ **CALVIN M. JOHNSON**, Jr., MD, FACS
Clinical Associate Professor
Department of Otolaryngology–Head and Neck Surgery
Tulane University School of Medicine;
Director
Hedgewood Surgical Center
New Orleans, Louisiana

■ **WILLIAM NUMA**, MD, FACS
Clinical Instructor
Harvard Medical School
Massachusetts Eye and Ear Infirmary;
Director
Beacon Facial Plastic Surgery
Boston, Massachusetts

ELSEVIER
SAUNDERS

SAUNDERS

1600 John F. Kennedy Boulevard
Ste 1800
Philadelphia, Pennsylvania 19103

Library of Congress Cataloging-in-Publication Data

Master techniques in rhinoplasty / [edited by] Babak Azizzadeh ... [et al.].—1st ed.
    p. ; cm.
  Includes bibliographical references and index.
  ISBN 978-1-4160-6262-2 (hardcover : alk. paper) 1. Rhinoplasty—Technique. I. Azizzadeh, Babak.
  [DNLM: 1. Rhinoplasty—methods. MV 312]
  RD119.5.N67M29 2011
  617.5'230592—dc22

                                                    2011008709

Acquisitions Editor: Stefanie Jewell Thomas
Developmental Editor: Lisa Barnes
Editorial Assistant: Sheila Smith
Publishing Services Manager: Pat Joiner-Myers
Designer: Lou Forgione

Printed in China

Last digit is the print number: 9 8 7 6 5 4 3 2 1

Contributors

Editors

Babak Azizzadeh, MD, FACS
Director
The Center for Advanced Facial Plastic Surgery;
Associate Clinical Professor
David Geffen School of Medicine at UCLA;
Attending Surgeon
Cedars-Sinai Medical Center
Beverly Hills, California
Mandibular Implants, Middle Eastern Rhinoplasty, Nasal Airway Obstruction

Mark R. Murphy, MD
Director
Palm Beach Facial Plastic Surgery
Palm Beach Gardens, Florida

Calvin M. Johnson, Jr., MD, FACS
Clinical Associate Professor
Department of Otolaryngology–Head and Neck Surgery
Tulane University School of Medicine;
Director
Hedgewood Surgical Center
New Orleans, Louisiana
Surgical Anatomy and Physiology of the Nose, Primary Open Structure Rhinoplasty

William Numa, MD, FACS
Clinical Instructor
Harvard Medical School
Massachusetts Eye and Ear Infirmary;
Director
Beacon Facial Plastic Surgery
Boston, Massachusetts
Surgical Anatomy and Physiology of the Nose, Primary Open Structure Rhinoplasty, Mestizo Rhinoplasty

Contributors

Peter A. Adamson, MD, FRCSC, FACS
Professor and Head
Division of Facial Plastic and Reconstructive Surgery
Department of Otolaryngology–Head and Neck Surgery
University of Toronto;
Staff Surgeon
Toronto General Hospital–University Health Network
Toronto, Ontario, Canada
The Psychology of Rhinoplasty: Lessons Learned from Fellowship, Postrhinoplasty Nasal Lobule Deformities: Open Approach

Kamal A. Batniji, MD, FACS
Attending
Hoag Memorial Hospital Presbyterian
Department of Otolaryngology–Head and Neck Surgery
Newport Beach, California
Repair of Acute Nasal Fracture

Rami K. Batniji, MD, FACS
Attending
Hoag Memorial Hospital Presbyterian
Department of Plastic Surgery
Department of Otolaryngology–Head and Neck Surgery
Newport Beach, California
Repair of Acute Nasal Fracture

Daniel G. Becker, MD, FACS
Clinical Associate Professor
Department of Otolaryngology–Head and Neck Surgery
University of Pennsylvania
Philadelphia, Pennsylvania;
Clinical Associate Professor
Otolaryngology–Head and Neck Surgery
University of Virginia
Charlottesville, Virginia
Reducing Complications in Rhinoplasty

Madeleine A. Becker, MD
Associate Director of Consultation-Liaison Psychiatry
Thomas Jefferson University Hospital
Department of Psychiatry and Human Behavior
Philadelphia, Pennsylvania
Reducing Complications in Rhinoplasty

William J. Binder, MD, FACS
Associate Clinical Professor
Department of Head and Neck Surgery
UCLA School of Medicine;
Attending Surgeon
Department of Head and Neck Surgery
Cedars-Sinai Medical Center
Los Angeles, California
Mandibular Implants

Jason A. Bloom, MD
Facial Plastic and Reconstructive Surgeon
Otolaryngology–Head and Neck Surgery
New York University Langone Medical Center
New York, New York
Reducing Complications in Rhinoplasty

Kevin Brenner, MD, FACS
Attending Plastic Surgeon
Cedars-Sinai Medical Center
Department of Surgery, Division of Plastic Surgery
Los Angeles, California;
Attending, Plastic Surgery
Box Clinic for Aesthetic and Reconstructive Surgery
Department of Plastic Surgery
Beverly Hills, California
Rib Grafting Simplified, Saddle Nose Deformity

Michael J. Brenner, MD, FACS
Assistant Professor of Surgery
Division of Otolaryngology–Head and Neck Surgery
Southern Illinois University School of Medicine;
Facial Plastic and Reconstructive Surgeon
Otolaryngology–Head and Neck Surgery
Saint John's Medical Center
Springfield, Illinois
*Evaluation and Correction of the Crooked Nose, Thin Skin
Rhinoplasty: Aesthetic Considerations and Surgical Approach*

Jay Calvert, MD, FACS
Private Practice
Beverly Hills, California;
Cedars-Sinai Medical Center
Los Angeles, California;
Hoag Hospital
Newport Beach, California
Rib Grafting Simplified, Saddle Nose Deformity

Mack L. Cheney, MD
Professor
Department of Otology and Laryngology
Harvard Medical School;
Division of Facial Plastic and Reconstructive Surgery
Massachusetts Eye and Ear Infirmary
Boston, Massachusetts
Calvarial Bone Grafting in Rhinoplasty

Robert J. Chiu, MD
Private Practice
Today's Cosmetic Surgery & Laser Center
Pittsburgh, Pennsylvania
The Management of Alar–Columellar Disproportion

Chia Chung, MD
Division of Plastic and Reconstructive Surgery
University of California San Francisco School of Medicine
San Francisco, California
Suturing Techniques to Refine the Nasal Tip

Roxana Cobo, MD
Chief
Private Practice
Service of Otolaryngology
Centro Medico Imbanaco
Cali, Colombia
Mestizo Rhinoplasty

C. Spencer Cochran, MD
Clinical Assistant Professor
Department of Otolaryngology–Head and Neck Surgery
University of Texas Southwestern Medical Center at Dallas
Dallas, Texas
Secondary Rhinoplasty via the External Approach

Marc Cohen, MD
Assistant Clinical Professor
Division of Head and Neck Surgery
David Geffen School of Medicine at UCLA
Los Angeles, California
Nasal Septal Perforation Repair

Minas Constantinides, MD, FACS
Director of Facial Plastic and Reconstructive Surgery
Department of Otolaryngology–Head and Neck Surgery
New York University School of Medicine;
Attending Physician
Department of Otolaryngology–Head and Neck Surgery
New York University Medical Center
New York, New York
The Large Nose

Ted A. Cook, MD
Professor
Department of Otolaryngology–Head and Neck Surgery
Division of Facial Plastic and Reconstructive Surgery
Oregon Health and Science University School of Medicine;
Department of Otolaryngology–Head and Neck Surgery
Division of Facial Plastic and Reconstructive Surgery
Oregon Health and Science University Hospitals
Portland, Oregon
The Middle Vault: Upper Lateral Cartilage Modifications

Richard E. Davis, MD, FACS
Director
The Center for Facial Restoration
Miramar, Florida;
Professor of Otolaryngology (Voluntary)
The University of Miami Miller School of Medicine
Miami, Florida
The Thick-Skinned Rhinoplasty Patient

Raffi Der Sarkissian, MD, FACS
Assistant Clinical Professor
Division of Facial Plastic Surgery
Boston University School of Medicine;
Staff Physician
Division of Facial Plastic Surgery
Massachusetts Eye and Ear Infirmary;
Staff Physician
The Boston Center for Plastic Surgery
Boston, Massachusetts
Cartilage Grafting in Rhinoplasty and Nasal Reconstruction

Brian W. Downs, MD
Evergreen ENT and Facial Plastic Surgery
Morganton, North Carolina
The Middle Vault: Upper Lateral Cartilage Modifications

Frank P. Fechner, MD
Instructor
Department of Otology and Laryngology
Harvard Medical School;
Assistant
Facial Plastic and Reconstructive Surgery
Massachusetts Eye and Ear Infirmary
Boston, Massachusetts;
Active Medical Staff
Department of Otolaryngology
University of Massachusetts Medical Center;
Affiliate
Department of Otolaryngology
University of Massachusetts Medical School
Worcester, Massachusetts
The Large Nose

Kenton Fong, MD
Division of Plastic and Reconstructive Surgery
Stanford University School of Medicine
Stanford, California
Suturing Techniques to Refine the Nasal Tip

Andrew S. Frankel, MD
Associate Professor
Department of Otolaryngology
Keck School of Medicine
University of Southern California
Los Angeles, California;
Private Practice
Lasky Clinic
Beverly Hills, California
Nasal Analysis

Alvin I. Glasgold, MD, FACS
Clinical Professor
Surgery
University of Medicine and Dentistry of New Jersey
Robert Wood Johnson Medical
New Brunswick, New Jersey;
Private Practice
Glasgold Group Plastic Surgery
Highland Park, New Jersey
The Mobile Tripod Technique: A Universal Approach to Nasal Tip Modification

Robert A. Glasgold, MD, FACS
Clinical Assistant Professor
Department of Surgery
University of Medicine and Dentistry of New Jersey
Robert Wood Johnson Medical
New Brunswick, New Jersey;
Private Practice
Glasgold Group Plastic Surgery
Highland Park, New Jersey
The Mobile Tripod Technique: A Universal Approach to Nasal Tip Modification

Ryan M. Greene, MD, PhD
Fellow
Department of Otolaryngology–Head and Neck Surgery
Division of Facial Plastic and Reconstructive Surgery
University of Miami
Miami, Florida
A History of Modern-Day Rhinoplasty; Rhinoplasty in the Aging Patient

Ronald P. Gruber, MD
Division of Plastic and Reconstructive Surgery
Stanford University School of Medicine
Stanford, California;
Division of Plastic and Reconstructive Surgery
University of California, San Francisco
San Francisco, California
Suturing Techniques to Refine the Nasal Tip

David Gudis, MD
Resident
Department of Otorhinolaryngology–Head and Neck Surgery
University of Pennsylvania Health System
Hospital of the University of Pennsylvania
Philadelphia, Pennsylvania
Reducing Complications in Rhinoplasty

Jack P. Gunter, MD
Clinical Professor
Department of Otolaryngology–Head and Neck Surgery
Department of Plastic Surgery
University of Texas Southwestern Medical Center at Dallas
Dallas, Texas
Secondary Rhinoplasty via the External Approach

Tessa A. Hadlock, MD
Associate Professor
Department of Otology and Laryngology
Harvard Medical School;
Director of Facial Nerve Center
Department of Otology
Massachusetts Eye and Ear Infirmary
Boston, Massachusetts
Calvarial Bone Grafting in Rhinoplasty

Peter A. Hilger, MD, FACS
Professor
Department of Otolaryngology
Division of Facial Plastic Surgery
University of Minnesota;
University-Fairview Hospital
Minneapolis, Minnesota;
Regions Hospital
St. Paul, Minnesota
Evaluation and Correction of the Crooked Nose, Thin Skin Rhinoplasty: Aesthetic Considerations and Surgical Approach

Raj Kanodia, MD
Staff Member
Department of Otolaryngology
Hollywood Community Hospital
Los Angeles, California;
Camden Surgery Center
Beverly Hills, California
Endonasal Rhinoplasty: Transcartilaginous Approach

Sanjay P. Keni, MD
Director
Keni Facial Plastic Surgery Center
Palos Heights, Illinois, and Chicago, Illinois;
Active Medical Staff
Department of Surgery
Division of Otolaryngology
Atlanticare Regional Medical Center
Atlantic City, New Jersey
The Mobile Tripod Technique: A Universal Approach to Nasal Tip Modification

William A. Kennedy, III, MD
Attending Surgeon
Department of Head and Neck Surgery
Albert Einstein University;
Attending Surgeon
Department of Head and Neck Surgery
North Shore/LIJ Hospital
New York, New York
Mandibular Implants

Michael M. Kim, MD
Assistant Professor
Department of Otorhinolaryngology
Mayo Clinic Arizona
Phoenix, Arizona
Short Nose

Russell W. H. Kridel, MD, FACS
Clinical Professor and Director
Department of Otolarygology–Head and Neck Surgery
Division of Facial Plastic and Reconstructive Surgery
University of Texas Health Sciences Center, Houston
Houston, Texas
The Management of Alar–Columellar Disproportion

Samuel M. Lam, MD, FACS
Director
Lam Facial Plastic Surgery Center & Hair Restoration Institute
Willow Bend Wellness Center
Plano, Texas
Asian Rhinoplasty

Babak Larian, MD, FACS
Assistant Clinical Professor of Surgery
University of California, Los Angeles
Los Angeles, California;
Director
Cedars-Sinai Head and Neck Cancer Center
Beverly Hills, California
Nasal Airway Obstruction

Arnold Lee, MD
Director
Facial Plastic and Reconstructive Surgery;
Assistant Professor
Otolaryngology–Head and Neck Surgery
Tufts Medical Center
Boston, Massachusetts
Nasal Reconstruction

Kimberly Lee, MD
Assistant Clinical Professor of Surgery
Division of Head and Neck Surgery
David Geffen School of Medicine at UCLA;
Attending Physician
Division of Head and Neck Surgery
Cedars-Sinai Medical Center
Los Angeles, California;
Director
Beverly Hills Facial Plastic Surgery Center
Beverly Hills, California
Nasal Airway Obstruction

Robin W. Lindsay, MD
Assistant Professor of Surgery
Department of Otolaryngology–Head and Neck Surgery
Uniformed Services University of the Health Sciences;
Attending Surgeon
Department of Otolaryngology–Head and Neck Surgery
National Naval Medical Center
Bethesda, Maryland
Calvarial Bone Grafting in Rhinoplasty

Jason A. Litner, MD, FRCSC
Private Practice
Profiles Beverly Hills
Beverly Hills, California
The Psychology of Rhinoplasty: Lessons Learned from Fellowship,
Postrhinoplasty Nasal Lobule Deformities: Open Approach

Grigoriy Mashkevich, MD
Assistant Professor
Otolaryngology–Head and Neck Surgery
New York Medical College
Valhalla, New York;
Assistant Professor
Otolaryngology–Head and Neck Surgery
Division of Facial Plastic Surgery and Reconstructive Surgery
New York Eye and Ear Infirmary
New York, New York
Middle Eastern Rhinoplasty

Kate Elizabeth McCarn, MD
Resident Physician
Otolaryngology–Head and Neck Surgery
Oregon Health and Science University
Portland, Oregon
The Middle Vault: Upper Lateral Cartilage Modifications

Umang Mehta, MD
Department of Otolaryngology–Head and Neck Surgery
Keck School of Medicine
University of Southern California
Los Angeles, California;
Lasky Clinic
Beverly Hills, California
Nasal Analysis

Sam P. Most, MD, FACS
Associate Professor
Chief, Division of Facial Plastic and Reconstructive Surgery
Department of Otolaryngology–Head and Neck Surgery
Stanford University School of Medicine
Stanford, California
Nasal Osteotomies

Paul S. Nassif, MD, FACS
Assistant Clinical Professor
Department of Otolaryngology
Division of Facial Plastic and Reconstructive Surgery
University of Southern California School of Medicine;
Attending Physician
Cedars-Sinai Medical Center
Department of Ear, Nose, and Throat
Los Angeles, California
African American Rhinoplasty

Gilbert Nolst Trenité, MD, PhD
Professor Doctor
Ear, Nose, and Throat Department
Academic Medical Center
Amsterdam, The Netherlands
Correction of the Pinched Nasal Tip Deformity

Aric Park, MD
Fellow
Facial Plastic and Reconstructive Surgery
University of Southern California
Los Angeles, California
Nasal Reconstruction

Amit Patel, MD
Assistant Professor
Facial Plastic and Reconstructive Surgery
Department of Surgery
University of Kentucky
AB Chandler Medical Center
Lexington, Kentucky
*Primary Endonasal Rhinoplasty: Double-Dome Technique via
Intercartilaginous Dome-Delivery*

Anand D. Patel, MD
Facial Plastic Surgeon
Devenir Aesthetics
Austin, Texas
The Management of Alar–Columellar Disproportion

Santdeep H. Paun, FRCS
Consultant Surgeon
Nasal and Facial Plastic Surgery
Departmental Lead Clinician
St. Bartholomew's Hospital
London, England
Correction of the Pinched Nasal Tip Deformity

James M. Pearson, MD
Clinical Assistant Professor
Department of Otolaryngology
University of Rochester;
Department of Otolaryngology
Stone Memorial Hospital
Rochester, New York
The Underprojected Nose and Ptotic Tip

Stephen W. Perkins, MD
Clinical Associate Professor
Department of Otolaryngology–Head and Neck Surgery
Indiana University School of Medicine;
President
Meridian Plastic Surgery Center;
President
Meridian Plastic Surgeons
Indianapolis, Indiana
*Primary Endonasal Rhinoplasty: Double-Dome Technique via
Intercartilaginous Dome-Delivery*

Annette M. Pham, MD
Fellow
Department of Otolaryngology–Head and Neck Surgery
Division of Facial Plastic and Reconstructive Surgery
University of Miami
Miami, Florida
A History of Modern-Day Rhinoplasty

Vito C. Quatela, MD, FACS
Clinical Associate Professor
Department of Otolaryngology
University of Rochester;
Department of Otolaryngology–Head and Neck Surgery
Strong Memorial Hospital
Quatela Center for Plastic Surgery
Rochester, New York
The Underprojected Nose and Ptotic Tip

Jeffrey D. Rawnsley, MD
Clinical Associate Professor
Director, Facial Aesthetic Surgery
Division of Head and Neck Surgery
David Geffen School of Medicine at UCLA;
Attending Surgeon
UCLA Division of Head and Neck Surgery
Ronald Reagan Medical Center
Los Angeles, California
Nasal Septal Perforation Repair

Anthony P. Sclafani, MD, FACS
Professor
Department of Otolaryngology
New York Medical College
Valhalla, New York;
Director of Facial Plastic Surgery
Department of Otolaryngology
The New York Eye and Ear Infirmary
New York, New York;
Attending Surgeon
Institute for Aesthetic Surgery and Medicine
Northern Westchester Hospital Center
Mount Kisco, New York
Alloplasts in Nasal Surgery

Anil R. Shah, MD, FACS
Clinical Instructor
Otolaryngology–Head and Neck Surgery
University of Chicago
Chicago, Illinois
Endonasal Rhinoplasty: Transcartilaginous Approach

Robert L. Simons, MD, FACS
Clinical Professor
Department of Otolaryngology–Head and Neck Surgery
Division of Facial Plastic and Reconstructive Surgery
University of Miami;
Medical Board Chairman
The Miami Institute for Age Management and Intervention
Miami, Florida
A History of Modern Day Rhinoplasty

Peyman Solieman, MD
Private Practice
Profiles Beverly Hills
Beverly Hills, California
Postrhinoplasty Nasal Lobule Deformities: Open Approach

Jacob Steiger, MD
Boca Regional Hospital
Steiger Facial Plastic Surgery
Boca Raton, Florida
Reducing Complications in Rhinoplasty

Ravi S. Swamy, MD, MPH
Department of Otolaryngology–Head and Neck Surgery
Stanford University School of Medicine
Stanford, California
Nasal Osteotomies

Jonathan M. Sykes, MD, FACS
Professor and Director of Facial Plastic and Reconstructive Surgery
Department of Otolaryngology
University of California Davis Medical Center;
Faculty
Department of Otolaryngology
Mercy San Juan
Sacramento, California;
Faculty
Department of Otolaryngology
Sutter Roseville
Roseville, California
Cleft Lip Rhinoplasty

Wyatt C. To, MD
Director
Facial Plastic Surgery
The Cosmetic and Skin Surgery Center
Frederick, Maryland
Primary Open Structure Rhinoplasty

Dean M. Toriumi, MD
Professor
Division of Facial Plastic and Reconstructive Surgery
Department of Otolaryngology–Head and Neck Surgery
University of Illinois, Chicago
Chicago, Illinois
Rhinoplasty in the Aging Patient

Tom D. Wang, MD
Professor
Department of Otolaryngology–Head and Neck Surgery
Division of Facial Plastic and Reconstructive Surgery
Oregon Health and Science University
Portland, Oregon
The Middle Vault: Upper Lateral Cartilage Modifications, Short Nose

Preface

When deciding to embark on this project, we set out to delineate a comprehensive book demonstrating conventional as well as alternative and competing techniques and concepts in rhinoplasty.

This text compiles a number of different rhinoplasty techniques from those who do it best. We have selected contributing authors from different backgrounds based on their accomplishments and expertise in rhinoplasty. Only time-tested techniques are being presented in the text to ensure that both young and experienced surgeons can master the essentials and subtleties of aesthetic and functional rhinoplasty.

Some techniques described in this book will be more technically challenging to execute than others, and some may require more patience, skill, or practice. Some techniques will be more predictable and leave less of the final surgical outcome to the seemingly capricious nature of the contracture associated with the cicatricial healing process, and yet some others may even fall into disfavor with time because of dissatisfaction with their long-term outcome after a seemingly excellent short-term result. However, all the techniques described in this book and in all subsequent publications by any authors that follow us and those who precede us, constitute an integral part of the constant learning process associated with becoming students with voracious appetites for the art and science of rhinoplasty. We hope reading this book will elicit a healthy exchange of information enriching our collective experience, rather than generate a reflexive reaction toward any given technique we happen to be less familiar with. Our apprentices will become our teachers and vice versa several times over.

Once the reader assimilates the foundations of the applied basic sciences, the different surgical techniques, personal preferences, and, most important, the rationale for those preferences, the surgical process is described in detail through text, illustrations, intraoperative photographs, and a highly detailed comprehensive surgical atlas on DVD. By providing these components, we hope to inspire the next generation of master rhinoplasty surgeons.

Babak Azizzadeh
Mark R. Murphy
Calvin M. Johnson, Jr.
William Numa

Acknowledgments

We would like to thank the numerous friends, family, and colleagues who have contributed to the completion of this text. Foremost, we need to acknowledge those who have introduced us to this fine art, our mentors, Calvin Johnson, Norman Pastorek, Tessa Hadlock, Vito Quatela, Keith Blackwell, Mack Cheney, Mark Varvares, Daniel Deschler, and Anthony Labruna. You have been both patient and demanding. By constantly insisting on the pursuit of perfection and providing reassurance during its humbling path, we owe our sincere gratitude.

To our colleagues Babak Larian, Guy Massry, Paul Nassif, Robert Glasgold, and Samuel Lam. Your constant, honest communication has helped us continue to move the field forward where our mentors left off.

We also need to thank those whose tireless efforts have made possible the completion and production of this text, Lisa Barnes, Rebecca Gaertner, Stefanie Jewell-Thomas, Alex Baker, the wonderful staff at Elsevier, and the AAFPRS and its audiovisual department staff.

And to those who have inspired us to pursue this wonderful career, Robert Murphy, Dr. Siamak Daneshmand, and Dr. Amiro Tamara.

Finally, we must also acknowledge our patients who have trusted us in the most personal way. It is for them and future patients that this text attempts to serve.

Babak Azizzadeh
Mark R. Murphy
Calvin M. Johnson, Jr.
William Numa

Contents

CHAPTER ONE

A History of Modern-Day Rhinoplasty

Robert L. Simons • Annette M. Pham • Ryan M. Greene

INTRODUCTION

From the *Edwin Smith Surgical Papyrus* to the Sushruta legacy to early nasal surgery techniques, the roots of modern-day rhinoplasty stem from the early beginnings of nasal reconstruction. Early on, it was recognized that the nose was a complex structure, a prominent and central feature of the face that was susceptible to disfigurement by trauma, infection, tumors, and even punishment. For this reason, mutilation, deformity, or an unattractive nose was linked to a social stigma, which then supported the necessity for the development of nasal reconstructive techniques. Understanding the complexities of the nose through reconstruction allowed pioneers in nasal surgery to embark upon the exploration of corrective surgery, or cosmetic rhinoplasty, for aesthetic purposes. It is this journey through time that will be traced to understand the history of contemporary rhinoplasty.

EARLY BEGINNINGS

The oldest known surgical treatise is known as the *Edwin Smith Surgical Papyrus*. While the exact dating is controversial, it is believed to have dated back to around 1600 BC.[1,2] In 1862, the treatise was discovered and purchased in Egypt by an American egyptologist, Edward Smith. It was later translated from its ancient hieroglyphic script in 1930.[1]

The treatise describes the diagnosis and surgical management for 48 cases. Among these cases, three involved the management of different types of nasal fractures. The treatment was simple—nasal manipulation with placement of external splints, such as those made from thin wood padded with linen, and nasal packing made of lint, swabs, or plugs of linen.[1,3] Thus, it is apparent that even in early civilizations, the importance of the basic principles of fracture stabilization after manipulation as well as internal lining support with packing was well recognized and documented.

THE SUSHRUTA LEGACY AND THE INDIAN METHOD

The art and science of total nasal reconstruction are thought to have originated in India with the work of a prominent figure, Sushruta, whose name literally meant "the one who is well heard" or "the one who has thoroughly learned by hearing."[4] Although his precise age is controversial, Sushruta probably lived around 1000 to 800 BC, a period known as "The Golden Age" in ancient India.[4] His greatest contribution to surgery was his description of nasal reconstructive surgeries, using different methods for a variety of nasal defects. One method, in particular, used skin from the forehead as a pedicled flap, which later was referred to as the "Indian method."

THE ITALIAN METHOD

The knowledge of nasal reconstructive surgery then spread from India to Arabia to Persia and finally to Europe. This undoubtedly occurred as the world became smaller and different civilizations had greater communication and contact through wartimes and invasion by leaders such as Alexander the Great. However, this period of shared information came to a halt when religious leaders forbade medical discoveries and exploration, as a manual occupation such as surgery was considered beneath respectable men and even borderline heretic.

With the revival of scholasticism in Europe during the fifteenth and sixteenth centuries, an interest in reconstructive plastic surgery was renewed. Nasal reconstruction was again revisited, and this time, for reconstruction of a nasal defect, the Branca family of Sicily described the use of an arm flap.[2] Although first described by them, this "Italian method" of reconstruction was credited to Gasparo Tagliacozzi (1546–1599), a professor of anatomy at Bologna. He wrote scientifically and philosophically on the subject in his treatise entitled *De Curtorum Chirurgia per Institionem, Libri Duo*.[1]

THE DEVELOPMENT OF CORRECTIVE RHINOPLASTY

Ultimately, one must be reminded that tracing the journey through time from Egypt to India to Europe is relevant in understanding that the roots of corrective rhinoplasty stem from reconstructive surgery. With the development of reconstructive techniques, surgeons began to better understand the complexity of nasal structure, form, and function. The basic principles of reconstruction became established with emphasis on the importance of a proper *nasal framework*, *endonasal lining*, and *external skin covering*. As a result, surgeons became free to explore how best to correct nasal deformities.

In 1818, the highly esteemed German surgeon Carl von Graefe (1787–1840) became the first to coin the term "rhinoplasty" when he published his major work entitled *Rhinoplastik*. von Graefe detailed in his book three successful rhinoplasties—the first using the Indian method with a forehead flap technique; the second, the Tagliacotian method; and the third, a modified free arm graft that he called the German method.[1] The textbook itself was 208 pages long and listed 55 previous books and articles, the most recent being that of a British surgeon named Joseph Carpue (1764–1846).[3] In an 1816 article, Carpue had described two successful nasal restorations using the Indian method originally described by Sushruta.[1]

Thus far, with all of the nasal reconstructive techniques, surgeries were described with great attention to detail and illustrations. An underlying theme throughout the description was a stated need to strike a balance between the need for the surgery in order to correct a deformity with the willingness of the patient to withstand the "barbaric" procedures without a reliable form of anesthesia. However, the inception of aseptic technique mainstreamed by Lister in the 1840s and the introduction of anesthetics, including the use of topical cocaine, brought about a new era in plastic surgery—corrective, or cosmetic, surgery. The background was now set for surgeons to explore methods for correction of more than an obvious deformity secondary to trauma, infection, or tumors; rather, to embark upon the task of corrective surgery for aesthetic purposes.

In 1845, the background was thus set for the renowned Berlin professor Johann Friedrich Dieffenbach (1792–1847) to introduce the idea of revision surgery on the reconstructed nose to improve the cosmetic outcome.[3] It was he who wrote, "The nose is man's most paradoxical organ. It has its root above, its back in front, its wings below, and one likes best of all to poke it into places where it does not belong."[5]

In addition, Dieffenbach is credited with making surgery more tolerable with the use of anesthesia. He wrote a comprehensive textbook entitled *Operative Chirurgie* and described the use of external incisions as well as excisions to correct nasal deformities (Figure 1-1). It is interesting to note that in that time period, surgeons were preoccupied with external approaches, even for placement of dorsal augmentation grafts (via longitudinal and glabellar incisions) for correction of saddle-nose deformities, as described by Israel and von Mangold.[5]

As a result, it was almost unheard of to perform a proper rhinoplasty with a completely intranasal approach until 1887, when John Orlando Roe (1849–1915) (Figure 1-2), an otolaryngologist from Rochester, New York, produced his landmark paper, "The Deformity Termed Pug Nose and Its Correction by a Simple Operation."[5] In this paper, Roe described the first endonasal rhinoplasty to

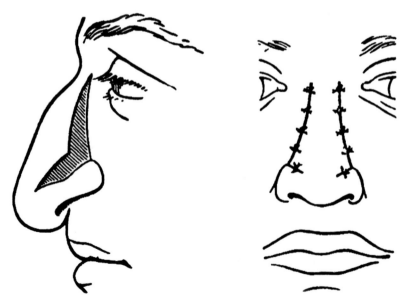

Figure 1-1 Dieffenbach's method of external excisions to alter the size of the nose. (From Davis JS. Plastic surgery: its principles pand practice. Philadelphia: P. Blakiston's Son & Co., 1919.)

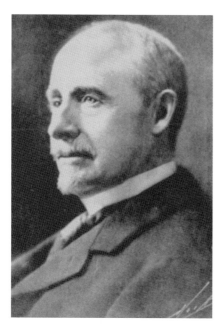

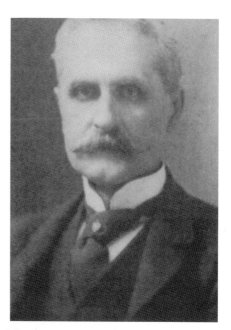

correct the tip in a patient with a "pug nose." Following this, in 1891, he published another paper discussing an aesthetic rhinoplasty in which the entire nose was addressed, including refinement of the tip and reduction of a prominent dorsal hump.

The following year, in 1892, Robert Weir (1838–1927) (Figure 1-3) published his data on using grafts to restore "sunken noses," or the saddle-nose deformity.[1] He also described a case of a corrective rhinoplasty performed in separate stages. He used Roe's endonasal technique for reducing the dorsal hump and narrowing the nose. Then, in another, separate procedure, he reduced the width of the nasal tip as well as the nasal alae by wedge resections, which to this day are still referred to as "Weir incisions."[1]

THE FATHER OF MODERN RHINOPLASTY

Chronologically, although the two American surgeons, Roe and Weir, were the first to describe their work in corrective rhinoplasty, the man who is credited with the title of "father of modern rhinoplasty" is Jacques Joseph (1865–1934) (Figure 1-4). In 1898, Joseph, then an orthopaedic-trained surgeon, presented to the Berlin Medical Society the case of a young man who had an extremely large nose and who had suffered from social ridicule. Joseph successfully reduced the nose using external incisions. More important, Joseph presented his idea that the effects of successful aesthetic surgery were not only manifest on the patient's physical appearance but also on the patient's emotional psyche.

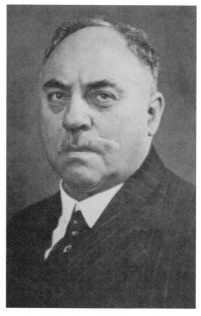

From this point, Joseph became immersed in the study of plastic surgery. During World War I, Joseph was chief of the Section of Facial Plastic Surgery in the ENT Department of the Charité Hospital in Berlin, where he was given the title of professor in 1918.[1] He analyzed and classified different nasal deformities—developing different surgical techniques to address them. In addition, he

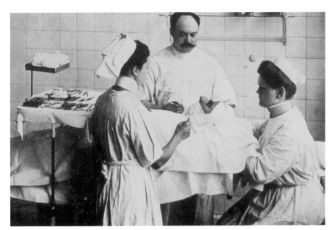

developed surgical instruments to carry out his operations. Eventually, his artistic skill (as evidenced by his own drawings) and documentation of his operations were produced in a comprehensive textbook entitled *Nasenplastik und Sonstige Geischtsplastik* in 1928, which was followed by a second edition in 1931.[1]

After World War I, Joseph, often referred to as "Joseph Noseph," continued at Charité Hospital for a few years before opening his own clinic, where he developed an enormous practice in facial plastic surgery.[6,7] With his reputation at its zenith, Joseph began offering a few apprentice positions (Gustave Aufricht from Hungary was one) and, to a greater number of international surgeons, a fee-set opportunity to watch the master operate (Figure 1-5).

STUDYING THE ART OF RHINOPLASTY

Among the foreigners who came to study under Joseph, three men, in particular, stand out in contributing to how the art of rhinoplasty is studied and taught today. Joseph Safian (1886–1983) and Gustave Aufricht (1894–1980) both deserve credit for introducing Joseph's methods to the United States in the 1930s.[5] In 1935, Safian's textbook entitled *Corrective Rhinoplastic Surgery* shed light on the different techniques that Joseph had described as the textbook was written in basic English terms, allowing the medical community to easily adopt Joseph's methods.

Aufricht similarly introduced Joseph's methods to the English-speaking world by describing Joseph's techniques in multiple papers. In 1940, his significant contribution was introducing the use of a dental compound splint (of which the basic design and principle remain in use today) as opposed to Joseph's method of postoperative splinting using only adhesive and gauze dressings, which had resulted in an occasional hematoma complication.[5] Safian and Aufricht, although both known for their rhinoplasties

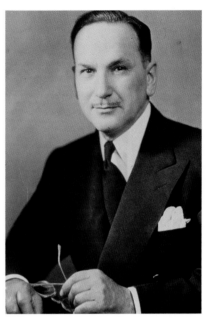

in New York City as well as for their written contributions to the art of rhinoplasty, were not known for their teaching.

In contrast to Safian and Aufricht, who were both plastic surgeons, Samuel Fomon (1889–1971) (Figure 1-6) had no surgical experience and no private practice, and he did not treat patients. Instead, he was an academician, a teacher of anatomy at the University of Illinois, one who prepared young physicians for their state board examinations.[7,8]

In the late 1930s, Fomon identified facial plastic surgery and rhinoplasty in particular as subjects lacking in depth of understanding or teaching, and he set about to fill the gaps.[8] He researched the literature, traveled extensively in Europe, and, speaking German, spent meaningful time with Joseph in Berlin. In 1939, he published his treatise entitled *Surgery of Injury and Plastic Repair*.[9] The extensive material on the nose mirrored to some extent Joseph's earlier text, but the information was now more widely available to Americans, and generally well-received by the medical community.

Fomon's interest was not to produce a library reference but rather to provide a practical guide for physicians who wanted to perform rhinoplasty. With wartime and travel injuries on the rise and the advent of antibiotics leading to a decrease in prior surgical procedures, for many surgeons the time was right to explore new territories.

In 1940, Fomon offered a course on rhinoplasty and otoplasty to interested otolaryngologists in Boston. As interests in what he was teaching grew, Fomon expanded his courses to include cadaveric laboratory dissections, as

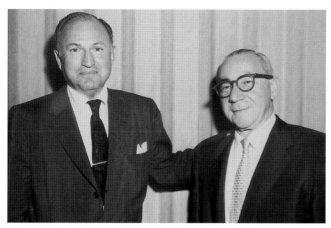

Figure 1-7 Irving B. Goldman, M.D. (*left*) and Joseph Safian, M.D. (*right*), two prominent rhinoplasty surgeons in New York City. (Photograph courtesy of Robert L. Simons, M.D.)

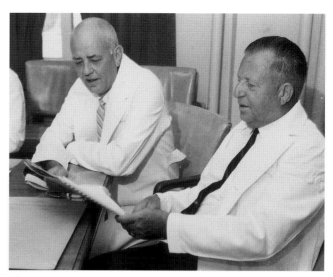

Figure 1-8 William C. Huffman, M.D. (*left*), and Dean M. Lierle, M.D. (*right*). (Photograph courtesy of Richard Farrior, M.D.)

well as live surgery to provide physicians with a practical guide and hands-on learning experience with rhinoplasty techniques. Patients were brought to Fomon by the students, and as one student stated, "Dr. Fomon taught us a lot of theory, and in turn we taught him surgical technique."[8]

Seeking a larger forum, Fomon moved his headquarters to the Manhattan General Hospital in New York City in 1942. At its inception, the Fomon course was of 6 weeks' duration—early morning lectures, followed by two live surgeries, afternoon lectures, and then evening cadaver dissections. Students, 50 to 75 in a class, crowded the amphitheater, observing procedures as best they could through binoculars.

In the early 1940s in New York City, a few surgeons, including Aufricht, Safian (Figure 1-7), as well as Jacques Malianac and Eastman Sheehan, had studied with Joseph in Germany and were known for their proficiency in rhinoplasty but not necessarily their teaching. Fomon's course at Manhattan General was the one place where students were welcome despite an environment in which neither the newly formed plastic surgery organization nor the older otolaryngology establishment endorsed the courses.

It took two prominent otolaryngologists to give credence and official recognition to Fomon's efforts. One was Dr. George Coates of Philadelphia, professor at the University of Pennsylvania and the long-term editor of the *Archives of Otolaryngology*. The other was Dean Lierle, chairman at the University of Iowa. For many years the secretary of the American Board of Otolaryngology (ABO), Dean Lierle, was known as "Mr. Otolaryngology."[7,8] His residency was a model for broad, in-depth head and neck training. A prominent member of his faculty, Bill Huffman, who was double board-certified in otolaryngology and plastic surgery, was sent to study with Fomon for 6 months (Figure 1-8). When Fomon was invited to teach at Iowa,

otolaryngologists throughout the country were encouraged to attend his courses.

THE FOMON TEACHING MODEL CONTINUES

For a legacy to grow, the teacher needs students to spread the gospel. Seated in the front row, four seats from Fomon in that first 1942 course in New York City was Irving B. Goldman (Figure 1-9). Goldman (1898–1975), who would become the first president of the American Academy of Facial Plastic and Reconstructive Surgery (AAFPRS), visited Europe prior to studying and teaching with Fomon and then began his own course and society at New York Mt. Sinai Hospital in the early 1950s.[7,8]

Similarly motivated was another early Fomon student and instructor, Maurice H. Cottle (1898–1981) (Figure 1-10). His home base was Chicago, and by 1944 he was offering his own course at the Illinois Masonic Hospital (Figure 1-11). This annual course was then given at Johns Hopkins University in 1954 when the American Rhinologic Society was organized. Its dedicated message about fundamental functional requirements in nasal surgery had been forcefully reinforced through the years by many Cottle disciples, including Pat Barelli, Robert Hanson, Raymond Hilsinger, and Kenneth Hinderer, and none more passionate than Eugene Kern, who served as professor of rhinology and facial plastic surgery at the Mayo Clinic in Rochester, Minnesota.

Cottle and Goldman both used the Fomon teaching model: morning operations, afternoon lectures, and evening cadaver dissections. Manuals accompanied didactic sessions. Without television, videotapes, or CDs available, students strained to see what was happening at the

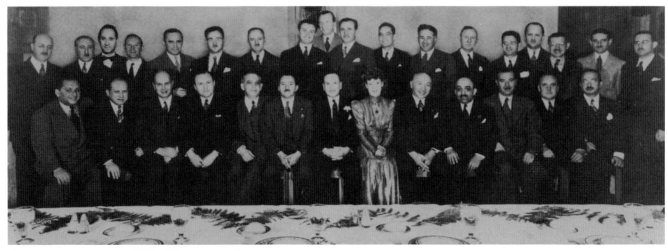

Figure 1-9 Testimonial dinner given for Samuel Fomon at the course on April 24, 1942. In the front row, Irving B. Goldman and Samual Fomon are seated fourth and seventh from the left, respectively. (Photograph courtesy of Simons RL: Coming of age: a twenty-fifth anniversary history of the American Academy of Facial Plastic and Reconstructive Surgery. New York: Thieme Medical Publishers, 1989.)

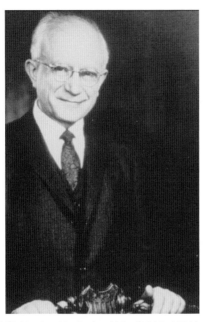

Figure 1-10 Maurice H. Cottle, M.D. (1898–1981). (Photograph courtesy of Simons RL: Coming of age: a twenty-fifth anniversary history of the American Academy of Facial Plastic and Reconstructive Surgery. New York: Thieme Medical Publishers, 1989.)

operating room table or in other instances invited the masters or their designated appointed instructors to visit (Figures 1-12 and 1-13).

Goldman and Cottle had similar teaching protocols but vastly different didactic philosophies and textural content. Cottle emphasized rhinology and the maintenance of nasal function; Goldman stressed aesthetics rather than just physiology. Fomon, Cottle, and Goldman were all mesmerizing teachers who demanded allegiance from their growing number of societal members.

THE GROWTH OF STUDENTS

One of Fomon's most successful students was one of his earliest, Howard Diamond from New York City (Figure 1-14). Diamond's reaction to the first rhinoplasty procedure he saw perhaps differs little from that of most people. In his own words: "It scared the hell out me," although he found that the instant resultant change fascinating.[8] As Diamond recalled, "Fomon was a very sharp, organized guy, but what a production: '7000 instruments and 14 nurses.'"[8]

For Diamond, rhinoplasty worked best when it was simple and uncomplicated. He really believed that "if you make it look easy it will always look good."[8] Diamond's popularity in the New York City area was unparalleled. Every morning, he had four to five cases, with the intra-cartilaginous approach becoming his trademark for quickly defining the nasal tip.

Another early student of Fomon's was Ira Tresley from Chicago (Figure 1-15), a man who shared Diamond's love for the operation and the desirability of distilling its essence to a few instruments and as little manipulation of the tissues as possible. Viewed by many at the time as the most technically skillful of rhinoplasty surgeons, Tresley, like Diamond, had a sufficiently large number of people seeking his service that he could pick and choose his cases. Diamond and Tresley both eschewed formal teaching, but their surgical ways influenced many of the teachers to come.

In the late 1940s and then into the 1950s, either directly or indirectly, Fomon's teaching ignited spheres of rhinoplasty activity. Morey Parkes, who trained at New York's Harlem Eye and Ear Hospital, once said, "It wasn't until I heard a lecture and took a course from Dr. Fomon that I became really inspired."[8] Not long after, he took his

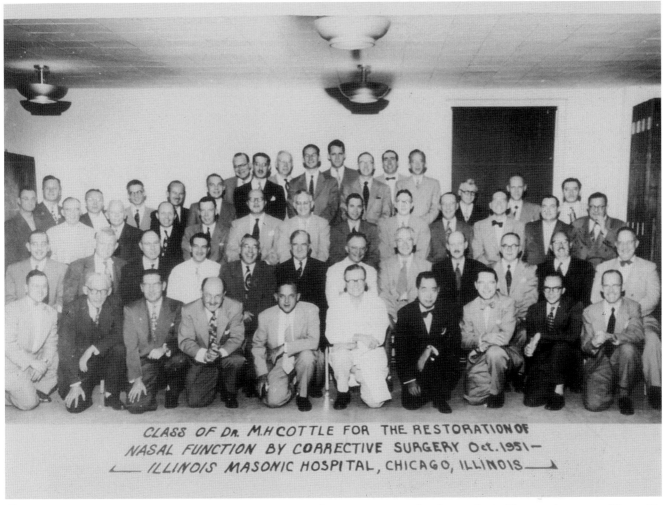

Figure 1-11 Participants of the Cottle rhinoplasty course in 1951 at Illinois Masonic Hospital in Chicago, Illinois. (Photograph courtesy of Simons RL: Coming of age: a twenty-fifth anniversary history of the American Academy of Facial Plastic and Reconstructive Surgery. New York: Thieme Medical Publishers, 1989.)

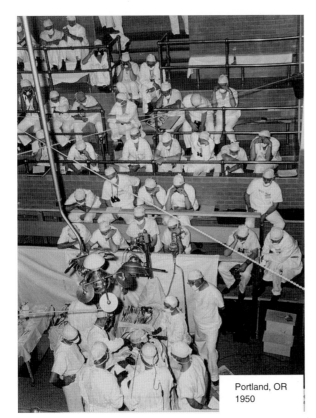

Portland, OR
1950

Figure 1-12 Maurice H. Cottle in the operating theatre at a 1950 course in Portland, Oregon. (Photograph courtesy of Robert L. Simons, M.D.)

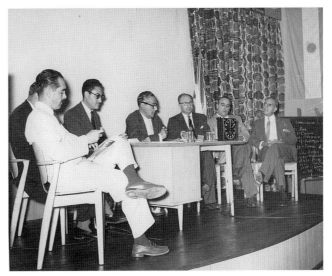

Figure 1-13 Irving B. Goldman *(3rd from right)* at an invited course in Cuba in 1951. (Photograph courtesy of Sidney Feuerstein, M.D.)

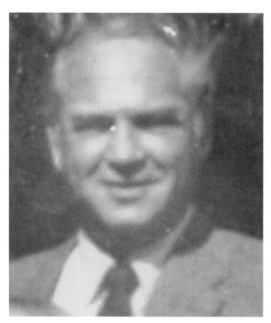

Figure 1-14 Howard Diamond, M.D. (Photograph courtesy of Robert L. Simons, M.D.)

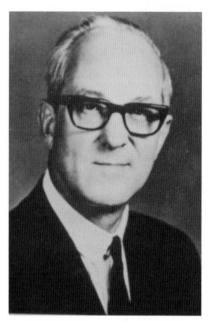

Figure 1-16 John T. Dickinson, M.D. (1918–1978). (Photograph courtesy of Simons RL: Coming of age: a twenty-fifth anniversary history of the American Academy of Facial Plastic and Reconstructive Surgery. New York: Thieme Medical Publishers, 1989.)

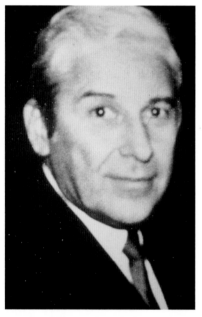

Figure 1-15 Ira Tresley, M.D. (Photograph courtesy of Simons RL: Coming of age: a twenty-fifth anniversary history of the American Academy of Facial Plastic and Reconstructive Surgery. New York: Thieme Medical Publishers, 1989.)

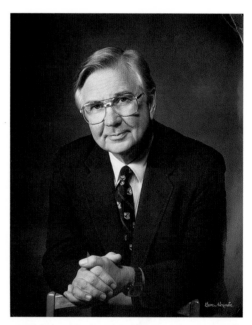

Figure 1-17 Richard Farrior, M.D. (Photograph courtesy of Simons RL: Coming of age: a twenty-fifth anniversary history of the American Academy of Facial Plastic and Reconstructive Surgery. New York: Thieme Medical Publishers, 1989.)

practice to the West Coast and joined Jesse Fuchs, Ed Lipsett, and then Wally Berman, who had finished a 3-year fellowship with the renowned double–board–certified chairman of plastic surgery, John Marquis Converse in New York. Together, Fuchs, Lipsett, Berman, and Parkes pioneered Los Angeles' fertile territory in facial plastic surgery.

Similarly inspired were successive senior residents at the University of Iowa in 1949 and 1950—namely John

Dickinson (Figure 1-16) and Richard Farrior (Figure 1-17), who would make their marks in Pittsburgh, Pennsylvania, and Tampa, Florida, respectively.

Back in New York, Goldman's course was taking hold and also making its mark. Early assistants, or lieutenants as they were called, returned year after year to listen to Goldman and to teach his methodology. Among them were

Irvin Fine, Samuel Bloom, Sidney Feuerstein, Trent Smith, Jan Beckhuis, and Lionello Ponti from Rome, who were all superb teachers in their own right.

But one of best student-teacher stories to be told involves a tall young man captured in two group shots taken at courses given in New Orleans. The first, a Fomon course in 1957 (Figure 1-18), followed a year later by a Goldman course in 1958 (Figure 1-19). His name was Jack Anderson. Early in his career, Anderson attended a meeting in Houston, Texas, called the Southern Graduate Assembly.[8] Samuel Fomon, a guest speaker, had an exhibit that included wax moulages of all the stages of rhinoplasty. "It was just gorgeous," Anderson recalled.[8] It was created for Fomon by Walt Disney Studios and was reported to cost $30,000, which in today's economy would be 10 times as much. Enthralled with what he heard and saw, Anderson went to take Fomon's course in New York City in 1952[8] (Figure 1-20).

He returned to New Orleans with an undying enthusiasm for rhinoplasty, which he characterized as the "queen of operations."[8,10] He soon became an active member of Fomon's Society—now organized as the

American Otolaryngologic Society for the Advancement of Plastic and Reconstructive Surgery. It was this organization, together with Goldman's American Facial Plastic Society, that amalgamated into the AAFPRS in 1964.[6,7]

THE QUEEN OF OPERATIONS FUELS FURTHER TEACHING AND ORGANIZATIONAL EFFORTS

In the formative years, the fuel that powered the educational and organizational efforts of AAFPRS leaders was that "queen of operations"—rhinoplasty. The early officers of this organization were known for their work in rhinoplasty (Figure 1-21).

Anderson, along with Richard Farrior and John Dickinson, started a Plastic Surgery Study Club.[10] The group included Oscar Becker and Ira Tresley of Chicago; Louis Feit, Joseph Gilbert, Abe Silver, Bennie Rish, and Irving Goldman from New York; Jesse Fuchs and Morey Parkes from Los Angeles, William Wright from Houston; and the latest member in 1963, a plastic surgeon from Boston,

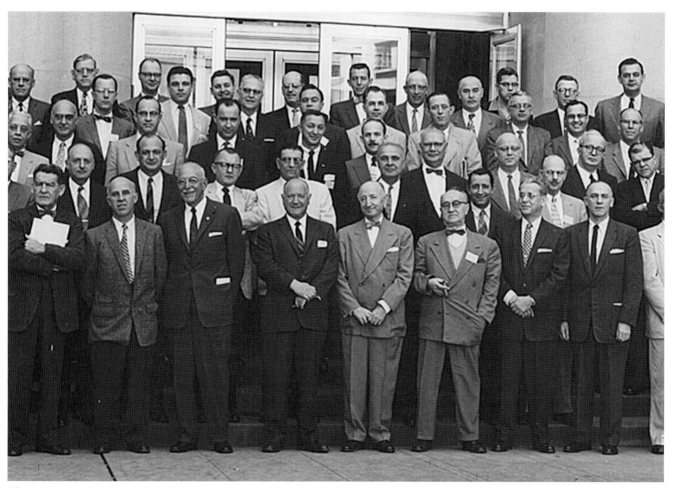

Figure 1-18 Fomon course held in New Orleans, Louisiana, in 1957. Dr. Jack Anderson is seen standing at the extreme right in the back row. (Photograph courtesy of Jack Anderson, M.D.)

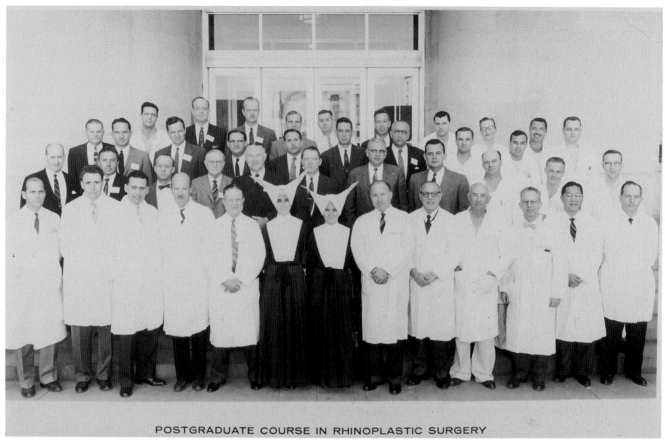

POSTGRADUATE COURSE IN RHINOPLASTIC SURGERY

Figure 1-19 The 1958 Goldman postgraduate course in rhinoplasty held in New Orleans under the auspices of Tulane University. Goldman stands eighth from the left in the front row, and Jack Anderson is fourth from the right in the second row. (Photograph courtesy of Simons RL: Coming of age: a twenty-fifth anniversary history of the American Academy of Facial Plastic and Reconstructive Surgery. New York: Thieme Medical Publishers, 1989.)

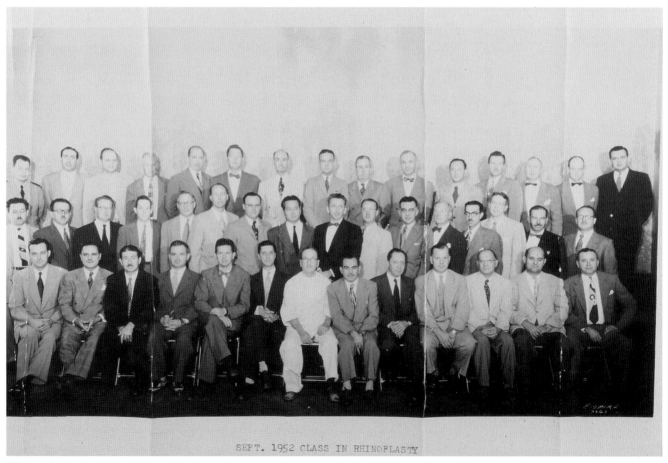

SEPT. 1952 CLASS IN RHINOPLASTY

Figure 1-20 Fomon course held in New York City in 1952. Fomon is seated in white in the front row, and Jack Anderson is standing at the far right in the back row. (Photograph courtesy of Jack Anderson, M.D.)

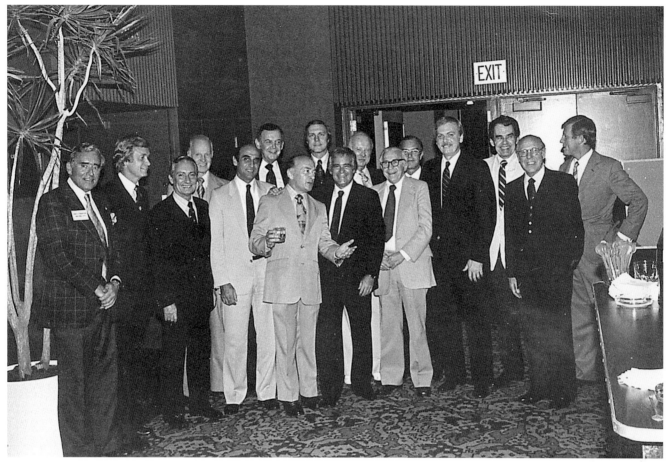

Figure 1-21 Rhinoplasty teachers gather for a course in Key Biscayne in 1980. Standing from left to right are Sidney Feuerstein, M. Eugene Tardy, Lionello Ponti, Jan Beekhuis, Frank Kamer, Jack Anderson, Leslie Bernstein, Gaylon McCullough, Bob Simons, Trent Smith, Richard Webster, Claus Walter, Charles Gross, William Wright, Irvin Fine, and Tony Bull. (Photograph courtesy of Robert L. Simons, M.D.)

Richard Webster (Figure 1-22). They were men with different backgrounds from across the country. Men who would meet periodically to watch one another operate and then question and criticize what they saw but always with the desire to better understand the operation, and in so doing they became better teachers—a capsule of the ethos that would successfully drive the newly organized AAFPRS.

Anderson's enthusiasm for rhinoplasty was contagious. As an active teacher at Tulane University, he drew the undivided attention of such young residents as Jack Gunter, Fred Becker, Calvin Johnson, and later, Wayne Larrabee and Mack Cheney. Always placing value on training and youthful input, Anderson spearheaded the academy's fellowship program, which began in 1974.[7] His first fellow was David Ellis, closely followed by another outstanding student teacher, Gaylon McCullough (Figure 1-23). Ellis was from Toronto, Canada—a place that joins New York, Chicago, Iowa, Los Angeles, and New Orleans as important landmarks in the American rhinoplasty journey.

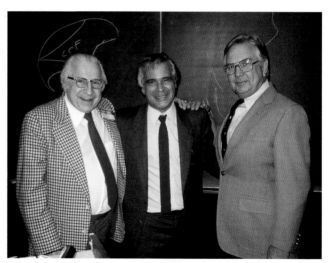

Figure 1-22 Richard C. Webster, M.D., on the *left*, convincing Bob Simons (*center*) and Richard Farrior (*right*) of his tip philosophy. (Photograph courtesy of Robert L. Simons, M.D.)

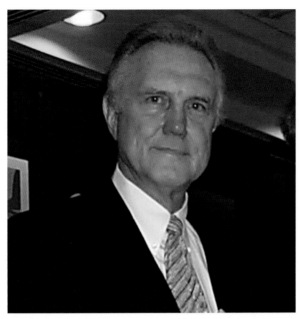

Figure 1-23 Gaylon McCullough, M.D. (Photograph courtesy of Robert L. Simons, M.D.)

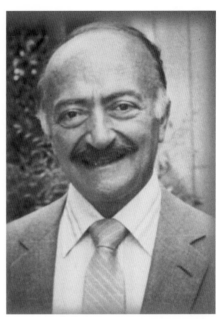

Figure 1-24 Leslie Bernstein, M.D. (Photograph courtesy of AAFPRS archival files.)

THE IOWA EXPERIENCE

In the early 1960s, a highly talented and focused teacher named Leslie Bernstein (Figure 1-24) joined the faculty at the University of Iowa. Trained in South Africa and London, Bernstein brought a background in dentistry and oral maxillofacial surgery and began his own courses in 1963. He was invited to write the chapter on nasal trauma in Fomon's 1970 rhinoplasty text. The forward in that book was penned by another esteemed facial plastic surgeon, John Conley, who writes of Fomon, "His original school in the 1940s opened the doors for the study of these techniques, removing it from occult position into the professional arena of the interested specialist and supraspecialist."[8]

Bernstein's rhinoplasty course, emphasizing the importance of anatomy, cadaver dissections, and artistic skills, has an unparalleled 45-plus—year run. Ultimately, the Iowa experience propelled the careers of men like Chuck Krause, Roger Crumley, Marc Connelly, Karl Eisbach, and Shan Baker. Bernstein's persistent teaching presence, first at Iowa and then in Sacramento and San Francisco, provided a platform for teaching and learning to many, including Richard Goode, Trent Smith, Robert Simons, Corey Maas, William Silver, and others.

THE GOLDMAN COURSE

It is important to remember that prior to fellowships in the mid-1970s, residency training in rhinoplasty was variable. Exposure to the operation prior to videotapes

was limited. The ongoing annual-based courses provided the introduction and graduate education for many students. Thus, a bonus for the residents at New York's Mt. Sinai Hospital was Goldman's annual June Course. A group picture taken at the 1965 course is evidence of Robert Simons' early involvement, as well as that of an equally young and enthusiastic Tony Bull from London (Figure 1-25).

Irving Goldman was the primary teacher and surgeon at the course from 1953 to 1969. After that, it was led by Sidney Feuerstein, Samuel Bloom, and Robert Simons, with William Lawson taking charge during the later part of its more than 40-year existence. A partial list of the second- and third-generation teachers receiving their baptism at Mt. Sinai included Frank Kamer, William Friedman, Harold Deutsch, Sid Sattenspiel, Mark Krugman, William Lawson, William Binder, Charley Gross, William Silver, Alvin Glasgold, Steve Pearlman, and Geoff Tobias.

Ongoing courses developed their own traditions if not mystique. At Mt. Sinai, the endonasal approach, marginal incisions for delivery of the alar cartilages, and vertical division of the dome and reposition, rather than excision of cartilages to control tip projections, were part of the normal operation. These tenets were gospel to the Mt. Sinai crowd while blasphemy to others.

CHICAGO COURSES

In Chicago, interest in rhinoplasty was equal to that in New York City. A different experience, more eclectic and

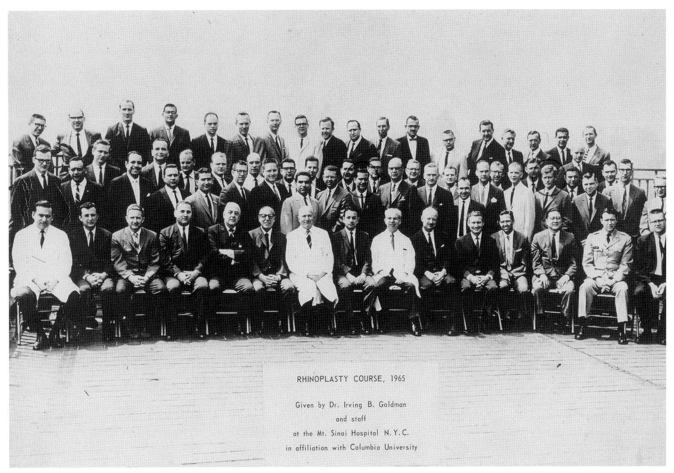

Figure 1-25 Goldman rhinoplasty course in 1965 at Mount Sinai Hospital in New York City. Circled are Bob Simons (*left*) and Tony Bull (*right*). (Photograph courtesy of Robert L. Simons, M.D.)

not as controlled as that of Goldman's course, occurred annually at Cook County General Hospital.

One of the primary beneficiaries was a young University of Illinois resident, M. Eugene Tardy (Figure 1-26). Tardy had first seen rhinoplasty as an intern at Tampa General Hospital where he met Richard Farrior. As a resident helping to organize cadaver dissections at the Cook County courses, his knowledge grew as he listened and learned from people like Richard Webster, William Wright, Jack Anderson, John Conley, Carl Patterson, Lou Tenta, Jack Kerth, and John Dickinson. Dickinson also brought to the course an ex-Tulane resident named Jack Gunter. Although it was several years prior to the official academy fellowships, Gunter spent a year (1968–1969) with Dickinson in Pittsburgh in a facial plastic surgery fellowship granted and funded by the National Institutes of Health and arranged with the help of Dean Lierle. This subsequently led to Gunter's teaching involvement with the academy, especially in its early soft tissue courses.

Among Tardy's mentoring influences, however, the most significant was Ira Tresley. Tardy was intrigued after watching Tresley's normal three cases on a Saturday morning by "how he made the operation look so easy, but

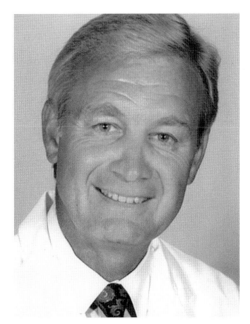

Figure 1-26 M. Eugene Tardy, M.D. (Photograph courtesy of M. Eugene Tardy, M.D.)

it wasn't so easy" (personal communication). With superb technique and communications skills, Tardy continued to raise the level of rhinoplasty teaching. His use of photographic diagrams and cadaver dissections, along with his high-quality operative demonstrations, made him a highly sought-after teacher both at home and abroad.

In fact, one can look at Chicago's rhinoplasty history and easily make a case that Tardy anchors a very strong "T" line. Starting from the early days, there were Tresley, Tenta, Tardy, Thomas, Toriumi—with Tardy separating the prefellowship and postfellowship years.

Another of today's outstanding teachers from Illinois and now in New York is Norman Pastorek, who was 2 years Tardy's junior at Illinois and who gives tremendous credit to Tresley and Tenta for his early training. And then there were the two residents in the Chicago program at Cook County Hospital in the early 1960s prior to the training of Tardy and Pastorek. One was an otolaryngology resident named Jack Kerth, who was associated in practice with Dr. Tresley when the renowned surgeon died in 1971. More important in our historic journey was Kerth's later enthusiastic mentoring at Northwestern University, which helped to inspire a talented band of men who would go on to make their mark in the rhinoplasty world. Within a 5-year period in the 1980s, the group of graduates from Northwestern included W. Russell Ries, Vito Quatela, Jonathan Sykes, Tom Wang, and Dean Toriumi.

The other example of the early "Chicago Influence" was a resident in plastic surgery at Cook County in 1962, Jack Sheen. Sheen's first exposure to rhinoplasty during his residency was, in his own words, "the damndest procedure you ever saw."[8] His job was to stand by and monitor the blood loss, and when the figure hit 1500 mL, the case was stopped (personal communication). Lacking sound aesthetic training while in his residency program, Sheen observed Tresley operate on a Saturday morning. Like others who had observed Tresley, this experience was once described as, "an epiphany—on the table the cases looked great. It was like watching a magician."[8]

Sheen began his practice where demand and competition were high—Beverly Hills, California. His observations about rhinoplasty slowly made a mark in the plastic surgery world.[11] He moved from a reductive to a more balanced augmented approach. He perceived rhinoplasty as changing structure rather than reducing it. His suggestions about augmenting the radix and middle vault, creating internal stress in the tip with cartilage grafts, and preoperatively recognizing short nasal bones or malpositioned alar cartilages challenged the current-day rhinoplasty concepts. His book, first published in 1978 and then reedited in 1987, was an eye opener.[11]

A CHANGE IN RHINPLASTY CONCEPTS—THE EXTERNAL APPROACH

In 1970, at the first AAFPRS International Symposium held in New York City, a tremendous impact on traditional rhinoplasty concepts occurred. A relatively unknown surgeon from Yugoslavia named Ivo Padovan (Figure 1-27) was given 10 minutes to present his experience and that of his teacher, Dr. Ante Sercer, regarding the external approach to rhinoplasty. The paper was generally dismissed by all 1000 present at the Waldorf Astoria Hotel

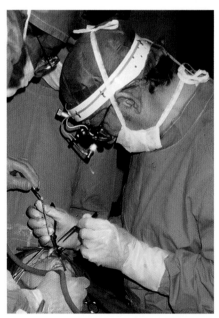

Figure 1-27 Ivo Padovan demonstrating his external approach to rhinoplasty. (Photograph courtesy of Richard Farrior, M.D.)

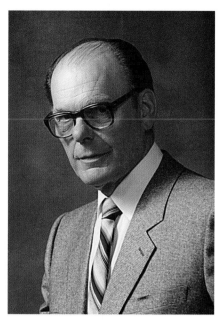

Figure 1-28 Wilfred Goodman, M.D. (Photograph courtesy of Canadian archival files.)

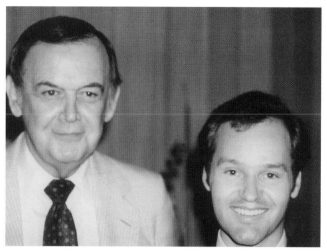

Figure 1-29 Jack Anderson, M.D. (*left*), with his fellow Peter Adamson, M.D. (*right*), in 1980. (Photograph courtesy of Peter Adamson, M.D.)

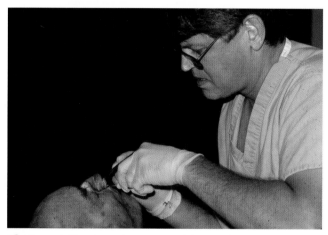

Figure 1-30 Calvin Johnson, M.D. (Photograph courtesy of Calvin Johnson, M.D.)

in New York City, except for two men from Toronto, Canada: Wilfred Goodman and David Bryant. By the next International Symposium in 1975 in Chicago, Goodman (Figure 1-28) was able to present 250 cases using the external transcolumellar approach, extorting the advantages of visualization and versatile management. Further reinforcing the message that the external approach was advantageous, he applied it to all patients.

The new approach intrigued Jack Anderson. His interest peaked even more following a postmeeting plane ride discussion with his good friend, David Bryant. Further assurances were received from a former fellow of Wilfred Goodman's in Toronto, Kris Conrad, who replied to Anderson, "No" when asked, "Is anybody suing you for opening these noses in Canada?"[8]

Once satisfied as to its safety and acceptance, Anderson began using the external approach and encouraged his scientifically motivated colleague, William Wright from Houston, Texas, to do the same. Fellows helped with the transition of their mentors. Calvin Johnson was associated with Anderson in 1980 when Peter Adamson came for a fellowship from Toronto with first-hand experience in the external approach (Figure 1-29). Wright received encouragement from his first fellow, Russell Kridel, who would later join his practice.

There are very few people in the history of facial plastic surgery to match Jack Anderson, when it came to motivating people or initiating action. With his initial report of success in 100 successive cases in the early 1980s followed by publication of his monograph, "Rhinoplasty: Emphasizing the External Approach" in 1986, the word spread and the rhinoplasty revolution regarding approach had begun. Surgeons and students thought that they could

see and treat more accurately. The pendulum of preference for endonasal versus external swung widely to the latter.

To better understand this cataclysmic change, it is interesting to examine the personal evolutions of two of today's outstanding rhinoplasty teachers: Calvin Johnson (Figure 1-30) and Jack Gunter (Figure 1-31). They were both initial students of Anderson with his early transcartilaginous endonasal approach and tripod theory. Both men expressed early frustration with knowing exactly what Anderson was doing with his knives or feeling secure in what they could see or achieve on a regular basis with this endonasal approach.

For Johnson, the operation remained intolerably unpredictable until the nuances and the finer points of the external approach were clarified by Anderson and Adamson. Armed with a better understanding of the external approach and with an appreciation of what grafts could achieve in a structural look as portrayed in Sheen's

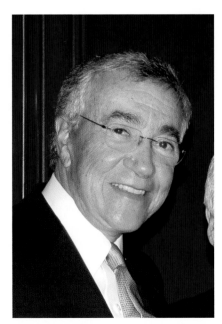

text,[11] Johnson sought to develop the concepts of the open structured rhinoplasty.

The promotions and clarification of his thinking culminated in the publication of his textbook *Open Structure Rhinoplasty* in 1990. Two of his fellows, both residents from Northwestern University, contributed to the development of the textbook. First, in the early stages there was help offered by Vito Quatela. Then in 1988 during his 6-month fellowship with Johnson, Dean Toriumi truly took control of the book's organization and timely publication.

For Jack Gunter, there was a similar lack of confidence and excitement about rhinoplasty until he went to a Triological Society meeting in Ft. Worth, Texas, in 1980 to listen to his old teacher, Anderson, talk of his 100 consecutive cases using the external approach. Gunter, who had taken a residency at Michigan in plastic surgery and who would soon be double board-certified, started to use the external approach in all of his secondary rhinoplasties. He wrote a paper on the open approach of revision rhinoplasty in the late 1980s[12] and certainly was instrumental in introducing the new approach to the plastic surgery world, a world that had been familiar with the rhinoplasty teachings of John Marquis Converse, Ralph Millard, George Peck, Tom Rees, and Jack Sheen. What was missing was a sustained forum for the unique needs of nasal surgery education.

Much to his credit, Gunter pioneered the annual rhinoplasty course for plastic surgeons in Dallas, Texas, in 1983. Over the past quarter-century, it provided a launching pad for the thoughts of surgeons such as Mark Constantian, Ron Gruber, John Tebbetts, Steven Byrd, Rollin Daniel, Rod Rohrich, Bahman Guyuron, Tony Wolf, and

Nicholas Tabbal—familiar names and figures because of their participation at various academy courses and meetings. An ecumenical presence to which the names of four other fine plastic surgeons—Gary Burget from Chicago, Frederick Menick from Arizona, Gilbert Aiach from France, and Ivo Pitanguy from Brazil—should be added. Gunter also introduced diagrammatic templates (Figure 1-32) for recording surgical procedures and became an ardent supporter of the use of grafts for the maintenance of nasal contour.

A LEGACY OF RHINOPLASTY TEACHING CONTINUES

Thus, Johnson and Gunter were two examples of personal educational evolutions. Each of their fellowship trainings extended beyond its first teachings, as they developed and taught new thought processes, concepts, and practices. This pattern continued as the legacy of rhinoplasty teaching was evidenced in the careers of three of the early AAFPRS fellowship graduates in the 1970s.

There was Fred Stucker (Figure 1-33), who left his naval command to study with Tardy and Beekhuis and who then went on to teach scores of residents and fellows at the Philadelphia Naval Hospital and then Louisiana State University. His latest achievement is a recently compiled rhinoplasty experience with more than 8000 cases.

Another was Gaylon McCollough, who spent his fellowship years with Jack Anderson, Richard Webster, and Wally Berman, developing ideas about domal sutures. More important, McCollough contributed to initiating the training of such current teachers as Devinder Mangat, Steve Perkins, Keith La Ferriere, Wally Dyer, Donn Chatham, William Beeson, Randy Waldman, and Daniel Russo.

Furthermore, there was Ted Cook, longtime director of Facial Plastic Surgery in Portland, Oregon. He trained with Richard Farrior and Richard Webster before infusing rhinoplasty goals and standards into a cadre of talented surgeons and teachers such as Richard Davis, Vito Quatela, Stephan Park, Craig Murakami, Tom Wang, Oren Friedman, and David Kriet.

Overall, Stucker, McCollough, and Cook played major roles in contributing to the legacy of rhinoplasty teachings. In addition to this group of esteemed players, Tardy's first fellow, Regan Thomas, should be added as he also played a role in the teaching legacy. Ultimately, they were all instrumental in strengthening spheres of rhinoplasty activity not just at home but also abroad.

FORMING AN INTERNATIONAL ALLIANCE

As formal teaching and courses in America developed, European surgeons and teachers also made their

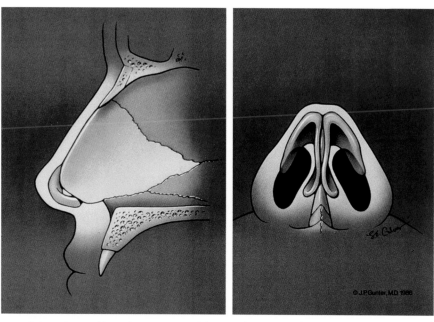

Figure 1-32 Rhinoplasty worksheet designed by Jack Gunter, M.D. (Photograph courtesy of Jack Gunter, M.D.)

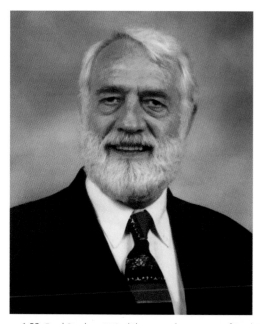

Figure 1-33 Fred Stucker, M.D. (Photograph courtesy of Fred Stucker, M.D.)

the way, Europe's academy, the Joseph Society, was born. In Italy, first Valerio Michelli Pelligrini, then Georgio Sulcenti, and currently Pietra Palma arranged instructional sessions. In Mexico, Efrain Davalos, a former student of Cottle, asked leaders of the AAFPRS to come to Moralia for an annual course in facial plastic surgery. In Bogota, Colombia, Fernando Pedroza, who had trained with Anderson and Webster, invited similar teachers to come motivate and educate.

The rhinoplasty universe was expanding with stars in Europe, South America, Mexico, Australia, the Middle East, South Africa, and Asia. A new vibrant galaxy called the International Federation of Facial Plastic Surgery Societies (IFFPSS) with members from the United States, Canada, Mexico, Colombia, Brazil, Australia, and Europe, now led by Drs. Gilbert Nolst-Trenite from the Netherlands and Roxana Cobo from Colombia, had arrived.

THE GROWTH OF MODERN-DAY RHINOPLASTY CONTINUES

The story of growth in modern-day rhinoplasty might be most purely appreciated in a genealogic sense when recalling fatherly figures like Jerome Hilger, who taught about internal osteotomies in the 1960s, or Richard Farrior, who mentored so many (including his son) and then followed the tracks of their offspring. With Peter Hilger, the past president of the AAFPRS, and Edward Farrior, a co-director of the most recent Advanced Rhinoplasty Course, a proud legacy is evident.

However, to understand and put this story of growth in proper prospective, it is relevant to return to Chicago

contributions, sharing their experiences to develop and bring new concepts to their own practices. They included Tony Bull from London, Lionello Ponti from Rome, Rudi Myer from Switzerland, and Claus Walter with his composite and spreader grafts from Germany. In addition, another German, an otologist named Horst Wullstein, along with John Conley and Richard Farrior were instrumental in promoting the first facial plastic surgery courses in Europe.

As in this country, with history repeating itself, courses produced group interest. And with Bull and Walter leading

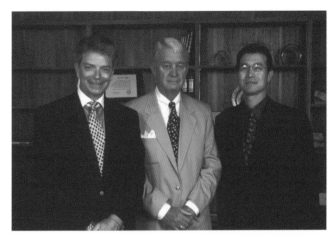

Figure 1-34 M. Eugene Tardy, M.D., flanked by J. Regan Thomas, M.D., and Dean M. Toriumi, M.D. (Photograph courtesy of M. Eugene Tardy, M.D.)

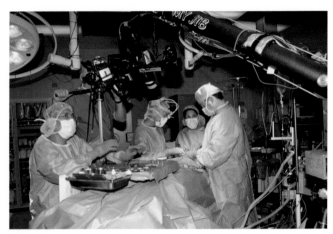

Figure 1-35 Dean Toriumi being videotaped in the operating room. (Photograph courtesy of Chuck Cox, photographer of AAFPRS.)

where the student-teacher-student planetary rotation is most clearly visible. In 1979, Regan Thomas was Eugene Tardy's first official fellow. Then in 2002, he returned to Chicago as chairman of the Department of Otolaryngology–Head and Neck Surgery at the University of Illinois, essentially becoming Tardy's boss. On faculty at the time of his return is a young rhinoplasty star, Dean Toriumi (Figure 1-34). Toriumi had benefited from the tutelage and relationship with Tardy, spending the last 3 months of his Northwestern University residency with Tardy and then, following his fellowship with Calvin Johnson and Wayne Larrabee, devoting a decade of rhinoplasty teaching and study in Tardy's world at the University of Illinois. With Thomas, the former pupil of Tardy, understanding well the needs of a student and a star, he afforded new departmental support for Toriumi.

With all cases now documented on videotape, the replay ability to see what was done, what worked, and what did not provided monumental strides in teaching and decision-making (Figure 1-35). The clarity of Toriumi's message and his use of large grafts to stabilize the nasal framework are compelling. The younger member of the Chicago trio today shines brightly.

CONCLUDING THOUGHTS

In tracing this journey through time, the history and development of rhinoplasty from early nasal reconstructive techniques to modern-day corrective rhinoplasty provide a story of growth and evolution. It is a story necessitating a coordinated alignment of all the aforementioned pioneering rhinoplasty surgeons, or cast of characters—in essence, an "alignment of the stars." However, the "cosmic changes" should come as no surprise to the veteran star gazers. Expected are continuing bursts of radiant light, somewhere or somehow in our forever changing world of rhinoplasty.

Certainly it was predicted by Samuel Fomon over six decades ago, when speaking at the first annual meeting of the American Otolaryngologic Society for the Advancement of Plastic and Reconstructive Surgery in New York City in 1943. He concluded his remarks on the role of plastic surgery in the field of otolaryngology by stating, "I envisage the appearance of a galaxy of outstanding names in this society which will sparkle through the pages of history along with those of the masters of the past."[8]

To which I add, let the names and contributors of the past become recognized makers, markers, and milestones as we continue our steady ascent into the future.

REFERENCES

1. Eisenberg I. A history of rhinoplasty. *S Afr J*. 1982;62:286–292.
2. Snell GED. A history of rhinoplasty. *Can J Otolaryngol*. 1973;2:224–230.
3. Whitaker IS, Karoo RO, Spyrou G, Fenton OM. The birth of plastic surgery: the story of nasal reconstruction from the *Edwin Smith Papyrus* to the twenty-first century. *Plast Reconstr Surg*. 2007;120:327–336.
4. Sorta-Bilajac I, Muzur A. The nose between ethics and aesthetics: Sushruta's legacy. *Otolaryngol Head Neck Surg*. 2007;137:707–710.
5. Rogers BO. Early historical development of corrective rhinoplasty. In: Millard DR Jr, ed. *Symposium on corrective rhinoplasty*. St Louis: CV Mosby; 1976:18–31.
6. Simons RL, Hill TS. Facial plastic surgery: subspecialty helps otolaryngology define its boundaries. *Otolaryngol Head Neck Surg*. 1996;115:1–14.
7. Simons RL. *Coming of age: a twenty-fifth anniversary history of the American Academy of Facial Plastic and Reconstructive Surgery*. New York: Thieme Medical Publishers; 1989.
8. Simons RL. Aligning the stars: the history of modern rhinoplasty. *Video presentation at the American Academy of Facial Plastic and Reconstructive Surgery meeting*. Washington, DC, September 2007.

9. Fomon S, Bell J. *Rhinoplasty: new concepts, evaluation and application*. Springfield, IL: C C Thomas; 1970.

10. Anderson JR. The dynamics of rhinoplasty. In: *Proceedings of the Ninth International Congress in Otorhinolaryngology. Excerpta Medica, International Congress Series 206.* Amsterdam: Excerpta Medica; 1969.

11. Sheen JH, Sheen AP. *Aesthetic rhinoplasty*. St. Louis: Mosby; 1978.

12. Gunter JP, Rohrich RJ. External approach for secondary rhinoplasty. *Plast Reconstr Surg.* 1987;80:161–174.

CHAPTER TWO

Surgical Anatomy and Physiology of the Nose

William Numa • Calvin M. Johnson, Jr.

Rhinoplasty surgery requires a robust understanding of the surgical anatomy and physiology of the nose and nasal airway. Only by building on this solid foundation can a rhinoplasty surgeon adjust and tailor surgical techniques to fit unique individual patient needs. By balancing the patient's concerns with the surgeon's diagnosis after a complete examination, the surgeon can determine which set of techniques are most suitable to accomplish the surgical goals set out for each individual patient.

There is valuable information to be gained from inspection and palpation of the patient's nasal structures, including the skin, cartilage, bone, and dynamic interplay of these structures in animation during the preoperative assessment. There are features of each individual nose that the surgeon will want to preserve; it may be the dorsal height for one patient or the ala–columellar relation for another. The preoperative analytical and diagnostic aspects of rhinoplasty surgery are at least as important as the execution of any given technique outlined in the remainder of this book.

The scope of this chapter is to serve as a practical clinical reference to applied surgical anatomy and physiology as related to rhinoplasty. For the purposes of clarifying preferred directional anatomical references, these have been depicted in Figure 2-1.

The skin and soft tissue envelope drapes the nasal skeleton, composed of the nasal bones, corresponding to the upper third of the nasal pyramid, and the lower two thirds, represented by the paired upper lateral cartilages (ULCs), paired lower lateral cartilages (LLCs), and septum in the midline. It is through the modification of these supporting structures that the rhinoplasty surgeon will be able to build the foundation onto which the skin and soft tissue envelope (S-STE) will rest, giving a pleasant appearance. Careful consideration should be given to the structural integrity of this foundation, as it will need to overcome both the natural aging process and the contractile forces associated with the cicatricial healing process following surgery. No compromises on nasal function need to be made in the name of accomplishing an aesthetically pleasing result.

THE SKIN AND SOFT TISSUE ENVELOPE

The thickness, elasticity, and general characteristics of the S-STE can be confirmed by palpation of the nose. However, clues to its thickness are present on inspection. The presence of acne or adnexal structures such as fine hair in the supratip region, as seen in some patients, will provide

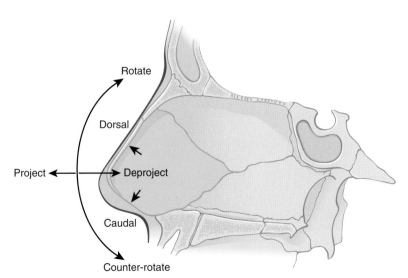

Figure 2-1 Preferred directional anatomic references pertaining to rhinoplasty.

insight into the skin thickness and the vascular supply that accompanies it. Topographic analysis of the nose is useful to discuss and accurately describe different anatomic landmarks[1,2] (Figures 2-2 through 2-6).

When divided into upper, middle, and lower thirds, the middle third of the nose, or that part covering the rhinion (osteocartilaginous juncture of the nose), will be the thinnest. In adults, the upper third of the S-STE will be the thickest, followed by the lower third. Adolescents and patients of ethnicity other than Caucasian will tend to have thicker S-STE on the supratip region of the lower third of the nose. However, the area of skin overlying the nasal domes will typically remain very thin. This underscores the importance of concentrating on avoiding irregularities to the middle third and around the area of the domes of the nose, so as to prevent its long-term collapse or irregularities, after soft tissue swelling subsides and the aging process ensues. The skin thickness of the soft tissue envelope of the nose will play a significant role in the degree of postoperative edema seen. Thin-skinned patients are found to have less edema that resolves faster than the greater, persistent edema found in patients with thicker skin.

The importance of these anatomic issues is evident when making surgical decisions. A straight-line removal of a nasal hump can result in an overreduced profile.

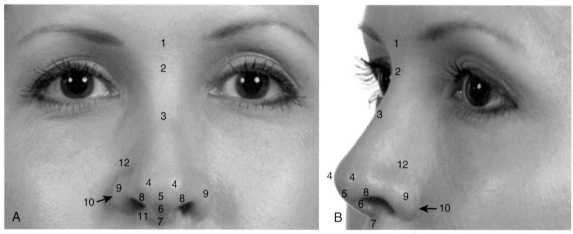

Figure 2-2 Topographic key landmarks on (**A**) frontal and (**B**) oblique views of the nose. *1,* Glabella; *2,* nasion; *3,* rhinion; *4,* tip-defining points; *5,* infratip lobule; *6,* columella; *7,* nasolabial angle; *8,* soft tissue triangles (facets); *9,* alar lobules; *10,* alar–facial groove; *11,* nasal sill; *12,* supraalar crease.

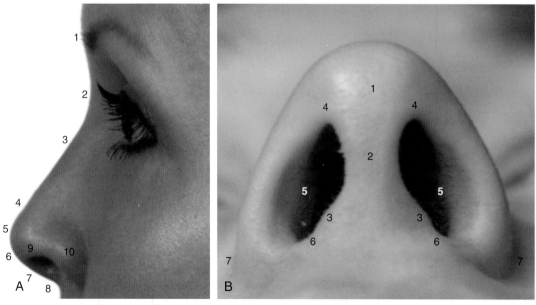

Figure 2-3 Topographic key landmarks. **A,** Lateral view of the nose. *1,* Glabella; *2,* nasion; *3,* rhinion; *4,* supratip break; *5,* tip-defining point; *6,* infratip lobule; *7,* columella; *8,* nasolabial angle; *9,* soft tissue triangle (facet); *10,* alar-facial groove. **B,** Base view of the nose. *1,* infratip lobule; *2,* columella; *3,* medial crural footplate; *4,* soft tissue triangle (facet); *5,* recurvature lower lateral cartilage; *6,* nasal sill; *7,* alar-facial groove.

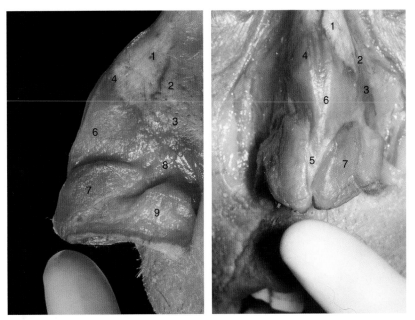

Figure 2-4 Cadaveric dissection demonstrating principal components of the nasal anatomy. *1,* Nasal bones; *2,* nasomaxillary suture line; *3,* ascending process of the maxilla; *4,* osteocartilaginous junction (rhinion); *5,* anterior septal angle; *6,* upper lateral cartilage (ULC); *7,* lateral crus of the lower lateral cartilage (LLC); *8,* sesamoid cartilage; *9,* alar lobule (fibrofatty tissue).

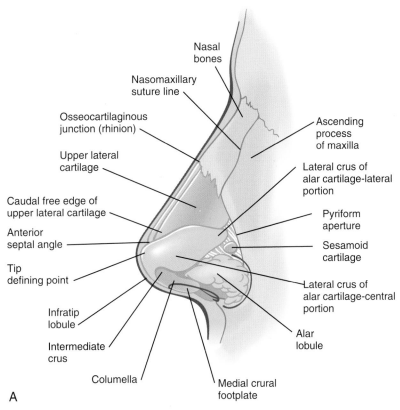

Figure 2-5 A, Nasal anatomy, lateral view.

Continued

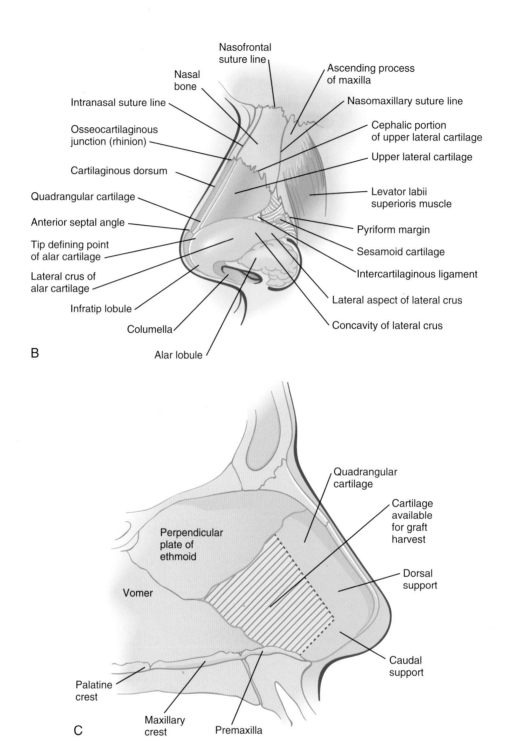

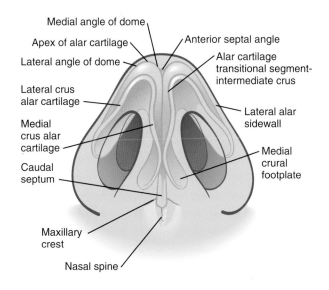

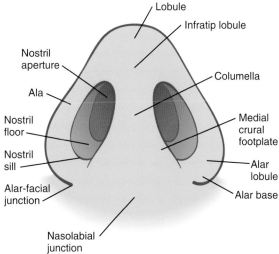

Figure 2-6 Nasal anatomy, base view.

Differential reduction of the cartilaginous and bony profile must be calibrated depending on the individual thickness of the overlying S-STE (Figure 2-7). It is equally important to adequately analyze the depth of the radix, as it can provide a natural balance to the nose. Significant deepening of the radix will accentuate any dorsal prominence. Conversely, in a carefully selected setting, a radix graft will balance the nasal profile, decreasing the amount of resection necessary to balance the nasal dorsum (Figure 2-8).

The nasal ala is composed of fibrofatty tissue and is devoid of cartilaginous structure, except for its attachments with the sesamoid cartilages through which it relates to the ULC, LLC, and the pyriform aperture.

THE NASAL SUPERFICIAL MUSCULOAPONEUROTIC SYSTEM

The major mimetic muscles of the nose include the levator labii superioris–alaeque nasi, depressor septii nasi, alar nasi, and transverse nasalis muscle. These are encased and interconnected throughout by a fibrous fascia referred to as the nasal superficial musculoaponeurotic system (SMAS). Maintaining the integrity of this vascularized layer is important when placing grafts and implants to maximize engraftment and minimize infections. Significant ptosis of the nasal tip or deformity occurring during animation will respond to addressing these muscles by either Botulinum toxin use or by surgical ablation.

THE BONY FRAMEWORK

The bony nasal pyramid is composed of the nasal bones and the nasal process of the maxilla. The nasal bones are in direct relation with the perpendicular plate of the ethmoid. In the crooked nose deformity secondary to trauma, these structures are commonly deviated together. Particular attention to the varying degrees of thickness and length of the bone should be kept in mind when planning and executing medial and lateral (and occasionally intermediate) osteotomies. Lateral osteotomies can predispose to nasal airway collapse secondary to compromise of the internal and/or external nasal valves, if care is not taken to perform these osteotomies at the level of the attachment of the inferior turbinate. The majority of the trajectory of the osteotomy takes place within the thicker maxillary process, with the exception of the cephalic end of the osteotomy, where the lateral osteotomies converge at the nasal bones (Figure 2-9).

The nasal bones overlap the cephalic margins of the ULCs. Surgeons should keep in mind that most nasal dorsal hump deformities are composed of the cartilaginous dorsum in continuity with the medial extension of the ULCs. Consequently, the bony component of the dorsal hump is often of lesser magnitude.[1,2]

THE CARTILAGINOUS FRAMEWORK

Conforming the two lower thirds of the nose, the cartilaginous nasal framework contributes important factors to nasal appearance and function. Intrinsic to the anatomic description of the cartilaginous framework of the nose is the description of the tip support mechanisms (Table 2-1).

Three major tip support mechanisms have been described[2]: (1) the size, shape, and resiliency of the LLCs, (2) the fibrous attachments of the medial crura to the caudal septum, and (3) the scroll, a fibrous recurvature attaching the cephalic border of the LLCs to the caudal

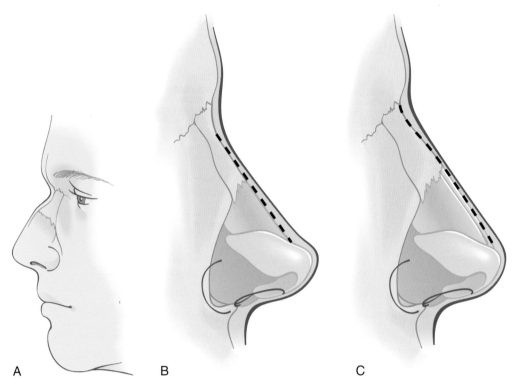

Figure 2-7 A, Dorsal profile of a large bony and cartilaginous hump. **B,** Dorsal profile reduction (bony and cartilaginous) with more aggressive resection at the rhinion. **C,** Dorsal profile reduction demonstrating the importance of the thickness of the skin and soft tissue envelope in the upper, middle, and inferior third of the nose while carrying out a dorsal reduction.

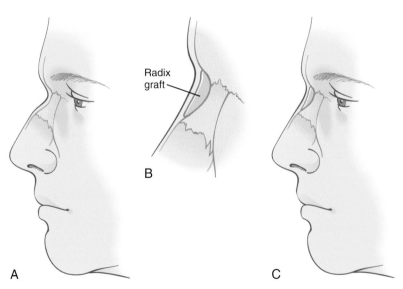

Figure 2-8 A, Deep radix accentuating dorsal hump. **B,** Radix graft. **C,** Correcting apparent dorsal hump by addressing radix depth with radix graft.

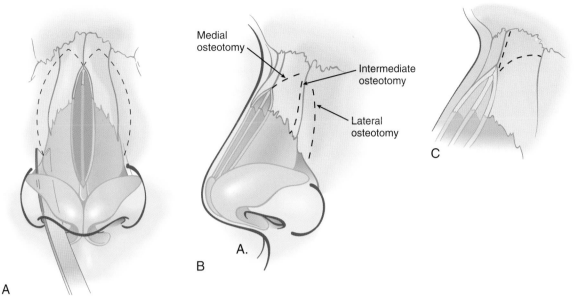

Figure 2-9 A, Medial and lateral osteotomies, correcting open roof deformity following cartilaginous and bony dorsal reduction. **B,** Medial, lateral, and intermediate osteotomies. **C,** Designing medial fading osteotomy.

Table 2-1 Major and Minor Tip Support Mechanisms

Major Tip Support Mechanisms

1. Size, shape, and resiliency of the lower lateral cartilages (LLCs)
2. Fibrous attachments of the medial crura to the caudal septum
3. Scroll, a fibrous recurvature attaching the cephalic border of the LLC, to the caudal border of the upper lateral cartilages (ULCs)

Minor Nasal Tip Support Mechanisms

1. Dorsal cartilaginous septum (anterior septal angle)
2. Interdomal ligament.
3. Membranous (caudal) septum
4. Nasal spine
5. Sesamoid complex
6. Attachment of LLC to the skin and soft tissue envelope

border of the ULCs. Six minor nasal tip support mechanisms have been described: (1) dorsal cartilaginous septum (anterior septal angle), (2) interdomal ligament, (3) membranous (caudal) septum, (4) nasal spine, (5) sesamoid complex, and (6) LLC's attachment to the S-STE.

The LLC contributes, in a great degree, to the characteristics of the size and shape of the lower third of the nose. In the area of the nasal domes, its caudal margin courses just under the level of the skin (Figure 2-10). The LLC can be followed posteriorly, superiorly, and laterally into the middle third of the nose. As the LLC is followed laterally, the caudal edge of the LLC will curve away from the nasal alar rim[2] (see Figure 2-5A).

In the frontal view, the LLCs will flare out at an angle not usually more acute than 40 degrees from the midline.[3] The ULCs form a significant part of the middle third of the nose, also know as the middle vault (Figure 2-10B). Their attachment to the LLC through the recurvature between them (also known as the scroll) will be responsible for part of the degree of upper and lower mobility of the LLC. The internal nasal valve is composed of the angle created between the ULC and the cartilaginous septum. Weakness of the ULC, short nasal bones, and/or an overly aggressive resection of the cartilaginous dorsal hump without reconstruction using spreader graft placement can predispose this area to collapse. The LLCs have been described as a tripod[4] where their medial crura correspond to the base of the tripod (Figure 2-11). Modification of the length of the tripod's leg length and support can affect the nasal structure, shape, function, and appearance.[4-6]

THE NASAL SEPTUM

The septum can be conceptually divided into a cartilaginous (quadrangular) portion and a bony portion. The bony portion is composed of the perpendicular plate of the ethmoid posterosuperiorly, the maxillary crest inferiorly, and the vomer posteriorly. When a septoplasty is performed, be it in isolation, as part of a septorhinoplasty, or as a means to harvest septal cartilage for any grafting purposes, care must be taken to preserve at least one centimeter of caudal and septal cartilage in the form of

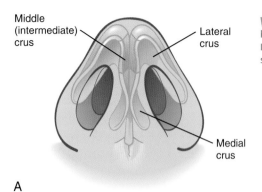

Middle (intermediate) crus

Lateral crus

Medial crus

A

Figure 2-10 A, Nasal base view demonstrating lower lateral cartilages including medial, lateral, and intermediate crura. **B,** Nasal bones, upper lateral cartilage and lower lateral cartilage. Internal nasal valve corresponds to the angle bound by the septum and the upper lateral cartilage seen on the right inset.

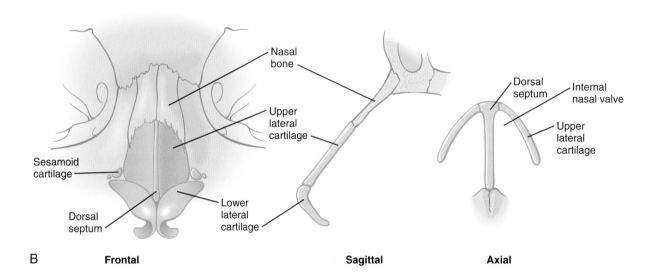

Nasal bone

Upper lateral cartilage

Sesamoid cartilage

Dorsal septum

Lower lateral cartilage

Dorsal septum

Internal nasal valve

Upper lateral cartilage

B   **Frontal**   **Sagittal**   **Axial**

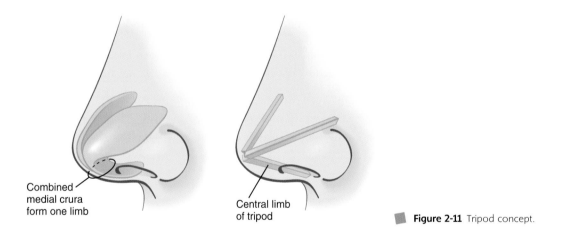

Combined medial crura form one limb

Central limb of tripod

Figure 2-11 Tripod concept.

an "L strut" to ensure an adequate degree of nasal dorsal and tip support (Figure 2-12).

PHYSIOLOGY OF THE NOSE

Nasal function includes olfaction, resonation of speech, humidification, as well as being the first line of defense in the respiratory tract by serving as a filter to particulate matter and the initial anatomic response site to inhaled antigens. The turbulent airflow within the nose is funneled around the warm, moist turbinates humidifying and preparing the air for its passage into the lower airway. Coursing through the nasal airway, the temperature of the air is regulated and aerosolized particles come in contact with chemoreceptors generating afferent responses accounting for olfaction. Therefore, olfaction can be altered with changes in nasal airflow. Significant alterations in intranasal anatomy and nasal airflow can affect the resonating characteristics mediated by the nose on

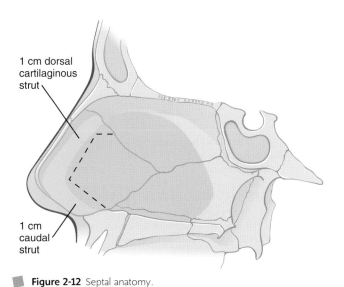

Figure 2-12 Septal anatomy.

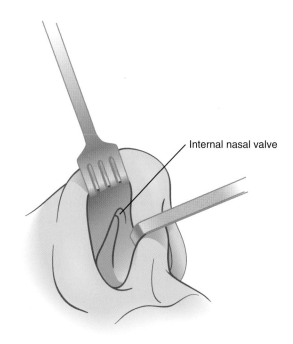

Figure 2-13 Internal nasal valve.

speech. Vasomotor responses (allergic and nonallergic) can be elicited by antigenic exposure, temperature changes, exertion, and trauma. Nasal airflow ushers aerosolized particles toward the olfactory neuroepithelium at the cribriform plate and the superior portions of the septum and lateral nasal wall.[10]

Nasal function relies on constant airflow. The nose provides the greatest resistance to airflow, contributing approximately 50% of the total airway resistance during quiet respiration.[11,12] Within the adult nose, the internal nasal valve area constitutes its narrowest portion and is thus the major flow-limiting segment.[2,3] The nasal valve area is bound superolaterally by the caudal border of the ULC, by the quadrangular cartilage medially, by the pyriform aperture inferiorly, and by the anterior portion of the inferior turbinate posteriorly (Figure 2-10B and 2-13).[7-9] Alterations within this critical area of the nose may have severe consequences in nasal resistance and airflow.

While performing rhinoplasty, certain structures may be altered, ultimately affecting nasal airflow resistance. The entire nasal cavity shares in the formulation of the airflow pattern during inspiration and expiration. Negative pressure is generated during inspiration and positive pressure during expiration. The normal nasal vestibule is designed to withstand expected nasal pressures experienced during normal breathing. However, during deep inspiration, negative pressure generated via the Venturi principle and Bernoulli effect may force the ULCs medially onto the septum, reducing the area of the nasal valve and resulting in a temporary obstruction of the nasal airway.

Weakness or deformity of the ULCs may result in nasal valve collapse and subsequent nasal obstruction even during normal inspiration. Weakened ULCs can also result in collapse of the lateral nasal wall at the juncture between the middle and lower nasal third, giving the nose

a pinched appearance. If both the ULCs and LLCs are weak or deformed, the entire cartilaginous wall may collapse, causing the nostrils to resemble narrow slits. The integrity of the nasal valve area depends on several factors: (1) the integrity and resilience of the ULCs, (2) attachments of the ULCs, and (3) intrinsic nasal musculature. The alar muscles are the least important of these factors.[13] Therefore, the ULCs and their attachments are critical in the preservation of the integrity of the internal nasal valve area and maintaining normal nasal airflow.[14]

EFFECT OF SPECIFIC SURGICAL MANEUVERS ON NASAL PHYSIOLOGY

When performing a rhinoplasty, a septoplasty is often performed to straighten the nasal septum or harvest septal cartilage for grafting purposes. In most cases, the septoplasty improves the nasal airway and therefore the nasal airflow.

Infracture of the nasal bones can affect the nasal valve area if the lateral osteotomies disrupt the caudal edge of the ULC and move it toward the nasal septum. Not only is the airway narrowed in dimension, but also the nasal valve area is disturbed, which can result in collapse of the internal nasal valve with normal inspiration. By performing lateral osteotomies at the pyriform aperture, at about the level of the attachment of the inferior turbinate, a segment of caudal nasal bone is preserved along the maxilla. When this segment of caudal nasal bone is preserved, the widely patent portion of the nasal airway and the external nasal valve are left undisturbed.

Removal of a bony dorsal hump usually has little effect on nasal airway resistance because this maneuver affects only the most superior region of the nasal airway and does not usually change the airway itself. However, care must be taken when reducing the cartilaginous portion of a dorsal hump as excessive manipulation or resection of the ULCs can compromise the internal nasal valve region and can result in collapse and increased nasal resistance. Scar contracture or adhesions in the region of the internal nasal valve can result in severe nasal obstruction that is difficult to correct. When the ULCs collapse medially onto the nasal septum, using spreader grafts,[15] medial ULC "flap" grafts, or suturing the ULCs back onto the nasal septum restores stability to the middle vault.

Resection or weakening of the LLCs can result in alar collapse on inspiration. If the LLCs must be divided, the resected ends should be sutured to one another, restoring their integrity, with or without alar onlay grafts to provide additional support. Reductive surgery of the lower third of the nose can also compromise the integrity of the nasal valve region by disrupting the interdomal ligament (intercartilaginous membrane). This ligament also plays a role in the patency of the nasal valve by providing a caudal attachment of the ULC to the LLC.

Finally, overaggressive alar base reduction may excessively reduce the nostril size, thus compromising the nasal airway. Obstruction at the level of the nostrils can be a significant problem, as these can collapse in a valve-like fashion on inspiration. If reductive surgery is undertaken, the underlying nasal infrastructure must be reconstructed to prevent airway collapse and disruption of normal nasal physiology. Dynamic collapse of the external nasal valve can be reconstructed by implanting alar onlay (Batten) grafts. However, once overreduced, the alar base is difficult to reconstruct.

When performing rhinoplasty with a knowledgeable command of the nasal anatomy and physiology, preoperative and intraoperative observations can be used to predict and identify structural problems, addressing them without compromising the structural integrity or cosmetic appearance of the nose.

REFERENCES

1. Tardy ME. *Rhinoplasty: the art and the science*. Philadelphia: WB Saunders; 1997.
2. Tardy ME, Toriumi DM. Philosophy and principles of rhinoplasty. In: Cummings CW, Fredrickson JM, Harker LA, et al., eds. *Otolaryngology: head and neck surgery*. 2nd ed. St. Louis: Mosby–Year Book; 1993.
3. Toriumi DM. New concepts in nasal tip contouring. *Arch Fac Plast Surg*. 2006;8(3):156–185.
4. Anderson JR. A reasoned approach to nasal base surgery. *Arch Otolaryngol*. 1984;110(6):349–358.
5. Whitaker EG, Johnson CM Jr. The evolution of open structure. *Rhinoplasty Arch Fac Plast Surg*. 2003;5:291–300.
6. Soliemanzadeh P, Kridel RW. Nasal tip overprojection: algorithm of surgical deprojection techniques and introduction of medial crural overlay. *Arch Fac Plast Surg*. 2005;7:374–380.
7. Rice DH, Kern EB, Marple BF, Mabry RL, Friedman WH. The turbinates in nasal and sinus surgery: a consensus statement. *Ear Nose Throat J*. 2003;82(2):82–84.
8. Leopold DA, Holbrook EH. Physiology of olfaction. In: Cummings CW, Flint PW, Haughey BH, et al, eds. *Otolaryngology: Head and neck surgery*. 4th ed. Philadelphia: Mosby Elsevier; 2005:chap 37.
9. Johnson CM Jr, Toriumi DM. *Open structure rhinoplasty*. Philadelphia: WB Saunders; 1990.
10. Leopold DA, Hummel T, Schwob JE, Hong SC, Knecht M, Kobal G. Anterior distribution of human olfactory epithelium. *Laryngoscope*. 2000;110(3):417–421.
11. Butler J. Work of breathing through the nose. *Clin Sci*. 1960;19:55–62.
12. Speizer F, Frank R. A technique for measuring nasal and pulmonary flow resistance simultaneously. *J Appl Physiol*. 1964;19:176–178.
13. May M, West JW, Hinderer KH. Nasal obstruction from facial palsy. *Arch Otolaryngol*. 1977;103:889–891.
14. Kern EB. Surgical approaches to abnormalities of the nasal valve. *Rhinology*. 1978;16:165–189.
15. Sheen JH, Sheen A. *Aesthetic rhinoplasty*. 2nd ed. St. Louis: CV Mosby; 1987.

CHAPTER THREE

Nasal Analysis

Andrew S. Frankel • Umang Mehta

INTRODUCTION

Nasal analysis in the setting of the preoperative consultation is undoubtedly one of the most critical elements of the rhinoplasty process. This is the time in which the patient and surgeon communicate expectations, build rapport, and mutually decide whether to proceed with surgery. In addition, it provides an opportunity for the surgeon to analyze the patient's anatomy and personal aesthetics, thereby developing a surgical plan leading to the most sought-after result: a satisfied patient. A well-executed surgery and beautiful result from the surgeon's perspective will be frustrating for both parties if the patient's desires are not considered. This chapter will examine the various components of nasal analysis, including patient history, nasal proportions, the tripod concept, nasal subunits, physical examination, photography, and imaging.

PATIENT HISTORY

A proper preoperative history must begin with the patient's demographic data, comorbidities, previous surgery (particularly any prior nasal surgery or other cosmetic surgeries), medications, prior hospitalizations, medication allergies, and family/social history and a thorough review of systems. The patient should complete a list of medications, including over-the-counter medications, herbal supplements, and vitamins. The use of nasal steroid sprays, antihistamines, and decongestant sprays such as oxymetazoline (Afrin) and phenylephrine (Neo-Synephrine) should be documented. A history of tobacco, alcohol, and drug use should be obtained. Components of the social history, such as profession and marital status, can provide a more complete picture of the patient as a whole and offer some clues regarding the patient's expectations of surgery and support system. The age of the patient is also important, as a 55-year-old patient is less likely to tolerate a dramatic change in appearance than is a 16-year-old. It is important in teenagers to ascertain just where they are along their growth curve so as to render a result that ultimately balances with the other facial features. In teenage females, our rule is to wait at least until 2

years following menarche before performing elective rhinoplasty—typically sixteen years old. In teenage males, we typically wait until the age of 17.

After reviewing the general history, we begin the assessment of the nose by asking the open-ended question, "What is it that you don't like about your nose?" This allows the patient to describe, in his or her own words, the specific aspects of the nose that are most bothersome to them. It is helpful to note the order in which patients mention these features, as this typically reflects the degree to which they are bothered by each aspect. This exercise is also very useful in getting a preliminary sense of the patient's own aesthetic sense and expectations, as well as his or her attention to detail. Such information can help determine at this early stage the chance for a successful outcome.

This is followed by the question, "How long have you been bothered by your nose?" At this stage, any history of nasal trauma or prior nasal surgery is elicited and discussed in more detail. The desire for a rhinoplasty should generally be one that has been present for some time, and persons who have recently decided to have the operation, on a whim, should be counseled and asked to return several months later once they have given it further thought. The motivation for seeking nasal surgery is revealed at this time. Patients are spurred to consider a rhinoplasty for a variety of reasons and the specific factors may impact the surgical plan. For example, a patient seeking a rhinoplasty to erase physical signs resulting from past domestic abuse may benefit from a more profound change than would a 55-year-old attorney who has recently noted that her nasal tip is drooping with age. The surgeon must also carefully assess whether the patient exhibits signs of body dysmorphic disorder. Patients who fixate on their nose in an unhealthy manner or who have unreasonable expectations regarding the impact that the nose will have on their life (e.g., promotion at work) are likely to be persistently unhappy after rhinoplasty.

Functional issues such as nasal obstruction, allergic rhinitis, or chronic rhinosinusitis are extremely pertinent in rhinoplasty. The surgeon should ascertain if one side of the nose is more difficult to breathe through than the other and assess the severity of the breathing difficulty. Sleep habits such as snoring, the use of nasal breathing strips, and sleeping on one side must be documented. It is also worth documenting whether the symptoms are seasonal, positional, or related to certain foods. Patients should be asked about symptoms such as recurrent epistaxis as well. Computed tomography (CT) scan of the sinuses is often useful for patients with functional concerns.

Any prior history of nasal surgery, including previous rhinoplasty, septoplasty, or functional endoscopic sinus surgery, should be discussed. Prior operative reports can be quite useful in formulating a surgical plan, although it is important to recognize that these notes are not always accurate. The timing of the most recent rhinoplasty is important to consider because the nose will continue to change over 12 or more months as postoperative edema resolves and wound contracture takes place. The surgeon must also question the patient about previous breast surgery when considering harvest of costal cartilage. Similarly, prior otoplasty or ear surgery is pertinent when auricular cartilage may be needed.

The patient's ethnic background can provide insight into their particular cultural aesthetic. A patient from South America, for example, will likely have a different idea of what constitutes an attractive nose than a similarly aged patient of Middle Eastern descent. This sort of consideration is essential for delivering a surgical result that the patient desires, even if it varies from the surgeon's own inclination. Additionally, appreciation for cultural differences helps with the process of preoperative imaging and facilitates development of a sense of trust with the patient.

NASAL ANATOMY

An understanding of the anatomy of the nose is obviously quite crucial for the rhinoplasty surgeon. The underlying structural framework of the nose consists of the paired nasal bones superiorly and the five major nasal cartilages caudally. The nasal bones are attached to the frontal bone superiorly, the lacrimal bones superolaterally, and the ascending processes of the maxilla inferolaterally.

The bony septum is composed of the perpendicular plate of the ethmoid posterosuperiorly and the vomer posteroinferiorly. The quadrangular cartilage, which can vary dramatically in size among different ethnic groups, provides the structure for the anterior portion of the septum. This cartilage is the predominant support of the dorsal and caudal portions of the lower two-thirds of the nose.

The upper portion of the quadrangular cartilage flares along its dorsal edge and is fused between the upper lateral cartilages. This is particularly relevant in the setting of profile reduction, as this flared segment is the excised portion. This can lead to narrowing and collapse of the middle vault if not properly supported. The internal nasal valve is comprised of the angle formed by the septum, the upper lateral cartilage, and the head of the

inferior turbinate. The paired lower lateral cartilages sit caudal to the upper lateral cartilages. The lower lateral cartilages are divided into three segments—the medial, intermediate, and lateral crura. The medial crura overlap the caudal edge of the septum. The region between the lower lateral and upper lateral cartilages is called the scroll, which is the recurvature of the upper lateral cartilages. This scroll can be prominent in some individuals.

The skin and soft tissue envelope overlying the bony-cartilaginous framework of the nose must also be understood. The skin of the nose varies in thickness significantly. The upper third is moderately thick but tapers into a thinner region over the rhinion or mid-dorsum. The skin over the lower third of the nose is more sebaceous and thick and tends to hypertrophy with age. Below the skin lies the nasal superficial musculoaponeurotic system, or nasal SMAS. There are four major groups of nasal muscles: dilators, compressors, elevators, and depressors. The dilators are the dilator naris anterior and dilator naris posterior. The sole compressor is the transverse nasalis. Elevators include the procerus and levator labii superioris alaeque nasi while the depressors are the depressor septi nasi and alar nasalis.

NASAL PROPORTIONS

A thorough discussion of the rhinoplasty consultation must first begin with a consideration of nasal proportions. The *nasofrontal angle* is defined as the angle between a line tangent to the nasal dorsum and a line tangent to the glabella through the nasion. This should measure between 115 and 135 degrees[1] (Figure 3-1). An obtuse nasofrontal

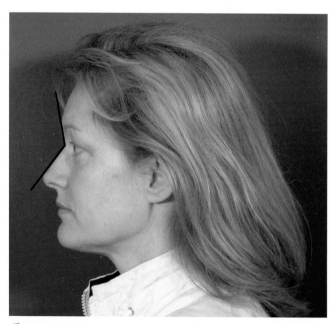

Figure 3-1 The nasofrontal angle should measure between 115 and 135 degrees.

angle gives the illusion of a very long nose on frontal view, as the patient lacks a well-defined nasal starting point (Figure 3-2).

The nasolabial angle is composed of the angle formed by a line from the subnasale to the most anterior point of the columella and a line connecting the labrale superius to the subnasale. This angle should ideally measure 90 to 95 degrees in men and 95 to 110 degrees in women (Figure 3-3). As a general rule, individuals with shorter stature can tolerate a more obtuse nasolabial angle as there will be less visible nostril when viewed from the front by average-statured individuals.

Less frequently discussed angles include the nasofacial angle and nasomental angle. The *nasofacial angle* represents the angle formed by a vertical line from the glabella to the pogonion, as it intersects with a line from the nasion to the nasal tip. This angle can vary from 30 to 40 degrees (Figure 3-4). The *nasomental angle* describes the angle between the nasion-tip line and the line from the tip to the pogonion. The range of this angle is from 120 to 132 degrees (Figure 3-5).

A significant relationship exists between the nose and chin and the two must be considered in conjunction with one another. The chin should ideally reach a vertical line

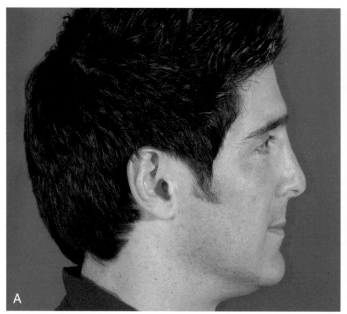
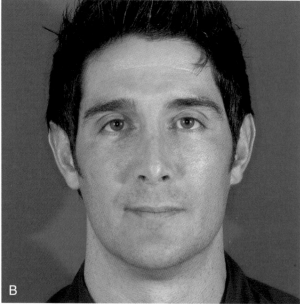

Figure 3-2 A shallow nasofrontal angle of nearly 180 degrees (**A**). On AP view, this obtuse angle causes the nose to appear excessively long (**B**).

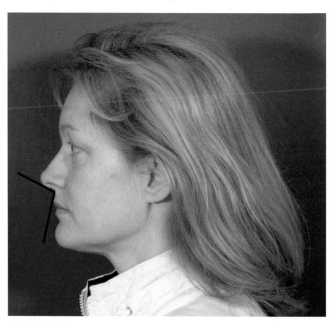
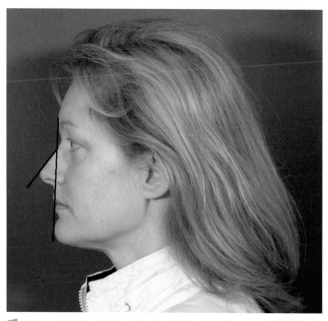

Figure 3-3 Nasolabial angle. Normal range is 95 to 110 degrees for females and 90 to 95 degrees for men.

Figure 3-4 Nasofacial angle, ideally 30 to 40 degrees.

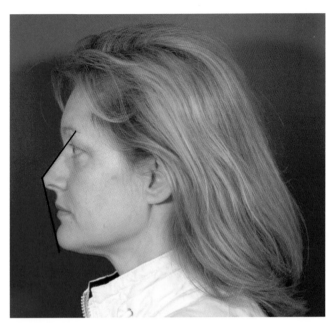

Figure 3-5 Nasomental angle, 120 to 132 degrees.

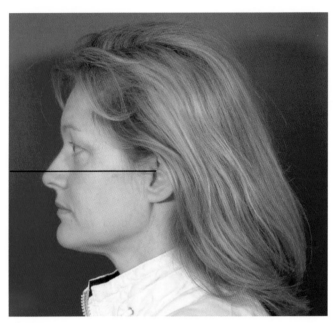

Figure 3-6 The Frankfort horizontal plane: a line drawn between the superior edge of the tragus and the infraorbital rim should parallel the floor.

drawn from the nasion, perpendicular to the Frankfort horizontal plane. The Frankfort horizontal plane represents the line drawn from the superior edge of the tragus to the infraorbital rim, which should be parallel to the ground in standard photographs (Figure 3-6). An underprojected chin must be discussed with the patient, as this can give the illusion of an overprojected nose. The option of chin augmentation should be offered in these situations.

The ideal projection of the nose has been described by Crumley as a 3:4:5 right triangle. The shorter side of the triangle represents the tip projection, the distance from the alar crease to the tip. The ratio between this measurement and the distance between the nasion and tip-defining point should be 0.6.[2] This tip projection ratio was previously described by Goode, with the ideal ratio between 0.55 and 0.6[1] (Figure 3-7).

On base view, the ratio between the tip complex (infratip) and columella should be 1:2, with symmetric, ovoid-shaped nostrils that are thinner at the apex than the base (Figure 3-8). On lateral view, the ideal ala to tip lobule ratio is 1:1. The extent of columellar show is also a significant consideration. It is recommended by most authors that the columellar show be between 2 and 4 mm, although in our experience, most patients favor between 2 and 3 mm.[3]

The width of the nose, as it relates to the overall width of the face, is another important consideration. The concept of "vertical fifths" has been well established, with the width of the nose from the lateral edge of one ala to the other approximating the width from the medial to lateral canthus. This should be equal to one-fifth of the overall width of the face. Therefore, the medial canthus

and lateral edge of the ala should align in a vertical line. The face can also be divided into horizontal thirds. The trichion to glabella portion represents the upper third; glabella to subnasale, the middle third; and subnasale to menton, the lower third[4] (Figure 3-9). Overresection of the caudal septum shortens the nose and can decrease the length of this middle third of the face. This also can lead to the appearance of an overly long upper lip. The width of the dorsum is important and should create a smooth curved line from the medial brow to the nasal tip.

TRIPOD CONCEPT

The nasal tip can be conceptualized as a tripod, where the lateral crura constitute the superior legs and the combined medial crura conform the third leg. Any maneuver that changes the shape of one leg of the tripod will cause a corresponding tilt in the nasal tip.

Following the tripod concept, shortening the inferior leg (combined medial crura) would counterrotate the nasal tip and decrease projection. Conversely, increasing the length of this leg, through the use of a columellar strut, for example, can increase rotation and projection. Alternatively, increasing the length of the superior legs of the tripod (the lateral crura) causes counterrotation and increased projection, whereas decreasing the length of the superior limbs leads to increased rotation but decreased projection. Lengthening all three limbs of the tripod would increase tip projection (without significant rotation), whereas a decrease in all three limbs would decrease projection.

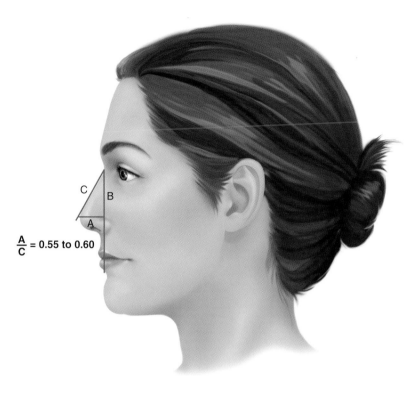

$\dfrac{A}{C}$ = 0.55 to 0.60

Figure 3-7 Goode's ideal tip projection: 0.55 to 0.6 of the length of the nose, from tip to nasion.

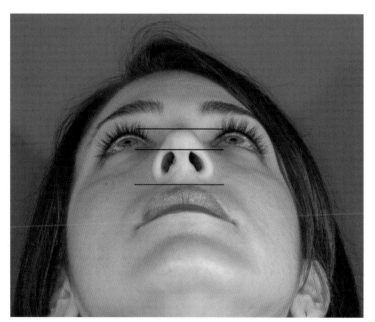

Figure 3-8 Ideal base view. Tip should be one-half the height of the columella.

The interrelation of the tripod complex with the septum must not be disregarded, however, and some authors advocate a tripod-pedestal concept. In this analysis of tip dynamics, the septum comprises the pedestal against which the tripod rests. This approach offers insight into the manner in which changes in the anterior septal angle or suturing of the lower lateral cartilage complex to the septum can result in powerful changes in tip rotation and projection.[5] A newer model for understanding tip dynamics is the "M-Arch," proposed by Adamson. This concept involves the visualization of the lower lateral cartilages as independent arches, with the lateral limb of

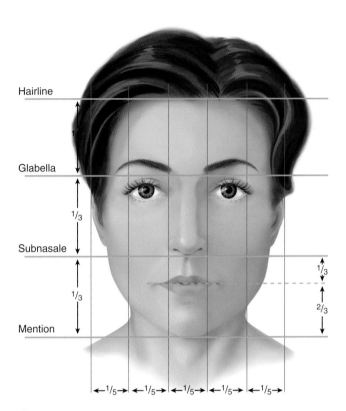

Figure 3-9 Vertical fifths and horizontal thirds.

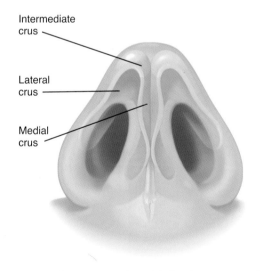

Figure 3-10 Adamson's M-Arch model of tip dynamics, note the intermediate crus.

each arch cephalically positioned. This model represents advancement in our understanding of the nasal tip because it considers the importance of the intermediate crura of the lower lateral cartilages, which are not included in the tripod concept[6] (Figure 3-10).

NASAL SUBUNITS

The subunit concept in facial plastic surgery is instrumental in planning nasal surgery, particularly in nasal reconstruction. The aesthetic unit of the nose is divided into nine subunits, based on convexities and concavities of the nasal surface. The reflection of light in a disparate manner from these areas of convexity and concavity creates predictable areas of light and shadows over the nose. This gives the illusion of borders between subunits, providing optimal locations for incision placement. Scars across a particular subunit tend to be more noticeable.

The nine subunits of the nose are the dorsum, paired lateral nasal walls, paired soft triangles, paired alar subunits, tip, and columella[7] (Figure 3-11).

PHYSICAL EXAMINATION

A systematic examination of the nose begins with an assessment of the thickness of the skin and soft tissue envelope. In thin-skinned individuals, changes to the bony-cartilaginous framework are more readily seen, which can be positive in terms of making the intended changes to the appearance of the nose. The obvious disadvantage of a thinner envelope is that underlying grafts and irregularities will be more readily palpable and visible. Thick skin limits the amount of refinement that is achievable and may result in more protracted swelling postoperatively. It is important to note the sebaceous nature of the tip skin and to discuss this finding with patients so as to manage expectations appropriately.

The bony pyramid is carefully palpated and examined to check for any deviation or bony prominences. The length of the nasal bones is an important predictor of potential postoperative problems. Short nasal bones in conjunction with a long middle nasal vault can lead to collapse of the upper lateral cartilages, if the middle nasal vault is not supported with spreader grafts and reconstitution to the dorsal septum. In addition to the deviation of the pyramid as a whole, concavity or convexity of each individual nasal bone can be palpated. Excessively curved nasal bones may, in rare cases, necessitate intermediate osteotomies. The most common complaint in patients seeking rhinoplasty is the removal of a dorsal hump. The nature of this procedure should be planned during preoperative nasal dorsal palpation, determining whether the area of concern is predominantly bony or cartilaginous.

The height of the radix, nasofrontal angle, and nasal starting point should also be noted. These can be important measurements to review with the patient during the imaging portion of the consultation as most patients are unaware of the aesthetic implications of this portion of the nose.

Examination of the septum involves both external and internal assessment. Externally, a C-shaped deformity of

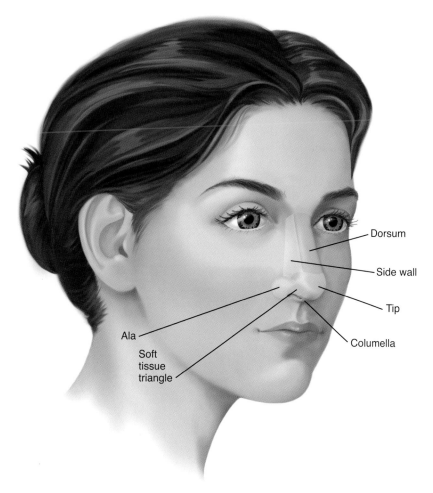

Dorsum

Side wall

Tip

Columella

Ala

Soft
tissue
triangle

Figure 3-11 Nasal subunits.

the dorsal septum is quite common and gives the nose a twisted shape, particularly on the overhead, bird's-eye view. Palpation and inspection of the anterior septal angle can reveal excess in this area, particularly in the setting of a Pollybeak deformity (Figure 3-12). Palpation of the caudal septum is another critical portion of the examination, especially for revision cases. An overly shortened caudal septum can lead to retraction of the columella and a short-appearing nose. At the same time, the nasal spine is palpated. A prominent nasal spine in conjunction with a large quadrangular cartilage may cause an overprojected, or "tension," nose deformity (Figure 3-13).

Intranasal examination with a headlight and nasal speculum is of significant value in assessing the integrity of the septum and the degree of septal deflection. In patients who have had previous nasal surgery, we carefully palpate the septum with a cotton-tipped applicator to determine how much, if any, of the septum has been resected and how much remains for grafting. This also allows the surgeon to assess if the dorsal and caudal portions of the septal L-strut are adequate for nasal support. Any septal perforations, intranasal synechiae, and contact

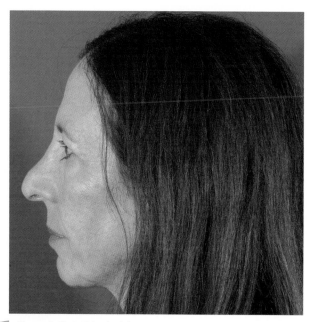

Figure 3-12 Pollybeak deformity.

points with the turbinates are documented. The size of the inferior turbinates and quality of the nasal mucosa can provide insight into the cause of the patient's nasal obstruction. A fiberoptic examination of the nasal cavity should be undertaken when the patient notes a history of nasal obstruction.

Collapse of the internal nasal valve due to inferomedial displacement of the caudal edge of the upper lateral cartilage is easily identified intranasally. The upper lateral cartilage can be manually displaced with a Q-tip while asking the patient to inhale and exhale through the nose. Improvement in nasal breathing via this maneuver or the modified Cottle maneuver is indicative of internal

valve-related nasal obstruction. Externally, upper lateral cartilage collapse can give the middle vault a pinched appearance or inverted-V deformity[8] (Figure 3-14). Examination of the lateral crura will yield causes of external valve stenosis, resulting from profound curvature, subluxation, overresection or excessive thickness. Dynamic collapse of the external nasal valve should be evaluated in inspiration and expiration (Figure 3-15).

Analysis of the nasal tip should begin with an assessment of the general shape. While examining and palpating the nose, the surgeon should perform the mental exercise of visualizing the underlying cartilages to determine their shape and contribution to the nasal tip. It is critical to

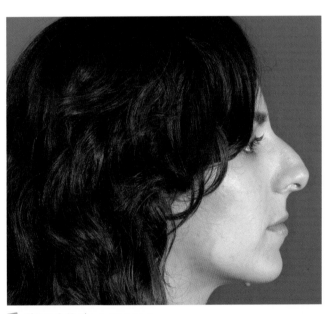

Figure 3-13 The tension nose.

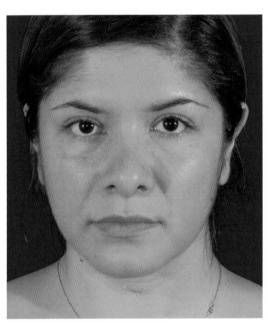

Figure 3-14 Inverted-V deformity. Note the washout of the brow-tip aesthetic line in the middle third of the nose.

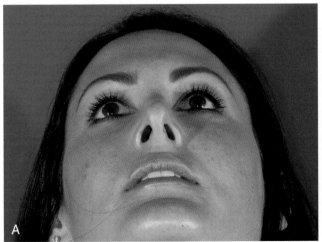

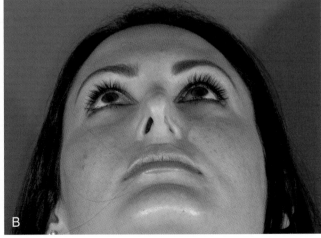

Figure 3-15 Collapse of the external valve. Note the patency on expiration (**A**) but collapse on inspiration (**B**).

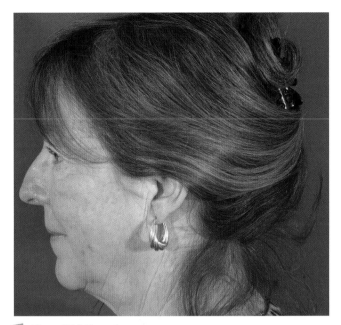

Figure 3-16 The aging nose.

consider the multitude of factors at play in creating the appearance of the tip. Consider, for example, the boxy, poorly defined, and wide nasal tip. This particular shape can occur as a result of a number of factors: (1) fullness in the region of the scroll, (2) prominent cephalic margins of the lower lateral cartilages, (3) cephalically malpositioned lateral crura, (4) convexity of the lower lateral cartilages, and (5) obtuse angles of divergence at the intermediate crura. There exist a multitude of tip forms that can impart an undesirable appearance to the nose, the discussion of which lies outside the scope of this chapter.

Palpation of the nasal tip allows the surgeon to assess the stiffness of the lower lateral cartilages and the other major and minor mechanisms of tip support. With aging, fibrous attachments of the scroll weaken, resulting in separation of the lower lateral cartilages from the upper lateral cartilages. In addition, the interdomal ligament weakens, causing splaying of the domes and additional loss of support. The overall effects of aging include ptosis of the tip, the appearance of lengthening of the nose, and valve collapse (Figure 3-16). The tip should be observed in animation, as this can further accentuate tip ptosis, due to the action of the depressor septi nasi muscle (Figure 3-17). Bossae at the tip can result from prominent knuckles at the dome and are almost always due to loss of integrity of the alar cartilages from overresection or division.

On lateral view, important considerations include nasal tip projection, the degree of columellar show, supratip break, nasolabial angle, and double break in the infratip region. There is frequently an asymmetry of the lower lateral cartilages that causes the profile view of the tip to differ dramatically from one side to the other. The thickness of the lateral alar skin and soft tissue is another common complaint of patients, particularly in certain ethnic groups. Patients must be counseled regarding the anatomy of these areas and the limitations in changing their shape. One should also document the depth of the alar grooves and projection of the premaxilla.

On base view, some important considerations include alar base symmetry, ratio of the infratip to the columella, projection of the caudal septum or medial crura into the airway, and presence of a previous transcolumellar scar.

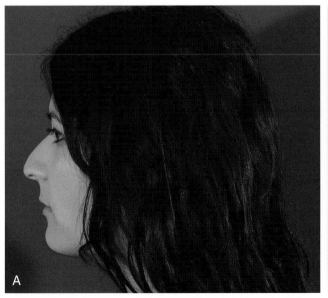

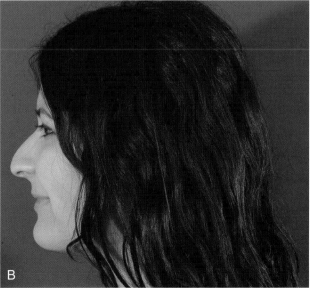

Figure 3-17 Tip ptosis (**A**). The degree of ptosis is often accentuated with smiling (**B**).

The shape and location of the prior transcolumellar incision must be noted. A poorly healed incision should be palpated to check for a step-off immediately underneath the incision so it can be addressed intraoperatively. Causes of this step-off include the edge of a shield graft or the division of the medial crura.

Revision rhinoplasty consultations necessitate a few additional points to consider. First, the overall quality of the skin and soft tissue envelope changes with each revision. Typically, the skin becomes increasingly translucent and its vascularity increases, which may lead to reddish and purple discolorations. Second, a paucity of internal lining and membranous septum resulting from previous surgery may be limiting factors in attempting to lengthen a nose, so it is important to evaluate these factors when considering such a plan. Third, the patient's ears should be closely examined and palpated to determine the presence and quality of the cartilage in the conchal bowls. Patients who have undergone prior otoplasty or cartilage harvest may not be candidates for additional harvest, necessitating a discussion regarding rib cartilage.

PHOTOGRAPHY

The importance of proper photographic documentation in plastic and reconstructive nasal surgery cannot be overstated. The benefits of photography include patient counseling, surgical planning, self-assessment, and documentation for insurance and medicolegal reasons.

Digital photography now allows for immediate viewing of patient photographs, and this is extremely helpful during an initial consultation. By viewing the photographs together, the surgeon and patient are able to identify desirable and undesirable features of the nose in an organized and detailed fashion. Any preexisting asymmetry should be pointed out to patients preoperatively as they will certainly notice such details as they scrutinize their nose after surgery. Patients often ask for hard or electronic copies of these photographs to share with family members after the consultation so as to aid with the decision of whether to proceed with the rhinoplasty. Also, patients may request to view photographs of other patients who have undergone surgery to determine if they like that particular surgeon's aesthetic. While viewing a photograph album may seem like a marketing issue, it is actually quite helpful in identifying patients who may want a result that is not typical of that surgeon. In the postoperative period, the preoperative photographs can be helpful in pacifying a patient who is unhappy with the result or is fixated on a small imperfection or asymmetry, by reminding the patient of the preoperative appearance. The use of computer imaging, which will be covered in the next section, obviously necessitates the taking of standardized, reproducible photographs.

The availability of photographs preoperatively allows the surgeon to generate a plan of expected surgical maneuvers. Intraoperatively, the photographs are very useful in reminding the surgeon of the patient's baseline nose as the infiltration of local anesthesia, elevating the skin-soft tissue envelope, and edema can distort the nasal appearance. From a self-assessment standpoint, the careful and honest comparison of preoperative photographs to those taken postoperatively is an invaluable yet humbling process. In our practice, we have found that even when patients are ecstatic with their surgical result, there are aspects of the nose that we wish could be slightly different. The rhinoplasty surgeon should be his or her own toughest critic, as this process promotes tremendous self-improvement over the course of one's career.

The equipment required for photography begins with the digital camera. The surgeon should carefully shop for a single-lens reflex camera that allows for the use of variable lenses. We find a 105-mm macro lens to be optimal for our purposes. Standardized distance and lighting are vital for elucidating subtle irregularities and asymmetries. Although there may be limitations based on your particular office space, care should be taken in aligning your flashes to minimize shadows yet maximize the details. Depth of field and other settings should be determined by trial and error until you are satisfied with the images. We currently use an aperture priority setting of F-16, an ISO of 200, and shutter speed of 1/60. A stool should be provided that allows the patient to rotate freely. It is helpful to place fixed markers to which the patient can face for the profile and three-quarter views. A flat blue or green background is most useful, as it is pleasing to the eye and provides more depth of field. Storing the digital photographs within a secure network is mandatory.

The standard views taken in rhinoplasty should include the anterioposterior (AP) view, right and left profiles, right and left three-quarter views, and base view. In many patients, we photograph a bird's-eye overhead view, to illustrate twisting of the nose. Additionally, we often shoot profile views with the patient smiling, to accentuate tip ptosis. Photographs should be taken precisely in the Frankfort horizontal plane. Care should also be taken on profile views to ensure that patients are not rotated more or less than 90 degrees from the camera, as this may distort the appearance of the nose significantly. Surgeons disagree over the precise definition of the three-quarter view, with some favoring lining up the dorsum with the medial canthus and others the nasal tip with the contralateral cheek. We advocate the latter.

IMAGING

The use of computer imaging to alter preoperative images ("morphing") has become an integral part of our rhinoplasty practice. The improvements in technology over the past decade and the ability to create and store multiple high-resolution images of patients have facilitated this exercise. There are a number of available imaging software programs, each with a variety of features, the discussion of which lies outside the scope of this chapter.

At the initial consultation, photographs are taken of the patient, and the photographs are uploaded into our database. The images are reviewed as is, often comparing the two profiles to one another to note asymmetries and other differences. Next, the surgeon uses the morphing software in the patient's presence to illustrate the changes that the surgeon believes would be warranted. The concepts of what would be done in surgery are discussed during this process and limitations are brought to the forefront. Once the surgeon is satisfied with the result, he or she offers the patient an opportunity to make changes

to suit the patient's individual taste. This is a crucial component of the consultation because it allows the surgeon insight into what the patient desires. Together the surgeon and patient then reach a consensus about the optimal end result, and these images are saved and brought into the operating room for reference during surgery. It should also be noted that imaging is typically most useful in the profile views. In the AP view, it is challenging to accurately morph the lights and shadows to illustrate expected changes in the nose. We find it quite helpful to compare our morphed photos to the actual postoperative photographs 12 months after surgery; this is an extremely educational, yet often humbling exercise (Figure 3-18).

For the process to realize its potential, the surgeon must use the morphing tools in a responsible manner and be realistic about the limitations of his or her skills. For example, a patient with an extremely thick soft-tissue

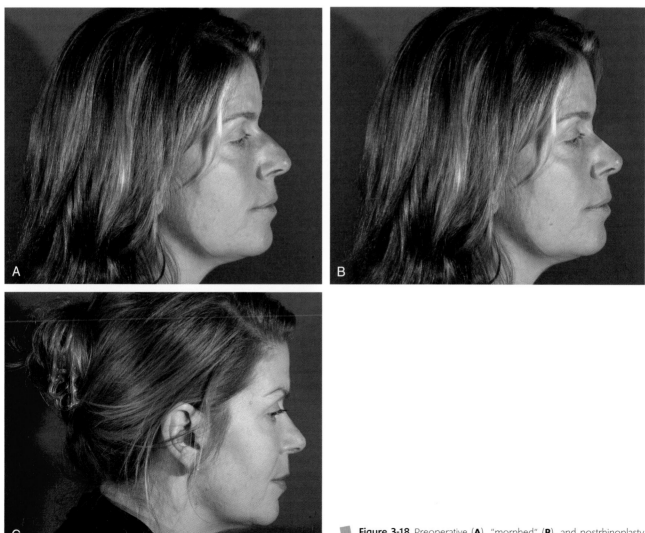

Figure 3-18 Preoperative (**A**), "morphed" (**B**), and postrhinoplasty (**C**) photographs.

envelope should not be shown an unrealistically delicate tip with clearly visible underlying anatomy. As a general rule, imaging should be used as a communication tool rather than as a marketing tool. A conscientious surgeon must explain the limitations of preoperative imaging with the patient and explain that the images reflect the surgical goal, rather than a guarantee of results. There certainly are medicolegal implications in imaging, which necessitate honest and clear communication between surgeon and patient regarding the role of imaging in the consultation.

For the patient, the chance to provide input into the generation of these images gives a sense of control and builds trust in the surgeon. Imaging also promotes an understanding of the interrelation of various aspects of the nose. For example, the surgeon can demonstrate that by increasing projection of the tip, one can reduce the degree to which the dorsum needs to be taken down in profile reduction. Patients frequently arrive at the rhinoplasty consultation with magazine clippings, asking for a specific celebrity's nose. We find it very useful to redirect patients to their own images created during the imaging exercise.

CONCLUSION

There is an oft-repeated tenet in rhinoplasty: It is far better to have a well-conceived surgical plan, based on an accurate assessment of the patient's particular anatomy and aesthetic, and to execute this plan with average surgical technique than it is to have a mediocre plan, with little or no consideration of the patient's wishes, and to carry it out exquisitely. The process of nasal analysis is fundamentally important in generating this plan and achieving the goal of satisfying the patient.

REFERENCES

1. Powell N, Humphreys B. *Proportions of the aesthetic face*. New York: Thieme-Stratton; 1984.
2. Crumley RL, Lanser M. Quantitative analysis of nasal tip projection. *Laryngoscope*. 1988;98(2):202–208.
3. Tardy EM. *Rhinoplasty, The art and the science*. Philadelphia: WB Saunders; 1997.
4. Friedman O. Changes associated with the aging face. *Fac Plast Surg Clin N Am*. 2005;13:371–380.
5. Johnson CM, To WC. *A case approach to open structure rhinoplasty*. Philadelphia: Elsevier Saunders; 2005.
6. Adamson PA, Litner JA, Dahiya R. The M-Arch model: a new concept of nasal tip dynamics. *Arch Fac Plast Surg*. 2006;8(1):16–25.
7. Burget GC. Aesthetic restoration of the nose. *Clin Plast Surg*. 1985;12:463.

CHAPTER FOUR

The Psychology of Rhinoplasty

Lessons Learned from Fellowship

Peter A. Adamson • Jason A. Litner

> *This above all: to thine own self be true,*
> *And it must follow, as the night the day,*
> *Thou canst not then be false to any man.*
> Polonius' advice to his son, Laertes, Shakespeare's *Hamlet*, 1603

Starting a practice in cosmetic facial surgery is daunting. Every new facial plastic surgeon is eager to make his or her mark and to put into practice his or her numerous years of training, although, in truth, the real education is only just beginning. The true value in having completed a fellowship is in acquiring a lifetime of lessons in what really matters to a cosmetic practice. Of course, what interests the young surgeon is to be technically excellent and to master the latest in techniques. Few surgeons, especially neophytes, jump to the topic of this chapter with enthusiasm, yet psychology is as germane to a successful rhinoplasty practice as is any other topic in this book, if not more so. Aesthetic surgery, more than almost any other branch of medicine short of psychiatry, is really a study of human relations. A patient's happiness has to do with so much more than just the technical proficiency and the surgical result. Recognition of this fact is a critical component underpinning all that we do. This chapter will attempt to encapsulate some of the most useful aphorisms a cosmetic facial plastic surgeon would do well to keep in his or her breast pocket at all times. It will also elucidate the warning signs that herald the potential for a maladaptive response to surgery and an unsatisfying situation for both the patient and surgeon.

Patients choose our services based on so many real and intangible factors. They do not really "need" us but they simultaneously hope we have something to offer them that will satisfy one of their most basic desires—to feel valued by themselves and by others. Most rational, healthy people do not actually want to have surgery. They understand, though, that surgery is the step that must be taken to reach their desired level of self-fulfillment. While they may not have decided on the surgeon or on an exact procedure, most patients have already taken the leap and decided to have surgery before they visit us. The objective of the consultation in their eyes is to determine if we are the right

surgeons for them. Likewise, many young surgeons believe they must "sell" their abilities. Instead, the surgeon should concentrate on determining patients' suitability to his or her practice based on his or her skills, personality, and comfort level while interacting with the patient. That critical assessment is the focus of this chapter.

A great deal has been written about the psychology of patients seeking aesthetic surgery, but this subject has never been more topical than in the past few years. Now that aesthetic surgery has entered the mainstream, prospective patients are treating it much like any other luxury purchase. The "retail-ification" of cosmetic surgery has advantages and disadvantages for both patients and surgeons. On the positive end, aesthetic improvements have become more accessible to a host of people who would not otherwise have had the chance to benefit from these procedures. On the negative end, the decision to undergo aesthetic surgery may be less deliberate than it had been in years past. The selection of a surgeon may be more impulsive and the preoperative rapport developed between patient and surgeon may be less than ideal. In addition, the number and types of practitioners who are providing these services have expanded immeasurably, and not all share the same level of training and proficiency. Market conditions have led to the commoditization of even invasive procedures such as rhytidectomy, where franchises are owned and operated by business people and surgeons are being used as technicians. Intensive marketing, competition, and mass media coverage of cosmetic surgery have trivialized operations and overidealized outcomes. Patients are also now led to believe that they can obtain a surgical rhinoplasty result with the use of injectable fillers alone. These factors increase the possibility that a rhinoplasty patient may encounter a poor outcome and, what may be worse, be ill-equipped to assimilate it.

Against this backdrop, it is ever more important that surgeons understand and embrace a rhinoplasty patient's psychology. Psychology is arguably more relevant to rhinoplasty than it is to other facial plastic surgical procedures, because patients seeking aging face procedures are not in search of a change so much as they are in pursuit of a return to a previously favorable self-image. Rhinoplasty patients, on the other hand, have often been living since puberty with the insecurity attached to their nose. This uneasiness has usually been a formative part of their body image. They are more apprehensive about the changes proposed since they often possess a clear vision of their preferred self-image, although they may have a hard time articulating that ideal. The failure of a rhinoplasty procedure to harmonize with this desired self-image can meet with profound anxiety. This is especially true for revision rhinoplasty patients who carry the added burden of already having experienced an overwhelming disappointment.

The gravity of this reality should not be underestimated. Physical violence against surgeons is rare but real. In the decade from 1995 to 2005, five plastic surgeons in the United States were killed by former patients. We all possess a dominant personality type and we tend to use it as a filter in response to our surroundings. In times of stress, this response mechanism becomes exaggerated.[1] Some of us weather the storms of our lives with little fanfare. Some withdraw and retreat into ourselves. Others strike out with aggression. A patient's personality type can be of prime importance in determining how he or she will interact when faced with an unexpected surgical result.

WHAT MAKES PATIENTS UNHAPPY

Treatises on the subject of patient unhappiness usually focus on patient factors that may contribute to this unfortunate situation and tend to deemphasize the discussion on surgeon-related factors as a possible cause. Since surgeon factors are the only ones we can really influence, it makes sense to explore these more in depth. You may find it hard to admit that, more often than not, patients are justifiably unhappy because you failed to meet their expectations. With any luck, this happens very infrequently but, as the saying goes, if you do not have any surgical problems, you are probably not operating enough. Even the most meticulous and accomplished among us has a measurable revision rate. Having a very low revision rate, however, does not by itself declare you a great surgeon. Your unhappy patients may simply be taking your revisions elsewhere.

Patient expectations may have been unfulfilled for several reasons that may or may not fall within your control. The surgical outcome may have been truly subpar. The patient may be the inauspicious recipient of a complication despite your best efforts at avoiding one. You

may have unwittingly misled the patient as to what you could accomplish with the proposed procedure. You may not have given the patient the time and attention he or she deserved. You may have talked the patient into having a chin implant because you thought it would improve her rhinoplasty result, even though she expressed no interest in this procedure. You may have been insensitive when she was airing her postoperative concerns. You may have accepted a patient who was a decidedly poor candidate for rhinoplasty. Most of these factors are avoidable. A patient's happiness with the procedure is arguably as much dependent on your attitude and conduct toward the patient as it is on the technical result itself and on the patient's personality features.

To be sure, many patient factors play a role in this interaction, and these will be examined. Yet, a survey by the American Academy of Facial Plastic and Reconstructive Surgery showed that the most common reason for patient unhappiness, more than all others combined, was a breakdown of rapport (51% of cases). The rapport developed preoperatively is most indicative of the direction of the postoperative dynamic. A strong preoperative bond will usually be reinforced under difficult circumstances when both the surgeon and patient are working toward a common goal of improvement. Likewise, a deficient relationship will usually decay under duress, sometimes beyond recovery. To fully understand and prevent problems pertaining to the surgeon–patient relationship, the microscope must be turned inward.

AVOIDING AND PREVENTING UNHAPPY PATIENTS

There is a kernel of truth in the old adage that the secret to a successful practice is first Affability, followed by Availability and, finally, by Ability. Yet, there is no getting around an undeniably flawed technical result. No amount of kindness on the part of the surgeon can fully compensate for this failure. Jack Anderson, M.D., was known to teach that it is not essential that you operate brilliantly; rather, you should strive to never operate badly. The best defense against unhappiness, then, is to consistently do good work. But, what of the majority of patients who encounter an "adequate" result, one that most people would describe as at least good, if not perfect? This result has the potential to produce an overjoyed patient, a mostly satisfied albeit mildly disappointed patient, or a hopelessly discontent one. This difference has mostly to do with perception. A patient who was given realistic expectations and who is treated with true caring will be inclined to overlook the minor imperfections associated with this outcome. A similar patient with the identical result will be given to chronic unhappiness if she was led to anticipate a far superior outcome or if she or he was treated unjustly. The following section takes a practical, rather than theoretical, approach to the discussion of what a surgeon may do to increase the chances for having patients fall into the former category. These truisms are not meant to be patronizing but, rather, to act as a gentle reminder that the surgeon very often controls the direction of the physician–patient dynamic. The fact that they are generally simplistic and even patently obvious does not diminish their value as good principles of patient management.

If you do not like the patient, do not operate. This seems self-evident, but you should follow the principle of performing surgery on happy patients that you like. This is probably the single most important tenet of patient selection. A small percentage of people have a negative outlook on virtually every aspect of their lives and there is no reason to expect that your surgery will be any different. These are pessimists who exaggerate the negative impact of a majority of their life circumstances. Many harbor a general mistrust of physicians. As a result, they are unlikely to be fully satisfied with even an excellent outcome. Thankfully, these patients are relatively easy to identify during the preoperative consultation. Happy people, in general, are more likely to remain happy with their results, to accept imperfection, and to refer their like-minded friends and colleagues. This way, you will continue to attract happy people to your practice.

Take yourself out of the equation. Understand, first and foremost, that you do not matter as much as you might think. We call what we do preoperatively "patient selection" when, in fact, the truth is that you do not choose the patient; the patient chooses you. You are the gatekeeper of your practice. At best, you can refuse a patient. It matters not what you think of your surgical results. It matters only what your patients think; theirs is the measure of your success.

Work at keeping your patients happy. When patients agree to have you perform surgery, they are excited and optimistic. They want to enjoy a fulfilling and productive relationship with you. Contrary to popular belief, most cosmetic surgery patients are usually happy, well-adjusted, and committed people who are interested in self-improvement. Testing has repeatedly shown that cosmetic surgery patients are in the normal range for self-esteem, although most have a low self-image for the particular feature of concern.[2] They are not typically unreasonable, discontent, disordered, experiencing chronic health concerns, or seeking secondary gain. Furthermore, most do not expect perfection. When they cease to be happy, it is usually because we have contributed to their displeasure by the way in which we have responded to them. A cosmetic practice is a little like a marriage in that happiness does not appear out of thin air. With that in mind, you should undertake every interaction with the philosophy that your foremost purpose is in helping your patients to achieve happiness.

Explore patients' motivations. If you have concerns that a patient may have a generalized low self-image or

is undertaking the procedure for some reason other than his or her personal satisfaction, you should consider not doing the surgery. A patient responding to external motivators is far more likely to be discontent even with an outstanding result. Unhealthy motivation and poor self-image often combine to increase the chances of psychological instability and dissatisfaction after surgery. By the time you agree to schedule surgery, you should be absolutely sure of the patient's sincere motives for self-betterment. Occasionally, surgery is not the answer and patients deserve to know that at the outset. Otherwise, you will discover a patient who continues to be dissatisfied despite obtaining a good technical result.

Listen more. It can be tempting during your consultation to launch into a discourse on what patients need and how fortunate they will be to benefit from your formidable talents. Spend more time listening than speaking during the consultation. A patient's questions can be as revealing as can their omissions. If the consultation becomes more about you than about the patient, you will have missed your chance to truly evaluate his or her suitability.

Be honest about your own motivations. External motivators play a complicating role when deciding on whether to operate on a potentially problematic patient. Experienced surgeons have the benefit of a more finely tuned "sixth sense" coupled with a motivation to avoid accepting patients who are at higher risk for being dissatisfied. A younger surgeon is more driven to accept every patient early in his career because he or she can ill-afford to lose a case. He or she wants every potential patient to choose him or her and will often ignore the little voice of unease that says this patient may not be right for him or her. Good judgment can easily be obscured by needs pertaining to the ego or to the pocketbook. An unselfish commitment to the patient's best interests in every situation may necessitate some short-term sacrifice, in the form of refusing surgery where appropriate, but will undoubtedly have the long-term rewarding effect of growing your practice.

Recognize and respect your limitations. It is more important to tell the patient what you cannot do rather than what you can. Check your ego at the door. You cannot be an expert at everything. The most respected giants in our field often do no more than four or five operations most of the time. They accumulate mastery of a technique. That is not to say that all learning should cease after training; quite the opposite is true. But, be cognizant of your place on the learning curve. If you are incorporating an emerging technology that you just discovered at a recent meeting, tell the patient that the potential benefits are not entirely clear. Ask yourself if this new technology is really likely to make your patient happier with the result. If a patient would most benefit from a rib graft, which you perform once a year, consider referring him or her to a trusted colleague who has more experience if you believe that to be the best procedure for that particular patient. A fourth time revision is perhaps not one you wish to include among your first 50 rhinoplasties. In general, a spirit of conservatism and prudence should prevail if you wish to minimize the number of unhappy patients you inherit. This is especially true early in your career where a single unhappy patient can wreak havoc on your budding practice.

Undersell the benefits. When you give your patients an expectation of the result preoperatively, whether by computer imaging or by other means, underpromise so that you can overdeliver, exceeding patient expectations. The authors make a habit of imaging a less than ideal result. We tell our patients that surgery is imperfect but we know that if they can be happy with the imaged "average" result, then we can almost assuredly do better for them. Be cautious of the rhinoplasty patient who also needs a chin implant. Do not push the patient to have a procedure that you think would be more beneficial. The level of unhappiness with a less than perfect result is far greater when the procedure was suggested by you rather than by the patient. Instead, be honest in your appraisal and dissuade patients from pursuing a procedure if they would not benefit optimally. Your integrity will be most welcome and will often result in a successful relationship in the future.

Do not let your head overrule your gut. Your gut instincts are not always right, but they often are. Your impression of the patient in the first 5 minutes of your interaction is usually an accurate preview of how this interaction will play out postoperatively. In the book *Blink*, the author Malcolm Gladwell describes that subcognitive perception enables us to make rapid assessments that have greater precision than those judgments that result from extensive analysis. The patient you initially think might present a problem after surgery often does live up to those expectations. Most physicians are often influenced by their urge to "do good." The hope that your technically good procedure will engender a joyful disposition in a patient who is psychologically unsuitable for surgery is rarely realized. If you are unsure about a patient's suitability, spend more time with him or her. If your doubts are reinforced, you will have made better use of your time in deciding not to proceed with surgery than in spending countless hours with an unsatisfied patient after surgery. Remember, though, that the more time spent with some personality types, the more psychologically healthy they may appear.

Inform your patients properly. There is a saying among experienced surgeons, "What you tell patients before surgery is an explanation … what you tell them afterwards is an excuse." It is true that patients hear only a small fraction of what you tell them during the consultation. So, make a habit of eliciting questions, speaking slowly, repeating often, and imparting information in more than one format. The authors routinely see patients for a second visit prior to surgery, partly to further gauge

their fitness for our practice but also to convey information at a time when they are more relaxed and more likely to be receptive. The authors ask patients to sign a document stating that they have received, read, understood, and agreed to abide by all of the preoperative and postoperative instructions. By doing so, patients grasp that they are partners in this endeavor.

Tell a patient about the possibility of a revision. It is easy to gloss over possible complications because this discussion is uncomfortable and many patients do not even wish to have it. This temptation should be avoided. Patients should be given information along with an explanation of the surgical consent both verbally and in writing. The authors send patients home with a sheaf of literature that is more inclusive rather than exclusive of instructions on preoperative and postoperative care in addition to potential risks of the proposed procedures. Patients should be given time to review this information so they have a chance to digest it quietly at home within their comfort zone. That way, you are not springing something new on them in the follow-up period at a time when they will view new information with suspicion.

Respect your patients. Be likable and courteous. Do not keep patients waiting and apologize when you do. Schedule enough time to answer their questions. Patients are more inclined to be happy with you if you show them you actually care about them personally. Although you cannot forge a successful practice just by being nice, a cordial nature can produce inestimable dividends. If you come off as distant, dismissive, or arrogant, your patient is likely to form the impression that you treat every aspect of his care or her with the same lack of concern, inclusive of the surgery. You are more likely to end up with a practice full of patients who point out your minor failings rather than be accepting of the minor imperfections they encounter.

Save your patients added expense, time commitment, and inconvenience. Do not put them through unnecessary tests. If there will be added expense in the event of a revision, spell these out for them ahead of time. Sometimes a patient is justified in being unhappy with the result. Consider what you are willing to do for them in that event.

WARNING SIGNS OF POTENTIAL PATIENT DISSATISFACTION

The patients described earlier in this chapter are those we seek for our practices. These are patients who have clear and sensible motivations and reasonable expectations. They understand the risks entailed by surgery and accept that there is no guarantee of a perfect result or of absolute satisfaction. They have divergent features of real concern but they are not excessively preoccupied with them. Their goals are reachable in our hands. They are courteous, pleasant, earnest, and dependable. They accept their share of the responsibility for their actions and decisions. They are not looking for nor expecting a radical, life-altering change. They desire an outstanding result but would be pleased with a good one. In short, these are generous, happy, and well-balanced people who constitute the majority of cosmetic surgery candidates.

We would all like to believe that every patient fits this description, but not all prospective patients do. These are not terrible people but they possess personality and psychodynamic traits and coping mechanisms that place them at an unhealthy risk for dysfunction following aesthetic surgery. They are more likely to be unhappy with any result. We owe it to our patients to remember our oaths and to make recommendations that will most benefit them. For some of these patients, surgery is not the appropriate recommendation and we should make every effort to save them and us the hardship of dealing with an unhappy outcome. Unfortunately, poor candidates for cosmetic surgery do not wear warning signs on their chests. Some of these maladaptive traits take time to become apparent and still others masquerade as wolves in sheep's clothing, only to surface after the procedure. What follows is an accounting of the common warning signs to which surgeons should be attuned in the preoperative period that will allow them to appropriately counsel patients not to proceed with surgery. These have been previously published in detail by the senior author (P.A.A.) under the moniker "The Dangerous Dozen" and can be further subcategorized as extrinsic or intrinsic factors.[3-5]

EXTRINSIC FACTORS

Patients Experiencing A Life Crisis

Sometimes patients request cosmetic surgery after a divorce, job loss, bereavement, accident, or illness. Alternatively, some patients wish to have surgery before a wedding or graduation. Be careful of operating on patients in the midst of a major life event, whether positive or negative, as these may be significant stressors. It is ever more important in these situations to analyze a candidate's rationale. It is true that someone who possesses improved self-esteem and confidence, as can be achieved through cosmetic surgery, may in turn have greater success finding a new mate or a new job. However, a decision made under pressured circumstances or situational stress may have unwanted consequences. Patients who thought surgery was the answer to their problems may perceive otherwise after these life stressors have settled. Patients should ideally possess a state of mind that will permit them to focus their energies on recovery. A more considered decision could often be made when life conditions have been stable for some time. Evidence points to the likelihood that patients who are motivated intrinsically to

undergo surgery, rather than by expectations relating to external factors, are more likely to view their surgical results as successes. So, while cosmetic surgery may sometimes bring about secondary gains in the way of positive life changes, these desired gains should not be the sole motivation for surgery.

Patients with Culturally Rooted Concerns

Some patients face possible disapproval from family members for their desire to alter the "family nose." For patients of specific ethnic backgrounds, their desire to even consider undergoing rhinoplasty may be met with condemnation by others sharing their ethnicity. Those close to them may perceive patients as rejecting their racial heritage. However, in our experience most ethnic rhinoplasty patients wish to achieve a more balanced nasal aesthetic while maintaining a strong ethnic identity. If possible, the family should be made aware of this motivation, as they will be more likely to be supportive of the patient's decision. Nevertheless, the negative influences of family members and friends may unduly taint a patient's postoperative perspective. Therefore, it is important to counsel patients with delicacy when they face such a situation if you wish to avoid having the patient's frustration with this scenario transferred to you. In addition, patients who have some ethnic-specific features must accept the inherent limitations presented, in that they may achieve a result that is shy of what they wish. Thicker skin may restrict the amount of definition and refinement achieved. Very low nasal height may permit less than desired augmentation. Darker skin may likewise render scars that are more visible. On the positive side, patients should also be apprised of the advantages inherent to some ethnic characteristics, such as superior graft concealment.

INTRINSIC FACTORS

The following descriptions relate general psychological states and behavior patterns that put patients at risk for postoperative dissatisfaction. These are not meant to be unkind to patients nor should they substitute for a referral for definitive diagnosis and treatment of a categorical mood, anxiety, or personality disorder. While a surgeon cannot take the place of a psychiatrist, he or she should be attuned to detection of these traits, regardless of whether they meet criteria sufficient for diagnosis, as they can impact the patient's postoperative temperament.

Mood Disorders

Depression. In any given year, 9.5% of the U.S. population, suffer from a depressive illness, with women being affected twice as often as men.[6] Preoperative depressive symptoms are the best predictors of postoperative depression, more so than other psychological aspects of surgery.[2] Rarely, this postoperative decompensation can be severe, even manifesting with psychotic symptoms. Postoperative depressive illness appears to occur more frequently after rhinoplasty. So, it is incumbent upon the surgeon to address this issue in the preoperative period. Patients with a history of depression should be informed of the increased risk for impaired coping in the postoperative period. The patient's counselor should be involved during the preoperative assessment to ensure that management of this illness is optimized prior to undertaking surgery. Extra care should be taken to ensure that these patients have the support they need to endure the stresses associated with postoperative healing.

Anxiety Disorders

Generalized anxiety disorder. Anxiety affects up to 18% of the U.S. population and often occurs coincidentally with depression.[7] People suffering from generalized anxiety have chronic, nonspecific worry that is difficult to control. Although they may be good surgical candidates, these patients usually need extra attention and care. They are pessimistic by nature and may tend to fret over even normal postoperative healing. Stressful events such as surgery may cause an exacerbation of symptoms. Nevertheless, reassurance and care will often allow these patients to appropriately frame their results and to obtain postoperative satisfaction.

Body Dysmorphic Disorder

Body dysmorphic disorder (BDD) is an uncommon but severe psychiatric disorder in which the affected person is excessively preoccupied with a minor or even imagined physical defect. People suffering from BDD are generally of normal or even highly attractive appearance, yet believe themselves to be so hideous as to inhibit normal social interaction. It is estimated that between 1% and 2% of the general population is affected, although the incidence of a milder phenotype may be as high as 5% to 15% among cosmetic surgery patients.[8,9] The nose is the third most frequently associated body area after the skin and hair.[10] Thus, facial plastic surgeons must maintain a high index of suspicion for this disorder with all patients seeking rhinoplasty.

BDD is linked to the obsessive-compulsive spectrum of disorders and affects men and women equally. Personality types that are more susceptible to this disorder include introverted, perfectionist, dependent, and avoidant personalities who are highly sensitive to criticism. They tend to be secretive, even reclusive, and reluctant to admit to the severity of the disorder or to seek help for fear of rejection. Psychological comorbidity is prevalent, including social anxiety, obsessive-compulsive disorder, and depression. Suicidal ideation is present in about 80% of sufferers, and the completed suicide rate is more than double that of those with clinical depression and 45 times the rate of the general population.[10] These patients should be identified preoperatively and dissuaded from

undergoing surgery since it is destined to failure in that it will not diminish appearance-related concerns. The disorder is likely to persist or worsen despite surgical alteration. Thankfully, effective treatment is usually possible in the form of selective serotonin reuptake inhibitors and cognitive-behavioral therapy.

Personality Disorders

Personality disorders are the psychological disturbance most commonly encountered in patients seeking cosmetic surgery.[11] The following descriptions summarize those specific personality types who are best deterred from considering cosmetic surgery.

Psychologically estranged personalities. If you encounter a patient who displays slightly odd thought or behavior patterns and with whom you have difficulty establishing a meaningful connection, you should consider this personality type. In the initial consultation, it is not uncommon to feel like "there is something missing" in the interaction. It just "does not feel right." Pay attention to these instinctive reactions, as persons having this personality type may appear more "normal" as you spend more time with them. These are patients who may exhibit some paranoid, schizoid, or schizotypical traits. They tend to have suspicious thoughts and are guarded about their histories and motivations. They may be eccentric in their mannerisms. They may also appear to be emotionally withdrawn and excessively serious and may react inappropriately to conversation. Patients who fit this category have trouble giving you their trust and fall into the generally unhappy group of patients. Plastic surgeons should avoid operating electively on patients with this personality type. In the postoperative period, psychologically estranged patients are more likely to be unforgiving and prone to anger and even aggression. Since surgeons can never truly be able to develop a rapport with patients of this personality type, it will be nearly impossible to deal with them effectively after surgery. Thankfully, these high-risk patients are rare.

Borderline personalities: The Goldilocks syndrome. Borderline personalities are unstable in many areas of their lives, including interpersonal relationships, thoughts, mood, behavior, and self-image. More often female, they are often very bright, manipulative, and beguiling and, for that reason, may escape detection in the initial consultation. Be wary of patients who appeal to your vanity with premature and excessive familiarity or praise. Frequently heard expressions include, "I just knew a surgeon with your talents could help me" and "You're the first one to understand me perfectly." This personality type's tendency to impulsive extremes and absolutes results in the phenomenon known as "splitting." While you may be idealized preoperatively, you may be vilified postoperatively with comparable ease.

The Goldilocks syndrome is a manifestation of the borderline personality with histrionic characteristics.

These patients function at a high level but tend to use their ample social skills in the service of manipulating others in their quest to become the center of attention. Like the protagonist of the children's story after which this patient is named, they will never be fully satisfied unless everything is "just right." She often fails to see her personal situation realistically and tends to overly dramatize her problems while shifting the blame for her disappointments to you. All of these factors, along with instability of self-image, predispose this patient to greater risk for development of dissociative tendencies, crisis involving loss of identity, and depressive states after rhinoplasty.

Patients with loss of identity will complain that their rhinoplasty changes, no matter how subtle, have caused them to no longer "look like themselves." When probed for details, they are vague, evasive, unfocused, and unable to give any more specific descriptions. This frustrates both patient and surgeon and may lead to inappropriate outbursts of anger by the patient. Somatic complaints are frequently associated with the nose, including airway obstruction, pain, and tenderness, especially at the rhinion. Borderline personalities typically become more apparent as the extent of the interaction increases, so ample time should be invested during the preoperative period. If in doubt, one should not operate on patients showing this personality type. Their unstable behavior and fluctuating self-image make these patients prone to isolation, unhappiness, and unpredictable and self-destructive behavior.

Narcissistic personalities: The exceptionalism syndrome. This personality type is excessively preoccupied with issues of personal adequacy, power, and prestige. Often, these patients are successful in their chosen industry and exhibit a pervasive pattern of grandiosity combined with a lack of empathy. These patients are easy to recognize and often will frustrate your front office staff by their blatant egocentrism starting as early as through the first telephone contact. The overriding message projected by this personality type is that his time is valuable while yours is expendable. He is often late, cancels appointments frequently, takes telephone calls in the office, and demands to see the physician immediately upon arrival because he has an important meeting afterward. These patients' overinflated sense of self-importance extends to their interactions as well. They hold the belief that no one but persons of high status are deserving of their attention and, very often, they will attempt to bypass any dealings with nurses, associates, or other staff members. While a patient with exceptionalism syndrome may treat the surgeon with deference, at least initially, difficulties often arise later. He is usually inconsiderate of the viewpoint of others and does not listen during the preoperative consultation. If the patient will not make time for the consultation or cancels for trivial reasons without the courtesy of notice or apology, you can be sure he will not have much patience for you after surgery nor is he likely to follow your postoperative directions. Since he is unwilling to accept a share of the responsibility for his decision, he is also unlikely to be forgiving of an imperfect result. You should try to identify and avoid this personality type early in the consultative process.

Antisocial personalities: The "my theory" syndrome. While the extreme antisocial personality can be characterized as a true psychopath, a milder phenotype is occasionally seen among aesthetic surgery candidates. These are patients having a superficial charm that masks an inflated self-appraisal and lack of empathy. They may be deceitful, withhold information, and fail to conform to office standards. They may have a history of drug seeking and substance abuse. There may also be a component of antagonistic behavior, including a disregard for financial obligations and a history of lawsuits against previous surgeons. Conduct is characterized by agitation, bouts of aggression, and impulsivity. The "My theory" syndrome patients display a variant of this personality type that blends obsessive and antisocial traits. These patients have little respect for the surgeon's viewpoint and have little interest in listening to what the surgeon has to say. Instead, they are only interested in advancing their own theories of what is wrong with their noses and what must be done to fix them. They are usually extensively well read and often present with scientific articles and detailed drawings or alterations of their own images. They believe they know exactly what surgical maneuvers are needed to achieve the improvements they seek. "My theory" patients frequently interrupt the consultative process, dominate the interaction, solicit information already provided, and react with veiled hostility when presented with an explanation or recommendation that does not support their own conclusions. Extra care must be taken to ensure that these patients are adequately informed of the risks and realities of surgery. If it appears that a "my theory" patient is unwilling to surrender his beliefs and to entrust his care to his surgeon, it would be wise to advise against surgery. Any patient who demonstrates hostility in the preoperative period or who breaks the "sacred trust" should be avoided altogether.

A more radical version of this personality is the well-described SIMON syndrome (*s*ingle, *i*mmature, *m*ale, *o*bsessive, and *n*arcissistic).[12-14] This syndrome has received singular attention in the literature because of the dangers involved. Patients falling into this category possess a multiplicity of maladaptive traits that dispose them to both dissatisfaction and potentially threatening behavior. As a result, surgeons should proceed with extreme caution when considering rhinoplasty in such patients.

Obsessive-compulsive personalities: The "package of pictures" syndrome. Compulsive personalities are high-achievers but they are rarely fully satisfied with their achievements and may have a deflated self-image. They are often orderly, punctual, and dependable. You can rely on these patients to follow instructions to the letter. Yet, while they can be reliable patients, they also tend to be excessively cautious and detail-oriented, making it difficult for them to make a decision. They may need to see you numerous times to review the imaging or surgical plan before agreeing to surgery. The "package of pictures" syndrome may be a specific manifestation of the obsessive personality type. Patients presenting with a package of pictures often have unrealistic expectations. They may present preinjury or presurgical photographs of themselves or photographs of models demonstrating the very clear and specific improvements they desire. Very often, these desired changes are unattainable for that patient. This does not mean that every patient in this category is at high risk for postoperative disappointment.

To stratify patients' risk in this scenario, it is necessary to ascertain to what degree they cling to their expectations. The trouble with obsessive patients lies in their inflexibility. You will be able to differentiate the obsessive personalities by their inability to "let go" of their excessively optimistic demands. If a patient is simply uninformed, he or she will be able to alter his or her expectations after careful explanation of the limitations and realities of cosmetic surgery. These are favorable surgical candidates who understand that the goal of surgery is improvement. If, however, a patient is unable or unwilling to reframe his or her too-lofty expectations and continues to demand unrealistic assurances of any kind, the surgeon should decline to operate. These patients manifest attributes of BDD and obsessive-compulsive personalities and are at very high risk for postoperative unhappiness. They are not dangerous per se, but they will often be troubled with the operative result. Postoperatively, they will perseverate over minor or barely perceptible defects and will find themselves unable to acknowledge the overall improvement or to derive enjoyment from their good surgical result.

Avoidant personalities: The unfocused syndrome. Avoidant personalities are socially inhibited and are preoccupied by feelings of inadequacy. They consider themselves to be personally unappealing and, rather than facing possible rejection, they choose to preempt this risk by consigning themselves to self-imposed isolation. This personality is associated with perceived or actual rejection by parents or close peers during the formative years and, thus, they have an intense desire for intimacy in relationships. This intense need can often be inappropriately displaced onto unrealistic hopes for the surgical outcome. The avoidant personality's interactions are distinguished by intense monitoring of their own internal reactions along with those of others. This constant monitoring produces in them extreme tension that manifests as hesitant speech and taciturn behavior. Surgeons should look for symptoms of self-loathing, extreme shyness, mistrust, emotional distancing, and loss of identity. They are often unfocused and may show a reluctance or incapacity for

identifying a specific complaint about their noses. Instead, they may shift the burden of decision and action to you. This indecision may be expressed by such phrases as, "I've never liked my nose but I cannot say why." Surgical planning is compromised in that surgeons bear the sole responsibility for an undesirable outcome. Patients in this situation are at risk for postoperative dissatisfaction. These will usually manifest as vague complaints, such as, "I do not know what it is, but I just do not like how the surgery turned out." Preoperative counseling should focus on gaining the patient's trust, encouraging him or her to identify specific concerns and to challenge his or her exaggerated negative beliefs. If that is successfully accomplished, then a satisfying operative experience is made possible.

Dependent personalities: The "exhausted surgeon" syndrome. As the name suggests, patients exhibiting this personality characteristic have exhausted themselves and every surgeon they have seen. They are the quintessential "doctor shoppers," spending inordinate amounts of time researching and visiting surgeons. This behavior pattern has arisen from a general lack of confidence in their own judgment, abilities, and capacity to make good decisions. Dependent personalities often require disproportionate amounts of advice and reassurance from spouses, friends, relatives, and even strangers, such as visitors to online rhinoplasty forums.

Like the avoidant personality, dependent patients would prefer for you to direct the consultation. When asked about her nose, this patient may demonstrate her need for you to assume responsibility with statements such as, "You're the expert. What do you think I should do to my nose?" They may have difficulty expressing open disagreement with your suggestions. When they are finally able to commit to surgery, these characteristics continue to guide the postoperative dynamic. This patient may go to excessive lengths to ensure your unwavering support and nurturance such as through elaborate gift-giving and excessive praise. Yet, they will probably not voice their disappointments and instead will eventually seek another surgeon when events do not go exactly as planned. Frequently, this syndrome is accompanied by anxiety, insomnia, and depression, as a result of the stress associated with perceived powerlessness and indecision. Not infrequently, it may affect aesthetic surgery patients who work in the medical or paramedical field. These patients meet the description of "maximizers" put forth by Barry Schwartz, author of *The Paradox of Choice.* Unlike "satisficers," who make quick and confident purchasing decisions and are satisfied by "good enough," "maximizers" are preoccupied by hypothetical "what if's." They are unable to commit to a decision without first exploring every avenue and making comparisons. They suffer from "paralysis of analysis," holding out for the absolute best conditions and surgeon, taking years to reach a decision. Because of the expectations heaped on this choice, patients with "exhausted surgeon" syndrome often suffer from buyer's remorse. They cannot help but compare their results to those of others, think of the alternatives, and wonder whether that other surgeon would have done any better. According to *The Paradox of Choice*, these patients could be happier if they gained insight into their struggles, enacted voluntary constraints on their freedom of choice, lowered their expectations, accepted good enough rather than perfect, and they stopped comparing their experiences to others. This advice is reminiscent of the surgeon's adage, "Perfect is the enemy of good." Comparably to the "maximize," we need to bear in mind that although perfection is our relentless pursuit, it is unattainable.

DEALING WITH UNHAPPY PATIENTS

Thankfully, patient dissatisfaction is uncommon in plastic surgery. Nevertheless, it can be a source of great stress to a practice, not to mention the distress experienced by the patient. It can be easy to characterize an unhappy patient as "difficult." Even when it may be justified, this attitude will not put you in the right mindset to deal with the situation most effectively. Rather, the overriding question should be how you can best help your patient beyond his or her current level of distress. To do this, you must learn to always gain control of your emotions and to overcome your instinct toward self-protectionism. That way, you can approach every interaction with the patient's best interests at heart and operate with the knowledge that you are "doing right" by the patient.

Embrace your complications. A most memorable lesson offered by Joseph V. Arigo, M.D., to his residents during their training was the turn of phrase, "Embrace your complications." This surgeon, who had never been sued in over 40 years of practice, was convinced that the secret to his success was not his technical prowess but his extraordinary care of occasional patients who had suffered setbacks during their course of healing. According to his philosophy, unhappy patients or those suffering complications should be contacted and seen in the office twice as often as was necessary or routine for an uncomplicated course. Where many surgeons go wrong is in following the impulse to retreat from "problem" patients. We all wish to avoid contentious situations. Yet, by rushing unhappy patients out of the office, refusing to listen or to let them vent their frustrations, and, in essence, disengaging from their care, we are only underscoring their misgivings that we perhaps did not do our best for them. You should take every opportunity to do the opposite. By showing the patient that his or her concerns are worthy of your time and caring, you are giving your patient much needed legitimacy. This simple act, by itself, can reduce the intensity of any negative feelings toward you.

Do not be overly defensive. One of the major pitfalls to avoid in dealing with unhappy patients is to take a defensive posture. Sure, it may help to bring out the preoperative photographs to demonstrate how much better the result is now. But, do not argue with unhappy patients. You would not make them happier. Be empathic and compassionate. Acknowledge their disappointment. Then, ask the patient what they are looking for to be happier with the result. Sometimes all they want is your empathy. If you think the result is good and you have done your best, tell them you do not think you can do any better for them. Try to understand the reasons for their disappointment even in the face of a good result. If the result is less than your best, admit to the fact that you see the problem. If there is something you think you can and should fix, then offer to do so at the appropriate time.

Say you are sorry. When something does not go as planned, say you are sorry. The prevailing culture among physicians is one of fear of apology for unexpected outcomes as this may be misconstrued as an admission of wrongdoing. Nondisclosure of medical errors is, in actuality, associated with a more negative emotional response, reduced patient satisfaction and trust, and increased likelihood of changing physicians or of seeking legal advice.[15,16] To encourage a policy of disclosure when there is a medical error involved, some states have now passed "apology laws" that allow providers to exclude statements of sympathy from evidence in a liability lawsuit. Although patient unhappiness does not constitute an error as such, patients facing a disappointment following cosmetic surgery are experiencing emotions similar to those facing a medical error claim. An expression of your empathy can go a long way toward attenuating a patient's sense of resentment without constituting an admission of wrongdoing. Often, this position can strengthen your rapport with your patient and permit you both to endure the outcome together. Of interest, the act of apology appears more important even than monetary restitution, as in one study an offer to waive costs was not associated with a statistically significant impact on patient responses.[15]

Do not lecture to or blame your patient. Labeling patients as "problems" or as "difficult" is self-defeating and sometimes unfair. This is pejorative defensive posturing that does not improve the situation and sets an antagonistic stance that risks alienating both the patient and the surgeon. It is easy to castigate a patient for not following instructions. But, it is the rare case where a poor outcome can be attributed solely and completely to a patient's noncompliance. Dealing with unwanted results really boils down to how people relate to one another. A patient that you see as a "problem" might have a completely different experience with another surgeon, and the opposite is true. We cannot relate perfectly to everyone. The objective of patient selection is to find the right fit. If the fit was not quite right, acknowledge that privately and try to make the best of the situation. By providing yourself this constant reminder, you will avoid having the interaction evolve into a far less constructive one.

Do not try to solve the problem. Surgeons are problem-solvers by nature. We tend to be overly analytical. When faced with an unhappy patient, resist the urge to solve the problem. The majority of patients experiencing postoperative concerns with healing are looking for understanding and acceptance of their worries, and for support and reassurance. This applies to every scenario. If the patient is experiencing distress around a normal course of healing, she or he wishes reassurance that all will be satisfactory. If a patient, on the other hand, has experienced a complication or a flawed result, she or he wishes honest disclosure and reassurance that you will do your best to support her or him through the problem. Depending on the circumstance, this may mean doing nothing but listening and providing support, returning her or his investment if you believe in that practice, revising the procedure if you can and if you feel it warranted, or referring the patient to a colleague if so desired. If you take a stance of partnership in the early period of distress, you are likely to cultivate a sense of collaboration rather than opposition. Patients' reactions rarely become litigious unless and until you have also escalated your oppositional behavior in response.

Resist the urge to rush to intervention. This caution is similar to that just given. Sometimes, you may have an inkling that a revision will be necessary in the future. However, time heals many concerns, so make a policy of watchful waiting. Waiting at least 6 months before offering a revision is a good strategy. This has several favorable effects. The early inflammatory response will have had time to settle, rendering the revision easier to accomplish. The patient's initial anxiety response associated with the outcome will also likely have diminished somewhat. Finally, the problem may resolve to the extent that neither the patient nor the surgeon believes a revision is necessary. An exception to this rule would be a case in which you expect that the problem will worsen or will not improve sufficiently over time.

Do not let the patient talk you into an unnecessary revision. If the result is not completely satisfactory, then you and the patient can agree that a revision may be advisable. Obviously, you will do your best to correct any problems. However, if the patient is overly concerned by a barely perceptible problem, you will not be doing the patient a service by trying to improve upon your good result. Remember the law of diminishing returns. The closer you get to an ideal result, the harder each incremental improvement is to achieve. If you agree to a revision, do not alter your surgical plan or add procedures at the final moment. This applies to the primary procedure as well.

Involve the patient's family or friends. If a patient is open to involvement of her or his family members or friends, this can sometimes help greatly in easing tensions. Rather than limiting the contact to the patient and surgeon, this scenario returns the communication to more of a discourse. This person may help to articulate the patient's concerns in a more constructive way. By introducing at least some measure of objectivity, this person may also ease the patient's agitation about the outcome. When the surgeon tells a patient she has had a good result, the surgeon will appear self-serving. When the patient's friend tells her that she has had a good result, the patient is more likely to be responsive.

An important aspect of this interaction is the family's attitude toward the patient. Some family members reject patients experiencing a difficult postoperative course, censuring them for failing to heed initial warnings not to undergo surgery. This lack of support can deepen the patient's sense of guilt and isolation. In this case, efforts to reach out to the family may help to bolster support for the patient and to facilitate her recovery.

Involve your staff. Experienced staff members are an invaluable part of a plastic surgeon's practice. Respect your staff's intuition. A well-attuned staff can alert you to potential problems with prospective patients and even save you from yourself at times. Staff can sometimes elicit greater information about a patient's history, motivations, expectations, coping strategies, and postoperative complaints than the patient is willing to express directly. This should inform your decision of whether to welcome the patient into your practice. Think twice about whether to operate on a patient who treats your staff far differently than he or she treats you.

Your staff should be trained to present themselves as a cohesive unit. You can hire the most wonderful individuals, but they must learn to work together effectively. Model the behavior that you wish them to exhibit. Since the patient experiences the practice in its entirety, one unpleasant note can sour the whole impression of your office. Your staff can be particularly helpful in dealing with unhappy patients. While dispensing medical advice is your prerogative, your staff can provide an air of availability, a listening ear, and an empathic voice. This does not mean they should jointly descend on an unhappy patient to convince him or her of his or her good result. This type of behavior will only raise a patient's suspicions. Rather, patients coping with postoperative difficulties will welcome a sense of staff receptiveness and responsiveness to help assuage their anxieties.

Involve your colleagues. Develop referral patterns with supportive colleagues early on in your practice. Having trustworthy colleagues with whom you can "float" your concerns and anxieties around unhappy patients can have a tremendously positive effect on your ability to manage these stressful situations. Sometimes, referring your dissatisfied patient to a colleague for an objective opinion can help to settle the patient's worries about the result. Give your patient several names of reputable physicians to whom you would entrust his or her care. You should understand that a distrusting patient will look upon your referral with wariness, suspecting that you and your colleague are in cahoots. This pattern of thinking will be discouraged if your overriding attitude is one of concern for your patient's well-being. Your patient will be more likely to be accepting of the fact that you are doing your best to satisfy her or his expectations.

Involve your medical liability insurance carrier. If it appears that a patient remains very angry and upset with the result despite the passage of time and your best efforts at resolution, you should consider involving your malpractice carrier or your institution's risk management unit once it appears the relationship is deteriorating. Your carrier may choose to intervene to help defuse the situation before it escalates beyond control. The company may also provide useful advice on how to conduct yourself in this situation. Finally, if you are considering a touch-up revision or a return of the patient's fees, you should look into obtaining a waiver of liability from the patient.

SUMMARY

Cosmetic surgery, and especially rhinoplasty, is different from other types of surgery by virtue of the whirlwind of emotions and expectations concerned and by the extraordinary weight attached to them. Attempting to displace the role of the psychiatrist in the assessment of rhinoplasty candidates is not only misguided but dangerous. That is by no means the purpose of this chapter. However, those surgeons who naively dismiss the impact of psychology on the rhinoplasty candidate's belief system do so at their own peril. The material offered here is designed to help the surgeon to understand both patient and surgeon factors that increase the chances for patient unhappiness.

In the current litigious climate in which we practice surgery, it can be easy to approach this topic from the perspective of self-preservation. Yet a surgeon is able to better develop a solid rapport and ultimately to satisfy his or her patients' desires if the surgeon approaches his or her practice with a spirit of beneficence. Emphasis should be placed on a caring and comprehensive approach to patient education that stresses the realistic goals, risks, results, and limitations of rhinoplasty. To ensure optimal outcomes and to minimize the number of unhappy patients under his or her care, a proactive approach needs be taken to refine the patient selection process. The question facing surgeons during the consultative process should be shifted from, "Can I achieve a good result for this patient?" to "Will I be able to satisfy this patient?" This nuanced shift in thinking not only takes into account the technical probabilities at hand but also marries these to the patient's characteristics and expectations within the context of the overall patient–physician relationship.

To make this change effectively, a surgeon must look outward to identify and steer clear of potential at-risk personalities but also look inward to identify his or her distinct style of behavior in reaction to various personality types. By combining these factors with experience, a surgeon can best resolve to determine which rhinoplasty candidates should or should not meet the threshold for admission to his practice. While patient dissatisfaction is an unpleasant reality imposed by the imperfect art of aesthetic surgery, as surgeons we should learn to minimize the impact of these uncertainties on our practice to create a legacy of contentment among patients and in our professional life.

REFERENCES

1. Littauer F. *Personality Plus.* Grand Rapids, MI: Fleming H. Revell Co; 1994.
2. Goin JM, Goin MK. *Changing the body: Psychological effects of physical surgery.* Baltimore: Williams and Wilkins; 1981.
3. Adamson PA, Chen T. The dangerous dozen: Avoiding potential problem patients in cosmetic surgery. *Fac Plast Surg Clin North Am.* 2008;16(2):195–202.
4. Adamson PA, Litner JA. Psychologic aspects of revision rhinoplasty. *Fac Plast Surg Clin North Am.* 2006;14(4):269–277.
5. Adamson PA, Strecker HD. Patient selection. *Aesthet Plast Surg.* 2002;26(suppl 1):S11.
6. Robins LN, Regier DA, editors. *Psychiatric disorders in America, the epidemiologic catchment area study.* New York: The Free Press; 1990.
7. Kessler RC, Chiu WT, Demler O, et al. Prevalence, severity, and comorbidity of 12-month DSM-IV disorders in the National Comorbidity Survey Replication. *Arch Gen Psychiatry.* 2005;62(6):617.
8. Wilson JB, Arpey CJ. Body dysmorphic disorder: Suggestions for detection and treatment in a surgical dermatology practice. *Dermatol Surg.* 2004;30:1391–1399.
9. Veale D. Body dysmorphic disorder. *Postgrad Med J.* 2004;80:67–71.
10. Phillips KA. *The broken mirror: understanding and treating body dysmorphic disorder.* New York: Oxford University Press; 2005.
11. Wright MR. Management of patient dissatisfaction with results of cosmetic procedures. *Arch Otolaryngol.* 1980;106:466–471.
12. Ely JF. Less is more: A conservative approach to male rhinoplasty. *Aesthet Plast Surg.* 1996;20:23–28.
13. Gorney M. Cosmetic surgery in males. *Plast Reconstr Surg.* 2002;110:719.
14. Rohrich RJ, Janis JE, Kenkel JM. Male rhinoplasty. *Plast Reconstr Surg.* 2003;112:1071–1085.
15. Mazor KM, Reed GW, Yood RA, et al. Disclosure of medical errors: what factors influence how patients respond? *J Gen Intern Med.* 2006;21(7):704–710.
16. Wei M. Doctors, apologies, and the law: An analysis and critique of apology laws. *J Health Law.* 2007;40(1):107–159.

Primary Open Structure Rhinoplasty

William Numa • *Calvin M. Johnson, Jr.* • *Wyatt C. To*

There are no shortcuts to quality.
Ernest and Mary Hansen

Founders of Hansen's Sno-Bliz, New Orleans, LA

PRIMUM NON NOCERE

The first goal during rhinoplasty, as with all other aspects of medicine and surgery, is to do no harm, and it pertains to both nasal function and aesthetics. Moreover, every rhinoplasty patient will present with a set of positive nasal functional or aesthetic features that need be preserved. Capitalizing on years of training and cumulative experience while paying close attention to the patient's stated concerns, surgeons should prioritize the nasal features to be surgically addressed and, in some ways even more important, those that need to be preserved both functionally and aesthetically.

Paradigms of beauty are somewhat subjective and variable, and may shift gradually with time. Some models considered beautiful today may have not been considered as such in different time periods throughout history. However, timeless concepts such as balance, symmetry, and general guidelines of facial and nasal proportions can help lead us with the certainty and conviction of knowing the surgical goal will be aesthetically pleasing and natural-appearing decades after accomplished.

An ideal surgical result is based on excellent nasal function as well as a proportioned, balanced, natural-appearing, aesthetically pleasing nose. Conceptually, a great rhinoplasty result deemphasizes the nose to allow the casual observer to look past it, focusing on the subject's eyes, appreciating the entire face in context, without specific distractions. Each rhinoplasty is different, in as much as a person's nose should befit their gender, ethnicity, and surrounding facial features as well as their underlying facial skeletal structure.

The rhinoplasty surgeon's mindset should be to carry out every measure possible to ensure that the current rhinoplasty procedure is the patient's last one. Having said that, some patients seek and subsequently undergo revision rhinoplasty. Surgeons should strive for a revision rate that approximates zero but should be able to tolerate one approximating 5%.

PREOPERATIVE EVALUATION AND DIAGNOSIS

A separate chapter is specifically dedicated to this critically important topic. Throughout the initial consultation, a complete medical history and head and neck physical examination is carried out, with particular attention being directed to the nasal anatomy and function. The patient's stated functional and aesthetic concerns are documented in the medical record and standardized digital photodocumentation takes place. An open conversation clarifying realistic expectations of what can be accomplished with rhinoplasty is carried out in light of the functional and aesthetic priorities discussed by both patient and surgeon.

The columellar scar is next to imperceptible if meticulous suturing techniques are used, and by itself it should not be a critical factor in deciding whether an endonasal or an external approach is carried out.

ANESTHESIA

The meticulous and detail-oriented nature of open structure rhinoplasty requires the use of general endotracheal anesthesia or deep intravenous sedation. Appropriate anesthesia will aid in hemostasis, amnesia, and analgesia during and after the case.

Prior to arrival at the surgical facility, the patient is instructed to take an antiemetic (aprepitant 40 mg) for postoperative nausea, along with an anxiolytic (lorazepam 1 mg) as needed for anxiety. An intravenous line is initiated, and the patient is administered a dose of anxiolytic and narcotic for sedation (typically midazolam 1 mg) (Sublimaze [fentanyl] 50 micrograms). Additional doses of midazolam and fentanyl may be administered throughout the duration of the surgery, titrating to appropriate levels of analgesia, amnesia, and sedation. Preoperative antibiotics with broad-spectrum gram-positive coverage are dosed intravenously.

Monitoring includes continuous pulsoximetry, electrocardiography, blood pressure, and end-tidal CO_2. General anesthesia can be induced with a propofol bolus in conjunction with a short- or intermediate-acting, nondepolarizing muscle relaxant such as atracurium. After intubation, general anesthesia is typically maintained with sevoflurane, which is favored for its fast onset and offset, its favorable cardiovascular profile, and its lower incidence of nausea, vomiting, and airway reactivity.

Use of a preformed endotracheal oral RAE tube allows the anesthesia tubing to run toward the patient's feet, away from the surgical field. Care is taken to avoid undue traction of the mouth and nose with the endotracheal tube to minimize traction and asymmetries, which can mislead the surgeon.

PATIENT POSITION AND SURGICAL PREP

The patient is placed in the supine position on the surgical bed, the head of which is tapered to allow the surgeon access to the head and neck region. Sufficient padding is layered underneath the patient, preventing pressure points and positioning-related injuries. After the induction of general anesthesia, the hair is taped or otherwise secured away from the face, and the face and nose are prepped and draped using standard sterile technique. Cotton-tipped applicators are used to clean the nasal vestibules. Eye lubrication is important to prevent corneal injuries.

OPEN STRUCTURE RHINOPLASTY: THE BASIC TECHNIQUE

A detailed description of the basic technique of open structure rhinoplasty is described in this chapter. This includes operative steps that are performed in most of our rhinoplasty procedures, such as the injection of local anesthetic, septal cartilage harvesting, skin and mucosal incisions, and dissection of the skin–soft tissue envelope (SSTE) from the underlying bony–cartilaginous framework.

We begin with analysis of the preoperative photographs (Figure 5-1). A high dorsum can be seen with a mild to moderate bony–cartilaginous dorsal hump. The tip is ptotic, blunt, and underrotated. The tripod is larger than ideal. The medial crura are prominent, while the lateral crura are bulbous and convex. A larger than ideal pedestal overprojects the tripod. A caudal septal deflection

deviates the nasal pyramid to the right. The caudal septum pulls the lip forward, blunting the nasolabial angle. The thickness of the SSTE can be described as thin to medium thickness.

PREOPERATIVE CONSIDERATIONS

1. The size and shape of the tripod must be optimized — notably, the bulbosity of the lateral crura and the bifidity of the medial crura.
2. As the anterior septal angle is reduced and the tip deprojected, the height of the dorsum will seem even higher. Thus, the bony–cartilaginous hump will require reduction.

OPERATIVE PROCEDURE

1. Marks are made in the midline of the glabella, the midline of the tip, and the midline of the upper lip to serve as reference points. Note that the nose is deviated to the right.
2. The nasal cavity is packed loosely with Nu-Gauze/cottonoid pledgets moistened with a solution containing 4% cocaine. This is left in place for several minutes and removed prior to injecting the local anesthetic.
3. An equal mixture of 1% lidocaine with 1 : 100,000 epinephrine and 0.5% bupivacaine with 1 : 200,000 epinephrine is used for injection. The bupivacaine is included for its longer duration of action, which helps to reduce the amount of inhalational and parenteral anesthetic agents needed to maintain an adequate level of anesthesia during the procedure. The septum is injected using a 27-gauge needle on a 12-mL offset port syringe. The offset port allows easier visualization of the nasal cavity during injection. The septum is injected in a subperichondrial/subperiosteal plane with the bevel facing the septal cartilage, elevating, hydrodissecting, and causing blanching of the mucosa. The local anesthetic provides hydrodissection, vasoconstriction, and hemostasis. Both sides of the septum are injected with multiple needle sticks in a posterior-to-anterior fashion.
4. The membranous septum is not injected directly to prevent distortion of the columella and tip. Instead, the caudal edge of the septum is injected and the local anesthetic is allowed to diffuse into the area of the membranous septum on its own.
5. The pyriform aperture and anterior nasal floor are injected at multiple sites.
6. The lateral walls of the nose are injected via an intercartilaginous approach just superficial to the nasal bone periosteum. Injection is done as the

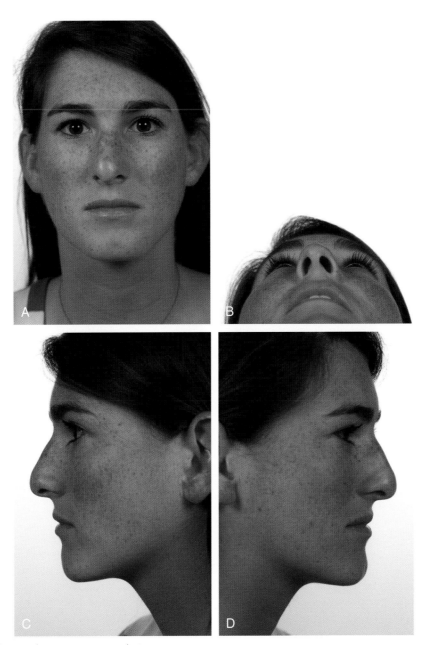

Figure 5-1 Photographs providing preoperative analysis.

needle is withdrawn, thereby avoiding injecting intravascularly.

7. The planned marginal incision is then injected at the caudal margin of the lower lateral cartilage (LLC). Multiple small injections are performed using a ½-inch 30-gauge needle. The nasal tip is manipulated between the thumb and index finger to evert the nostril and expose the caudal edge of the LLC.

8. The columella is then injected, with the needle just off the caudal edge of the medial crus. Only a very small amount (0.2 to 0.3 mL) is infiltrated to prevent tip distortion.

9. The interdomal region is injected with a very small amount of local anesthetic.

10. The cocaine-soaked nasal packing is left inside the nose while the patient is prepped and draped.

11. A limited amount of local anesthesia is injected, perhaps 7 to 8 mL in the septum and 1 to 2 mL in the tripod/lateral nasal walls. More injected anesthetic may distort the nasal structure, making the true appearance more difficult to judge. No local anesthesia is injected into the nasal dorsum to avoid distortion.

12. Tip projection can be measured with the projectimeter, which uses the bony points of the

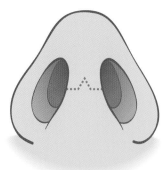

Figure 5-2 The midcolumellar incision is placed at an area where the underlying cartilage is closest to the skin.

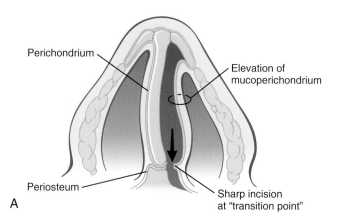

A

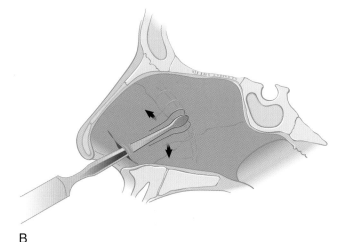

B

Figure 5-3 **A, B,** The perichondrium is incised and the flap is raised in the subperichondrial plane.

patient's forehead and maxilla as fixed landmarks to provide a reproducible assessment of tip projection. Projection can be measured at various points during the surgery.

13. The open approach to the nose involves a mid-columellar inverted-V transverse incision with bilateral marginal incisions (see Figure 5-2). The mid-columellar incision is designed to break up the scar line avoiding cicatricial contracture. It is placed at an area where the underlying cartilage is closest to the skin, thus minimizing the risk of creating a depressed scar. If the incision is placed too low in the columella, where the skin is not as closely supported by the underlying medial crus, indentation of the scar can occur. Placement of the incision too high near the apex risks scar contracture, which can deform the nostrils.

14. The septum can be addressed first to correct deformities in this area and to obtain appropriate grafting material. A full transfixion incision is usually used to allow access to the caudal septum and nasal spine. This incision is made as close as possible to the caudal edge of the septum so as to maintain the integrity of the membranous septum, which will serve as part of the pocket for the columellar strut. The incision may be extended to the nasal spine if necessary. If caudal septal work is not required, a Killian incision may be used.

15. The perichondrium is incised, and the subperichondrial plane identified. The cartilage may be lightly cross-hatched with the No. 15 blade, then abraded with a dental amalgam packer, a Woodson elevator, or a cotton-tipped applicator to raise the perichondrium.

16. The mucoperichondrial flaps are raised bilaterally with the elevator, taking care to elevate past the borders of the septal cartilage and the perpendicular plate of the ethmoid, vomer, and maxillary crest (Figure 5-3).

17. The cuts in the septal cartilage are made with a No. 15 blade leaving at least 15 mm at the caudal and dorsal struts for support (Figure 5-4). The cartilage graft is then freed from its attachments to the bony septum using the dissector to atraumatically remove the cartilage from between the maxillary crest and vomer. Care must be taken to ensure the graft remains intact during the harvesting process. The harvested cartilage is stored in sterile saline or antibiotic solution.

18. The thickness of the cartilage graft varies depending on the location, and we use this to our advantage. The columellar strut is usually designed from the maxillary or dorsal portion of the graft, areas that are of relatively uniform thickness. When a shield graft is used, the thickened portion of the septum near the bony–cartilaginous junction is used for the distal end of the tapered tip graft (Figure 5-5). Other grafts (alar, apex, spreader, etc.) can be made from the remaining cartilage.

19. Loss of projection may be seen after septoplasty, due to the transfixion incision, as this can divide one of the major tip support mechanisms.

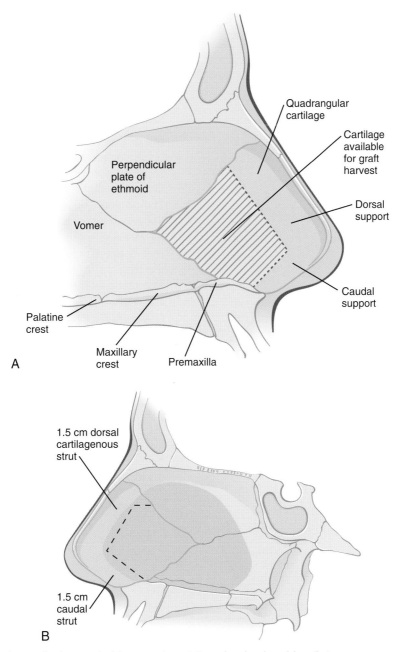

Figure 5-4 **A, B,** Septal cartilage graft is harvested while preserving a 1.5 cm dorsal and caudal cartilaginous strut.

20. Quilting sutures are placed using 4-0 gut on a straight Keith needle in a running horizontal mattress fashion to reapproximate the mucoperichondrial flaps and obliterate the dead space. A short (~1 cm) incision is made through one of the flaps overlying the maxillary crest to allow drainage of blood and serum from the septoplasty site. Silicone/silastic septal splints can be sutured onto each other using a 2-0 silk suture. If spreader grafts are planned, the septoplasty can be performed through a an anterior (external) approach.

21. The inverted-V mid-columellar incision is made with a No. 11 or 15 blade, taking care to avoid cutting into the medial crus of the LLC (see Figure 5-2). The incision must be kept perpendicular to the skin surface to avoid beveling the flap. If a No. 11 blade is used, a sawing motion is carried out for this portion of the procedure.

22. The mid-columellar incision is joined to the marginal incisions, which are created with the No. 15 blade at the caudal edges of the LLCs (Figure 5-6). Medially, the marginal columellar incision is created approximately 2 mm behind the columellar rim. Laterally, the back edge of the blade can be used to palpate the caudal edge of the cartilage and guide the incision. The nostril is pinched between the 10-mm Joseph double hook and the surgeon's finger and is everted. This especially helps with exposure of the marginal incision near the apex of the domes. It is very easy to inadvertently cut the LLC. The lateral and medial marginal incisions are connected along the undersurface of the soft tissue triangle, taking care to avoid notching the rim, which may lead to distortion of the nostril apex.

23. The angled Converse scissors are used to elevate the columellar portion of the flap. Care is taken to elevate the entire corner (junction between the mid-columellar and marginal incisions) with the flap.

24. The plane of dissection while elevating the columellar flap is just superficial to the medial crus—we try to keep this portion of the flap as thick as possible.

25. This is especially important in the patient with a thin SSTE. The flap should be of uniform thickness across the columella—the soft tissue between the medial crura is not elevated with the flap.

26. Dissection is continued along the LLC, elevating the SSTE using three-point retraction (Figure 5-7). Two small skin hooks are held by the assistant, one on the skin flap and the second one along the undersurface of the medial crus. The surgeon uses

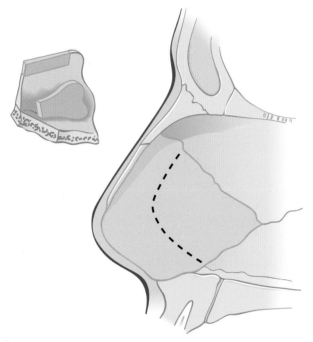

Figure 5-5 The thickened portion of the septum near the bony-cartilaginous junction is used for the distal end of the tapered tip graft. Other grafts such as alar, apex, and spreader grafts can be made from the remaining cartilage.

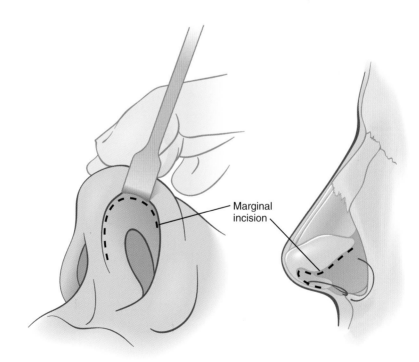

Marginal incision

Figure 5-6 Marginal incisions are made at the caudal edges of the LLCs. The marginal columellar incision is created approximately 2 mm behind the columellar rim.

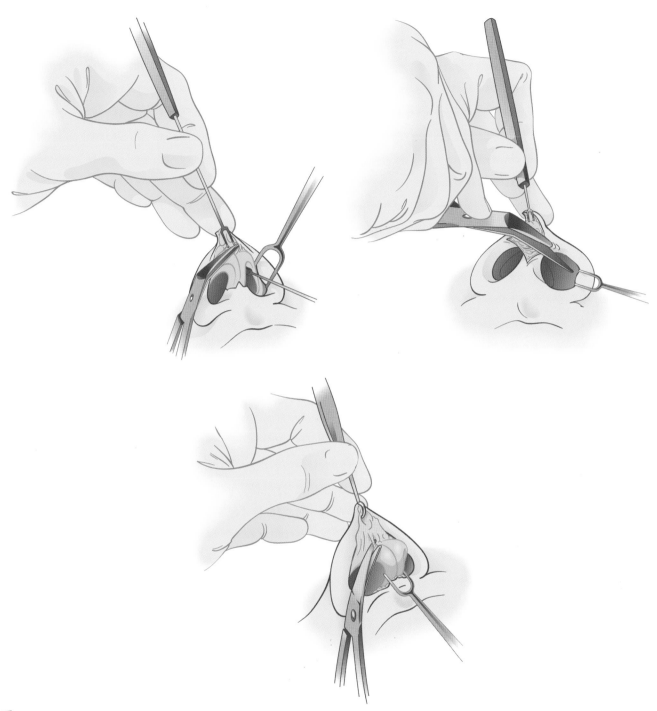

Figure 5-7 Dissection is continued along the LLC, elevating the SSTE using three-point retraction. The skin hooks are repositioned as necessary to optimize exposure by the principle of traction and countertraction.

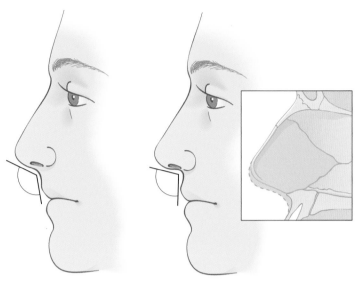

Figure 5-8 A, B, A pie-shaped segment of caudal septum can be excised. Varying the nature of the excision can help tailor the intended result (a wider excision at the posterior septal angle, will aid favoring tip counter rotation and make the nasolabial angle more acute).

the 10-mm double hook to retract the nostril rim. The skin hooks are repositioned as necessary to optimize exposure by the principle of traction and countertraction.

27. Dissection is carried out along the relatively avascular plane just superficial to the perichondrium, taking care to avoid injuring the cartilage. The lateral extent of dissection is to the region of the sesmoid cartilages bilaterally; the LLC are not detached from the overlying SSTE laterally.

28. In addition to dissection with the scissors, blunt dissection of the SSTE off the cartilage is performed using the cotton-tipped applicators.

29. The adherence of the SSTE to the cartilage varies between patients. The most adherent SSTE is found in young patients with very reactive, sebaceous skin.

30. Dissection between the domes is avoided while raising the flap.

31. Dissection progresses cephalad, exposing the upper lateral cartilage (ULC). A No. 15 blade is used to divide the perichondrium off the ULC, after which the flap is raised in a subperichondrial plane. A periosteal elevator is used to raise the flap over the nasal and frontal bones up to the nasofrontal angle. Staying in a subperiosteal plane while elevating the SSTE at the level of the nasal bones allows easy avoidance of the angular vessels.

32. Once the SSTE flap has been completely raised, the tip cartilages may be evaluated in situ, in their undisturbed, anatomic configuration.

33. A pie-shaped segment of caudal septum can be excised. Varying the nature of the excision can

help tailor the intended result (a wider excision at the posterior septal angle will aid favoring tip counter rotation and make the nasolabial angle more acute) (Figure 5-8).

34. An overly prominent nasal spine can be reduced to modify the nasolabial angle.

35. A Wright stitch is placed to affix the septal remnant in the midline. Superiorly, this suture incorporates the septal mucoperichondrium. Inferiorly, the suture goes through septal mucoperichondrium and maxillary crest periosteum (see Figure 5-9). Care must be taken, as this maneuver can further decrease tip projection.

36. We prefer to carry out nasal dorsal work prior to addressing the nasal tip as the latter can readily be modified to complement the dorsum.

37. The cartilaginous dorsum is reduced sharply with the No. 15 blade under direct vision, taking care not to violate the nasal mucosa (Figure 5-10).

38. When reducing a large bony hump, an osteotome is used to uncap the bony dorsum prior to rasping (Figure 5-11). When correcting a concurrent moderate to severe lateral deviation of the nasal dorsum, an off-balance osteotomy will help correct the deformity (Figure 5-12). If the rasp alone is used to reduce a large hump, a "floating" central remnant may result. The osteotome is positioned at the caudal border of the frontal bones. The osteotome must be directed toward the nasofrontal angle to prevent overresection of the lower bony dorsum and a resulting irregular dorsum.

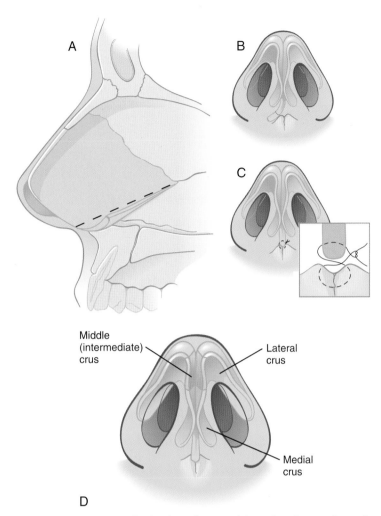

Middle
(intermediate)
crus

Lateral
crus

Medial
crus

A

B

C

D

Figure 5-9 A "swinging door" maneuver with excision of redundant inferior-caudal septal cartilage can be performed to correct any existing caudal septal deviations.

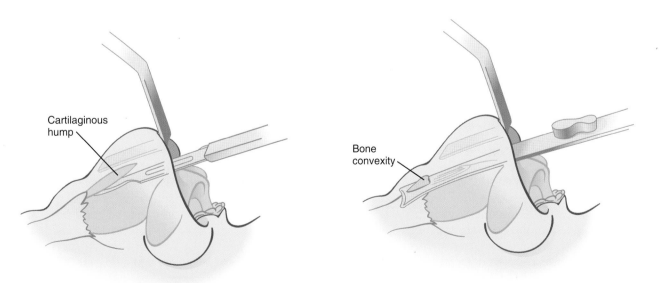

Cartilaginous
hump

Bone
convexity

Figure 5-10 Cartilaginous dorsum sharply reduced under direct vision.

Figure 5-11 When reducing a large bony hump, an osteotome is used to uncap the bony dorsum prior to rasping.

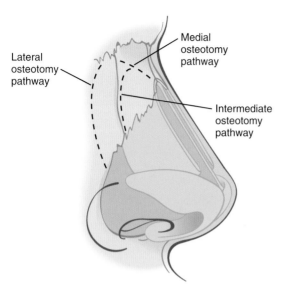

Figure 5-12 When correcting a concurrent moderate to severe lateral deviation of the nasal dorsum, an off-balance osteotomy will help correct the deformity.

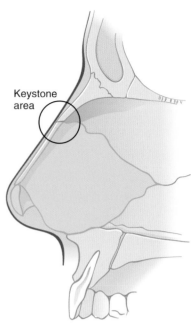

Figure 5-13 To obtain a straight dorsum, the bony–cartilaginous junction should be slightly higher than the rest of the dorsal skeleton.

39. A tungsten carbide rasp is used in a pulling fashion to reduce the bony dorsum in a graduated fashion. The bone of the cephalic bony dorsum near the nasion is significantly thicker than that of the caudal portion. It is thus easy to overreduce the caudal bony dorsum with rasping, leaving excess cephalic bone. To compensate for this, the rasp can be angled more perpendicularly than the intended plane of the dorsum by lifting up the handle, thus putting more pressure on the cephalic bony dorsum. The rasp must be used in the correct direction.

40. The rasps are cleaned frequently with a wire brush. We try to remove all the bony fragments from the nose, especially from the nasofrontal angle.

41. The reduced dorsum is visually inspected. This may be difficult to do due to swelling of the SSTE, especially during lengthy procedures. Additional refinement of the cartilaginous or bony dorsum is done as necessary.

42. The variable thickness of the SSTE must be taken into consideration while contouring the nasal dorsum. The skin is thickest over the nasion and supratip and thinnest over the bony–cartilaginous junction and tip. Consequently, to obtain a straight dorsum, the bony–cartilaginous junction should be slightly higher than the rest of the dorsal skeleton (Figure 5-13). A radix graft may also be helpful to fine-tune and deaccentuate a dorsal hump due to a deep radix (Figure 5-14).

43. At this point, either the middle vault or the nasal tip can be addressed.

44. The first step in addressing the lower third of the nose is the placement of a columellar strut to provide structure and support to the medial limb of the tripod (Figure 5-15). The columellar strut may also help lengthen and project the nose. The domes may also be narrowed slightly by lifting the domes up onto the strut. If the medial limb does not have sufficient strength by the end of the case, postoperative sagging of the medial crura and a hanging columella will result. A columellar strut is used in almost all our cases, except when additional support requires placement of a caudal septal extension graft.

45. The dorsal portion of the harvested septal cartilage used for the strut has a relatively uniform thickness. The strut is shaped and smoothed around the edges. Sufficient cartilage is reserved for other grafts.

46. A pocket is created between the medial crura for the columellar strut using the Converse scissors as a dissection instrument. Tissue is left between the medial crural footplates and the nasal spine to keep the strut in place. This pocket should not communicate with the transfixion incision. The strut is then gently inserted along the axis of the medial crura (Figure 5-16). It should not extend much past the medial crura and should not rest on the nasal spine or anterior septal angle. If the strut

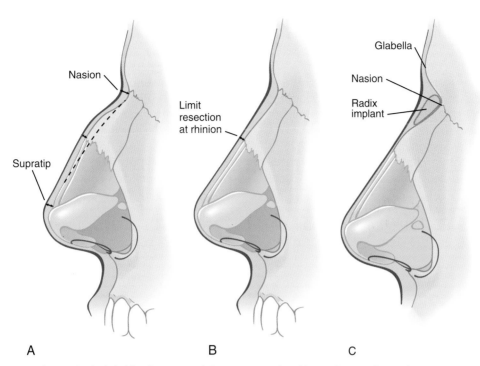

Nasion

Supratip

Limit
resection
at rhinion

Glabella

Nasion

Radix
implant

A   B   C

Figure 5-14 A radix graft may also be helpful to fine-tune and deaccentuate a dorsal hump due to a deep radix.

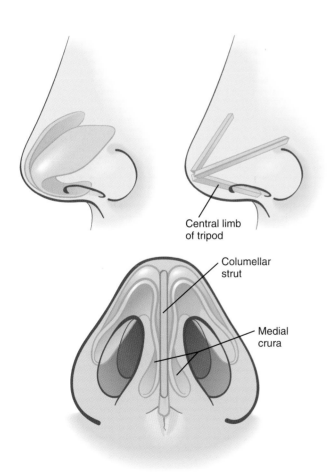

Central limb
of tripod

Columellar
strut

Medial
crura

Figure 5-15 The columellar strut may also help lengthen and project the nose by strengthening the central limb of the tripod.

rests on bone, it can tend to shift and "click" from one side to the other.

47. A horizontal mattress using a 4-0 gut on a Keith needle is used in a through and through fashion to secure the columellar strut (Figure 5-16 B and C). Placing the domes on slight tension with the skin hook may help. Care must be taken to avoid creating domal asymmetry while doing this.

48. Excision of a segment of the caudal septum can at times allow the tripod to settle in a cephalad fashion. Redundant mucoperichondrium along the transfixion incision can be excised in conjunction with the caudal septal excision to support the elevated tip position. Extreme caution must be exercised with this maneuver, as this can have a powerful effect which can be difficult to revert. The transfixion incision is repaired with 4-0 chromic gut, bringing the medial limb of the tripod up to the caudal septum.

49. On the nasal base view, the aim is to restore an ideal equilateral configuration to the nose (Figure 5-18, *A*) from a boxy (or trapezoidal) configuration or from an isosceles configuration in a tension nose deformity, where an overly lengthy septum typically overprojects the nasal tip, creating narrow nostrils as seen on the base view.

50. Prominent caudal medial crura can be responsible for the excess columellar show and the bifid

columella. To correct this deformity, the vestibular skin can be elevated off the cartilage, exposing the medial crura down to the crural footplates, after which the caudal septal margin can trimmed.

51. The LLCs can be shaped and reoriented using suturing ("cartilage-sparing") techniques including a series of domal and interdomal sutures as well as other maneuvers to bring the nasal domes together into the desired levels of symmetry, alignment, rotation, and projection. This technique will be covered in detail in another chapter (Figure 5-18).

52. Overly lengthy and wide lateral crura can be reduced with a medial cephalic trim extending between the domes. The cephalic trim is usually conservative and confined to the medial two thirds of the LLC, avoiding a full-length injury to the scroll (recurvature between the ULC and LLC) (Figure 5-19). At least 7 mm of LLC width is left to ensure adequate support. Carrying out a cephalic trim without reducing the excess LLC length can result in an even wider, bulbous tripod due to the resultant weakening of the lateral limbs of the tripod.

53. A mucosal apposition stitch is placed caudal to the anterior septal angle incorporating the mucosa only, bringing the mucosa near the domes together and slightly narrowing the tip. This maneuver provides additional domal support and decreases supratip dead space.

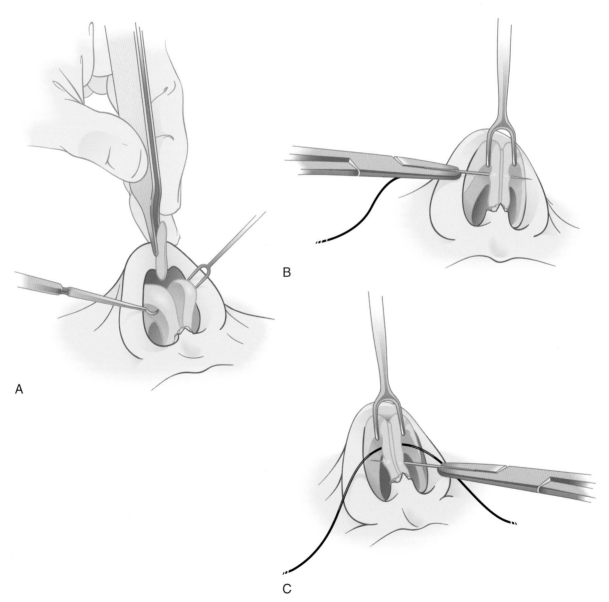

A

B

C

Figure 5-16 A-C, A horizontal mattress using a 4-0 gut on a Keith needle is used in a through-and-through fashion to secure the columellar strut. Placing the domes on slight tension with the skin hook may help.

54. To reduce the length of the lateral crus, a segment of cartilage can be excised or incised and subsequently overlapped. The segment excised may be from the intermediate or lateral crus depending on the area of excess and the appearance of the domes. A transverse incision is made with the No. 15 blade, after which the lateral edge is elevated in a subperichondrial plane. The lateral edge is allowed to overlap and the excess portion is excised, leaving the incised edges apposing one another without tension or a gap. Simple 6-0 nylon sutures are used to repair the edges.

55. Alar onlay grafts provide additional support to the incised segment. If a shield graft is used, it is designed first, and the remaining septal cartilage may be used for any additional grafts. The distal portion of the tip graft uses the thicker portion of the cartilage at the posterior bony–cartilaginous junction. Although templates to cut shield cartilage grafts have been used in the past, we prefer to fashion our own, thereby individualizing each nasal tip based on each patient's needs.

56. Alar onlay grafts are carved and beveled, then laid over the lateral crus, supporting the incised edges. The onlay grafts are sutured in place using 4-0 gut in a through-and-through manner. The edges are

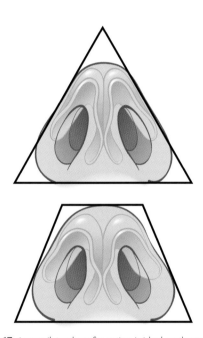

Figure 5-17 An equilateral configuration is ideal on the nasal base view.

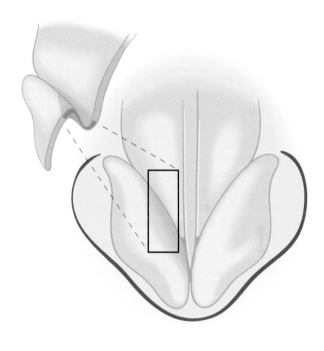

Figure 5-19 The cephalic trim of the LLC is limited to the anterior two thirds of the scroll.

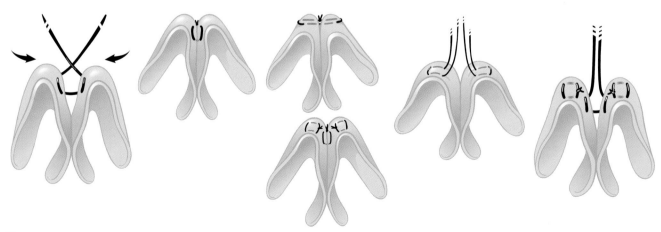

Figure 5-18 Various cartilage-sparing suture techniques can be used in an open rhinoplasty.

carefully beveled in vivo to ensure that they are not seen through the SSTE. This is done bilaterally with careful attention to symmetry.

57. A 2-0 Prolene transfixion suture is placed to hold the medial crus/columellar strut complex up to the membranous septum. This suture allows the medial limb of the tripod to heal in the rotated position. It is typically left in place for 2 weeks.

58. The shield tip graft is trimmed and carefully beveled (Figure 5-20). It is thicker and wider at the tip with a tapering base. The graft is sutured in place to the underlying domes and medial crura with 6-0 nylon suture (Figure 5-21). Precise placement of the tip graft to provide proper projection and definition is paramount. The graft must be flexible enough to follow the curvature of the medial crura. If the tip graft is too rigid it will be evident under the SSTE as a "gravestone" deformity. The tip graft extends slightly past the domes, and can serve to project, narrow, and define the tip, accentuating a supratip break (Figure 5-22).

59. The skin flap is re-draped and the nasal tip evaluated. Repositioning of the graft may be necessary, and patience during this portion of the case is required.

60. Sharp reduction of the bony dorsum will leave an open roof deformity requiring lateral osteotomies to close it. Medial osteotomies may also be necessary if the structure of the medial bony dorsum is too intact to allow a controlled infracture or outfracture depending on the desired effect. They are performed fading laterally towards the face (Figure 5-23). The thick bone of the nasofrontal angle is avoided. If an intermediate osteotomy is planned, it is best to carry out after the medial fading osteotomy to retain support of the attached nasal bone until the lateral osteotomy is performed last.

61. The pyriform apertures at the planned lateral osteotomy sites are reinjected with local anesthesia. A No. 15 blade is used to incise the mucosa at the pyriform apertures at the origin of the inferior turbinates. Scissors are used to enlarge the incision and start dissection in a subperiosteal plane. Dissection is completed with the periosteal elevator. In older patients, periosteal elevation is avoided to enable some residual soft tissue support.

62. The path of the planned osteotomy is demonstrated externally following a high–low–high course as demonstrated in Figure 5-23A. Note that the path is such that a triangular remnant of bone will be left at the pyriform aperture to prevent collapse at the apex of the osteotomy.

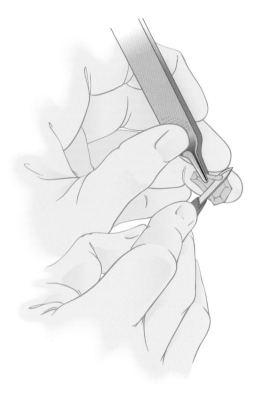

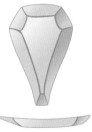

Figure 5-20 The tip graft is shaped and beveled to minimize visibility.

The final step of the lateral osteotomy is the controlled infracture or outfracture, performed by rotating the osteotome toward or away from the midline, as necessary.

63. The osteotome is guided through the incision and seated perpendicularly to the anterior margin of the pyriform aperture. The osteotome is advanced several millimeters in this vector until solid bone is encountered. The osteotome is then redirected cephalad, almost parallel to the anterior face, along the base of the bony nasal pyramid, gradually angling up towards the nasofrontal angle, until the level of the medial canthus, where the controlled fracture is performed.

64. A transcutaneous osteotomy using a 2-mm straight osteotome may be necessary if the infracture is incomplete to avoid a rocker deformity (Figure 5-23C).

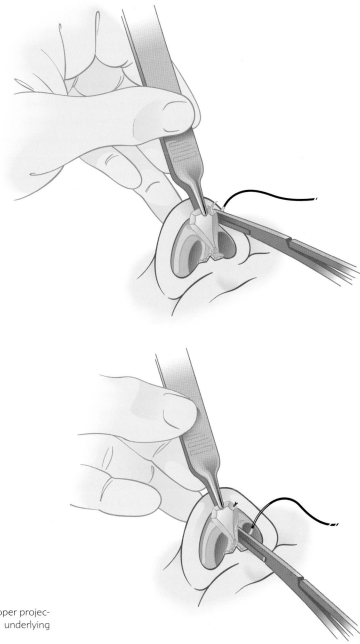

Figure 5-21 A, B, Precise placement of the tip graft to provide proper projection and definition is paramount. The graft is sutured in place to the underlying domes and medial crura using 6-0 nylon suture.

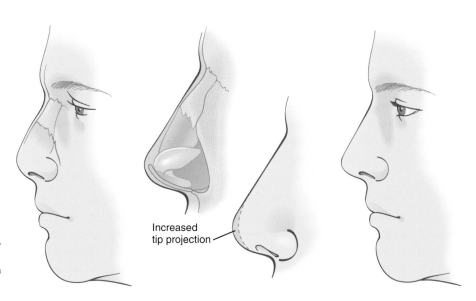

Increased tip projection

Figure 5-22 The tip graft extends slightly past the domes, and can serve to project, narrow, and define the tip, accentuating a supratip break.

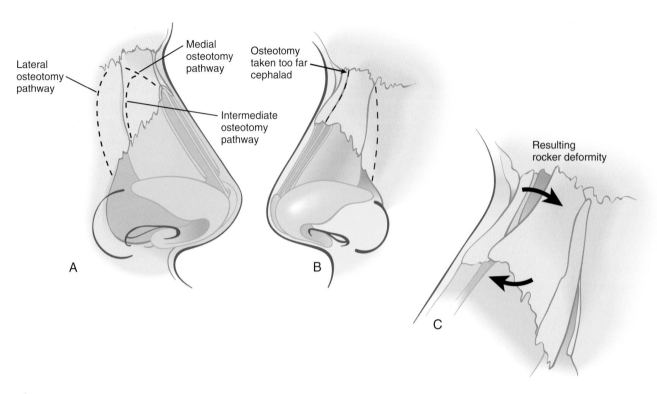

Lateral
osteotomy
pathway

Medial
osteotomy
pathway

Osteotomy
taken too far
cephalad

Intermediate
osteotomy
pathway

Resulting
rocker deformity

A   B   C

Figure 5-23 A, Osteotomy details (medial, intermediate, and lateral osteotomy). **B,** Osteotomy extended too far cephalad. **C,** Resulting rocker deformity.

65. The middle vault is an area that has appropriately received increased attention over the past decade, as it is critically important to restore an optimal nasal function. When the internal nasal valve (the angle formed by the septum and the ULC) is more acute than 15 degrees, or when short nasal bones exist, patients will often benefit from reconstructing the internal nasal valve. One of the most effective reconstructive methods is by the use of spreader grafts (Figure 5-24). This will be covered in detail in a separate chapter.

66. Near the end of the case, the SSTE flap is re-draped and the external nasal appearance is evaluated.

67. The tip graft is trimmed and beveled in situ, and the appearance reevaluated.

68. The bony–cartilaginous framework is carefully inspected and hemostasis is obtained.

69. The transcolumellar incision is closed with interrupted, simple 6-0 nylon suture, taking particular care to evert the skin edges. Precise placement of the corner stitch is particularly important to prevent notching. Sometimes, a vertical mattress suture can be used to obtain maximal eversion.

70. The marginal incisions are sutured using interrupted 6-0 chromic sutures. No attempt is made to close the marginal incision at the domes, as this has potential to distort the tip.

71. Projection can be measured at the end of the case. The tip is reprojected by the columellar strut and tip graft to achieve the intended nasal tip projection. Deprojection of the tip can cause an unintended widening of the alar base. To address this issue, and in some patients who intend to correct a widened alar base, certain alar base reduction techniques can be used and will be discussed in a separate chapter in more detail (Figure 5-25).

72. Alar batten grafts are onlay grafts aimed at stiffening the lateral nasal sidewall to prevent collapse of the LLCs with inspiration. They are positioned in a tight pocket created by dissecting superficial, lateral, and superior to the LLC and are positioned superficial to the pyriform aperture. They are typically fashioned from septal cartilage but can also be carved from conchal or costal cartilage (Figure 5-26).

73. Mastisol (Ferndale Labs, Ferndale, MI) is applied to the skin prior to application of elastic tape. The

elastic tape keeps gentle pressure on the SSTE, reducing the amount of postoperative edema. Tape is applied with gentle pressure from the nasofrontal angle to the supratip. A longer strip is placed around the infratip lobule as a sling, squeezing and supporting the tip in its intended level of rotation.

74. An Aquaplast splint (Aquaplast Corp., Wyckoff, NJ) is then applied. This material becomes soft and pliable when exposed to hot water, hardening as it cools off.

75. Bacitracin ointment is applied to both nares prior to placement of a moustache dressing (Figure 5-27).

POSTOPERATIVE COMMENTS

1. The dorsum and tip blend in better, improving the profile.
2. Overall projection has been increased by 1.4 mm.
3. Tip rotation has been increased, which along with a reduction of the columellar show, improves alar–columellar harmony.
4. Bifidity of the tip is corrected.
5. Nostrils are better defined and the nasolabial angle is more appropriate.
6. The strong chin balances the still slightly large nose; the patient has generally angular features, which go along well with the strong profile.

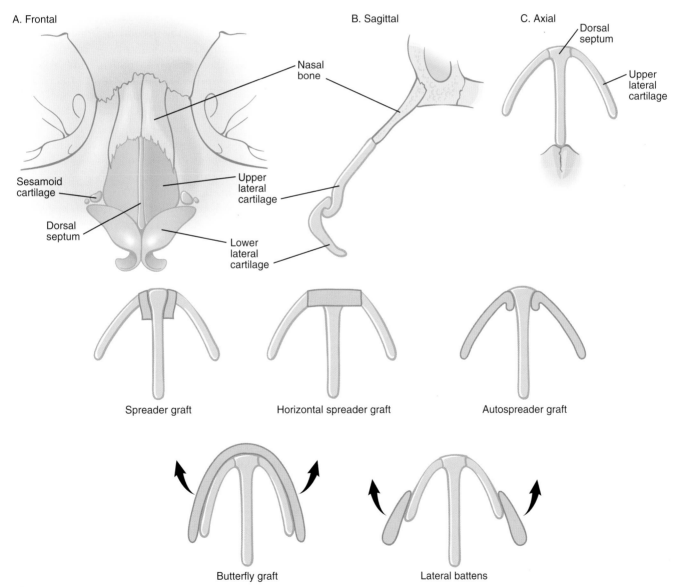

A. Frontal

Nasal bone

Sesamoid cartilage

Dorsal septum

Upper lateral cartilage

Lower lateral cartilage

B. Sagittal

Nasal bone

Upper lateral cartilage

C. Axial

Dorsal septum

Upper lateral cartilage

Spreader graft

Horizontal spreader graft

Autospreader graft

Butterfly graft

Lateral battens

Figure 5-24 The middle nasal vault is a critically important area to preserve and restore for optimal nasal function. There are a number of different ways to reconstruct the internal nasal valve.

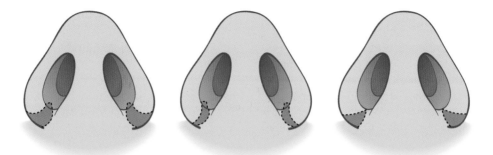

Figure 5-25 Alar base reduction.

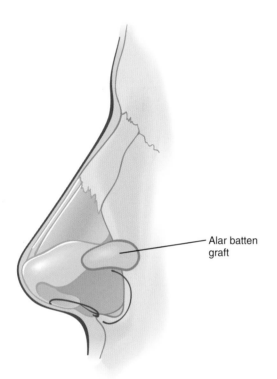

Alar batten graft

Figure 5-26 A, B, Alar batten grafts are onlay grafts aimed at stiffening the lateral nasal sidewall to prevent collapse of the lower lateral cartilages with inspiration. They are positioned in a tight pocket created by dissecting superficial, lateral, and superior to the LLC and are positioned superficial to the pyriform aperture. They are typically fashioned from septal cartilage but can also be carved from conchal or costal cartilage.

Another representative patient, in this case presenting with a tension tip deformity and a prominent nasal dorsal hump deformity (Figure 5-28).

POSTOPERATIVE CARE

Patients are given detailed postoperative instructions. The marginal and transcolumellar incisions are cleaned with peroxide and cotton swabs once a day, followed by application of topical Bactroban (2% mupirocin topical)

ointment (SmithKline Beecham Pharmaceuticals, Philadelphia, PA) to keep the incisions moist and infection free and to reduce crusting. The head is elevated during sleep, and the use of a humidifier is encouraged. The patient is allowed to shower on the second postoperative day, keeping the cast and tape dry with plastic wrap. Activity is limited during the first week; patients are asked to avoid heavy lifting and exertion. The level of activity is gradually increased, until all limitations are lifted at 4 weeks.

Alcohol and nonsteroidal anti-inflammatory drugs are avoided for 2 weeks postoperatively. A combination of 500 mg acetaminophen/5 mg oxycodone is used for pain control, but most patients can obtain adequate pain control with just acetaminophen after postoperative day 3. Zolpidem 10 mg is prescribed for insomnia. In revision cases, amoxicillin–clavulanate is prescribed as postoperative antibiotic prophylaxis.

Close follow-up is important to monitor the healing process and to reassure the patient. The first postoperative visit is on day 4, when the nasal passages are cleaned and inspected. The transcolumellar sutures are removed during this visit. The incision is then glued with Collodion (Paddock Laboratories, Minneapolis, MN) and taped with brown paper tape (3M Corp, Minneapolis, MN). On postoperative day 7, the cast and tape are removed using Detachol adhesive remover (Ferndale Laboratories Inc, Ferndale, MI) to loosen the adhesive and carefully lift the tape off from the skin while using a cerumen curette to keep down the SSTE. The skin of the nose is then cleaned with adhesive remover, and elastic tape is reapplied. The elastic tape is left on for an additional week, after which the nose is taped with the brown paper tape. Taping the nose helps decrease nasal swelling, maintain rotation, and support the tip while healing takes place.

Septal splints may be used in cases where a severe septal deviation is corrected or a septal perforation repaired. These are typically left in place for 1 to 2 weeks. If a Prolene transfixion suture was placed, then it is removed after a similar duration. Patients are occasionally instructed to perform nasal "exercises" if they have had

Text continued on p. 77

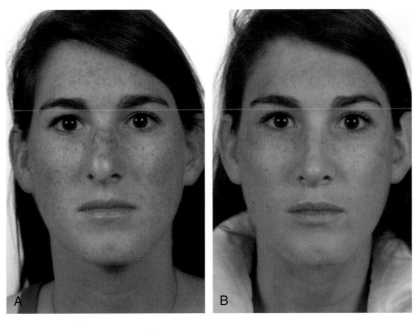

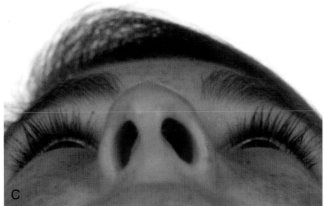

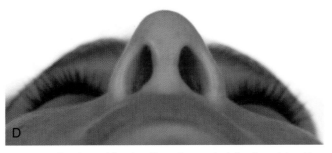

Figure 5-27 A–H, Young Caucasian, thin-skinned female with ptotic, poorly-defined nasal tip with moderately severe right-sided deviation of the nasal pyramid. Tip graft significantly aids to define her nasal tip.   *Continued*

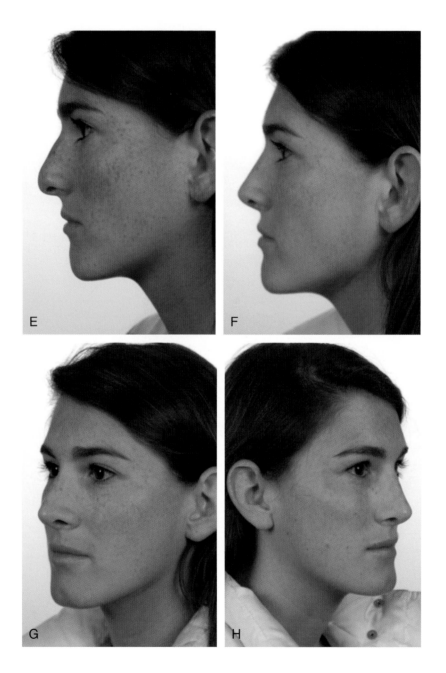

Figure 5-27, cont'd.

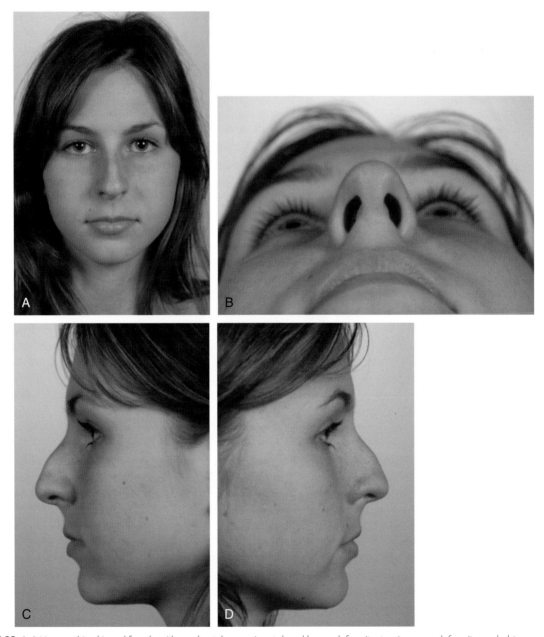

Figure 5-28 A-J, Young, thin-skinned female with moderately prominent dorsal hump deformity, tension nose deformity, and obtuse nasolabial angle.

Continued

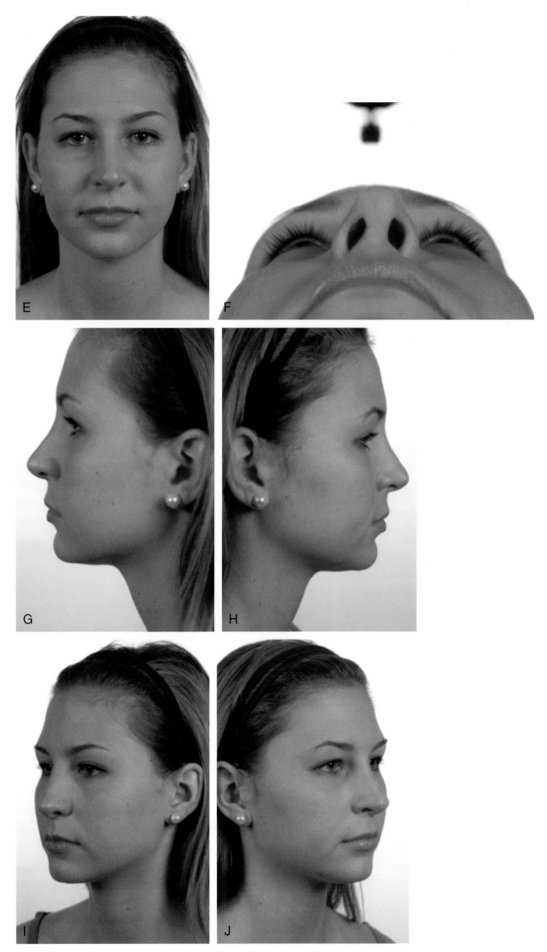

Figure 5-28, cont'd. Adequately corrected proportions of her nasal contour and features.

osteotomies to narrow the bony vault. Gentle pressure is applied to the upper third of the nose in a posterior and medial vector for 10 seconds several times each day. This maneuver helps the nasal bone fragments heal in the correct position and encourages the SSTE to settle down onto the bony–cartilaginous framework.

Swelling of the SSTE may take 1 year or longer to subside, and thus the final result may not be evident until that time. In patients with a particularly thick or swollen SSTE, minute amounts of Kenalog (triamcinolone HCl) 10 mg/mL may be injected using a 30-gauge needle and tuberculin syringe to decrease SSTE edema. This is especially useful in the supratip region. The steroid is injected beneath the dermis; if it is injected too superficially, skin atrophy may result. Gentle pressure is held for several minutes over the injected site. Injections may be repeated as necessary but no more frequently than once a month.

We never discharge a rhinoplasty patient from our care, preferring to see them on an annual basis after they are 1 year post surgery. This allows us to evaluate the long-term consequences of our surgery and perform touch-up procedures if necessary. Revisions are not considered any sooner than after 1 year postoperatively.

CHAPTER SIX

Primary Endonasal Rhinoplasty

Double-Dome Technique via Intercartilaginous Dome-Delivery

Amit Patel • Stephen W. Perkins

Surgical refinement of the nasal tip is considered by many to be one of the most challenging components of rhinoplasty. At the heart of the challenge is the need to not only adequately access and visualize but also control the complex three-dimensional architecture of the alar cartilages while being cognizant of tip support mechanisms and postoperative contracture. Although numerous approaches have been described throughout the literature, the endonasal delivery flap technique continues to be a workhorse in the armamentarium of surgical approaches for tip refinement. This chapter will focus on the beauty, versatility, and simplicity of endonasal tip surgery.

Tip rhinoplasty techniques have evolved substantially since Joseph first introduced cosmetic rhinoplasty in the late 1800s.[1] This evolution continues even to this day as discussions on the "ideal" surgical approach for nasal tip contouring ensue. The various incisions commonly used in rhinoplasty and their respective indications are illustrated in Figure 6-1. Four essential points must be kept in mind when choosing an approach for intermediate to advanced tip maneuvers: (1) the ability to adequately visualize the entire alar complex including all areas of the medial, intermediate, and lateral crura; (2) the ability to modify each alar unit separately and address asymmetries; (3) the ability to maintain or reconstitute tip support mechanisms; and (4) the ability to minimize resection of natural structural elements.

Next, we describe our philosophy, which is based on the creation of the double-dome unit as described by McCollough and English.[2] In our hands, this particular tip-sculpting technique has become a workhorse in tip modification as it nicely fulfills the above criteria. In fact, a 15-year review of the senior author's results with use of the double-dome unit procedure for tip rhinoplasty not only has proved the technique to be reliable with consistent results but also has shown it to carry a low rate of revision.[3] In this chapter, we will first describe our basic surgical technique for endonasal intercartilaginous dome-delivery via the double-dome technique, followed by a review of specific nasal tip deformities and steps utilized to correct these.

PREOPERATIVE ANALYSIS AND PATIENT SELECTION

It is critical to determine the exact tip deformities before creating a surgical plan. What is the aesthetic problem of the tip and what is one attempting to achieve? This begins with a detailed examination during the consultation period. Standardized forms are helpful for ensuring a complete examination as well as simplifying documentation (Figure 6-2). The tip shape should be described, such as *bulbous*, *twisted*, or *infantile*. Both the degree of rotation and the extent of projection should be evaluated. Skin thickness is critical to assess, and this issue alone may dictate the approach to be taken and/or the procedure to be performed. Palpation is helpful in determining the nature, volume, strength, and resiliency of the lobular cartilages as well as in evaluating tip support. Finally, it is important to note columellar abnormalities and their relation to the alar cartilages.

The ideal patient for these techniques has been described by Tardy.[4] The ideal patient has a slightly bifid or broad tip with dual-dome highlights. Thin skin and sparse subcutaneous tissue allow for more refined results from these endonasal techniques. The alar cartilages themselves must be firm and strong. Finally, the alar sidewalls should be thin and delicate, yet resist collapse and recurvature. By using the endonasal delivery approach along with a graduated approach to tip contouring, excellent aesthetic results can be achieved.

There are certain conditions, in our experience, that favor the use of the external columellar approach. It is often difficult to deliver, in a safe and adequate manner, alar cartilages in a patient with scar tissue in the lobule from previous surgery or trauma. Middle nasal vault deformities, in our experience, are more easily corrected

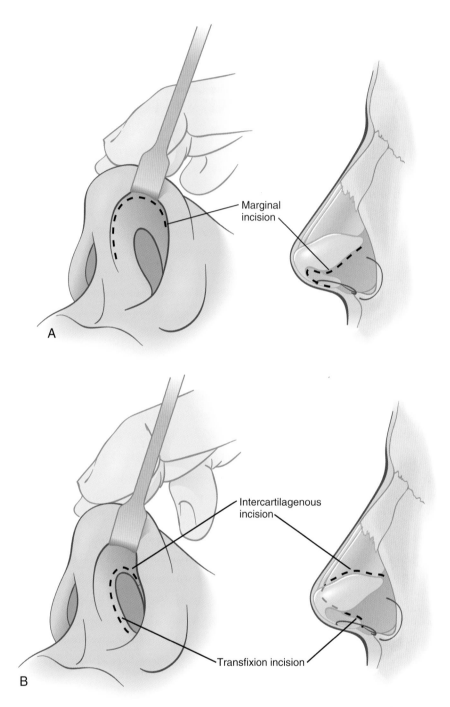

Marginal
incision

Intercartilagenous
incision

Transfixion incision

A

B

Figure 6-1 **A,** Marginal incision. **B,** Intercartilaginous incision. The intercartilaginous incision violates an important tip support mechanism, which must be considered when the tip is reconstructed. The double-dome suture helps to stabilize the tip complex.

through the external columellar approach. Patients with marked asymmetry in the nasal tip, with thin skin and bossa, may require camouflage tip grafting sutured in place. Also, marked twisting of the columella with significant discrepancies between the two medial crura may necessitate the use of an external columellar approach. Other indications for the external approach are extremely soft alar cartilages with no inherent support as well as

marked overprojection, overrotation, underprojection, and underrotation of the lobule.

All patients are initially seen in consultation with their selected surgeon. The consult room is designed to put the patient at ease while still maintaining a professional environment. The nasal analysis begins with the patient on a comfortable bar stool in front of a three-way mirror with the physician directly behind him or her.

Together they analyze the nose with the physician gently guiding the discussion. The three-way mirror not only allows the patient to get a more accurate view of the three-dimensional qualities of their nose but also relays specific concerns to the surgeon.

An in-depth nasal history is taken during the consult. Inquiries include any previous nasal trauma or surgery, difficulties breathing through the nose, any history of sinus disease or allergies, and present nasal medications.

The physician also reviews the more extensive complete history form, which is completed by the patient prior to consultation. An intranasal examination is performed at this time to detect deformities of the septum, enlargement of the turbinates, or other intranasal pathology. A preoperative rhinoplasty form is also completed to document the consultation findings as well as for later reference.

The procedure should be thoroughly discussed at this time and goals summarized with the patient. The

Meridian Plastic Surgeons   **Nasal History and Physical**

Patient:_____

__History of trauma to nose: _____
_____

__Previous surgery:_____
__Difficulty breathing: ☐R ☐L ☐Bilateral ☐Snoring ☐Mouth breathing
__Patient desires: ☐Straighter nose ☐Improved breathing
__Sinus disease
__Medications tried: _____
_____

━━━━━━━━━━━━━━━━━━ Functional abnormalities ━━━━━━━━━━━━━━━━━━

__Deviated nasal bones		__Traumatic dorsal hump	R__ L__
__Fractured nasal bones		__Dorsal saddling: Cartilage__ Bone__ Both__	
__C-shaped deformity R__ L__		__Angulated	R__ L__
__Irregular nasal bones		Dorsal ridge	R__ L__
__Nasal bones holding septum off center			

Pyramid	Drawing	Septum
R	L	R L

Septum deviated   R__ L__
Spurs   R__ L__
Caudal end deflected
blocking vestibule   R__ L__

__Floor obstruction   R__ L__
__Nasal valve collapse   R__ L__
  __Internal __Alar
__Middle vault narrowing or collapse R__ L__
__Loss of tip support
__Collapsed lobule w/ valve collapse R__ L__
__Avulsed/depressed ULC's   R__ L__
__Soft lobular cartilages

__Intranasal synechia(e)   R__ L__
__Inferior turbinate hypertrophy R__ L__
__Middle turbinate hypertrophy
  or concha bullosa   R__ L__
__Septal ulcer   R__ L__
__Septal perforation:
          Size:_____
          Location:_____
__Nasal polyposis   R__ L__
__Retraction of columella
__Acute nasolabial angle
__Premaxillary deficiency: R__ L__
          Complete____
__Cleft lip nasal deformity: R__ L__
          Bilateral_____

```
┌─────────────────────────────┐
│      % airway obstruction   │
│                             │
│         R___  L___          │
│ (60–65–70–75–80–85–90–95–100–105) │
└─────────────────────────────┘
```

Notes:_____
_____
_____
_____
_____
_____
_____
_____

Doctor: _____   Date: _____

Figure 6-2 Standardized forms used for ensuring a complete examination as well as simplifying documentation.

Continued

Meridian Plastic Surgeons   **Nasal History and Physical**

Patient:_____

__History of trauma to nose: _____
_____

__Previous surgery:_____
__Difficulty breathing: _____
__Patient desires: Improved tip: ☐ Smaller   ☐ More defined
              Improved dorsum: ☐ Straighter   ☐ Narrower   ☐ Hump removed

───────────────── Cosmetic abnormalities ─────────────────

__Deviated nasal bones   __Dorsal hump
__Fractured nasal bones   __Traumatic dorsal hump
__C-shaped deformity   R__ L__   __Dorsal saddling
__Irregular nasal bones   __Angulated   R__ L__
__Nasal bones holding septum off center   __Dorasl curved septum only   R__ L__
__Too short   __Dorsal ridge   R__ L__
__Too long: ☐ Whole lobule ☐ Infra tip lobule   __Avulsed/depressed ULC's
__Projection: ☐ Over ☐ Under   __Acute/deep N-F angle
__Soft lobular cartilages   __Obtuse N-F angle
__Rotation: ☐ Over ☐ Under   __Poor tip support

───────────────────────── Tip ─────────────────────────

__Supratip fullness: ☐ Soft tissue ☐ Cartilage   __LLC's asymmetric   R__ L__
__Bulbous tip   __Concave LLC   R__ L__
__Asymmetric tip   __Bossa   R__ L__
__Broad tip   __Retracted ala   R__ L__
__Bifid tip   __Nostrils wide: Horizontal   R__ L__
__Amorphous tip   Asymmetrical   R__ L__
__Infantile tip   __Wide alae   R__ L__
                                        __Alar base flare   R__ L__
                                        __Unusual cartilage bump   R__ L__

─────────────────────── Columella ───────────────────────

__Crooked   R__ L__   __MC buckle   R__ L__
__Show: Elongated septum   __Medial crural shift caudally   R__ L__
__Hanging   __Acute nasolabial angle _____%
__Retracted   (60–65–70–75–80–85–90–95–100–105)
__Short   __Bifid
__Long
__Twisted
__Short infratip lobule

───────────────────────── Dorsum ─────────────────────────

__Dorsal hump   Cartilage____   Bone____
__Dorsal irregularities   Cartilage____   Bone____
__Dorsal saddle   Cartilage____   Bone____
__Dorsum wide
__Open roof deformity ☐ Central ☐ Right ☐ Left
__Thick skin
__Thin skin
__Skin irregularities
__Weak chin

Doctor: _____ Date: _____

Figure 6-2, cont'd

physician reviews with the patient what to expect on the day of surgery, including the length of surgery, anesthesia, recovery, and discharge. Initial postoperative care and activity restrictions are also discussed. Finally, the limitations of the surgery, as well as possible complications, are given as part of the informed consent.

The consultation is then continued in the photography suite, where computer imaging is used to illustrate the planned aesthetic endpoint. This allows for confirmation that both the patient and the surgeon agree on the desired goals to be achieved. Following this, a full set of nasal images are taken for preoperative documentation.

The last phase of the consultation is spent with the scheduling nurse, where questions can be answered in what often is a more comfortable setting for the patient. Fees are reviewed with the patient, and signed copies of the procedures and fees are given to the patient. Any necessary lab work is arranged at this time.

Prior to surgery, all patients receive folders with detailed instructions for surgery, prescriptions, and a booklet reviewing postoperative healing and expectations. All patients start an oral antibiotic the day prior to surgery, most often either oral cephalexin (Keflex) or azithromycin (Zithromax), and continue this for 5 days.

SURGICAL TECHNIQUE

At 1.5 hours prior to surgery, patients are administered oral diazepam (Valium), promethazine (Phenergan), metoclopramide (Reglan), and dexamethasone (Decadron) as well as oxymetazoline nasal (Afrin Nasal Sinus) spray. In the operating room, deep sedation, typically using intravenous propofol, is instituted prior to infiltration of the local anesthesia. First, pledgets soaked in 4% cocaine are placed intranasally. After adequate time for decongestion, infiltration is started with 2% lidocaine (Xylocaine) with 1:50,000 epinephrine. No more than 7 to 8 mL is injected to minimize volume distortion.

The delivery approach is begun by making either a complete transfixion or a high septal transfixion incision depending on tip projection (Figure 6-3). Curved sharp scissors are then used to dissect up over the anterior superior angle and expose the upper lateral cartilages. Next, intercartilaginous and marginal incisions are made in a standard fashion (see Figure 6-1). Thin Metzenbaum scissors are then used to separate the overlying skin from the underlying lower lateral cartilages, nasal domes, and infratip lobule (intermediate crura). Finally, the alar cartilages are delivered with a single hook and supported with Metzenbaum scissors (Figure 6-4). In this fashion, each dome is assessed and recontoured individually.

The first step in achieving improved tip definition is the removal of fibrofatty tissue between the domes. This allows greater approximation of the two alar domes. An intact or a complete strip can be performed next by excising the cephalic portion of the lateral crura (Figure 6-5).

This achieves both volume reduction and improved supratip definition. It is essential to preserve at least a 7- to 9-mm width of cartilage. In a few select cases, this may be all that is required and the cartilages may be replaced in situ. In most cases, however, other techniques are required to achieve satisfactory tip definition and symmetry.

The ideal alar configuration has been described as being when the domal segment is convex, the adjacent lateral crura is slightly concave, and the overlying soft tissue is thin.[5] Occasionally, careful "pinching" of the individual dome cartilages can mold the cartilage into the ideal shape. Most often, however, individual dome treatment with suture is required. Prior to placing the single-dome suture, the vestibular skin is separated from the undersurface of the domal cartilage (Figure 6-6). A 5-0 absorbable synthetic polyglycolic acid (Dexon) mattress suture is placed at the junction of the lateral and medial

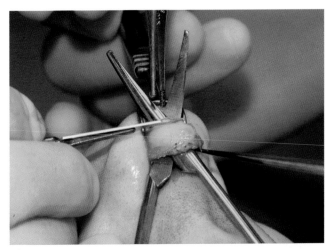

Figure 6-4 Delivery of lower lateral cartilage/Dome (LLC) with single hook and supported with Metzenbaum scissors.

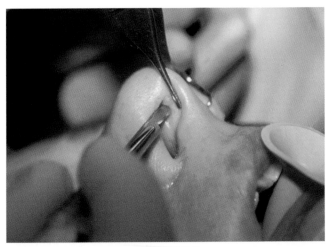

Figure 6-3 High septal transfixtion or complete transfixtion incision.

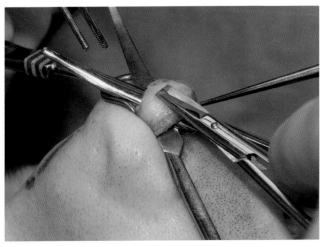

Figure 6-5 Cephalic trim.

crura. The knot is tightened to the point where the proper amount of domal definition is achieved (Figure 6-7).

If the individual domes remain asymmetric or improved supratip definition is desired, individual dome trimming can be performed. This involves "beveling" the cephalic portion of the single-dome unit (Figure 6-8).

With achievement of symmetric, aesthetically pleasing individual domes, the entire tip is reevaluated. Utilization of the endonasal approach allows this continual critiquing. A double-dome or transdomal mattress suture is next used to bring together the individually defined domes and stabilize these into one unit. Stabilization of the domes is the key to maintenance of long-term results. The suture is placed horizontally through the lateral and medial crura of both domes. We typically use a 5-0 clear polypropylene (Prolene) suture. The desired amount of lobular narrowing can be achieved by altering the tension of the stitch. With the domes replaced, the amount of

narrowing can be seen as one tightens the knot (Figure 6-9). It is important to avoid cinching down the suture and creating a unitip appearance.

The tip is then reevaluated. At this point, the decision is made on whether more aggressive steps will be required to achieve the desired tip aesthetics. This could include steps such as lateral crural flap, dome division, or the Lipsett maneuver. Marked disparity in length between the two medial crura is best corrected with the Lipsett procedure.[6] With this technique, the lengthier medial crura is delivered and dissected free from its attachments. An appropriate length of crura is resected to achieve equality in length between the medial crura. The two resected ends are then reapproximated with 6-0 monocryl (Figure 6-10). Removing or replacing the double-dome mattress sutures and addressing the anterior-posterior or caudal-cephalic placement of a suture in relation to the other dome may address minor asymmetries.

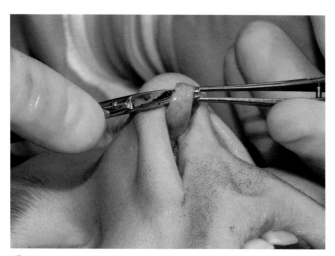

Figure 6-6 LLC/Dome separated from vestibular skin.

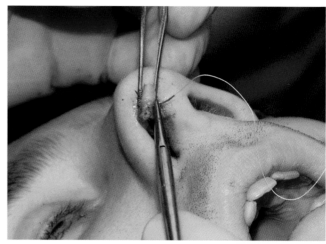

Figure 6-7 Suture is placed such that the knot is tied medial to both domes.

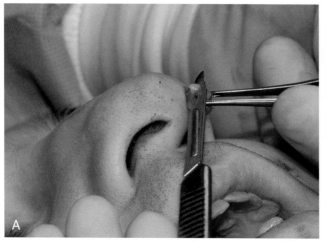

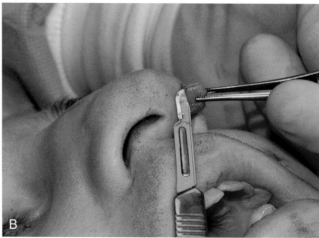

Figure 6-8 Asymmetries or abnormalities of the tip contour that persist after placement of the dome sutures can be corrected through a slight beveled trim at the cephalic border of a one-dome unit.

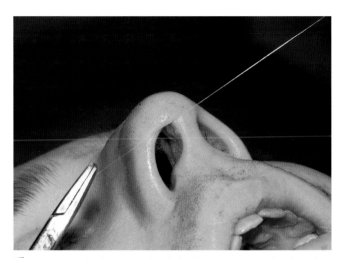

Figure 6-9 The knot is tied with both dome units replaced to their natural position. This allows a "real-time" assessment of the degree of narrowing that is achieved. Excessive narrowing should be avoided to prevent a "unitip" appearance.

Finally, correction of tip asymmetries may be more easily addressed with dome division, which can be performed medial to the dome, lateral to the dome, or at the mid-point of the dome (Figure 6-11). Dome division is used for a variety of situations when the described more conservative techniques have not been successful. Dome division can allow for more tip narrowing, which is especially required in those with thick skin. Furthermore, it can also be used to achieve upward rotation and increase or decrease tip projection.

Conservative upward rotation of the tip, on the other hand, is typically achieved by resection of an inverted triangle of caudal septum with corresponding vestibular skin and using a columellar strut to assist in "pushing" the lobule cephalically. If further rotation is required following this, the lateral crural flap technique can be used. This can involve a full incision of the lateral crura or simply a cephalic wedge excision (Figure 6-12). The

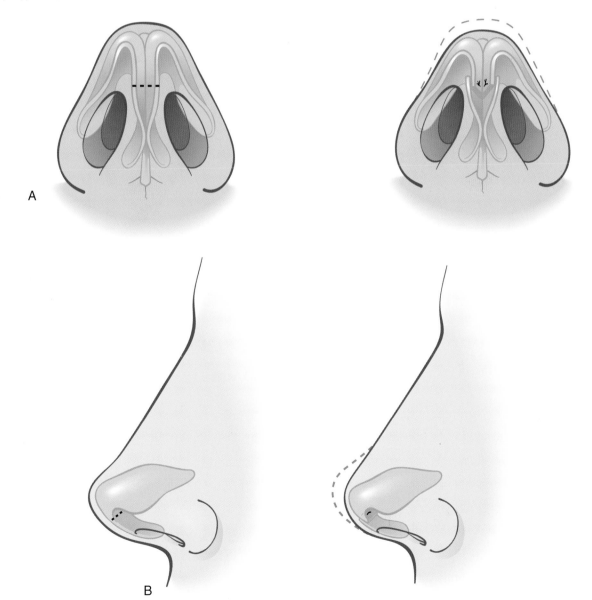

Figure 6-10 Lipsette maneuver to correct an overprojected tip or asymmetry in projection between the two dome complexes.

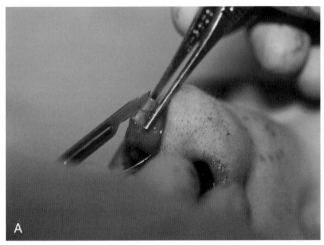
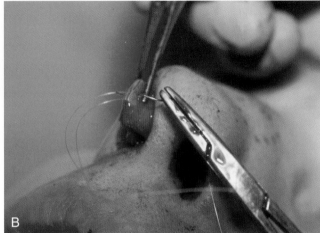

Figure 6-11 Vertical dome division.

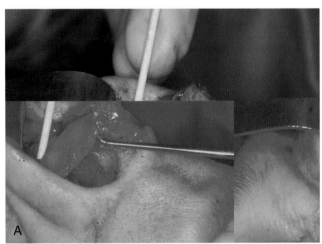
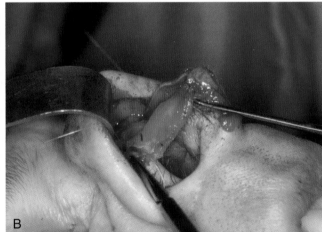

Figure 6-12 Lateral crura flap to increase rotation.

lateral crura can be overlapped and sutured to shorten their length and create upward rotation.

Following achievement of a symmetric and well-defined tip, attention is then turned to the septum, the dorsum and, last, osteotomies. A columellar strut fashioned from septal cartilage is placed between the medial crura and anterior to the nasal spine prior to osteotomies. Intranasal incisions are closed with 5-0 catgut. In closing the marginal incisions, it is important to avoid the lateral crura when suturing. Retraction of the lateral crura could lead to possible alar collapse and nostril asymmetries.

A small rolled piece of absorbable oxidized regenerated cellulose (Surgicel) is placed inside the nose within the vestibule of each newly constructed dome to add stability and prevent hematoma. Tan surgical tape (Micropore) along with an alloy metal splint is used for the external dressing that is removed at 1 week.

INDIVIDUAL CASE EXAMPLES

BROAD/WIDE TIP

Tips that demonstrate minimal deformity and minimally excess width can be addressed in the most conservative fashion. Single-dome suture treatment is often not required in these patients if the alar dome cartilages are delicate, thin, or soft. A conservative cephalic trim followed by a double-dome suture alone can often achieve the desired result (Figure 6-13).

BULBOUS/BOXY TIP

The bulbous tip requires individual treatment of the domes. This is most often addressed with a conservative cephalic trim and an individual single-dome mattress

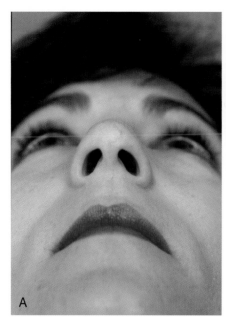 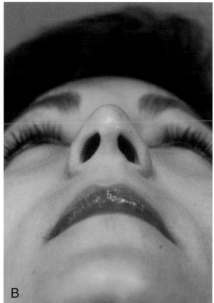

Figure 6-13 Broad/wide tip.

suture. Reconstitution of the double-dome unit with a 5-0 clear Prolene suture completes tip refinement (Figure 6-14). In the case of residual excess width, an alar spanning suture can be used to achieve further narrowing.

BIFID TIP

The bifid tip often requires both single-dome and double-dome mattress treatment of the tip complex. Occasionally, suture approximation of the tip alone will eliminate the bifidity. Most often, however, placement of either a non-sutured tip graft or a columellar filler graft is also required (Figure 6-15).

TRAPEZOID TIP

The trapezoid tip deformity is due to divergent intermediate crura (Figure 6-16). Cartilage splitting or transcartilaginous cephalic margin resection is unwise in these patients as both can lead to the late development of bossae. The alar cartilages have to be reoriented more caudally, or lateral alar batten grafts or possibly even alar struts must be added. This can be necessary if the lateral alar sidewalls are weak and tend to collapse or re-curve inward when the domes are brought together. Reconstitution of the interdomal ligament—single-dome and double-dome suture techniques—is required for correction. Tip grafting of the infratip lobule is also often necessary. Often, even when the earlier-mentioned aggressive techniques are used, an aesthetic tip cannot be achieved. In these more difficult cases, dome division is indicated to narrow the tip and straighten the lateral ala.

ASYMMETRIC TIP

A variety of techniques can be used to correct the asymmetric tip depending on the degree and the exact deformity. Minor deformities may be corrected with double-dome suture techniques alone. If asymmetry is due primarily to a disparity in medial crura length, the Lipsett procedure may be used. For marked asymmetry between the domes, dome division is used (Figure 6-17). Typically, the over-projecting dome is truncated and the double-dome unit is reconstituted. When the entire nose is overprojected, bilateral dome truncation may be performed.

COMPLICATIONS

BOSSA FORMATION

Knuckling of the lower lateral cartilages with healing can occur. Typically, this is due to weakening of the lateral crura secondary to either overresection or cartilage-splitting techniques. Patients with thin skin, strong cartilages, and nasal tip bifidity are at the highest risk for this. Bossae can be treated by resecting the deformed cartilage through a marginal incision. Further camouflage can be provided by either morselized cartilage or fascia.

ALAR RETRACTION

Retraction of the ala is usually due to either overresection of the lateral crura or excess resection of vestibular mucosa. Improper suture placement during closure of the

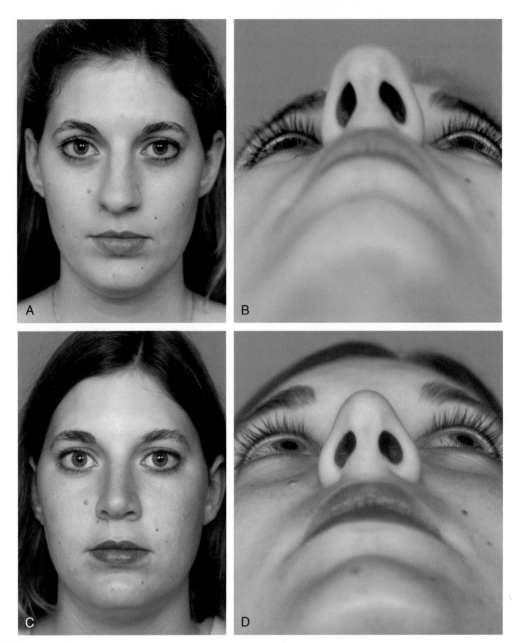

Figure 6-14 Bulbous/boxy tip.

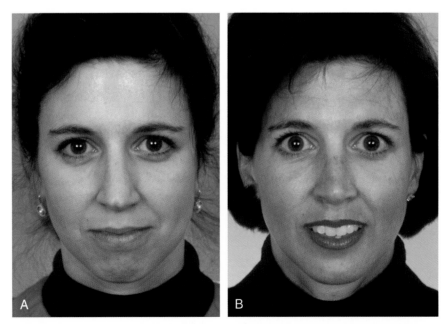

Figure 6-15 Bifid tip.

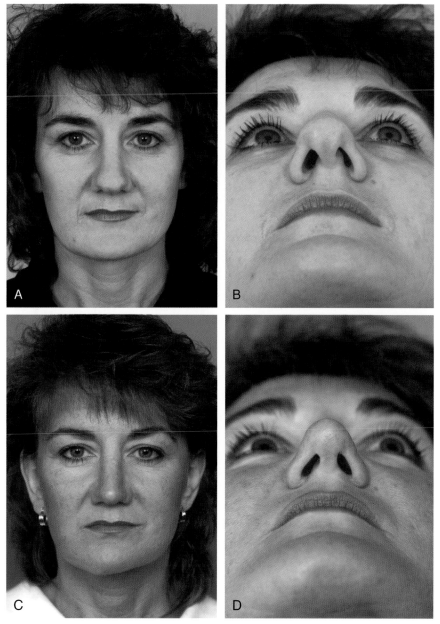

Figure 6-16 Trapezoid tip.

marginal incision can also retract the alar rim. Preservation of a complete strip of 8 mm or more in patients with a thin alar rim will help to prevent retraction.

Alar retraction can be corrected by taking a composite graft from the cymba concha of the ear.[7] A marginal incision is made in the area of retraction and a small pocket is corrected. The graft is then sutured into place, in effect pushing down the alar rim.

TIP ASYMMETRY

Postoperative asymmetry of the tip can have a variety of causes. Most often, this is due to uneven placement of the double-dome stitch. Healing forces can alter what was symmetric initially during the postoperative period. Minor

asymmetries not noted before surgery may become more obvious with a more overall symmetric nose. Preoperative identification of tip asymmetries and meticulous technique can help to prevent their occurrence.

IMPROPER PROJECTION

Intercartilaginous and transfixion incisions do lead to decreased tip support as well as decreased projection. This is usually counterbalanced by the increased strength of the medial crura with creation of the double-dome unit. Struts provide further strength and projection.

Most commonly, due to the inherent strength achieved with the double-dome unit, overprojection is the more common minor complication. Preoperative planning and

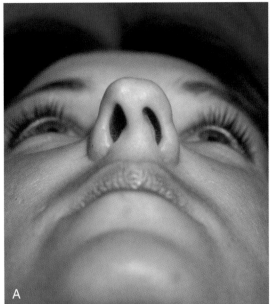 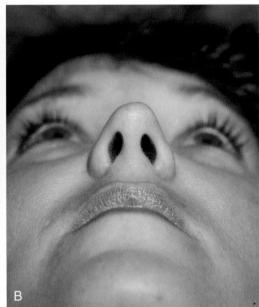

Figure 6-17 Asymmetric tip.

continual intraoperative assessment will help to avoid either overprojection or underprojection.

SUMMARY

The advantages that open rhinoplasty offers with increased exposure come with many downsides. The external incision itself can be a source of noticeable scarring, alar notching, or even trap door deformity. Patients are required to make a special visit for removal of the columellar sutures at postoperative day 5. This is both an inconvenience and a somewhat painful experience. Finally, resolution of tip edema is significantly prolonged with the external approach. For all of these reasons, our first choice is to use endonasal dome-delivery technique whenever possible.

Endonasal double-dome techniques, in particular, are based on the philosophy of utilization of the normal anatomic structures of the nasal tip (lobule). The merits of these techniques are many. Results of individual steps can continuously be reevaluated. Most of these incremental steps are reversible. Often, use of grafts can be avoided as well as the possibility of secondary deformities that come with them. The disadvantages of these techniques include the need for greater surgical finesse in delivering and suturing the alar cartilages. Also, techniques for the correction of certain deformities may be better addressed through the external approach. Nevertheless, for most primary cosmetic tip rhinoplasties, the beauty and expedient nature of the endonasal delivery flap approach with double-dome techniques provide consistent long-term results and few complications.

CONCLUSION

Variation in patient anatomy, aesthetic expectations, and tolerance for postoperative recovery time precludes the existence of a single technique. Additionally, differences in surgical training, philosophy, and comfort among rhinoplasty surgeons support the need for a variety of approaches. We, therefore, emphasize the importance of transcending beyond a "cookbook" philosophy toward tip rhinoplasty.

REFERENCES

1. Tebbets JB. Rethinking the logic and techniques of primary tip rhinoplasty: A perspective of the evolution of surgery of the nasal tip. *Clin Plast Surg.* 1996;23:245–253.
2. McCollough EG, English JL: A new twist in nasal tip surgery: An alternative to the Goldman tip for the wide or bulbous lobule. *Arch Otolaryngol.* 1985;111:524–529.
3. Perkins SW, Hamilton MM, MacDonald K. A successful 15 year experience in double-dome tip surgery via endonasal approach: Nuances and pitfalls. *Arch Fac Plast Surg.* 2001;3:157–164.
4. Tardy ME. Sculpturing the nasal tip. In: Tardy ME, ed. *Rhinoplasty.* The art and science. Philadelphia: WB Saunders; 1997:374–571.
5. Daniel RK. Rhinoplasty: creating an aesthetic tip: A preliminary report. *Plast Reconstr Surg.* 1987;80:775–783.
6. Lipsett EM. A new approach to surgery of the lower cartilaginous vault. *Arch Otolaryngol.* 1959;70:42.
7. Tardy ME Jr, Toriumi DM. Alar retraction: A composite correction. *Fac Plast Surg.* 1989;6(2):101–107.

CHAPTER SEVEN

Secondary Rhinoplasty via the External Approach

C. Spencer Cochran • Jack P. Gunter

The incidence of postoperative nasal deformities requiring secondary rhinoplasty varies from 5% to 12%.[1] The etiologies of postoperative nasal deformities (Table 7-1) are usually related to one or any combination of the following three problems: (1) displacement or distortion of anatomic structures, (2) underresection due to incomplete surgery, and (3) overresection due to overzealous surgery. Diagnosing these deformities and reconstructing the nasal osseocartilagenous framework form the foundation for obtaining consistent functional and aesthetic results in secondary rhinoplasty.

While adequate results may be attained with the endonasal technique in certain circumstances, the limited dissection and exposure offered by the endonasal approach often do not permit accurate assessment, intraoperative diagnosis, and appropriate treatment of complex anatomic problems. Open rhinoplasty techniques eliminate these restrictions imposed by the endonasal approach. We present a systematic approach to secondary rhinoplasty via the external approach that helps ensure consistent aesthetic and functional results in patients with both major and minor postoperative nasal deformities.

PREOPERATIVE ASSESSMENT AND PLANNING

A precise anatomic diagnosis is a key step to achieving optimal results in secondary rhinoplasty. The preoperative evaluation begins by defining the deformity, which is accomplished by a detailed history, physical examination, and complete aesthetic facial and nasal analysis. Starting superiorly, the nasofrontal angle height and depth are noted. The bony pyramid, upper lateral cartilages, and supratip are evaluated for their length, height, width, and symmetry. The nasal tip is evaluated in terms of its projection, rotation, symmetry, and position of the tip-defining points. The alae are inspected for increased width, collapse, or retraction. The columella is examined for increased or decreased show. The columellar-lobular and columellar-labial angles are evaluated to ascertain the desired angulation. The internal nasal examination

evaluates patency of the nasal valves, position and integrity of the septum, and state of the turbinates.

After the diagnosis is determined and the deformities are defined, the goals of the surgery are established, and a treatment plan is formulated. The operative goals are individualized for each patient according to the deformity. The goals may be to augment the nasofrontal angle, straighten the nasal dorsum, lower the supratip area, correct tip asymmetry and alar collapse, decrease columellar show, etc. If the existing osseocartilagenous framework is underresected, the amount and location of further reduction are determined. If the nasal framework has been overresected, it is determined what tissues are missing and where augmentation is needed. Secondary surgery is usually deferred until 12 months after the previous rhinoplasty.

GRAFTING ALTERNATIVES

A key component of the operative planning includes assessment of the grafting requirements and the potential source of grafting materials that will be required. While septal cartilage is generally the preferred grafting material in both primary and secondary rhinoplasty, severe deformities or a paucity of available septal cartilage requires an alternative source of grafting material. This is particularly true in secondary rhinoplasty when structural deformities resulting from previous procedures necessitate significant numbers of grafts.[2] Autogenous cartilage is preferred for any nasal framework replacement.

SEPTAL CARTILAGE

There are several advantages to using septal cartilage. A large amount of septal cartilage and septal bone can be harvested from the same operative field without the morbidity of an additional donor site. Compared to auricular cartilage, septal cartilage is more rigid, provides better support, and does not have convolutions. It is preferably used as a columellar strut, spreader grafts between the upper lateral cartilages and the septum, and lateral crural

Table 7-1 Etiologies of Postoperative Nasal Deformities

- Displacement or distortion of anatomic structures
- Underresection due to incomplete surgery
- Overresection due to overzealous surgery

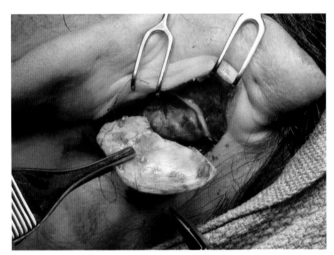

Figure 7-1 Intraoperative view of auricular cartilage graft harvested via a postauricular incision.

strut grafts to support or replace parts of the lower lateral cartilage complexes. When a sufficient quantity is available, it may also be used as a dorsal onlay graft for minimal amounts of dorsal augmentation.

AURICULAR CARTILAGE

The auricle can provide a modest amount of cartilage for nasal reconstruction.[3] Using a postauricular approach, the amount of harvested conchal cartilage can be maximized without compromising ear protrusion by preserving sufficient cartilage in three key areas: (1) the inferior crus of the antihelix, (2) the root of the helix, and (3) the area where the concha cavum transitions into the posterior-inferior margin of the external auditory canal. An incision is created longitudinally along the posterior aspect of the auricle, and dissection is carried down through the perichondrium. A 27-gauge needle dipped in methylene blue is percutaneously placed every 1 to 2 cm along the inner aspect of the antihelical fold to tattoo the cartilage along the planned excision path to ensure that sufficient antihelical contour is maintained. Dissection proceeds along both the anterior and posterior surface of the conchal bowl, and a kidney bean–shaped piece of conchal cartilage (Figure 7-1) is harvested while leaving sufficient cartilage at the aforementioned key areas for support.

Because of its flaccidity and convolutions, it is best used when these characteristics are desired. It is usually used for reconstructing the lower lateral cartilage complex,

for small onlay grafts, or for placement in the columella to provide tip support. However, it is a second choice to septal cartilage because of the inherent difficulty in obtaining and maintaining the desired shape and contour. While initial results of dorsal augmentation with auricular cartilage are often satisfactory, surface irregularities can become apparent with the passage of time. Furthermore, the irregular contour and limited supply of auricular cartilage often preclude its use.

COSTAL CARTILAGE

Because autogenous rib cartilage provides the most abundant source of cartilage for graft fabrication and is the most reliable when structural support or augmentation is needed, rib cartilage has been our graft material of choice for secondary rhinoplasty when sufficient septal cartilage is not available.[4,5]

The choice of which rib to harvest depends on the planned uses and grafting requirements because the amount of cartilage required dictates whether the cartilaginous segment is needed from one rib, one rib and a portion of another, or two ribs. In general, the surgeon should choose the cartilaginous portion of a rib that provides a straight segment as it is often possible to construct all required grafts from a single rib. For dorsal augmentation with a dorsal onlay graft, we prefer to harvest cartilage from the fifth, sixth, or seventh rib, depending on which rib feels the longest and straightest. If additional grafts are needed, a part or the entire cartilaginous portion of an adjacent rib may be harvested.

Rib cartilage may be harvest from either the patient's left or right side; however, harvesting from the patient's left side facilitates a two-team approach. In female patients, the incision is marked several millimeters superior to the inframammary fold and measures 5 cm in length (Figure 7-2). In males, the incision is usually placed directly over the chosen rib to facilitate the dissection.

The skin is incised with a scalpel, and the subcutaneous tissue is divided with the use of electrocautery. Once the muscle fascia has been reached, the surgeon palpates the underlying ribs and divides the muscle and fascia with electrocautery directly over the chosen rib. The dissection should be carried medially until the junction of the rib cartilage and sternum can be palpated. The most lateral extent of the dissection is demarcated by the costochondral junction. Identification of the junction is facilitated by the subtle change in color at the interface; the cartilaginous portion is generally off-white, whereas the bone demonstrates a distinct reddish-gray hue.

After exposure of the selected rib, the perichondrium is incised along the long axis of the rib. Perpendicular cuts are also made at the most medial and lateral aspects of the cartilaginous rib to facilitate reflection of the perichondrium.

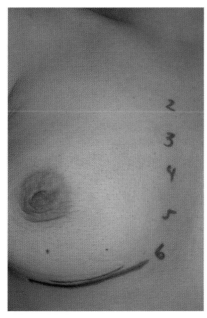

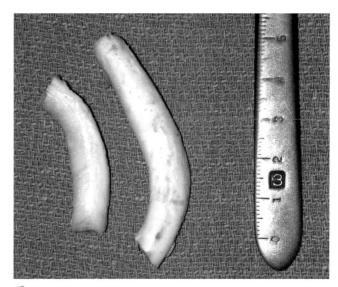

Figure 7-3 Right fifth and sixth rib cartilage segments.

Figure 7-2 The skin incision (thin line) for harvesting rib cartilage grafts in a female patient is placed several millimeters superior to the inframammary fold (thick line). The ribs are numbered according to their position.

A Dingman elevator is used to elevate the perichondrium superiorly and inferiorly from the cartilaginous rib. The subperichondrial dissection continues circumferentially as far posteriorly as possible until a curved rib stripper can be used to complete the posterior dissection. The curved rib stripper is slid back and forth along the rib, with care taken to remain between the cartilage and perichondrium until the undermining is complete.

The cartilaginous rib is cut near its attachment to the sternum and laterally where it meets the bony rib by making a partial-thickness incision perpendicular to the long axis of the rib using a No. 15 blade at the aforementioned junctions. The cartilaginous incision can then be completed with a Freer elevator using a gentle side-to-side movement. Once the cartilage segment is released both medially and laterally, the graft is easily removed from the wound and placed in sterile saline until the surgeon is ready to fabricate the grafts. If more grafting material is required, a portion of cartilage or the entire cartilaginous part of another rib is then harvested in a similar fashion (Figure 7-3).

The donor site is checked to ensure that no pneumothorax has occurred by filling the wound with saline solution and the anesthesiologist applies positive pressure into the lungs. If no air leak is detected, a pneumothorax can be excluded. A 16-gauge angiocath catheter is inserted through the skin and placed in the bed of the wound to allow instillation of a long-acting local anesthetic at the conclusion of the procedure. The wound may then be closed in layers using 2-0 Vicryl sutures. Particular attention should be directed at reapproximating the perichondrium. It is important to close the perichondrium, muscle,

and fascia layers tightly to prevent a palpable or visible chest wall deformity. A tight closure also helps "splint" the wound and reduce postoperative pain. Skin closure is carried out using deep dermal and subcuticular 4-0 Monocryl sutures.

If a pneumothorax has been diagnosed, this usually represents an injury only to the parietal pleura and not to the lung parenchyma itself. As such, this does not mandate chest tube placement. Rather, a red rubber catheter can be inserted through the parietal pleural tear into the thoracic cavity. The incision should then be closed, as previously described, in layers around the catheter. Positive pressure is then applied and the catheter is clamped with a hemostat until the surgeon is prepared for removal. At the end of the operation, the anesthesiologist applies maximal positive pressure into the lungs and holds this as the catheter is placed on suction and removed. A postoperative chest radiograph should be taken if there is any concern about the effectiveness of reestablishing negative pressure within the pleural space.

In older patients, ossification of the cartilaginous rib is a significant concern, and a limited computed tomography scan of the sternum and ribs with coronal reconstructions is recommended in those patients in whom there is a high index of suspicion. Despite appropriate preoperative screening, occasionally patients will present with premature calcification of the cartilaginous rib. Frequently, this is limited and occurs commonly at the junction of the osseous and cartilaginous portions of the rib. Small foci of calcification may also be found within the body of the rib cartilage itself. This can impair the preparation of individual grafts as well as act as a site of weakness often having a tendency to fracture during graft harvest. We have found that the use of a smooth diamond burr can also prove useful in contouring areas of calcification to salvage these uncommon circumstances. If the cartilage is unexpectedly found to be so extensively calcified at the time of the operation that it is unusable, we would then consider the use of irradiated donor cartilage, accepting the increased risks of progressive resorption over time. Irradiated homologous rib cartilage has been used successfully,[6] but problems with infection, absorption, and warping limit its routine use in dorsal augmentation (R. O. Dingman, personal communication, 1980).

OPERATIVE TECHNIQUE FOR SECONDARY RHINOPLASTY

A systematic approach to the open rhinoplasty technique is helpful for obtaining consistent results. While an individualized approach is applied to each case and variations in operative steps and sequence occur, the general steps of open secondary rhinoplasty (Table 7-2) proceed in the following sequence: incisions, skin elevation, intraoperative diagnosis and assessment of grafting requirements, septoplasty/septal cartilage harvest, dorsal modification, establishment of desired tip projection and reconstruction of the nasal tip complex, osteotomies, final tip cartilage positioning and shaping, wound closure, and application of splints and dressings.

INCISIONS AND ELEVATION OF THE SOFT TISSUE ENVELOPE

With the patient under general anesthesia, the external nose and septum are injected with 1.0% lidocaine with 1:100,000 epinephrine, and the internal nose is packed with gauze soaked with a vasoconstricting medication, such as oxymetazoline HCl. Bilateral marginal incisions along the caudal edge of the lower lateral cartilages are terminated medially at the narrowest part of the columella and connected with a transcolumellar incision. A straight-line incision is avoided by placing a broken-line incision across the columella, which allows precise wound closure.

Elevation of the soft tissue envelope is begun by dissecting the thin columellar skin off the caudal edges of the medial crura. The dissection continues over the lateral crura in either a medial-to-lateral or lateral-to-medial direction. Care should be taken to avoid unnecessary retraction or injury to the soft tissue envelope, and in particular, the columellar skin, as the blood supply may be tenuous due to previous disruption in prior surgeries. The normal tissue planes are frequently nonexistent, having been replaced with varying amounts of scar tissue, and the surgeon should be cautious not to perforate the skin overlying the lower lateral cartilage complexes.

As dissection continues over the tip, it is important to preserve the integrity of the domal segments when they are present as this will facilitate reconstruction of the tip complex. Once the tip is exposed, dissection continues over the dorsal septum and upper lateral cartilages. Once the nasal bones have been reached, a Joseph elevator is used to lift the periosteum off the nasal bones superiorly to the level of the nasofrontal angle. Retraction of the undermined area allows exposure of the entire osseocartilagenous framework.

INTRAOPERATIVE DIAGNOSIS AND ASSESSMENT OF GRAFTING REQUIREMENTS

After the soft tissue envelope is elevated from the underlying nasal framework, the nasal cartilages are evaluated and correlated with the preoperative diagnosis. The extent of the upper lateral cartilages and nasal tip deformity is determined, and any cartilages displaced or distorted by scar tissue are dissected free, but resection or final correction is delayed. Next, it is determined whether the tip projection needs to be altered since this will determine the height at which the dorsal profile line should be set. Any alteration of the dorsum should be performed with the final tip projection in mind.

Silicone sizers can be used to estimate the shape and size of the columellar strut and dorsal onlay graft when indicated. The silicone sizers are prefabricated by the surgeon from molds of anatomically shaped dorsal onlay grafts and columellar struts carved in a paraffin wax block in an assortment of shapes and sizes (Figure 7-4). RTV (room temperature vulcanizing) silicone is mixed, poured into the molds, and left for 24 hours to polymerize before trimming to their final form. The sizers are then sterilized before being placed in the operative field. With a columellar sizer in place, various dorsal sizers are then placed on

Table 7-2 Operative Sequence in Open Secondary Rhinoplasty

Incisions and elevation of the soft tissue envelope
- Dissection of displaced tip cartilages

Intraoperative diagnosis and assessment of grafting requirements
- Estimation of desired tip projection

Septal cartilage harvest/septoplasty

Dorsal modification
- Dorsal reduction (if indicated)
- Spreader graft placement
- Dorsal augmentation (if indicated)

Osteotomies

Tip reconstruction using the tripod concept
- Establishment of final tip projection
- Lateral crural reconstruction

Final inspection

Wound closure

Application of splints and dressings

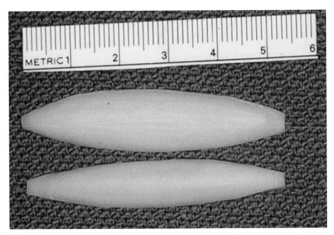

Figure 7-4 Silicone dorsal onlay graft sizers prefabricated by surgeon are helpful in estimating the desired graft size.

the dorsum and the skin is redraped until the desired combination is determined.

SEPTAL CARTILAGE HARVEST/SEPTOPLASTY

If septal work is required, the septum may be approached from above after the upper lateral cartilages have been divided from the septum. The upper lateral cartilages can be freed from the dorsal septum after submucoperichondrial tunnels are created bilaterally using an elevator beginning at the septal angle. Alternatively, the septum may be approached via a separate transfixion incision.

The mucoperichondrium is elevated on one side, and the appropriate septal modification or septal cartilage harvest is performed. If septal cartilage is to be harvested, care should be taken to preserve an "L-shaped" septal strut measuring at least 1 cm in width. If the caudal septum is deviated or dislocated from the maxillary crest or nasal spine area, it should be reduced to the midline and fixated with a figure-of-eight suture. It may be necessary to separate the medial crura to gain better exposure, but their attachment to each other, which aids in support of the tip, must be reestablished before the end of the operation.

DORSAL MODIFICATION

After the desired tip projection is estimated and septal work has been completed, the cartilaginous-bony dorsum is evaluated and any needed augmentation or reduction of the dorsum is performed. Reduction of the bony dorsum is usually performed with a rasp, and any remaining contour irregularities of the bony dorsum can be smoothed using a drill with a coarse diamond burr. The dorsal septum and upper lateral cartilages can then be trimmed to the desired height with a scalpel or sharp-angled scissors (Figure 7-5).

Frequently, secondary rhinoplasty patients require placement of dorsal spreader grafts. Spreader grafts are usually paired, longitudinal grafts placed between the dorsal septum and the upper lateral cartilages (Figure 7-6). They are used to straighten a deviated dorsal septum, improve the dorsal aesthetic lines, correct upper lateral cartilage collapse, and reconstruct an open roof deformity.[7] If the dorsal aspect of the septal "L-strut" has been weakened or overresected during previous surgery, dorsal spreader grafts placed along either side of the septum allow for stabilization and also provide a stable platform for dorsal augmentation.

The length and shape may vary depending on the indication. The grafts may extend above the level of the dorsal septum to slightly augment the dorsum or extend caudally beyond the septal angle as extended spreader grafts to lengthen the nose. The grafts should be suture-fixated to the septum prior to reapproximation of the upper lateral cartilages to the septum–spreader graft complex.

With the midvault reconstructed, the dorsum may then be augmented as necessary. Autogenous rib cartilage has been our graft material of choice for dorsal augmentation when sufficient septal cartilage is not available. Prior to graft preparation, the dorsum of the nose must be prepared to receive the dorsal graft. The recipient bed on the dorsum must be made as flat and smooth as possible to give the greatest surface area for the dorsal onlay graft to contact. A uniform surface of the dorsal recipient bed aids in the graft adhering solidly to the osseocartilagenous framework. This prevents postoperative movement of the graft after healing is complete, as is often seen in grafts placed in soft tissue envelopes.

The major disadvantage in using rib cartilage is its tendency to warp (Figure 7-7). In response to this, the senior author (J.P.G.) devised a technique in which the larger costal cartilage grafts, the dorsal onlay graft, and often the columellar strut are reinforced with a centrally placed Kirschner wire (K-wire) to decrease warping and provide a more stable and predictable result.[8] To avoid warping of smaller grafts, we follow the principle of carving balanced cross sections originally described by Gibson and Davis[9] and later substantiated by Kim et al.[10]

The harvested rib segment that is selected for the dorsal onlay graft is manually stabilized in a specifically designed K-wire guide jig, and a smooth 0.028-inch K-wire is drilled longitudinally through the center of the graft. The 0.028-inch K-wire is removed and replaced with a threaded 0.035-inch K-wire to better stabilize the graft and avoid migration of the K-wire. The same routine is used for placing an internal K-wire in the columellar strut if rib cartilage is used.

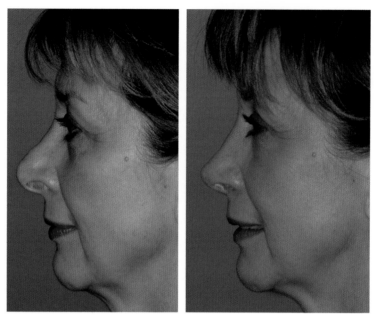

Figure 7-5 Preoperative (*left*) versus postoperative (*right*) photographs of a secondary rhinoplasty patient with a dorsal deformity resulting from inadequate resection of her dorsal septum during a previous rhinoplasty.

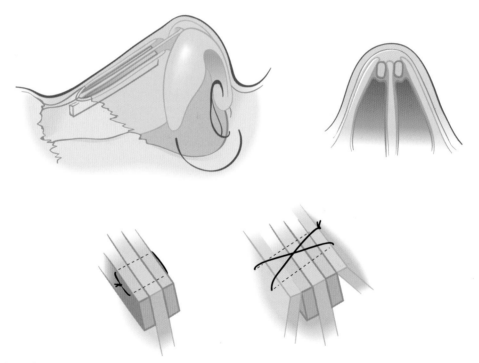

Figure 7-6 Spreader grafts are sutured along the dorsal septum.

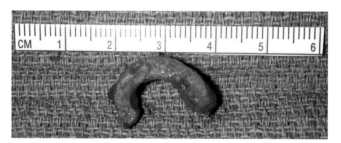

Figure 7-7 Rib cartilage graft (without K-wire stabilization) removed from a secondary rhinoplasty patient that exhibits significant warping.

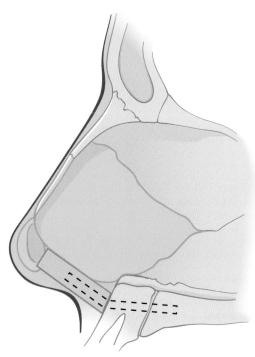

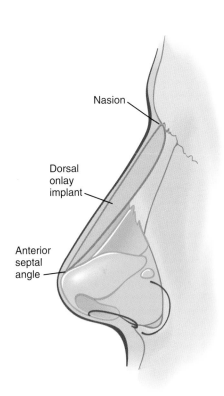

Figure 7-8 A columellar strut graft fashioned out of rib cartilage with internal K-wire stabilization is placed in a maxillary drill hole, which allows precise control of projection and rotation.

Figure 7-9 Rib cartilage dorsal onlay graft.

The cartilage grafts with the internal K-wires are then carved into similar but slightly larger shapes of the selected sizers. The K-wire in the dorsal onlay graft should be placed to within 2 to 3 mm of the cephalic end of the graft and cut flush with the caudal end. The K-wire in the columellar strut should extend three-fourths of the length of the graft with 8 to 10 mm of the K-wire left exposed at the graft base, which will be seated into a drill hole created in the maxilla (Figure 7-8).

The grafts are then placed in their anatomic position to determine what further shaping is required. Carving proceeds carefully from this point usually by scraping the grafts with the sharp edge of a No. 10 blade perpendicular to the graft surface until the exact desired size, shape, and contour are obtained. After the carving is completed, the K-wire placement can be adjusted if indicated.

Next, the dorsal onlay graft is placed and secured (Figure 7-9). Fixation of the cephalic end of the dorsal graft is achieved by placing a temporary 0.028-inch smooth K-wire percutaneously through the graft into the nasal root. This percutaneous K-wire is removed in the office with a wire twister 1 week postoperatively when the external splint is removed. Caudally, the graft is secured to the nasal dorsum by a suture that passes around or through the graft and through the upper lateral cartilages and nasal septum–spreader graft complex in the area of the septal angle. Any remaining tip work is then

completed as well as indicated osteotomies, if not previously performed.

TIP RECONSTRUCTION USING THE TRIPOD CONCEPT

Once the nasal dorsum has been addressed, attention is redirected to the tip, where the estimated tip projection is confirmed, final tip projection is established, and reconstruction of the tip cartilages is performed. The Tripod Concept, which relates nasal tip support and shape to the paired lower lateral cartilage complexes, is a useful premise for nasal tip reconstruction and for correcting deformed lower lateral cartilages. Each lower lateral cartilage complex consists of a medial crus (including the intermediate crus) and a lateral crus. These paired complexes can be visualized as a tripod (Figure 7-10), with each lateral crus forming a separate lateral (cephalic) leg and the adjoining medial crura forming the caudal third leg.[11] Using this concept to anatomically simulate the paired lower lateral cartilage complexes allows reestablishment of this tripod and is the goal for any nasal-tip reconstruction.

To be successful, the reconstructed tripod structure must have the strength to support the tip and prevent the alar sidewalls from collapsing and the shape to provide the nasal tip with an aesthetically pleasing, natural

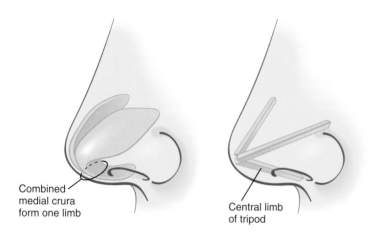

Combined medial crura form one limb

Central limb of tripod

Figure 7-10 The Tripod Concept. Each lateral crus makes up one of the lateral legs of the tripod and the paired medial crura make up the caudal leg.

appearance. Septal, auricular, and rib cartilage can all be used with each having its own inherent advantages and disadvantages.

The method used for rebuilding the tripod depends on several factors. The most important factors are (1) how much usable cartilage is present in the tip and (2) what cartilage (septal, auricular, or rib) is available for grafting. In minor tip deformities (Figure 7-11), when the lateral crura are present but collapsed or mildly deformed, lateral crural strut grafts fashioned from septal or auricular cartilage are the treatment of choice to reestablish the shape and stability of the lateral legs of the tripod.[12] Lateral crural strut grafts are grafts placed in an undermined pocket between the undersurface of the lateral crus and the vestibular skin and stabilized by suturing it to the crus (Figure 7-12). They are used to correct alar retraction, alar rim collapse, and concave, convex, or malpositioned lateral crura (Figure 7-13). The lateral crural strut grafts extend laterally to overlap the piriform aperture and end in an undermined pocket inferior to the alar groove. If the pocket is created superior to the alar groove, it will sometimes produce a visible bulge above the ala. We use a columellar strut in almost all cases of nasal-tip reconstruction to stabilize the caudal leg and thereby resist displacement by scar tissue contraction or swelling.

When the lateral crura are absent or so deformed that they cannot be used, correction is more challenging, and autogenous rib cartilage has proved to be the cartilage of choice. If the lateral crura are not usable but the medial crura and domes are intact, a columellar strut is sutured between the medial crura to strengthen the caudal leg of the tripod. Next, the vestibular skin is undermined off the undersurfaces of the domes. The lateral crural strut grafts are sutured to the undersurface of each dome to replace the missing lateral crura (Figure 7-14).

If both the medial and lateral crura are absent or unusable, autogenous rib cartilage is carved as a "shaped" columellar strut to act as the caudal leg of the tripod

(Figure 7-15). It is carved to simulate the contour of the caudal margins of the medial crura and medial portion of the domes along the columella-infratip lobule. The graft is stabilized with an internal 0.035-inch threaded K-wire that extends to within 4 or 5 mm of the tip.[13] Approximately 10 mm of the K-wire protrudes from the base of the graft and is placed in a 12-mm drill hole in the maxilla just off the midline in the nasal spine area after the spine is removed with a rongeur. The strut replaces the support of the missing medial crura. The drill hole should travel just below and parallel to the nasal floor so that it will not extrude through the nasal or palatal bony surfaces.

The lateral legs of the tripod are reconstructed in a fashion similar to that used when the domes are present. The only difference is that instead of suturing the medial ends of the lateral crural strut grafts to the undersurface of the domes, the surgeon sutures the grafts to the tip of the "shaped" columellar strut to replace the missing lateral crura (Figure 7-16). It is preferable and easier to suture the lateral crural strut grafts to the undersurface of the domes, assuming they are present, than to the tip of the columellar strut. In the event that the domes are absent, the "shaped" strut and the lateral crural strut grafts should be tapered. A soft tissue onlay graft of fascia or perichondrium is also an effective means of camouflaging irregularities of the tip cartilages and grafts edges.

WOUND CLOSURE AND SPLINTS

The skin is redraped after a final inspection of the nasal framework. The external appearance and nasal interior are evaluated, and the incisions are closed. After closure of the marginal incisions with interrupted 5-0 chromic sutures, the transcolumellar incision is meticulously closed with interrupted 6-0 nylon sutures. No subcutaneous sutures are necessary. If septal work has been performed, bilateral septal splints are placed and sutured in place with through-and-through 3-0 nylon sutures. Nasal

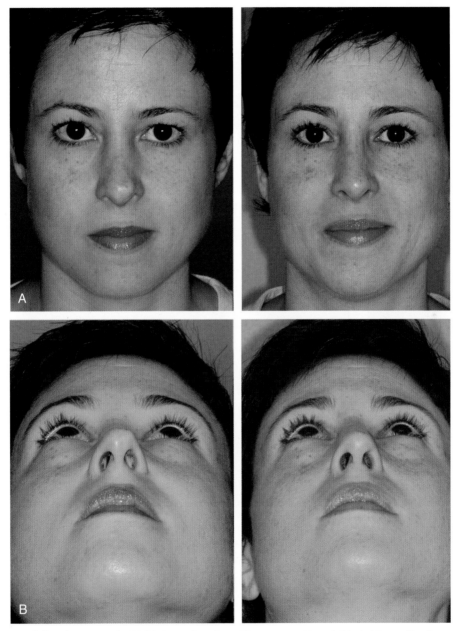

Figure 7-11 Preoperative (*left*) and postoperative (*right*) views of a patient with an asymmetric and distorted tip resulting from a previous surgery, which was corrected using septal and auricular cartilage to reconstruct her tip.

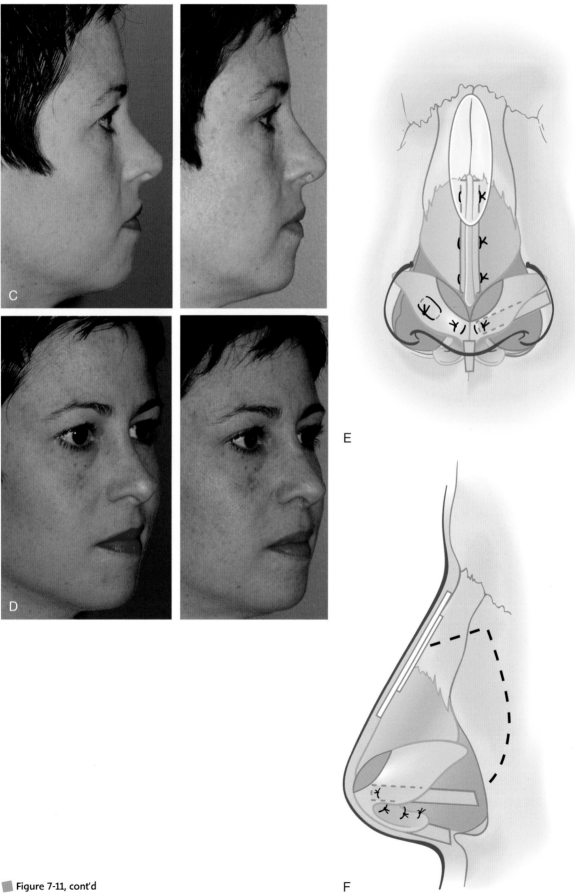

C

D

E

F

Figure 7-11, cont'd

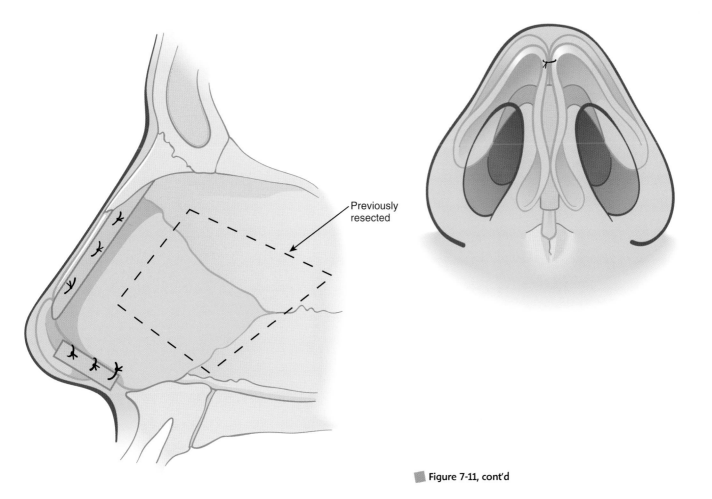

Previously
resected

Figure 7-11, cont'd

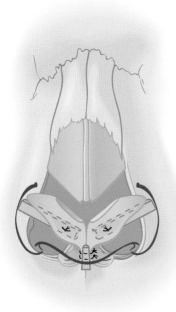

Figure 7-12 Lateral crural strut grafts are placed under the existing lateral crura when they are only minimally deformed.

packing is avoided if hemostasis is adequate. Steri-Strips and an aluminum cast are placed on the nose and remain for 1 week.

DISCUSSION

The major advantage of the open approach in the management of secondary nasal deformities lies in the complete, undistorted anatomic exposure of the nasal framework. This allows for a precise anatomic diagnosis and correction of the deformity with original tissues and supplemental cartilage grafts. The bony and cartilaginous structures can be continuously assessed intraoperatively. The final anatomic alignment and symmetry of the nasal framework become more predictable. Despite all the advantages of the open approach, it is not indicated for every secondary nasal deformity. Minor asymmetries or underresection can sometimes be corrected endonasally, but for major deformities, the open approach is preferred.

The major potential disadvantage of the open rhinoplasty technique is the transcolumellar scar. However,

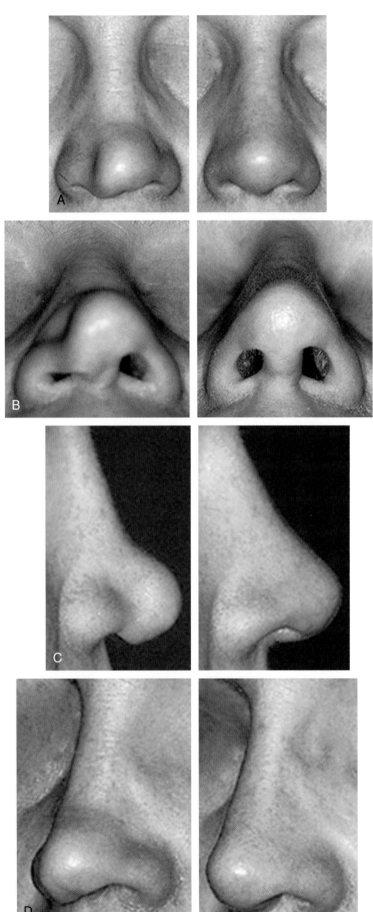

Figure 7-13 Preoperative (*left*) versus postoperative (*right*) views of a secondary rhinoplasty patient whose deformities were corrected with a dorsal onlay and columellar strut fashioned out of rib cartilage and reinforced with internal K-wires.

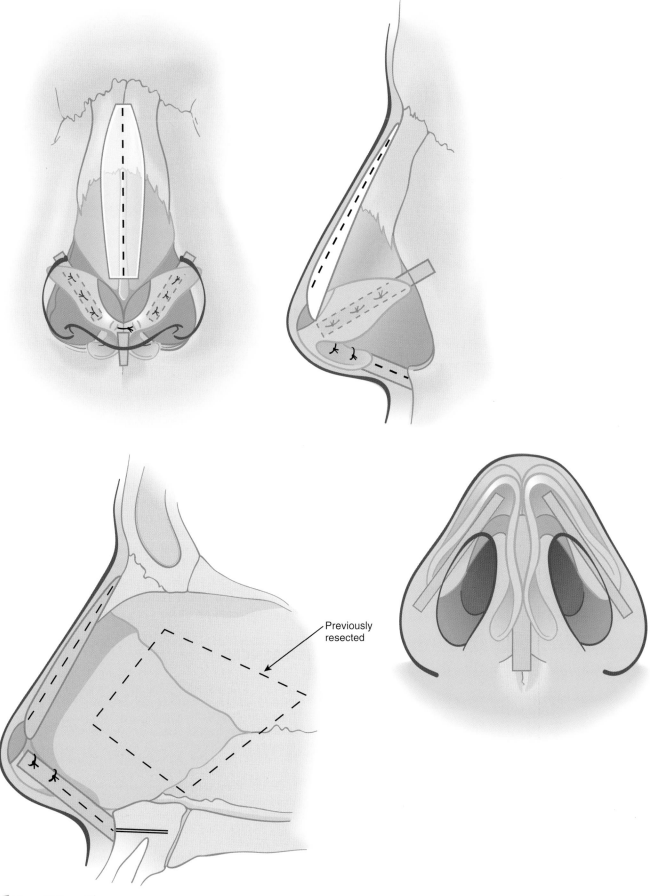

Previously
resected

Figure 7-13, cont'd

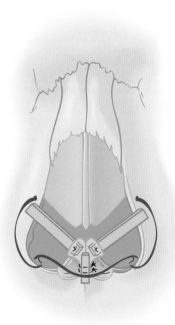

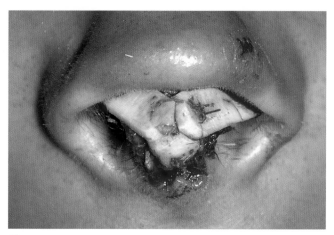

Figure 7-16 Intraoperative photograph showing lateral crural strut grafts sutured directly to the "shaped" columellar strut.

Figure 7-14 For lateral crura that have been completely resected or that are unusable, the lateral crural strut grafts are sutured to the undersurface of the domes.

using a broken line incision across the columella with strict attention to operative technique during closure results in a scar that is usually indistinguishable at conversational distances. Wound separation and delayed secondary healing are rare occurrences. The open approach also increases the operative time and may prolong tip edema. The increased operating time is necessary for the suture stabilization required for any grafting and repositioning of the anatomic structures and accurate closure of the transcolumellar incision.

Major postoperative nasal deformities having a distorted nasal framework with aesthetic and functional compromise are a difficult problem. The complexity of secondary nasal deformities requires strict adherence to the basic principles as outlined, an understanding of the individual's aesthetic nasal analysis, and a systematic treatment plan. Use of the open approach for major postoperative nasal deformities has produced more consistent aesthetic and functional results in the management of these multifaceted problems.

REFERENCES

1. Rees TD, Krupp S, Wood-Smith D. Secondary rhinoplasty. *Plast Reconstr Surg.* 1970;46:332.
2. Gunter JP, Rohrich RJ. Augmentation rhinoplasty: Onlay grafting using shaped autogenous septal cartilage. *Plast Reconstr Surg.* 1990;86:39.
3. Murrell GL. Auricular cartilage grafts and nasal surgery. *Laryngoscope.* 2004;114(12):2092–2102.
4. Gunter JP, Rohrich RJ. External approach for secondary rhinoplasty. *Plast Reconstr Surg.* 1987;80:161.
5. Gunter JP, Rohrich RJ. Augmentation rhinoplasty: Dorsal onlay grafting using shaped autogenous septal cartilage. *Plast Reconstr Surg.* 1990;86:39.
6. Clark JM, Cook TA. Immediate reconstruction of extruded alloplastic nasal implants with irradiated homograft costal cartilage. *Laryngoscope.* 2002;112(6):968–974.

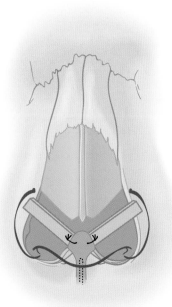

Figure 7-15 When both the medial and lateral crura have been resected or are unusable, the nasal tip tripod is reconstructed with lateral crural strut grafts that are sutured directly to a "shaped" columellar strut.

7. Sheen JH. Spreader graft: A method of reconstructing the roof of the middle nasal vault following rhinoplasty. *Plast Reconstr Surg.* 1984;73(2): 230–239.

8. Gunter JP, Clark CP, Friedman RM. Internal stabilization of autogenous rib cartilage grafts in rhinoplasty: A barrier to cartilage warping. *Plast Reconstr Surg.* 1997;100:162.

9. Gibson T, Davis WB. The distortion of autogenous cartilage grafts: its causes and prevention. *Br J Plast Surg.* 1958;10: 257.

10. Kim DW, Shah AR, Toriumi DM. Concentric and eccentric carved costal cartilage: A comparison of warping. *Arch Fac Plast Surg.* 2006;8(1):42–46.

11. Anderson JR. A reasoned approach to nasal base surgery. *Arch Otolaryngol.* 1984;110:349–358.

12. Gunter JP, Friedman RM. Lateral crural strut graft: Technique and clinical applications in rhinoplasty. *Plast Reconstr Surg.* 1997;99:943–952.

13. Gunter JP, Clark CP, Friedman RM. Internal stabilization of autogenous rib cartilage grafts in rhinoplasty: A barrier to cartilage warping. *Plast Reconstr Surg.* 1997;100(1): 161–169.

Endonasal Rhinoplasty: Transcartilaginous Approach

Raj Kanodia • Anil R. Shah

Rhinoplasty is one of the most challenging operations in plastic surgery. The three-dimensional nature of the nose, conformed by skin and soft tissue envelope (S-STE), and the shape and orientation of the nasal cartilages and bones are variables that, when grouped together, confer a nearly limitless number of different configurations seen in nasal appearance. Additionally, each of the constituent parts of the nose are intricately related to one another so that even small change in one component can lead to substantial changes elsewhere, thereby creating a large impact upon the nose. Another obstacle in rhinoplasty is the technical demands that the operation imposes. Nowhere else in plastic surgery is the margin upon which success hinges so slim, that a millimeter can spell the difference between a successful result or disappointment. Finally, manipulation of the form of the nose requires an artistic vision and sense of proportion and dimension. While there may be an aesthetic ideal for other operations, the ideal nose for one face may be completely different for another face, necessitating a keen aesthetic judgment by the surgeon.

Wide variations in technique, philosophies, and surgical results can be seen among rhinoplasty surgeons. Some surgeons use an "ideal nose strategy" for rhinoplasty. These surgeons have a vision of a perfect nose and focus their rhinoplasty efforts toward the creation of this idealized goal for every face. Unfortunately, the "ideal nose strategy" carries some inherent flaws. This strategy assumes that all parts of the nose that do not meet the criteria of this ideal nose need to be changed. The authors contend there is a wide range of features that may be deemed as attractive and must be considered in the context of the remainder of the facial features and nose. Surgeons who ascribe to the ideal nose strategy will often use more extensive radical procedures with extensive grafting in an effort to impart more dramatic changes to the nose. While the surgeon may be able to achieve their goal in changing one aspect of the nose, it often comes at the expense of unintended changes in the remainder of the nose. Another downside with the ideal nose mindset is that it will lead the surgeon to creating an imbalance between the nose and the corresponding facial features. A successful rhinoplasty operation is a marriage between the face and nose so that not only is the appearance of the nose improved but the remainder of the facial features are also enhanced.

PHILOSOPHY

Rather than purporting that all noses should appear similar (the ideal nose strategy), the senior author (R.K.) ascribes an approach that attempts to maximize the beauty within each nose. The senior author has developed a philosophy emphasizing a collection of subtle changes to the nose as a means to maximize both its function and natural appearance. A central tenet to this philosophy is to respect the complexities of the nasal anatomy. Each constituent part of the nose is interrelated, whereby seemingly small changes in one part of the nose may create untoward subsequent changes in other parts of the nose. The time factor can add another dimension of complexity where additional changes may manifest within the nose when long-term follow-up is undertaken.

This philosophy is based on 28 years of experience and more than 5000 rhinoplasty patients. The aesthetic goals of the operation are to create subtle, artistic refinements that will continue to improve during the healing continuum. While some surgeons may try to forcibly manipulate each nose to look like an "ideal nose," the authors contend that soft, subtle changes to the existing nose will lead to a more natural looking nose and harmoniously achieve facial balance. Many of these small changes will continue to improve with time, resulting in further refinement of the nose.

The senior author's approach to nasal tip definition is classified under the broad category of *transcartilaginous techniques*, where the lower lateral cartilages are shaped through direct excision and removal of excessive lower lateral cartilage bulk.[1] Traditionally, these techniques have been separated into two categories: retrograde excision of cartilage and direct excision. The transcartilaginous approach offers several distinct advantages. First, this technique is the least disruptive technique available. The only major tip supportive mechanism affected is the relationship between the lower lateral cartilages and the upper lateral cartilages.[2] However, the underlying anatomy of the nose, including the vestibular mucosa, is left for the most part undisrupted, which translates visually into results that maintain the natural features of the nose. While other techniques may leave behind a footprint of a rhinoplasty such as a columellar scar, asymmetry of the alar rim, or loss of the highlights of the soft tissue facets, the transcartilaginous approach we describe provides visual improvements while minimizing the usual surgical stigmata. When properly executed, the integrity of the lower lateral cartilage is preserved, providing a natural shape to the lower lateral cartilage. Over time, further nasal tip refinement is seen as the skin continues to mold.

ADVANTAGES/DISADVANTAGES

When a rhinoplasty surgeon decides to perform a particular surgical maneuver, consideration must be given to the serious, aesthetic consequences for the patient. For example, suture techniques can in some instances exacerbate internal recurvature of the lower lateral cartilages, creating potential airway obstruction. Over time, some suture techniques can result in bossae and knuckling or, if improperly executed, can also lead to nostril asymmetry, alar notching, loss of the soft tissue triangle facets, unnatural nasal contours, and alar depressions. Additionally, suture techniques can result in a pinched nasal tip, an obvious surgical stigma.

The transcartilaginous technique has the significant advantage of minimizing soft tissue edema. While the open technique and suture methods will require dissection over the nasal domes, the soft tissue of the nasal tip is left relatively undisturbed while using the transcartilaginous operation. The larger extent of supratip swelling associated with other techniques can lead to an undesired outcome. Many surgeons have attempted to compensate for this additional swelling by overprojecting the nose, making the entire nose larger. Most patients seeking primary rhinoplasty do not want their nose larger but instead are seeking a less extreme version of their existing nose.

One purported disadvantage of the transcartilaginous technique is the steep learning curve associated with it. This technique requires the ability to interpret the underlying lower lateral cartilage anatomy without direct visualization. A combination of visualization, palpation, and judgment are necessary tools to perform this technique. In addition, the surgeon must be able to determine if the amount of cartilage excised was symmetrical and exact in nature. Another obstacle in learning the transcartilaginous approach is the ability to make small changes to control nasal tip projection and rotation. Every surgical technique carries an associated learning curve; the authors believe the transcartilagionous technique significantly

limits potential complications compared to other more aggressive techniques.

PREOPERATIVE EVALUATION

All patients are evaluated in person by the physician. While the Internet and email are continuing to revolutionize the practice of medicine, electronic photographs cannot replace a thorough intranasal exam and palpation of the lower lateral cartilages and nasal tip support. Anterior rhinoscopy allows for evaluation of the nasal septum and any deflections which may need to be addressed during the operation. Palpation of the anterior portion of the septum can help determine the contribution of the septum to projection and rotation. During the initial consultation, an understanding between the surgeon and patient is necessary to ensure the patient and surgeon have a shared goal of what can be achieved.

OPERATIVE TECHNIQUE

PREOPERATIVE PREPARATION

Preoperative preparation of the patient plays a significant role in creating the setting of a successful operation. First, preoperative icing is performed on all patients. Ice acts as a natural and powerful vasoconstrictor of the nose, which significantly reduces edema, swelling, and bruising. Low doses of preoperative diazepam and meperidine can help patients relax and thereby release less stress hormones, which can lengthen the recovery process.

INJECTION TECHNIQUE

Cotton pledgets soaked with 2% tetracaine (Pontocaine) are placed against the intranasal mucosa to locally anesthetize the field. Patients are initially injected with a solution of 0.5% ropivacaine and 1% lidocaine with epinephrine 1:200,000 in a 1:1 mixture along the soft tissues of the nose and septal mucosa. The authors prefer to mix the epinephrine due to a perceived longer lasting effect intraoperatively and quicker onset of action than that seen when using premixed lidocaine and epinephrine. Care must be taken to ensure avoiding dosing mistakes when mixing these directly. Another common mistake to be avoided is using too much volume with local anesthesia, thereby obscuring the nasal form of the nose.

ADDRESSING THE SEPTUM

Initially, a modified hemitransfixion incision is made 5 mm posterior to the membranous septum. The posterior location of the incision conceals visibility of the scar from the lateral view. In addition, the farther posterior location is less likely to disrupt nasal tip support as opposed to a hemitransfixion or full transfixion incision. The septal mucoperichondrium is then retracted with a brown forcep and initially elevated with a Woodson elevator. If cartilage grafting is needed, septal cartilage can be harvested along the nasal floor just above the maxillary crest with a septal knife. Not uncommonly, septal deviations can cause airway obstruction and once removed will improve nasal airflow; these include deflections of the perpendicular plate and septal spurs along the nasal floor.

If manipulation of the anterior septum is required, a retrograde septal mucosal approach can be used with a spreading motion of the gooseneck dissecting scissors. If exposure of the nasal spine or depressor septi muscle is needed, a Parkes retractor can be utilized. Changes in projection and rotation of the nose can be performed by changing the length and shape of the caudal septum. Deprojection of the nose and rotation can be performed by precise resection of a portion of the anterior septal angle. Shaving the caudal septal region will in part lead to slight shortening of the nose, and can help rotate the tip if wedge-shaped portion is excised. Counterrotation can be performed by careful excision of the posterior septal angle.

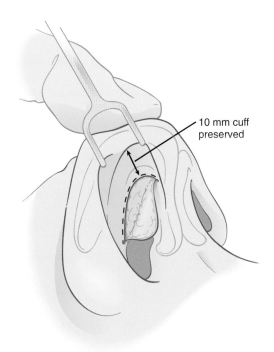

Figure 8-1 The vestibular mucosa is exposed and the excess cartilage is precisely sculpted to reshape the lower lateral cartilage.

ADDRESSING THE NASAL TIP

The lower lateral cartilages are addressed by a transcartilaginous approach. The surgeon must be able to accurately predict how much cartilage must be excised and how much is left in vivo to achieve the desirable aesthetic outcome and prevent untoward sequelae. A two-pronged retractor is used to retract the nostril, and the forefinger is used to present the lower lateral cartilage into view. An incision is first made through the vestibular mucosa only along the midportion of the lower lateral cartilage, 6 to 9 mm superior from the alar rim.

The vestibular mucosa is bluntly elevated superiorly during the excision, allowing for exposure of the lower lateral cartilage. An incision is then made with a No. 15 blade scalpel on the lower lateral cartilage, outlining the caudal extent to be resected. Gooseneck scissors are used to dissect the soft tissues from the lower lateral cartilage in a supraperichondrial plane to the cephalic edge of the lateral crus. The superior portion of the lower lateral cartilage, including a portion of the lateral, intermediate, and medial lower lateral cartilage, is excised. Once the cartilage has been excised, the lower lateral cartilages are inspected externally and visual changes of the shape of the nasal tip are inspected, preserving an intact strip of lower lateral cartilage (Figures 8-1 and 8-2). The lateral portion of the lower lateral cartilage is preserved, preventing potential alar collapse and unsightly alar pinching. Vestibular skin in this area is treated with the utmost care and is preserved.

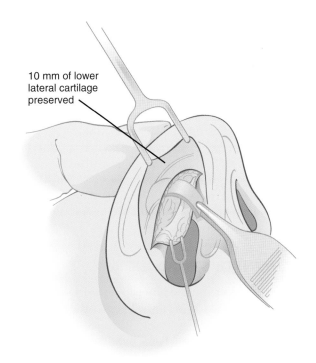

Figure 8-2 The cartilage is removed from the nose, preserving an intact strip of lower lateral cartilage.

Through the transcartilaginous incision, the scroll area can be visualized. Precise excision of the cephalic scroll allows for further definition of the nasal tip. In addition, doing so can allow for additional space for nasal tip rotation.

ADJUSTING THE NASAL DORSUM

Through the same transcartilaginous incision, the dorsum is skeletonized supraperichondrially and subperiosteally. The nasal dorsum is visualized with the aid of a Parkes nasal retractor. The dorsal septal cartilage is excised in a precise, deliberate manner using a No. 15 blade knife in a cephalic-to-caudal manner. Dorsal convexities can be addressed with a gouge. The overlying surface of the nasal bones is more dense cancellous bones, making it more resistant to nasal rasping. Precise removal of nasal humps with a gouge can be performed to "uncap" the nasal bones and allow for medial movement of the nasal bones. Different gouges can be used depending on the length and height of bone to be uncapped and opened.

An advantage that the endonasal technique offers over an external rhinoplasty approach is the dorsal profile adjustments. In external rhinoplasty, the soft tissues of the nose may have additional swelling, making minute changes of the dorsum difficult. When using endonasal techniques, it is crucial to expose the anterior septal angle to ensure that the supratip break can be visualized and manipulated.

CLOSING THE OPEN ROOF DEFORMITY

The osteotomy site is injected with local anesthesia 5 minutes prior to the procedure, allowing for additional vasoconstriction. A sharp soft tissue modified Parkes gouge is used to allow a passage lateral to the nasal bone for the osteotome and elevate the nasal periosteum. Osteotomies are performed with a guarded osteotome in a low manner. Osteotomies take place along the widest portion of the nasal bone to prevent a palpable and/or visual stepoff and create a natural contour to the nose. Incomplete osteotomies can be completed with a Quisling osteotome. After the osteotomies have been performed, the nose is evaluated. Ice is placed intraoperatively to allow for natural vasoconstriction intraoperatively.

PLACEMENT OF SPREADER GRAFTS

Spreader grafts are placed into precise mucosal pockets if there is anticipated potential weakness of the middle third of the nose. The grafts are best fashioned from the septal cartilage along the nasal floor, just along the maxillary crest. This portion of the septal cartilage is the strongest. Spreader grafts are placed by inserting the grafts in a precise pocket 2 mm from the dorsal aspect of the septum. Preservation of the dorsal mucosal cuff prevents the grafts from pushing out dorsally. The grafts are secured with a 3-0 chromic suture. If there is a mild septal deviation, asymmetric spreader grafts can be placed.[3] Typically, a larger spreader graft is placed on the side of the dorsal septal deflection, to reposition the nasoseptal pyramid over to the nondeviated side.

CARTILAGE SCORING

At the conclusion of the case, some patients may have excessive cartilaginous memory to the lower lateral cartilages. Vertical scoring incisions can be made using a No. 15 blade, weakening the lower lateral cartilage on the vestibular side while still preserving its overall natural contour. Vertical scoring is preferred because it reduces the spring of the lower lateral cartilages, allowing for convex cartilage shapes to become flatter over time. An important technical point with vertical cartilage scoring is symmetry in location and depth of the scoring maneuvers to allow for gradual symmetric reduction in the bulbosity of the nasal tip.

The mucosal incisions must be meticulously closed to prevent synechiae and potential alar retraction or notching. Preservation of the vestibular mucosa allows for a natural and physiologic nose. A thin sheet of compressed Gelfoam is placed along the dorsum to allow for even skin healing.

POSTOPERATIVELY

A small sheet of paper is placed against the dorsal surface of the nose in an effort to protect it from contact from the glue of the adhesive tape. Topical glues are avoided to prevent skin sloughing, swelling, and minimize breakouts to the nasal skin. Aquaplast is contoured to support the nasal bones and maintain their position for 1 week postoperative. Ice is applied for 48 hours.

DISCUSSION

A variety of techniques can be classified under the broad term of *cartilage splitting endonasal rhinoplasty* with pros and cons associated with each technique. The classic transcartilaginous approach creates a bipedicled flap based on an incision along the rim and a narrow blood supply. In the direct transcartilaginous approach, one incision is made along the vestibular skin and cartilage. Some authors have reported using percutaneous punctures to improve the accurate reshaping of the intermediate crus.[4] The authors report that visualization and palpation contribute to the ability to accurately assess the intermediate lateral crus region.

As many trends in rhinoplasty seem to come and go, the truest tests of any technique are time, predictability, and results. Open structure rhinoplasty and other techniques play a significant role and will continue to do so in rhinoplasty. Unfortunately, in our opinion some surgeons are "overtreating" patients who present for primary rhinoplasty surgery. It is important for novice surgeons to realize that a longer or more invasive procedure does not always necessarily translate into improved results and can in some instances expose patients to complications.

CONCLUSION

The transcartilaginous approach is a versatile primary rhinoplasty technique. It has the advantage of preserving the lower lateral cartilage shape and form, the natural features of the nose, maintaining the nasal anatomic integrity (Figures 8-3 through 8-15).

Endonasal rhinoplasty is a technique quickly becoming a lost art. A recent survey found that 50% of surgeons are now using the open approach more than 50% of the time.[5,6] While every rhinoplasty technique may have merit in specific situations, many surgeons are now aggressively treating primary rhinoplasty patients as revision cases. We make the case for condition-related approaches, avoiding resorting to the external approach for every nose.

As the field of facial plastic surgery advances, new techniques and trends are often welcomed with unbridled enthusiasm despite limited follow-up and experience. The field of rhinoplasty is no different. Many new purported advances have been mentioned, including alloplastic implants, autologous, and other grafts such as acellular human and porcine dermis, etc. However, the true measure of a technique is consistently achievable and long-lasting natural-appearing results.

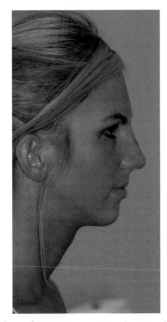

Figures 8-3 through 8-8 Preoperative photographs demonstrate an ideal candidate for finesse rhinoplasty. Her nose demonstrates overly strong features which overpower the rest of her face.

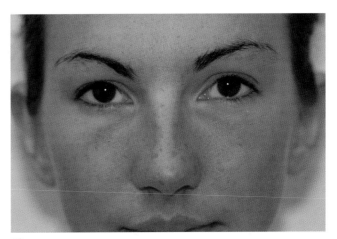

Figure 8-5

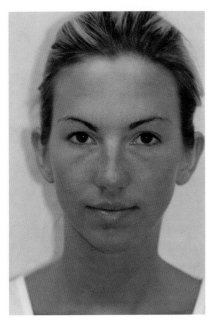

Figure 8-4

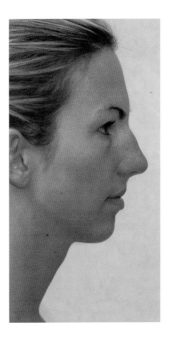

Figure 8-6

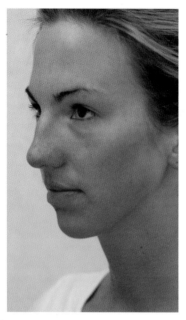

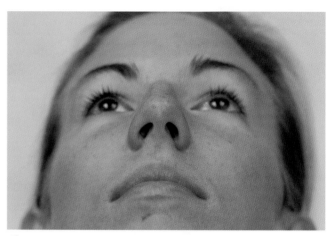

Figures 8-9 through 8-15 Postoperative result (surgery performed by Dr. Anil R. Shah) demonstrates improvement in overall shape of nose while still maintaining a natural appearance. The patient's nose retains a slight high point along the bridge so that her nose will have few, if any, stigmata of a rhinoplasty.

Figure 8-7

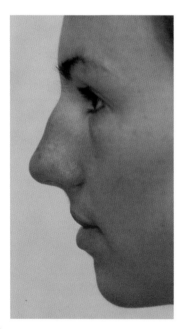

Figure 8-8

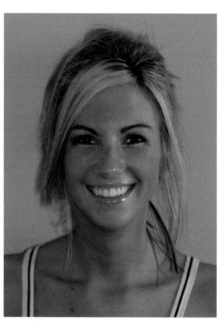

Figure 8-10

While each rhinoplasty surgeon may have a philosophy and artistic aesthetic sense, the senior author has chosen to focus on emphasizing the existing natural beauty of each nose, rather than trying to completely change its character. One of the central tenets to this approach in rhinoplasty is to preserve and enhance the existing nose. The character of the nose, the natural features of the nose, and the underlying structural integrity are all vital features that must be left undisturbed. The senior author makes changes in rotation, projection, and definition by a combination of several techniques that protect

the integrity of the lower lateral cartilages. Primary rhinoplasties only need refinement and finesse, not a changed rebuilt nose.

Many surgeons try to impose their vision of what is beautiful and in effect take away natural features of the face. Alar grafts, batten grafts, and radix grafts may have a place in secondary rhinoplasty, but in primary noses, they bulk up the nose. Furthermore, most grafts add a certain rigidity to the nose, taking away its natural feel and look. Although surgeons may be able to achieve the desired amount of change, they do so at the expense of

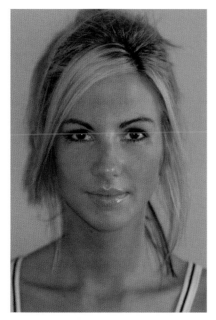

Figure 8-11

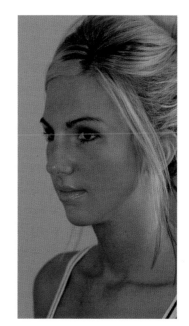

Figure 8-13

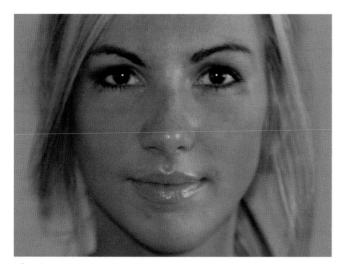

Figure 8-12

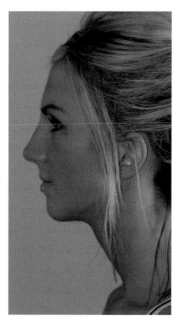

Figure 8-14

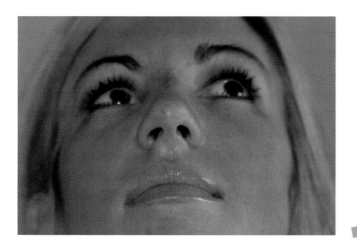

Figure 8-15

the appearance of the rest of the nose. Collective small changes can add up to a greater good, preserving natural beauty.

REFERENCES

1. Parkes MH, Kanodia R, Kern EB. The universal tip: a systematic approach to aesthetic problems of the lower lateral cartilages. *Plast Reconstr Surg.* 1988;81(6):878–890.
2. Ingels K, Orhan KS. Measurement of preoperative and postoperative nasal tip projection and rotation. *Arch Facial Plast Surg.* 2006;8(6):411–415.
3. Oliveria PW, Pezato R, Gregorio LC. Deviated nose correction by using the spreader graft in the convex side. *Rev Bras Otorrinolaringol.* (Engl Ed) 2006;72(6):760–763.
4. Neto JC, Coffler HJ. A new and simple marker for the transcartilaginous incision: The Cabas-Coffler marker. *Plast Reconstr Surg.* 2008;121(3):126e–127e.
5. Constantian MB. Differing characteristics in 100 consecutive secondary rhinoplasty patients following closed versus open surgical approaches. *Plast Reconstr Surg.* 2002;109(6): 2097–2111.
6. Adamson PAA, Galli SK. Rhinoplasty approaches: current state of the art. *Arch Facial Plast Surg.* 2005;7: 32–37.

CHAPTER NINE

Reducing Complications in Rhinoplasty

Daniel G. Becker • *Madeleine A. Becker* • *Jason A. Bloom* • *David Gudis* • *Jacob Steiger*

The nationally reported revision rate for primary rhinoplasty ranges from 8% to 15%.[1-9] Unfortunately, there will likely never be a shortage of patients requiring revision rhinoplasty. Experienced surgeons consistently achieve a high level of satisfaction among their patients. Still, complications can occur despite technically well-performed surgery. All surgeons have complications.

Success in rhinoplasty is based on well-developed judgment, wisdom, and accumulated knowledge and experience. Similar to most surgeries, rhinoplasty is a science and an art. Skill comes from experience and wisdom, combined with a measure of talent, and the surgeon must have a detailed understanding of the multiple anatomic variants encountered. The surgeon also must have accumulated the appropriate surgical techniques and experience. Specifically, the surgeon must acquire knowledge of the surgical alternatives, and how healing forces will affect the final surgical outcome. This skill set is only acquired by careful follow-up of patients operated over time.

There is no "standard" rhinoplasty. Each operation is unique in that it must be tailored to the specific anatomic components involved and the desires of the patient. By developing a consistent, meticulous routine in which the patient's nose is analyzed with regard to its anatomic components and their complex interrelationships, the surgeon can best select the appropriate incisions, approaches, and techniques for the patient's nose. These concepts are discussed in the first part of this chapter.

Having the opportunity in practice to examine numerous revision rhinoplasty patients from across the United States and around the world, the senior author has observed a wide range of problems. By carefully studying the problems encountered in a revision practice, the rhinoplasty student can improve their ability to address problems encountered during both primary and revision rhinoplasty. With this in mind, for the second part of this chapter the senior author selected problems encountered in the course of his revision practice which warrant highlighting. The selected problem patterns are either encountered frequently or illustrate specific surgical techniques that may be particularly useful in the rhinoplasty surgeon's armamentarium.

ANATOMY, NASAL ANALYSIS, AND NASAL EXAMINATION

Although the anatomy of the nose has been fundamentally understood for many years, only relatively recently has there been an increased understanding of the long-term effects of surgical changes upon the function and appearance of the nose. A detailed understanding of nasal anatomy is critical for successful rhinoplasty.[10] Accurate assessment of the anatomic variations presented by a patient allows the surgeon to develop a rational and realistic surgical plan. Furthermore, recognizing variant or aberrant anatomy is critical to preventing functional compromise or untoward aesthetic results.

The development of nasal and facial analysis skills is an important part of the effort to reduce the risk of complications. Nasal and facial analysis requires an understanding of the concept of the "aesthetic ideal." A nose that is considered "ideal" is one that is harmonious with a patient's other favorable facial features. This of course will vary to a certain degree depending upon a patient's gender and ethnicity. Indeed, our perception of beauty helps define what makes an ideal shape for a female or male nose, so there is also always a slight artistic element to this concept. While the "aesthetic ideal" cannot be completely boiled down to simple lines and numbers alone, guidelines or proportions do exist that represent an aesthetic ideal.[1,10] Examples include the nasolabial angle, the nasofrontal angle, the nasomental angle, and others. Artists have long made studies of beauty and aesthetic proportions and, today, facial plastic surgeons must similarly understand beauty in order to make changes that can enhance their patients' facial harmony and beauty. A detailed study of nasal and facial anatomy, and the ideal aesthetic proportions, is recommended.[1,10]

AESTHETIC NASAL EXAMINATION

Detailed anatomic analysis of the nose is an essential first step in achieving a successful surgical outcome. The study of nasal anatomy in the unoperated and in the operated nose is a lifetime learning endeavor. The surgeon constantly seeks to add to his or her knowledge of the anatomic variants, and the problems that can occur. The senior author's approach to nasal analysis in a primary and secondary rhinoplasty is described (Tables 9-1 and 9-2).[9,10] The preoperative analysis in revision rhinoplasty carries the additional layer of complexity of a prior surgical intervention, with subsequent distortion of the preexisting anatomy.

Studying all standard preoperative photographic views for rhinoplasty (frontal, base, lateral, oblique) allow a systematic, detailed anatomic analysis that complements the physical examination process.

Analysis begins by examining all four views and making an assessment of the overall stature of the patient, the facial skin quality, and the symmetry of the face. The principle of dividing the face into horizontal thirds and vertical fifths is a useful tool to obtain a general sense of any areas of the face that may play a key role in nasal appearance and the outcome of nasal surgery. It is essential that these incongruent areas or asymmetries be recognized and discussed with the patient preoperatively. Thickness and quality of the facial skin–subcutaneous tissue complex must be determined, as it plays a critical role in dictating the limitations of what can and cannot be accomplished with aesthetic nasal surgery.

After completing the general assessment, the surgeon should note and highlight the most striking characteristics of the nose. These are typically the characteristics that bring the patient for rhinoplasty, such as excessive size, deviation, or a dorsal hump. These primary patient concerns must be recognized, highlighted, and addressed above all else.

As the surgeon reviews each photographic image, the major aesthetic and technical points that can be evaluated on a given view are noted first. Subtleties in analysis are then addressed. It is important to recognize both the characteristics of greatest concern to the patient and the more subtle findings. The patient may not notice these other subtle abnormalities if they are left unaddressed by the surgeon. Postoperatively, the scrutinizing patient may notice and point out these abnormalities. Stepwise, methodical analysis of the patient and all photographic views allows the well-trained surgeon to identify key anatomic and aesthetic points to be addressed.[10]

As the preoperative analysis proceeds in revision rhinoplasty, a critical question that guides examination of each area is, "Was it underresected, overresected, asymmetrically resected, or appropriately treated?" Any unoperated areas of the nose are identified. Also, the presence of possible grafts or implants is considered throughout the examination. For a detailed discussion of analysis, further reading and study are recommended.[9]

FUNCTIONAL NASAL EXAMINATION

Anterior rhinoscopy should be undertaken in the rhinoplasty patient and may identify abnormalities such as deviated septum, inferior turbinate hypertrophy, synechiae or scar bands, septal perforation, and other abnormalities. Examination also includes nasal endoscopy when there are functional nasal complaints, such as nasal obstruction (Figure 9-1).[11,12] If indicated, a sinus computed tomography scan may also be obtained.

Pownell et al.[11] described diagnostic nasal endoscopy in the plastic surgical literature. They trace the historical development of nasal endoscopy, explain its rationale, review anatomic and diagnostic issues including the differential diagnosis of nasal obstruction, and describe the

Table 9-1 Analysis in Primary Rhinoplasty—Guide to Nasal Analysis

General
Skin quality: Thin, medium, or thick Primary descriptor (i.e., why is the patient here?): for example, "big," "twisted," "large hump"
Frontal View
Twisted or straight: Follow brow—tip aesthetic lines Width: Narrow, wide, normal, "wide—narrow—wide" Tip: Deviated, bulbous, asymmetric, amorphous, other
Base View
Triangularity: Good versus trapezoidal Tip: Deviated, wide, bulbous, bifid, asymmetric Base: Wide, narrow, or normal. Inspect for caudal septal deflection Columella: Columellar/lobule ratio (normal is 2:1 ratio); status of medial crural footplates
Lateral View
Nasofrontal angle: Shallow or deep Nasal starting point: High or low Dorsum: Straight, concavity, or convexity; bony, bony—cartilaginous, or cartilaginous (i.e., is convexity primarily bony, cartilaginous, or both) Nasal length: Normal, short, long Tip projection: Normal, decreased, or increased Alar—columellar relationship: Normal or abnormal Nasolabial angle: Obtuse or acute
Oblique View
Does it add anything, or does it confirm the other views?

Many other points of analysis can be made on each view, but these are some of the vital points of commentary.

Table 9-2 Nasal Analysis in Revision Rhinoplasty—Simplified Algorithm Visual and Manual Examination

General

Skin quality: Integrity, vascularity, mobility, skin thickness (thin, medium, or thick)
Identify primary concerns leading patient to seek revision
For each issue and anatomic area, is problem due to underresection, overresection, asymmetric resection?

Frontal

Width: Narrow, wide, normal, "wide–narrow–wide"
Dorsum: Twisted or straight: follow brow-tip aesthetic lines.
Open roof? Rocker deformity? Visible or palpable deformities? Prior osteotomies? If so, normal or abnormal?
Middle vault: Assess width. Inverted V? Underresected, overresected, asymmetric?
Tip: deviated, bulbous, asymmetric, amorphous. Symmetry, bossae? Tip support (palpate). Status of all prior incisions.
    Assess for presence of grafts. Alar side wall pinching or retraction?

Base

Tip: Deviated, wide, bulbous, bifid, asymmetric.
Symmetry, bossae? Status of caudal septum. Projection. Tip support (palpate). Status of all prior incisions. Assess for
    presence of grafts.
Triangularity: Good versus trapezoidal.
Base: Wide, narrow, or normal
Inspect for caudal septal deflection.
Assess status of all external incisions.
Columella: Columellar–lobule ratio (normal is 2 : 1 ratio)
            Status of medial crural footplates

Lateral

Nasofrontal angle: Shallow or deep
Nasal starting point: High or low
Dorsum: Straight, concavity, or convexity: bony, bony-cartilaginous, or cartilaginous (i.e., is convexity primarily bony,
    cartilaginous, or both?). Visible or palpable irregularities? Overresected, underresected, or both? Pollybeak? Saddle
    nose?
Nasal length: Normal, short, long
Tip: Projection (normal, increased, decreased), rotation (nasolabial angle), double break, alar-columellar relationship,
    bossae? Status of caudal septum. Tip support. Status of all prior incisions. Assess for presence of grafts.

Oblique

Does it add anything, or does it confirm the other views?

There are many other points of analysis that can be made on each view, but these are some of the vital points of commentary.

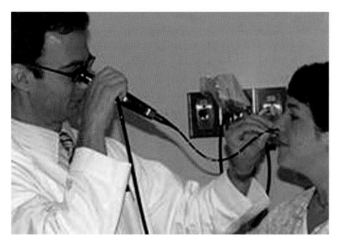

Figure 9-1 Nasal endoscopy may be performed with either a rigid or flexible telescope, and allows improved diagnosis in the evaluation of nasal obstruction.

selection of equipment and correct application of technique, emphasizing the potential for advanced diagnostic potential.

Levine[12] reported that 39% of patients with a complaint of nasal obstruction had findings on endoscopic examination that were not identified with traditional rhinoscopy. Many of Levine's patients had seen other physicians for this problem and had not received appropriate treatment.

Becker et al.[13,14] described that, in patients seeking cosmetic nasal surgery who also had nasal obstruction, nasal endoscopy allowed the diagnosis of additional pathology not seen on anterior rhinoscopy, including obstructing adenoids, enlarged middle turbinates with concha bullosa, choanal stenosis, nasal polyps, and chronic sinusitis (Figure 9-2). In their series, additional surgical therapy was undertaken in 28 of 96 rhinoplasty patients

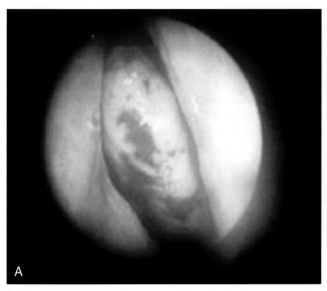 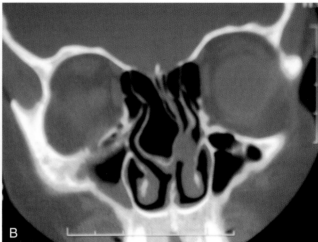

Figure 9-2 A patient seeking revision rhinoplasty had persisting nasal obstruction despite a history of prior septoplasty at the time of her rhinoplasty. Endoscopic examination was suggestive of a large concha bullosa (**A**). CT scan was confirmatory (**B**).

due to findings on endoscopic exam. Thirteen patients underwent endoscopic sinus surgery. Nine patients had a concha bullosa requiring partial middle turbinectomy. Three patients—all revision surgeries—had persisting posterior septal deviation requiring endoscopic septoplasty. Two patients underwent adenoidectomy. One patient required repair of choanal stenosis.

Static and dynamic nasal valve collapse are commonly encountered in revision rhinoplasty patients.[15–20] In Becker et al.'s report, 19 of 21 patients with nasal valve collapse reported a past history of rhinoplasty.[20]

Pinching of the nasal sidewall and alar retraction are hallmarks of nasal valve collapse. Observing the patient performing normal and deep nasal inspiration may lead directly to the diagnosis of nasal valve collapse (Figure 9-3). A "modified" Cottle maneuver, in which the lateral nasal sidewall is supported and elevated slightly with a cerumen curette or similar device, is strongly supportive of the diagnosis when the maneuver results in the patient's report of significant subjective improvement in nasal breathing.

INCISIONS AND APPROACHES

Incisions are methods of gaining access to the bony and cartilaginous structures of the nose and include transcartilaginous, intercartilaginous, marginal, and transcolumellar incisions. Approaches provide surgical exposure of the nasal structures including the nasal tip and include cartilage-splitting (transcartilaginous incision), retrograde (intercartilaginous incision with retrograde dissection), delivery approach (intercartilaginous and marginal incisions), and external (transcolumellar and marginal incisions). After analyzing the individual patient's anatomy, appropriate incisions, approaches, and tip-sculpturing techniques may be selected.[1,10,21]

The selection of the planned incisions, approaches, and surgical techniques for a particular patient is of course the central decision of the rhinoplasty process. An operative algorithm may provide a helpful starting point in selecting the incisions, approaches, and techniques used in nasal surgery.[1,10,21] In every case, the patient's anatomy dictates the selection of an appropriate technique. As the anatomic deformity becomes more abnormal, a graduated, stepwise approach is taken. However, other factors, such as the need for spreader grafts, complex nasal deviation, surgeon preference, and other factors may also appropriately affect the ultimate selection of approach.

The endonasal approaches may be generally preferred for patients requiring conservative profile reduction, conservative tip modification, selected revision rhinoplasty patients, and other situations in which conservative changes are being undertaken. Advantages of less invasive approaches include less dissection, less edema, and less "healing." However, less invasive approaches provide by their very nature less exposure, which in some cases may be a disadvantage.

Indications for external rhinoplasty approach[10,21–23] generally include asymmetric nasal tip, crooked nose deformity (lower two thirds of nose), saddle nose deformity, cleft-lip nasal deformity, secondary rhinoplasty requiring complex structural grafting, and septal perforation repair. Other indications may include complex nasal tip deformity, middle nasal vault deformity, and selected nasal tumors. Some surgeons prefer the open approach for less complex nasal tip deformities due to the precision that they believe it offers them, in their hands, compared to the endonasal approach.

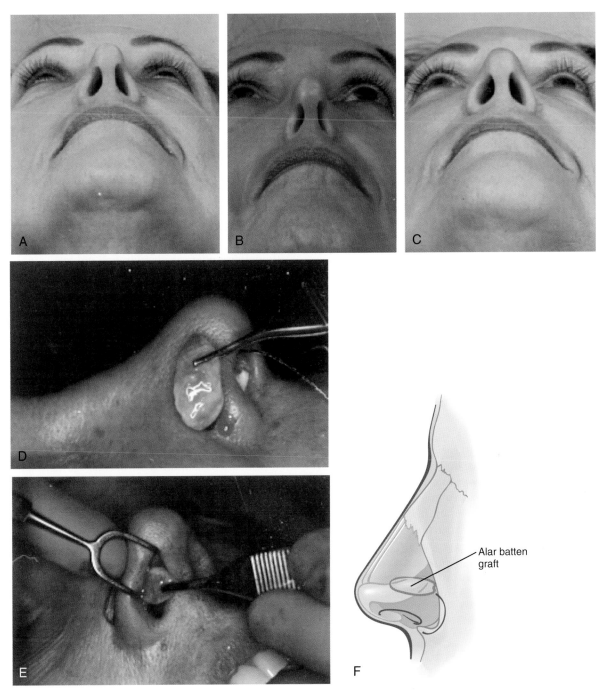

Figure 9-3 Nasal valve collapse may be apparent on normal inspiration, as seen here. Alar batten grafts may be placed via an external rhinoplasty approach, or into a precise pocket made through an endonasal incision as shown here. This graft is nonanatomic and is typically placed caudal to the lateral crura where there is maximal collapse of the lateral nasal wall and supra-alar pinching. If alar batten grafts are placed too far cephalic, excessive fullness over the middle vault will be noted. Patients should be told that there will be temporary fullness in the area of the graft. This fullness will typically decrease over 2 to 3 months. For maximal support, the alar batten graft should extend over the bone of the pyriform aperture. **A,** Preoperative; **B,** preoperative with normal inspiration; **C,** postoperative; **D, E,** intraoperative, endonasal approach; **F,** diagrammatic of alar batten graft.

Advantages of the external approach include the surgical exposure available, potentially allowing more accurate anatomic diagnosis. The external approach also provides the opportunity for precise tissue manipulation, suturing, and grafting. Disadvantages include the transcolumellar incision, wide field dissection resulting in potential loss of support, and nasal tip edema.

A central tenet of rhinoplasty decision-making has been the concept of a graduated approach.[10,21] This concept is based on the idea that achieving the desired goals with the least amount of surgical dissection provides the best chance of success. However, the critical issue is how much exposure is needed for reliable execution of any specific technical maneuver. Adamson[24] has astutely observed that there is no ideal approach—each surgeon will develop a unique approach based upon the concepts outlined and based on the techniques and experiences he or she has developed in the course of an eclectic training.

Perkins[25] describes an evolution in his personal philosophy that reflects some of the issues involved in this decision-making process and provides valuable insight into the evolution in the decision making that has occurred over the past 15 to 20 years. While the concept of a graduated approach to achieve a pleasing aesthetic result has been foremost in his personal philosophy, the evolving need to achieve more refined results and prevent late complications has resulted in his increased use of the open approach, which allows the opportunity to use certain grafting techniques. Perkins continues to strongly advocate the philosophy that the approach selected should provide the least intervention in the shortest time to achieve a satisfactory result and satisfy the patient's goals. However, his choice of approach has changed due to late complications that he has seen occur. The two areas where he finds most commonly occurring late complications in rhinoplasty are the midnasal pyramid and lateral alar sidewalls. He emphasizes the paramount importance of providing a structural foundation for the middle vault (i.e., spreader grafts). While issues such as these can be addressed using the endonasal approach, Perkins indicates that it is sometimes far easier to place structural grafts via the external approach. Also, he maintains that when marked reduction of overprojection is required, it is often easier to use the external columellar approach.

Regardless of approach, one must be mindful of the need to maintain appropriate structural support. When the approach is disruptive of tip support, countermeasures, such as the placement of a columellar strut, are warranted. When the support to the upper lateral cartilages has been disrupted, spreader grafts may be appropriate.

COMMUNICATION WITH PATIENT

It is important that the communication between patient and surgeon regarding the goal of surgery be a clear one. This is discussed in detail in other chapters in the book, as well as in other articles.[9] Clear and thorough communication between patient and surgeon is extremely helpful in reducing complications in rhinoplasty. The authors recommend that the rhinoplasty surgeon give considerable and careful thought to his or her approach during the office consultation, with the goal of optimizing communication with the patient about their proposed procedure.

With this in mind, computer imaging warrants specific discussion. Computer imaging is a "video game." It is simply a way to communicate a shared surgical goal. It does not generate an "after" picture. As the senior author

explains to patients, it is not a guarantee and should not be taken to offer even the slightest implication of a guarantee. The senior author does not provide the patient with printouts of the computer imaging.

Having said this, the senior author finds computer imaging to be extremely useful. He routinely prints out the preoperative photos and shared-surgical-goal photographs and has them for intraoperative reference point. The senior author reviews his notes and these photographs preoperatively and also throughout surgery to keep the goal of surgery foremost in his mind as surgery progresses.[9]

PSYCHOLOGY OF RHINOPLASTY

Although a separate chapter will address this specific topic, some points are worth mentioning. Patients seeking cosmetic rhinoplasty are generally healthy patients who are unhappy about the appearance of their nose. The psychology of human appearance and the psychological benefits of cosmetic surgery have been well studied. It is important for the surgeon to consider psychological factors when evaluating a patient for rhinoplasty.[26]

Although the rate of psychiatric disorders among cosmetic surgery patients is essentially unknown, it is probably safe to say that all of the major psychiatric disorders can coexist among patients who desire cosmetic surgery. Body dysmorphic disorder (BDD) is a psychiatric disorder that warrants mention here because it does appear to occur with increased frequency among rhinoplasty patients. BDD is defined by the *DSM-IV-TR* as a preoccupation with an imagined or slight defect in appearance that results in significant emotional distress or impairment in daily functioning.[27] Few studies have examined the rate of BDD among rhinoplasty patients.[26]

Psychological assessment of rhinoplasty patients is an important part of the preoperative evaluation. Efforts should be made to help determine whether patients' preoperative motivations and expectations are realistic, to identify the patients appearance concerns and whether they are proportionate to the abnormality, and to identify patients with psychiatric conditions that may contraindicate surgery. The reader is referred to an overview of this subject by Crerand et al.[26] for more detailed information on this important subject.

TECHNICAL OVERVIEW OF POTENTIAL COMPLICATIONS—SPECIFIC PROBLEMS TO AVOID

OVERRESECTION OF LATERAL CRURA

Overresection of the lateral crus is perhaps the most common problem seen in a revision rhinoplasty practice.[9,10,28–30] Overresection of the lateral crus leads to the

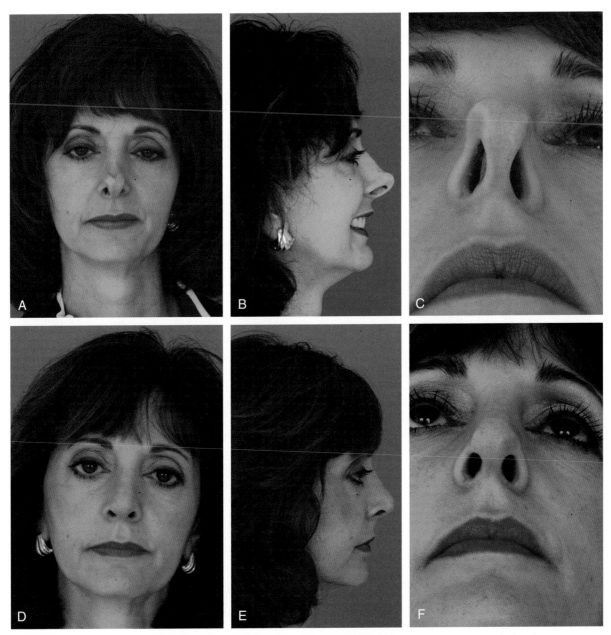

Figure 9-4 Overresection of the lateral crura in this patient resulted in the predictable, unfavorable changes described in the text. Reconstruction included bilateral alar batten grafts. The patient also required shortening of the persistently overprojected tip cartilages via vertical dome division with excision and suture reconstitution. **A–C,** preoperative; **D–F,** postoperative.

predictable changes of alar retraction, pinching, bossae, and tip asymmetry (Figure 9-4). Excision of vestibular mucosa in primary rhinoplasty also may contribute to scar contracture with alar retraction. A conservative approach to cephalic resection is warranted in rhinoplasty.

In many revision cases, the amount of lateral crus that remained seemed ample; that is, it falls within the "guideline" of 6 to 9 mm that typically is cited. In these cases, the scar contracture secondary to healing apparently overpowered the remnant cartilage. If the tip cartilages are soft and weak and if the scar contracture is profound, undesirable changes can occur.

In some cases, this situation can be anticipated. An anatomic study of the alar base recognized that in a normal patient population, 20% of patients had a thin alar rim. This anatomic variation must be recognized, and cephalic resection probably should be avoided or minimized in these patients to minimize the risk of inducing alar retraction or external nasal valve collapse.[29] These changes are not always predictable, however, and are not always avoidable.

For example, bossae are caused by a knuckling of lower lateral cartilage at the nasal tip owing to contractural healing forces acting on weakened cartilages. Patients with thin skin, strong cartilages, and nasal tip bifidity are especially at risk. Excessive resection of lateral crus and failure to eliminate excessive interdomal width may play some role in bossae formation.[9,10,29]

Understanding that the healing forces are not completely predictable, it is important to take a conservative approach when undertaking cephalic resection. Although risk cannot be eliminated, it can be reduced in this manner.

Alar batten grafts are the first-line treatment of alar retraction and nasal valve collapse[10,15,20,29] (see Figure 9-3). Batten grafts have been well described in the literature and are generally most effective in less severe cases (1- to 2-mm deficit).[10,15,20,29]

Auricular composite grafts commonly are used in more severe cases[9,30,31] (Figure 9-5). The skin and cartilage of the anterolateral surface, just inferior to the inferior crus, of the opposite ear (e.g. left ala, right ear) provide the best donor site and the best contour. When a smaller graft is needed, direct closure of the donor incision can be undertaken. When a larger graft is needed, a "revolving door" postauricular flap may be used to close the defect (Figure 9-6). For placement of the composite graft, an incision several millimeters from the nostril rim is followed by careful dissection freeing adhesions, creating a defect and displacing the alar rim inferiorly. Volume and support must be restored to hold the nostril rim in position. This role is fulfilled by the composite graft. The fashioned composite graft is sutured carefully into place.[9,30,31] Typically, the senior author uses 6-0 plain gut suture. A cotton ball or other light dressing is applied intranasally to apply light pressure for 1 to 3 days.

MINIMIZING COMPLICATIONS OF THE NASAL DORSUM

Sharp osteotomes are essential to provide a clean, precise bony hump excision. When the osteotome is dull, the chance of an asymmetric resection or overresection of the bony hump increases. Some surgeons have at least two sets of osteotomes and rotate them—one set is always out, being sharpened. Other surgeons sharpen their osteotomes manually, with a sharpening stone, during each case. Both approaches are effective.[9,10,31]

An anatomic approach is preferable. Detailed anatomic nasal analysis should guide surgery. When undertaking a hump reduction, the surgeon should examine the excised tissue, assessing its symmetry, and whether it was the desired excision (Figure 9-7). (If the bony dorsum is rasped, this of course is not possible.) Similar anatomic examination of the remaining cartilaginous and bony nasal dorsum also must be undertaken. It is expected that additional, calibrated refinement would be needed and should be undertaken with dogmatic adherence to the anatomic examination. Preoperative markings on the skin may be helpful to some surgeons for hump reduction and for osteotomies. Persistent irregularities of the bony dorsum may be addressed by rasping. The senior author finds that a powered rasp may be preferable to manual rasping in this situation (Figure 9-8).[9,32,33]

Larrabee has pointed out that while there is a tendency to treat the bony pyramid in an essentially closed fashion when using either the closed or open approach, the benefits of increased exposure to the dorsum available

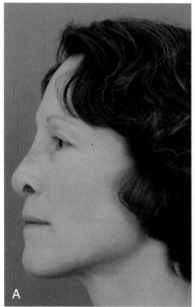
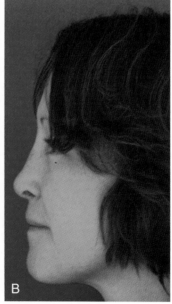

Figure 9-5 Composite grafts are useful in the treatment of severe alar retraction.

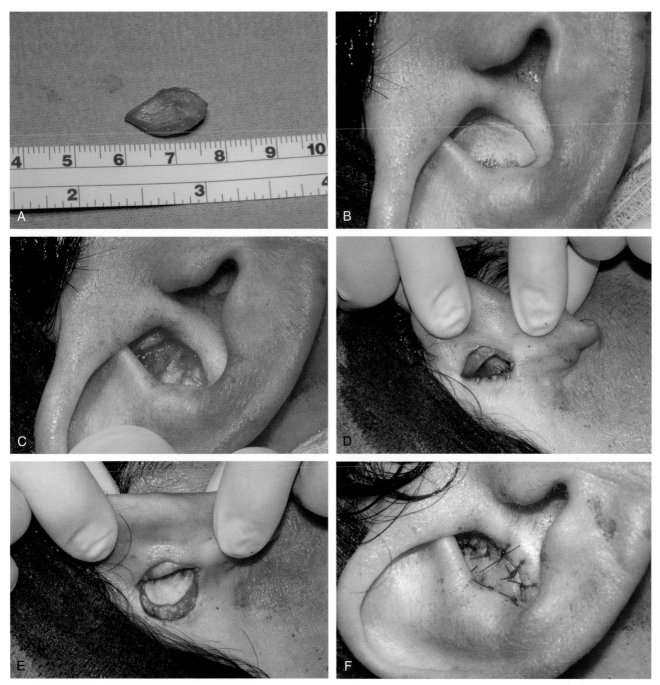

Figure 9-6 When composite graft harvest leaves a defect that is challenging to close primarily, a "revolving door" flap is a useful reconstructive option.

with the open rhinoplasty approach should be exploited whenever possible (Figure 9-9).[34]

In the senior author's experience, a closed approach has been reliable for addressing most bony profile problems. However, when performing an open rhinoplasty, the senior author now prefers to undertake hump reduction under direct visualization. When using an osteotome, an 8- to 10-mm nonguarded osteotome is generally used (wider osteotomes can create an injury to the skin–soft tissue envelope). While rasping during open rhinoplasty,

the senior author uses a powered rasp under direct visualization.[33,34]

THE POLLYBEAK DEFORMITY

Pollybeak refers to a specific problem of the nasal dorsum—postoperative fullness of the supratip region, with an abnormal tip–supratip relationship (Figure 9-10). This problem may have several causes, including failure to maintain adequate tip support (postoperative loss of tip

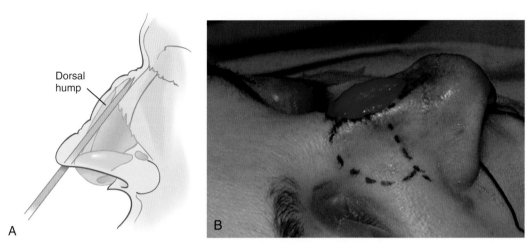

Figure 9-7 En bloc resection of the nasal hump allows careful anatomic examination as the surgeon assesses the need for additional, calibrated refinements of the nasal dorsum.

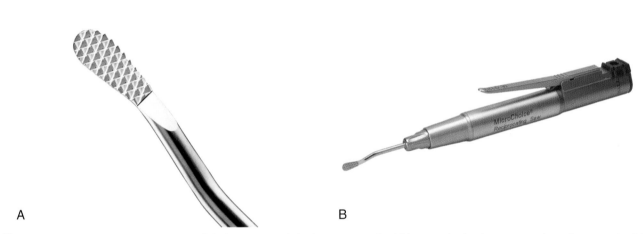

Figure 9-8 After creation of an "open roof" by hump removal, the bony margins should be smoothed with a rasp. Any bony fragments should be removed, ensuring that all obvious particles are removed from under the skin–soft tissue envelope. Failure to remove all fragments may lead to a visible or palpable dorsal irregularity. The powered rasp (Linvatec-Hall Surgical, Largo, FL) oscillates at speeds of 15,000 rpm with minimal back-and-forth excursion of only several millimeters. The senior author finds the powered rasp more precise and preferable to manual rasping.

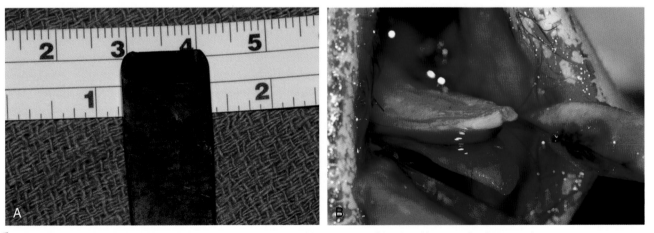

Figure 9-9 An unguarded osteotome of appropriate size allows en bloc resection of the dorsal hump under direct visualization.

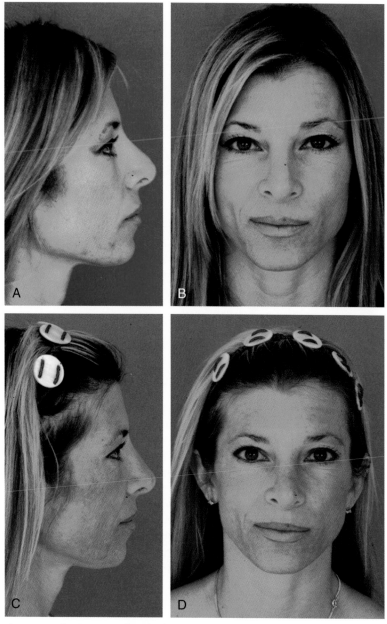

Figure 9-10 Patient with cartilaginous and soft tissue pollybeak after rhinoplasty. **A–B,** preoperative; **C–D,** postoperative.

projection), inadequate cartilaginous hump (anterior septal angle) removal, or supratip dead space or scar formation. Treatment of the pollybeak deformity depends on the anatomic cause.[9,35] The best treatment constitutes its avoidance. If the cartilaginous hump was underresected at the anterior septal angle, however, the revision surgeon should resect additional dorsal septum. Adequate tip support must be ensured; maneuvers such as placement of a columellar strut may be beneficial. If a pollybeak deformity is a result of excessive scar formation, triamcinolone (Kenalog) injection or skin taping in the early postoperative period should be undertaken before any consideration of surgical revision.

OVERRESECTION AND SADDLE NOSE

Saddle nose refers to the appearance of the nose after loss of support of the nasal vault with subsequent collapse (Figure 9-11). This deformity has been described after overresection of the septum, with failure to preserve an adequate septal "L-strut." A minimum of 15 mm of cartilage is recommended as a rule of thumb—if a dorsal hump resection is planned, this must be accounted for in planning adequate L-strut for nasal support. Other causes of saddle nose deformity include septal hematoma, septal abscess, and severe nasal trauma. Excessive dorsal hump resection also leads to saddle nose deformity.

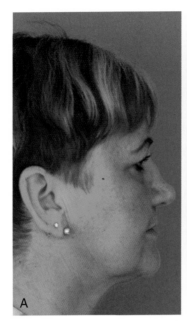
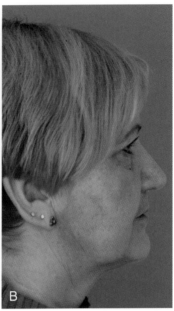

Figure 9-11 Precise pocket, triple layer cartilage onlay grafting effectively treated this patient's saddle nose deformity. **A,** preoperative; **B,** postoperative.

Onlay cartilage grafting can effectively camouflage and correct mild and moderate saddle deformities (see Figure 9-11). Single or multiple layers of septal cartilage, auricular cartilage are commonly used effectively.[36,37] Severe saddle nose deformity may require major reconstruction with cantilevered cartilage or bone grafts.[38-40]

Precise pocket grafting can be effectively used when this is an isolated problem[9] (see Figure 9-11). The pocket is dissected over the anterior septal angle, via bilateral limited marginal incisions. Bilateral incisions are used to ensure symmetry of the pocket, so that the graft will lie straight. Asymmetric dissection of the pocket can be a cause for graft shifting.

When a patient has thin skin, Alloderm or temporalis fascia may be used to provide some additional cushion. While it appears that this may provide some lasting benefit, the long-term fate of Alloderm is unknown.

ALLOPLASTS

The senior author's experience with alloplasts has been to remove them. The author has removed alloplasts for different indications including patient discomfort/pain, an unacceptable cosmetic result, infection, and because of extrusion into the nose and through the skin. There is disagreement among rhinoplasty surgeons regarding the use of alloplasts. The nose fulfills few of the requirements for use of alloplastic materials. If the alloplast extrudes through the skin, the skin–soft tissue envelope is permanently and irreparably damaged (Figure 9-12). The senior author discourages the use of alloplasts in primary and revision rhinoplasty.[9]

INVERTED-V MIDDLE VAULT COLLAPSE

In inverted-V middle vault collapse deformity, the caudal edges of the nasal bones are visible in broad relief. Inadequate support of the upper lateral cartilages after dorsal hump removal can lead to inferomedial collapse of the upper lateral cartilages and an inverted-V deformity (Figure 9-13).[41] Inadequate infracture of the nasal bones is another significant cause of inverted-V deformity. The anatomic cause of inverted-V deformity must be recognized. Osteotomies with infracture of the nasal bones, spreader grafts, or both should be performed when appropriate.

Narrowing of the middle nasal vault that occurs when the T configuration of the nasal septum is resected with dorsal hump removal may be problematic in the high risk patient.[10,41] Spreader grafts act as a spacer between the upper lateral cartilage and septum, preventing excessive narrowing in the high risk patient or correcting an over-narrow middle vault when it exists.

Use of spreader grafts in primary rhinoplasty is becoming much more common.[10,41] Spreader grafts can be effective in maintaining the contour of the middle vaults after hump reduction. While it may be technically easier to place spreader grafts via an external approach, spreader grafts can be placed via the endonasal or the external (open) approach.[10,25,39,41]

It should be noted that the use of the external rhinoplasty approach may lead to a greater need for spreader grafts to preserve the nasal valve and middle nasal width, which may be put at risk due to the loss of support to the upper lateral cartilages caused by more extensive skin undermining.

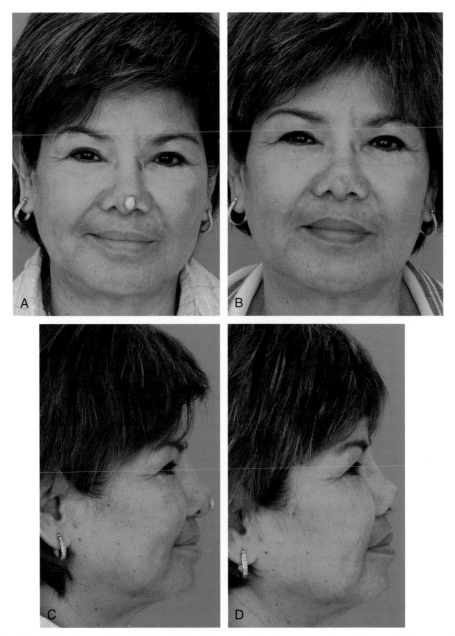

Figure 9-12 If the alloplast extrudes through the skin, the skin–soft tissue envelope is permanently and irreparably damaged. **A, C,** preoperative; **B, D,** postoperative after removal of alloplast.

TWISTED NOSE—NEWLY OR PERSISTENTLY TWISTED

The surgical treatment of a twisted nose can range from simple to complex. The numerous techniques described to address a twisted nose speaks to its complexity. A graduated, stepwise approach, guided by precise anatomic diagnosis, is recommended (Figure 9-14).[1,42]

Persisting deviation after rhinoplasty may occur at the upper third, middle third, or tip of the nose or may occur postoperatively in a previously straight nose. Preoperative anatomic diagnosis is a crucial component of successful treatment. Still, deviations may occur or persist despite accurate diagnosis and technically well-performed surgery. Persisting deviation of the nasal bones may occur because of greenstick fractures or other problems with osteotomies.[42,43] Inherent deviations in the cartilage of the middle nasal vault may prove especially challenging. Also, hump removal may uncover asymmetries that result in postoperative deviation where none existed previously. Tip asymmetry may be overlooked preoperatively, or it may due to asymmetric excision of lateral crura, asymmetric placement of a columellar strut, or placement of a overly long columellar strut, among other causes. Numerous surgical maneuvers are available to address the deviated nose.[42,43]

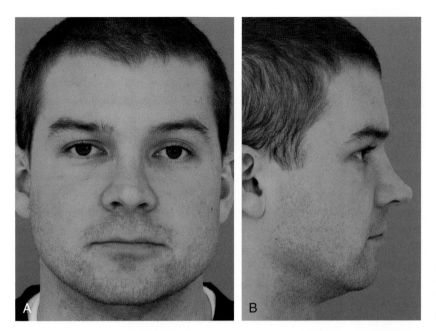

Figure 9-13 This patient had prior rhinoplasty in which it appears that the overprojection of the nasal tip and the need for support of the middle nasal vault was unrecognized. He presented for correction of his tip abnormalities and his inverted-V deformity.

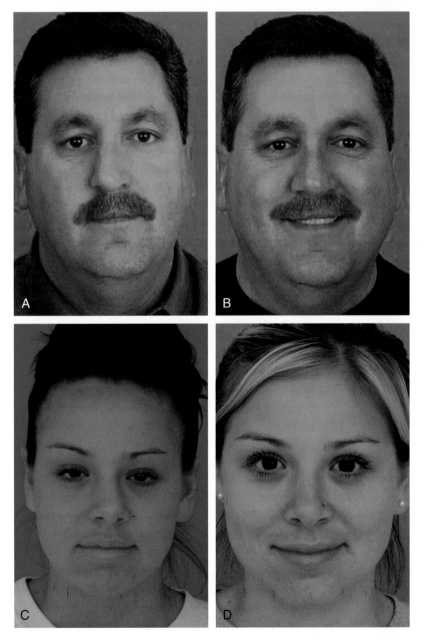

Figure 9-14 Treatment of the twisted nose requires precise anatomic diagnosis and a graduated, stepwise approach. **A, C,** preoperative; **B, D,** postoperative.

SKIN–SOFT TISSUE ENVELOPE

In the unoperated nose, the skin–soft tissue envelope has well-defined tissue planes in which avascular dissection may be undertaken. Vascular supply and lymphatics are found superficial to the nasal musculature.[44,45] Dissection in the proper tissue planes (areolar tissue plane, i.e., submusculoaponeurotic) preserves nasal blood supply and minimizes postoperative edema. Operating in the more superficial planes not only leads to a bloody surgical field but also risks damage to the vascular supply with potential damage to the skin. When the skin–soft tissue envelope is damaged, it can never be restored fully, creating an esthetically displeasing appearance.[9,44,45]

SUMMARY

The dedicated rhinoplasty surgeon continues to acquire throughout his or her career an increasingly detailed understanding of the anatomy and the problems that occur related to rhinoplasty and a growing armamentarium of techniques to achieve their improvement or correction. In addition to the study of the unoperated nose, much can be learned from the study of revision rhinoplasty that applies to both primary and revision rhinoplasty patients. This chapter outlines aspects of the authors' approach and discusses selected technical problems and approaches to minimize their occurrence. Focusing on the two essential goals—making patients happy and making their current procedure the patient's last nasal surgery—both primary and secondary rhinoplasty can be a uniquely rewarding experience for both patients and surgeons.

REFERENCES

1. Tardy ME. Rhinoplasty: The art and the science. Philadelphia: WB Saunders; 1997.
2. Kamer FM, Pieper PG. Revision rhinoplasty. In: Bailey B, ed. Head and neck surgery otolaryngology. Philadelphia: Lippincott; 1998.
3. Rees TD. Postoperative considerations and complications. In Rees TD, ed. Aesthetic plastic surgery. Philadelphia: WB Saunders; 1980.
4. McKinney P, Cook JQ. A critical evaluation of 200 rhinoplasties. Ann Plast Surg. 1981;7:357.
5. Thomas JR, Tardy ME. Complications of rhinoplasty. Ear Nose Throat J. 1986;65:19–34.
6. Tardy ME, Cheng EY, Jernstrom V. Misadventures in nasal tip surgery. Otolaryngol Clin N Am. 1987;20(4):797–823.
7. Simons RL, Gallo JF. Rhinoplasty complications. Fac Plast Surg Clin N Am. 1994;2(4):521–529.
8. Becker DG. Complications in rhinoplasty. In: Facial plastic and reconstructive surgery. 2nd ed. New York: Theime; 2009.
9. Becker DG. My personal philosophy of revision rhinoplasty. In: Becker DG, Park SS, eds. Revision rhinoplasty. New York: Thieme; 2007.
10. Toriumi DM, Becker DG. Rhinoplasty dissection manual. Philadelphia: Lippincott, Williams and Wilkins; 1999.
11. Pownell PH, Minoli JJ, Rohrich RJ. Diagnostic nasal endoscopy. Plast Reconstr Surg. 1997;99(5):1451–1458.
12. Levine HL. The office diagnosis of nasal and sinus disorders using rigid nasal endoscopy. Otolaryngol Head Neck Surg. 1990;102:370.
13. Becker DG. Septoplasty and turbinate surgery. Aesthet Surg J. 2003;23:393–403.
14. Lanfranchi PV, Steiger J, Sparano A, et al. Diagnostic and surgical endoscopy in functional septorhinoplasty. Fac Plast Surg. 2004;20:207–215.
15. Toriumi DM, Josen J, Weinberger MS, Tardy ME. Use of alar batten grafts for correction of nasal valve collapse. Arch Otol Head Neck Surg. 1997;123:802–808.
16. Constantian MB, Clardy RB. The relative importance of septal and nasal valvular surgery in correcting airway obstruction in primary and secondary rhinoplasty. Plast Reconstr Surg. 1996;98(1):38–54.
17. Goode RL. Surgery of the incompetent nasal valve. Laryngoscope. 1985;95:546–555.
18. Sheen JH. Spreader graft: A method of reconstructing the roof of the middle nasal vault following rhinoplasty. Plast Reconstr Surg. 1984;73(2):230–237.
19. Constantian MB. The incompetent external nasal valve: Pathophysiology and treatment in primary and secondary rhinoplasty. Plast Reconstr Surg. 1994;93(5):919–933.
20. Becker DG, et al. Alar batten grafts for treatment of nasal valve collapse. J Long-Term Effects Surgical Implants. 2003.
21. Tardy ME, Toriumi DM. Philosophy and principles of rhinoplasty. In: Cummings C, et al, eds. Otolaryngology—Head and neck surgery. 2nd ed. St Louis: Mosby–Year Book; 2003:278–294.
22. Johnson Jr CM, Toriumi DM. Open structure rhinoplasty. Philadelphia: Saunders; 1990.
23. Adamson PA. Open rhinoplasty. In: Papel ID, Nachlas NE, eds. Facial plastic and reconstructive surgery. St Louis: Mosby–Year Book; 1992:295–304.
24. Adamson PA. Nasal tip surgery in open rhinoplasty. Fac Plast Surg Clin N Am. 1993;1(1):39–52.
25. Perkins SW. The evolution of the combined use of endonasal and external columellar approaches to rhinoplasty. Fac Plast Surg Clin N Am. 2004;12:35.
26. Crerand CE, Gibbons LM, Sawrer DB. Psychological characteristics of revision rhinoplasty patients. In: Becker DG, Park SS, eds. Revision rhinoplasty. New York: Thieme; 2007:32–41.
27. American Psychiatric Association. Diagnostic and statistical manual of mental disorders. 4th ed. text rev. Washington, DC: American Psychiatric Press; 2000.
28. Tardy ME, Chang EY, Jernstrom V. Misadventures in nasal tip surgery. Otolaryngol Clin N Am. 1987;20(4):797–823.
29. Becker DG, Weinberger MS, Greene BA, Tardy ME. Clinical study of alar anatomy and surgery of the alar base. Arch Otolaryngol Head Neck Surg. 1997;123(8):789–795.
30. Tardy ME, Toriumi DM. Alar retraction: Composite graft correction. Fac Plast Surg. 1989;6(2):101–107.
31. Becker DG, Bloom J. 5 Techniques that I cannot live without in revision rhinoplasty. Fac Plast Surg. 2008;24(3):358–364.
32. Becker DG, Park SS, Toriumi DM. Powered instrumentation for rhinoplasty and septoplasty. Otolaryngol Clin N Am. 1999;32(4):683–693.
33. Becker DG. The powered rasp: Advanced instrumentation for rhinoplasty. Arch Fac Plast Surg. 2002;4:267–268.

34. Larrabee Jr WF. Open rhinoplasty and the upper third of the nose. *Fac Plast Clin N Am.* 1993;1(1):23–38.

35. Tardy ME, Kron TK, Younger RY, Key M. The cartilaginous pollybeak: etiology, prevention, and treatment. *Fac Plast Surg.* 1989;6(2):113–120.

36. Tardy ME, Schwartz M, Parras G. Saddle nose deformity: Autogenous graft repair. *Fac Plast Surg.* 1989;6(2):121–134.

37. Gunter JP, Rohrich RJ. Augmentation rhinoplasty: Dorsal onlay grafting using shaped autogenous septal cartilage. *Plast Reconstr Surg.* 1990;86(1):39–45.

38. Daniel RK. Rhinoplasty and rib grafts: Evolving a flexible operative technique. *Plast Reconstr Surg.* 1992;94(5):597–611.

39. Murakami CS, Cook TA, Guida RA. Nasal reconstruction with articulated irradiated rib cartilage. *Arch Otolaryngol Head Neck Surg.* 1991;117:327–330.

40. Fedok FG, Preston TW. Managing the overresected dorsum. In: Becker DG, Park SS, eds. Revision rhinoplasty. New York: Thieme; 2007:96–111.

41. Toriumi DM. Management of the middle nasal vault. *Oper Tech Plast Reconstr Surg.* 1995;2(1):16–30.

42. Toriumi DM, Ries WR. Innovative surgical management of the crooked nose. *Fac Plast Surg Clin North Am.* 1993;1(1):63–78.

43. Murakami CS, Bloom DC, Most SP. Managing the persistently twisted nose. In: Becker DG, Park SS, eds. Revision rhinoplasty. New York: Thieme; 2007:85–95.

44. Rettinger G, Zenkel M. Skin and soft tissue complications. *Fac Plast Surg.* 1997;13(1):51–59.

45. Toriumi DM, Mueller RA, Grosch T, et al. Vascular anatomy of the nose and the external rhinoplasty approach. *Arch Otol Head Neck Surg.* 1996;122:24–34.

CHAPTER TEN

Nasal Osteotomies

Ravi S. Swamy • Sam P. Most

In 1898, Jacques Joseph was one of the first surgeons to promote the concept of the nasal osteotomy as a way to reshape and reposition the bony vault.[1] The primary indications for osteotomies are to straighten a deviated nasal dorsum, narrow the nasal side walls, and close an open nasal vault. While the objectives remain clear, osteotomies continue to be a source of trepidation for rhinoplasty surgeons. Whether the approach to rhinoplasty is external or endonasal, osteotomies rely predominantly on a tactile sense rather than direct visualization. Its execution requires careful planning, intimate knowledge of the anatomy, and appreciation of the dynamics between the upper one-third bony vault and lower two-thirds cartilaginous framework as there is a fine line between inadequate and overmobilization of the nasal bones. We will review important anatomic principles and describe the different techniques of osteotomies to achieve better precision and consistency in attaining superior aesthetic results without compromising nasal function.

NASAL ANALYSIS

Achieving success in rhinoplasty is based on careful preoperative planning and assessment. The relationship of the nose to the face has been studied for centuries. Objective measurements of contour, angles, and proportions have been proposed and accepted to help provide the facial plastic surgeon with guidelines that define ideal standards of beauty and aesthetic facial harmony. One of these guidelines states that the aesthetically pleasing face can be divided equally into vertical fifths, with the nasal base width equal to the intercanthal distance.[2] The width of the upper two thirds of the nose should be approximately 75% of the width of the nasal base (Figure 10-1). The nasal dorsum should also follow a gentle curvilinear path from the medial brow to the nasal tip. The dorsum should also be perpendicular to a line drawn vertically from the midglabella to the menton (Figure 10-2). The

external contour of the upper third of the nose is defined by the two side walls: the dorsum and the nasofrontal angle. The nasofrontal angle is the external landmark identifying the deepest or most posterior portion of the nasal dorsum, and by this definition is synonymous with the radix, or *soft tissue* nasion. The *bony* nasion is the junction between the frontal and nasal bones. The rhinion is the osseocartilaginous junction of the nasal bones inferiorly with the superior edge of the upper lateral cartilages. The bony nasal vault and its intimate attachment to the upper lateral cartilages make it the main determinant of nasal width of the upper and middle third of the nose.[3] Precise manipulation of the bony pyramid is essential to provide balance with any nasal tip work and create overall aesthetic harmony. Failure to complete proper osteotomies can negate the effects of intricate tip maneuvers and leave the patient with a "washed-out" or poorly defined nose on frontal view, even though the patient may have an improvement on profile and oblique views.[4]

PERTINENT NASAL ANATOMY

The nasal bones are paired structures that attach superiorly to the frontal bone and laterally to the nasal process of the maxillary bones. Together, these bones form the bony nasal vault. The perpendicular plate of the ethmoid, a portion of the bony septum, attaches to the undersurface of the nasal bones in the midline. The nasal bones are thin inferiorly and become thick superiorly.[5,6] Figure 10-3 demonstrates this by transillumination of the skull. The variable thickness of the bony structures of the nose will influence osteotomy placement. The nasal septum supports the nose along its entire length. The septum serves to support the dorsal profile, and loss of this structure can result in the classic saddle-nose deformity. Preservation of adequate (>1 cm) dorsal and caudal septal struts is necessary to preserve support after any nasal surgery. The anterior nasal spine supports the caudal septum and the

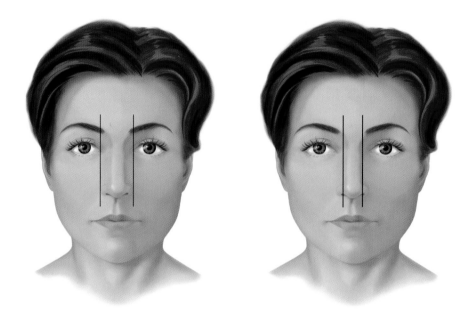

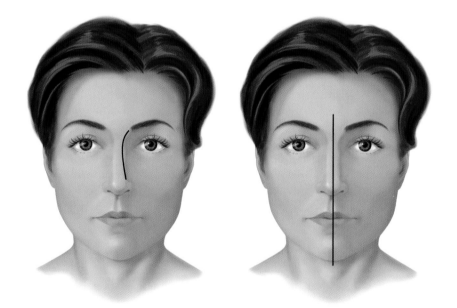

feet of the medial crura. When excessive in size, the nasal spine may actually blunt the nasolabial angle.[6]

The paired upper lateral cartilages are triangular and fused medially to the dorsal septum. The cartilages attach to the undersurface of the nasal bones at their superior extent and are connected to the frontal process of the maxilla by dense fibrous connective tissue. The paired lower lateral cartilages support the nasal lobule and nostrils. This fibrocartilaginous arch is supported medially by the caudal septum and nasal spine. Laterally, the arch is

supported by the lateral crura and a variable number of small accessory cartilages between the lateral crura and pyriform aperture.[6]

DORSAL HUMP REDUCTION

Prior to instituting maneuvers to mobilize and shift the bony nasal vault, it is critical to evaluate the contribution of the dorsal hump to the nasal profile and whether a

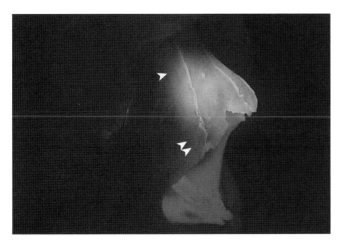

Figure 10-3 Transillumination of the skull reveals the variable thickness of the nasal bones, which are mobilized with osteotomies in rhinoplasty. The nasal bones are thicker superiorly (*arrowhead*) and thinner inferiorly (*double arrowheads*). (From Most SP, Murakami CS. A modern approach to nasal osteotomies. Fac Plast Surg Clin North Am. 2005;13:85–92.)

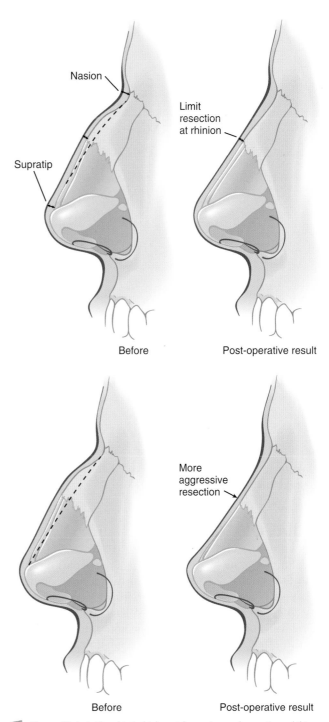

Figure 10-4 A, The skin is thicker at the nasion and supratip and thinner at the rhinion. Dorsal resection limiting resection at the rhinion will result in a straighter postoperative profile. **B,** A more aggressive dorsal resection that creates a straight orientation of the underlying cartilaginoskeletal framework will give a concave postoperative profile appearance due to the difference in thickness of the overlying skin. (From Toriumi DM, Hecht DA. Skeletal modifications in rhinoplasty. Fac Plast Surg Clin North Am. 2000;8: 413–423.)

hump reduction will be required.[7] To gain proper access to this area, sharp dissection of the midline raphe of decussating periosteal fibers should be completed up to the level of the nasofrontal angle. Care should be taken to stay midline to avoid lateral disruption of supportive soft tissue attachments to the nasal skeleton. It is also important to consider the variation of thickness of the skin soft tissue envelope over the nasal dorsum. The skin is thickest in the nasion and supratip areas and thinnest over the rhinion; therefore, resection of the dorsal hump at the rhinion should be performed with extreme care[8] (Figure 10-4). In fact, to achieve a straight soft tissue profile, the cartilaginoskeletal framework at the rhinion should be kept slightly convex.[6]

Several techniques are available to reduce the bony dorsum. An osteotome or a rasp can be used, depending on the surgeon's experience and preference. Most surgeons use an osteotome for larger humps and a rasp for smaller reductions and refinements. The dorsal septum and upper lateral cartilages can be reduced sharply with a scalpel. For removing larger humps, a conservative correction is performed with an osteotome (often double-guarded) and refinements are then made with a tungsten carbide pull rasp or scalpel.[6] It is critical not to violate the attachments of the upper lateral cartilages to the undersurface of the caudal margin of the nasal bones as lack of support of the cartilages may lead to inferomedial collapse and cause an inverted-V deformity[9] (Figure 10-5).

The orientation of the bony vault must be considered and evaluated before dorsal hump removal. If the vault is shifted toward one side, the hump removal should not be symmetric. Less bone should be excised from the side of the deviation[7] (Figure 10-6). Performing a hump reduction with this technique more closely approximates a midline vertical orientation of the lateral nasal bones and prevents excessive reduction in their height.[7] Dorsal hump

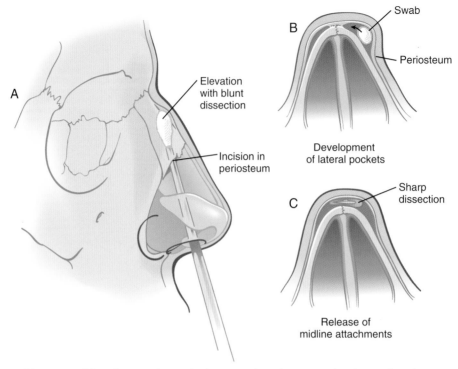

Figure 10-5 Elevation of the periosteal flap is begun with a Cottle elevator, and may be continued to the nasofrontal suture using the same instrument or a periosteal elevator. Care should be taken to preserve the lateral periosteal attachments as this will help reduce the risk of a flail bone.

reduction may lead to an open roof deformity that sets the stage for osteotomies.

MEDIAL OSTEOTOMIES

By definition, a medial osteotomy is a cut separating the nasal bones from the bony septum in the midline. This technique is used in conjunction with the lateral osteotomy to create a predictable site of back fracture for the lateral osteotomies. The medial osteotomy should be used in cases of an extremely wide or deviated nose, an iatrogenic open roof difficult to close with a lateral osteotomy, an increased bony width above the infraorbital rim, and in the presence of thicker nasal bones.[10] Medial osteotomies are generally difficult to perform and should be used judiciously. As previously described, the bony vault varies in thickness regionally, and the nasal skin in the midline tends to be the thin; therefore, bony irregularities can be more evident.

Typically, when performing a medial osteotomy, a small osteotome is placed at the caudal margin of the nasal bone just lateral to the septum. As the osteotome is driven upward, a slight lateral trajectory of 15 degrees should be taken to meet up with the planned superior extent of the lateral osteotomy (Figure 10-7). Several studies have shown more reliable and consistent results with this medial "oblique" osteotomy versus a more

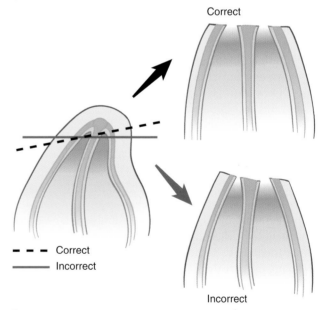

Figure 10-6 **A,** In crooked noses, the dorsal hump resection should be performed in a tangential plane by removing more bone and cartilage on the convex side (*dotted line*) rather than approaching it with a straight perpendicular cut (*solid line*). **B,** Illustration of the position and height of nasal bones after hump removal and osteotomies are performed to straighten the bone. *Note.* If the tangential plane was taken, the nasal bones will be more symmetric. (From Toriumi DM, Ries WR. Innovative surgical management of the crooked nose. Fac Plast Surg Clin North Am. 1993;1:63–78.)

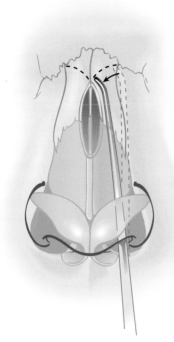

Figure 10-7 Medial osteotomy. Either a straight or a curved osteotome creates a controlled fracture adjacent to the septum and up to the transition to the thicker frontal bone. A straight path remaining midline or a more oblique angle of 15 degrees laterally can be taken and this will help with mobilization of the bone once the lateral osteotomy is completed. (From Most SP, Murakami CS. A modern approach to nasal osteotomies. Fac Plast Surg Clin North Am. 2005;13:85–92.)

straight medial osteotomy.[11] As nasal bone thickness increases from caudal to cephalic and from lateral to medial, there exists a curvilinear bone thickness transition zone. This transition in bone thickness provides a natural cleavage plane for the medial oblique osteotomy.[10] Less-angulated medial osteotomies can lead to cuts into the thicker frontal bone that could lead to a less desirable contour and higher likelihood of rocker deformities.

LATERAL OSTEOTOMIES

The lateral osteotomy is the workhorse osteotomy and will narrow the bony vault, improve contour of the brow-tip aesthetic line, and close an open roof deformity created by dorsal hump reduction.[10] When Joseph first described the lateral osteotomy in 1898, he described the technique of using a saw to make a low, continuous osteotomy.[1] The path of his osteotomy extended from the inferior pyriform aperture up into the nasal process of the frontal bone. The aggressive mobilization of the nasal bones by Joseph and other early surgeons revolutionized aesthetic rhinoplasty; however, any hope of preserving an adequate nasal passage for breathing fell by the wayside and resulted in high rates of postoperative nasal airway compromise. The recognition that preservation of the periosteum and lateral

suspensory ligaments of the lower lateral cartilage helped to lower the incidence of postoperative airway compromise has been an important positive technical modification.[6] Thus, modern techniques of osteotomy have evolved to consider the effects of bony repositioning on functional as well as aesthetic outcome. It was not until the introduction of the high–low–high lateral osteotomy in the late 1970s that an exceptional aesthetic outcome could be achieved in conjunction with sufficient nasal airway.[12] The terms "high" and "low" refer the path of the osteotomies along the nasal sidewall (Figure 10-8). "Low" means closer to the maxilla and "high" is towards the nasal dorsum. The lateral osteotomy can be completed in two ways: the linear (single-cut) technique or the perforating technique.

The linear osteotomy technique is completed entirely intranasally. First, the monopolar cautery is used to make an incision in the mucosa above the anterior attachment of the inferior turbinate, along the pyriform aperture. An osteotome is used to start the lateral osteotomy at or above the anterior end of the inferior turbinate and is initially directed at an angle perpendicular to the face (Figure 10-9). This starting point above the inferior turbinate helps protect a small triangle of bone at the base of the pyriform aperture from being disturbed.[13] This ensures preservation of the lateral attachments of the suspensory ligaments and the natural position of the inferior turbinate, thereby maintaining the patency of the nasal airway.[12,14] The osteotome is leveled off as it approaches the ascending process of the maxilla, and then the osteotomy is finished at the level of the medial canthus.

To help with mobilization of the nasal bones superiorly, several techniques may be used. With the osteotome still engaged near the medial canthus, medial rotation with digital pressure allows for completion of a greenstick fracture. A percutaneous transverse superior osteotomy may be necessary if the bones are thick. A 2-mm osteotome is used percutaneously midway between the nasal dorsum and the medial canthal region. Through a single skin puncture, the osteotome may be used to create three to four small perforating osteotomies, allowing the nasal bone to be mobilized without disrupting the overlying periosteal support. When more precision is necessary, the lateral osteotomy can be connected to a previously completed medial oblique osteotomy.[6] If medial and lateral osteotomies are taken too high into the thick frontal bone, the superior aspect of the osteotomized nasal bone may project laterally when the bone is infractured, thus causing a rocker deformity[9] (Figure 10-10).

PERFORATING OSTEOTOMIES

An alternative to the linear technique for lateral osteotomy is the perforating technique. Proponents of this technique assert that it provides a controlled, stable fracture

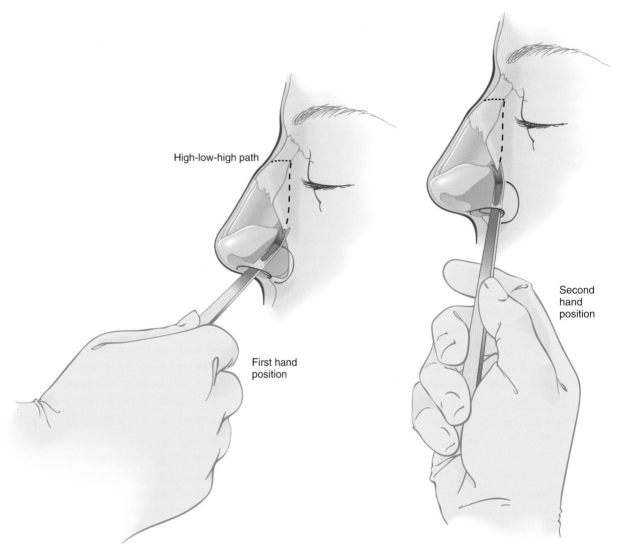

High-low-high path

First hand
position

Second
hand
position

Figure 10-8 Lateral osteotomy. The dashed line depicts high–low–high path along nasal side wall. "Low" refers toward the maxilla and "high" is toward the dorsum.

with less nasal airway narrowing, hemorrhage, edema, and ecchymosis.[15] Using a sharp 2-mm straight osteotome, a series of "postage stamp" perforations are placed along the desired fracture site using a transcutaneous approach. With the advent of small, sharp microosteotomes, more intense and efficient force can be applied onto the nasal bones. Moreover, less force will be required to cut the bone, resulting in less chance of an uncontrolled fracture line.[16] Given the direct nature of this technique on the skin, there is the advantage of more precise placement of the osteotomy. Studies have shown that there is less mucosal disruption and violation of branches of the lateral nasal and angular arteries, resulting in less bleeding and postoperative edema.[15,17] The perforating osteotomy, of course, necessitates incisions through the skin; however, these small incisions heal without significant scars and are undetectable in majority of cases.[17,18]

The "inside-out" perforating technique can also be used to widen the excessively narrow bony nasal pyramid, the cause of which may be congenital or secondary to previous trauma or surgery.[12,19] This technique is performed by making a series of osteotomies beginning inferiorly near the attachment of the inferior turbinate and proceeding superiorly. The direction of the force vector is directed laterally, which aids in proper displacement of the bony segment in the desired direction.[19] Studies have shown this technique to be more effective and provide greater preservation of the periosteal support of the bony segments than a continuous osteotomy.[19,20]

The perforating osteotomy can be effective in patients with short nasal bones as this technique prevents overmobilization of the delicate, short bones, and preserves maximal soft tissue support.[6] This is also true in difficult cases such as revision rhinoplasty or posttraumatic nasal

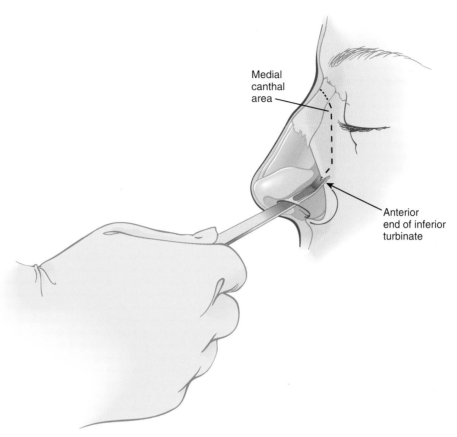

Figure 10-9 The lateral osteotomy is begun at the anterior end of the inferior turbinate and is first made perpendicular to the face. The surgeon should place his or her hand on top of the osteotome and, once seeded in the bone, supinate and grip the osteotome from below and proceed up the bone using the other hand to guide the osteotome toward the medial canthal area.

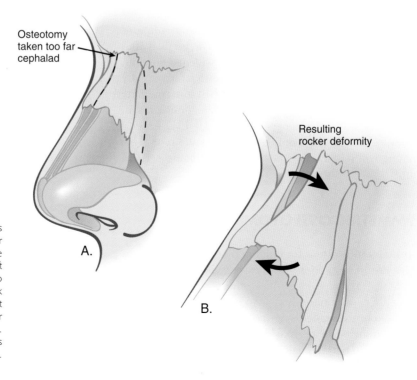

Figure 10-10 A, Medial and lateral osteotomies that are taken too high cephalically into the thicker frontal bone can cause a rocker deformity. **B,** The forces on the upper thicker bone cause a lateral shift and a fulcrum effect will force the lower segment to rotate medially. If the upper segment is pushed back medially, the lower segment may "rock" laterally out of position. A transverse osteotomy in the thinner nasal bone below will be needed to rectify this issue. (From Toriumi DM, Hecht DA. Skeletal modifications in rhinoplasty. Fac Plast Surg Clin North Am. 2000;8:413–423.)

surgery, in which maintenance of structural support is critical.[15] Cadaveric studies have demonstrated preservation of considerably more periosteal support with the perforating technique compared with the linear technique.[15,18] With increased accuracy and decreased morbidity, this is often the preferred technique, especially in inexperienced hands; however, patients with severe deviations and thickened nasal bones are more appropriately treated with the single-cut linear osteotomy technique.[13]

INTERMEDIATE OSTEOTOMIES

The intermediate osteotomy is essentially a bone cut along the nasal sidewall in a region between the medial and lateral osteotomy. The exact placement of the osteotomy may vary depending on surgical goals. The open rhinoplasty approach affords more precision with this technique due to direct visualization when setting the osteotome, while in a closed approach, an intercartilaginous incision is required and the osteotomy is completed with careful tactile feedback. These osteotomies are generally completed through exceedingly thin bone and require minimal force from the mallet to prevent an unintentional fracture line.[21] In situations where both intermediate and lateral osteotomies are required, the intermediate osteotomy should be performed prior the lateral osteotomy, as the intermediate cut cannot be made easily after the nasal bone is mobilized by a lateral osteotomy. Once again, it is imperative that the soft tissue attachments be maintained to the nasal bone for additional support and prevention of nasal collapse.

Bilateral intermediate osteotomies are frequently used in patients with a wide nasal dorsum. At the midline, the lateral nasal bones fuse with the perpendicular plate of the ethmoid bone. This union has both a vertical and transverse component. In patients with a widened dorsum, the transverse component is a contributing factor.[21] By completing medial osteotomies followed by intermediate osteotomies 4 mm lateral to the medial osteotomies, a thin strip of bone can be removed (Figure 10-11). Lateral osteotomies can then be completed to close the roof. This technique will narrow the apex without reducing vertical height.[22]

ASYMMETRIC OSTEOTOMIES

The primary indications for unilateral or asymmetric osteotomies are to straighten a severely deviated nose where one side wall is much longer than the other or to correct a markedly convex nasal bone. An asymmetric or unilateral osteotomy executed on the deviated side will help with recontouring of the nasal wall into a more normal curvature that better coincides with the opposite side.[8] Typically, the asymmetric osteotomy can be in the form

of intermediate osteotomy or lateral osteotomy. A single lateral osteotomy can be beneficial to medialize the convex side of the nose. The concave side can then be addressed with placement of onlay or spreader graft.[23]

A unilateral intermediate osteotomy may be effective on the deviated nasal bone at the area of maximal convexity[24] (Figure 10-12). In patients with history of extensive nasal trauma, there may be areas of fibrous unions along

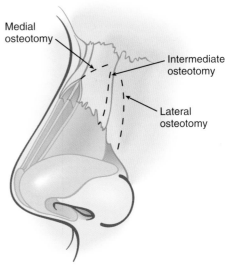

Figure 10-11 A single intermediate osteotomy can be placed on the convex side of the deviation between the medial and lateral osteotomies. The intermediate osteotomy should precede the lateral osteotomy as it would not be possible to complete the intermediate cut after the lateral cut has been made.

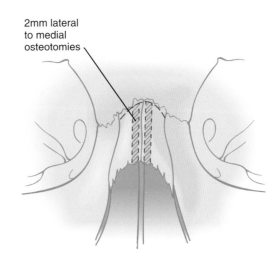

Figure 10-12 Medial osteotomies are made followed by intermediate osteotomies that are completed 2 mm lateral to them. The intervening thin strip of bone (*shaded area*) between the septum and paramedian osteotomies can be removed. Lateral osteotomies are then completed to close resulting open roof deformity. The nasal pyramid can be narrowed without losing dorsal height with this maneuver. (Adapted from Cochran CS, Ducic Y, Defatta RJ. Rethinking nasal osteotomies: an anatomic approach. Laryngoscope. 2007;117:662-667.)

the nasal bones where previous fractures have healed. The osteotome will tend to follow these fibrous connections because they offer less resistance than intact bone. In such cases, the surgeon must take extra care to guide the osteotome in the desired direction.[24]

Another technique calls for two lateral osteotomies on the more convex side, and is known as the "double lateral osteotomy." Proponents believe that part of the asymmetry is due to longer and often thicker nasal bones at the maxillary process on the convex side.[25] By completing two lateral osteotomies on the convex side, one can achieve better mobilization of this thicker bone and better symmetry with the opposite side. This technique will also decrease the chance of a palpable bony stepoff that may be encountered with an intermediate osteotomy completed at the site of maximal convexity.[25–27] These osteotomies can be accomplished as a linear cut or through the perforated technique.[26,27]

High septal deviations are commonly seen in patients with crooked nasal pyramids and should be identified and addressed appropriately. If the septal deviation is at the keystone area, care should be taken to completely mobilize the segments of the bony pyramid while maintaining the support attachments between the bony dorsum and the cartilaginous and bony portions of the septum[13] (Figure 10-13).

When approaching the severely crooked nasal vault, the sequence of osteotomies should commence on the concave side of the deviation (the opposite side of deviation), then move to the midline, and end on the convex (the deviated side). This is analogous to turning the pages of an open book, with the nasal walls and septum simulating the pages (Figure 10-14). This allows creation of a space in which to realign the deviation.[5,6] If the septal deviation persists in this area despite these maneuvers, delicate scoring of cartilage may be completed. Disruption of the keystone area, however, can lead to a postoperative saddle-nose deformity that can require extensive reconstructive surgery to correct.[13] Despite proper utilization of osteotomies, small deviations may persist, and while perfection may be the enemy of good, camouflaging grafts may be beneficial.

COMPLICATIONS

Complications of osteotomies can be aesthetic, functional, or both. The most common complication of osteotomy is likely continued or de novo creation of bony irregularities. Indeed, the term *complication* may be an inaccurate term.

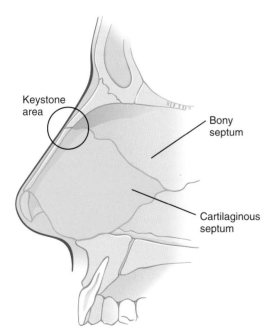

Figure 10-13 The keystone area. This is junction of the bony and cartilaginous septum with the bony dorsum. Septal deviations in this area can often contribute to a deviation in the dorsum and should be addressed with care not to disrupt these critical support attachments.

Keystone area

Bony septum

Cartilaginous septum

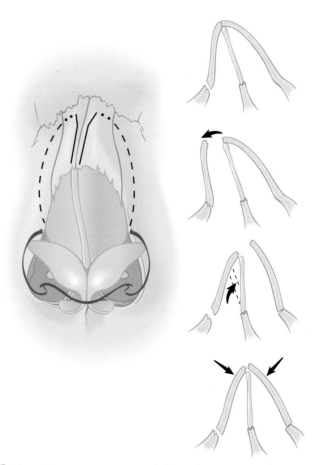

Figure 10-14 To correct a severely deviated nose, sequential osteotomies are performed in a fashion similar to opening a book. The osteotomies are begun on the concave side, beginning laterally and moving toward the opposite side. In this way, the depressed side is elevated and the convex side is deprojected.

as perfect symmetry of the bony vault is difficult to achieve, especially in cases of preexisting asymmetry. However, some contour deformities may be due to incorrect placement of or unexpected pathway of the osteotomy. In the case of the lateral osteotomy, this is most commonly the error of placing the osteotomy too medially along the nasal side wall, resulting in a palpable or visible deformity. Similarly, placement of the medial osteotomy too far laterally (away from the midline) can result in a high side wall or dorsal step-off deformity.

The most difficult complication of osteotomies is the creation of a flail segment of bone. In this case, overmobilization and/or failure to preserve periosteal attachments results in the nasal bone "falling into" the nasal cavity. In this case, it is important that the surgeon recognize this problem and take corrective action. Unfortunately, this is a difficult problem to correct and no simple solution exists. In the authors' experience, placement of a high nasal pack often fails as the pack tends to be displaced inferiorly. One alternative is to place a bolster and suture in the high nasal vault, beneath the flail bone, and suture this to the skin with a through-and-through suture until the external splinting is removed. Alternatively, one may immediately camouflage graft the area of the flail segment by dissection over the depressed area and placement of a suitable graft. Care must be taken to examine the airway intranasally to determine if the grafting worsens medial displacement of the bone.

Finally, nasal obstruction used to be one of the most common complications of osteotomies. In some cases, it may still occur. However, with careful planning prior to osteotomy placement, preservation of the inferiormost triangle of bone of the pyriform aperture, and avoidance of overmobilization, this has become more rare.

CONCLUSIONS

There are a variety of surgical maneuvers to narrow the nasal pyramid and overcome asymmetry of the upper third of the nose. Mastery of nasal osteotomies requires a detailed knowledge of nasal anatomy, sophisticated appreciation of nasal aesthetic harmony, and an erudite approach to each individual patient. Though frequently reserved for the conclusion of the surgical procedure, osteotomies are not the sine qua non to successful rhinoplasty but represent another set of tools in the surgeon's armamentarium and should be used judiciously. The surgeon must always consider the relationship between the bony and cartilaginous portions of the nose and recognize how their modification affects overall nasal function. Methodical preoperative planning, careful execution, and selective implementation are vital to achieving consistent success while avoiding complications.

REFERENCES

1. Joseph J. *Die Hypertrophie der starren Nase: Nasenplastik und sonstige gesichtsplastik über smammaplastik und einige weitere Operationen aus dem gebiete der ausseren Korperplastik.* Leipzig, Germany: Kabitzsch; 1931.
2. Orten SS, Hilger PA. Facial analysis of the rhinoplasty patient. In: Papel ID, ed. *Facial plastic and reconstructive surgery.* 2nd ed. New York: Thieme; 2002:361–368.
3. Most SP, Murakami CS. Management of the bony nasal vault. In: Papel ID, ed. *Facial plastic and reconstructive surgery.* 2nd ed. New York: Thieme; 2002:402–406.
4. Tardy ME. *Rhinoplasty: The art and the science.* Philadelphia: WB Saunders; 1997.
5. Most SP, Murakami CS. A modern approach to nasal osteotomies. *Fac Plast Surg Clin North Am.* 2005;13:85–92.
6. Most SP, Murakami CS. Nasal osteotomies: Anatomy, planning, and technique. *Fac Plast Surg Clin North Am.* 2002;10:279–285.
7. Toriumi DM, Ries WR. Innovative surgical management of the crooked nose. *Fac Plast Surg Clin North Am.* 1993;1:63–78.
8. Toriumi DM, Hecht DA. Skeletal modifications in rhinoplasty. *Fac Plast Surg Clin North Am.* 2000;8:413–423.
9. Becker DG, Becker SS. Reducing complications in rhinoplasty. *Otolaryngol Clin North Am.* 2006;39:475–492.
10. Harshbarger RJ, Sullivan PK. The optimal medial osteotomy: A study of nasal bone thickness and fracture patterns. *Plast Reconstr Surg.* 2001;108:2114–2119.
11. Gruber R, Chang TN, Kahn D, et al. Broad nasal bone reduction: an algorithm for osteotomies. *Plast Reconstr Surg.* 2007;119:1044–1053.
12. Larrabee WF. Open rhinoplasty and the upper third of the nose. *Fac Plast Surg Clin North Am.* 1993;1:23–38.
13. Larrabee WF, Murakami CS. Osteotomy techniques to correct posttraumatic deviation of the nasal pyramid: A technical note. *J Craniomaxillofac Trauma.* 2000;6:43–47.
14. Guyuron B. Dynamics of rhinoplasty. *Aesthet Plast Surg.* 2002;26:S10.
15. Rohrich RJ, Minoli JJ, Adams WP, et al. The lateral nasal osteotomy in rhinoplasty: An anatomic endoscopic comparison of the external versus the internal approach. *Plast Reconstr Surg.* 1997;99:1309–1312.
16. Becker DG, McLaughlin Jr RB, Loevner LA, et al. The lateral osteotomy in rhinoplasty: Clinical and radiographic rationale for osteotome selection. *Plast Reconstr Surg.* 2000;105:1806–1816.
17. Hinton AE, Hung T, Daya H, et al. Visibility of puncture sites after external osteotomy in rhinoplastic surgery. *Arch Fac Plast Surg.* 2003;5:408–411.
18. Gryskiewicz JM. Visible scars from percutaneous osteotomies. *Plast Reconstr Surg.* 2005;116:1771–1775.
19. Byrne PJ, Walsh WE, Hilger PA. The use of "inside-out" lateral osteotomies to improve outcome in rhinoplasty. *Arch Fac Plast Surg.* 2003;5:251–255.
20. Murakami CS, Larrabee WF. Comparison of osteotomy techniques in the treatment of nasal fractures. *Fac Plast Surg.* 1992;8:209–219.
21. Tebbetts JB. *Primary rhinoplasty: Redefining the logic and technique.* 2nd ed. Philadelphia: Mosby; 2008.
22. Cochran CS, Ducic Y, Defatta RJ. Rethinking nasal osteotomies: An anatomic approach. *Laryngoscope.* 2007;117:662–667.

23. Roofe SB, Murakami CS. Treatment of the posttraumatic and postrhinoplasty crooked nose. *Fac Plast Surg Clin North Am.* 2006;14:279–289.

24. Kim DW, Toriumi DM. Management of posttraumatic nasal deformities: The crooked nose and the saddle nose. *Fac Plast Surg Clin North Am.* 2004;12:111–132.

25. Bracaglia R, Fortunato R, Gentileschi S. Double lateral osteotomy in aesthetic rhinoplasty. *Br J Plast Surg.* 2004;57:156–159.

26. Parkes ML, Kamer F, Morgan WR. Double lateral osteotomy in rhinoplasty. *Arch Otolaryngol.* 1977;103:344–348.

27. Westreich RW, Lawson W. Perforating double lateral osteotomy. *Arch Fac Plast Surg.* 2005;7:254–260.

CHAPTER ELEVEN

Cartilage Grafting in Rhinoplasty and Nasal Reconstruction

Raffi Der Sarkissian

GENERAL PRINCIPLES

Maintaining or achieving structural integrity of the nasal form is a formidable task in rhinoplasty and nasal reconstruction. Maintaining the form and function of the nose is an equally important objective as creating a pleasing aesthetic contour. In this regard, numerous autograft, allograft, and synthetic materials have been proposed as the ideal replacement or augmentation matrix in nasal surgery. Despite trials of use of various synthetics such as Mersilene polyester fiber mesh, expanded polytetrafluoroethylene, porous high-density polyethylene, and numerous others, cartilage grafting remains the most reliable technique in providing nasal support, replacement of structural components of the nose, and augmentation for a variety of reasons.[1–5]

Because cartilage is a normal component of the native nasal structure, it is logical to use it to replace deficiencies and create structural, contour, and aesthetic enhancements. Cartilage grafts are equally suited for structural support of the nose as well as nonsupporting applications such as camouflage grafts. Grafts can be of variable rigidity based on site of harvest and how they are modified prior to use. A whole spectrum of graft strength, thickness, volume, and malleability can be achieved by use of septal grafts, auricular grafts, costal cartilage grafts, or combinations. Thick or rigid grafts are best suited for supporting applications. Thin grafts are useful when minimal visibility is desired as in areas of thin skin over the nasal dorsum or in revision cases. Stacked and sutured grafts can help create greater support or can be used in augmentation cases when significant augmentation is required. Morselized cartilage grafts can be applied in a camouflaging fashion and will tend to "drape" more smoothly over existing structures. Diced or crushed cartilage can be used as plumping grafts along the nasolabial junction or wrapped with Surgicel, acellular dermis or temporalis fascia to augment the dorsum.[6,7,11] Cartilage grafts can be modified to address the patient's particular need, whereas allografts are either solid and noncompressible or soft and nonsupportive. An additional benefit in using cartilage grafts is the ability to suture fixate the grafts, thereby creating less movement and a tendency for more rapid integration and vascularization.

As with any ideal implant, autologous cartilage is biocompatible and in its native state has a relatively minimal metabolic requirement allowing rapid integration. In addition, autologous cartilage is an ideal choice for compromised tissue vascularity as commonly seen in traumatic nasal deformity, revision rhinoplasty, and patients with collagen vascular disorders and diabetes.

A further advantage of use of cartilage grafting is the almost unlimited donor source such as septum, ear, and costal cartilage. Nasal septal grafts are the easiest to obtain in primary rhinoplasty or in secondary cases if the septum was not previously harvested. Auricular cartilage from one or both ears provides grafts of various shapes and sizes often suitable for camouflaging or low-volume augmentation grafting. Costal cartilage provides large volumes of material that can be carved and shaped into numerous grafting applications. Fortunately, donor site morbidity is quite minimal in harvesting cartilage from each of these sources. Donor sites for cartilage can be easily camouflaged. Septal grafts are harvested via an intranasal incision, auricular cartilage grafts can be approached through the post auricular sulcus or a well-concealed anterior incision, and costal cartilage can be obtained via an inframammary crease incision.

Multiple uses of cartilage grafts have been well described.[5,8] In general, it is helpful to define the purpose of the intended grafts. In so doing, the appropriate volume of graft material of adequate strength and rigidity can be harvested for the desired application. Areas suitable for augmentation grafts are the nasofrontal recess, dorsum, nasal tip, and columella. Replacement grafts are common along the lateral crura of the lower lateral cartilages and along the caudal margin of the upper lateral cartilages. Structural grafts are commonly used in the columella in the form of struts between the medial crura and in extended tip graft configuration. Functional applications include alar replacement grafts, lateral crural strut grafts, batten grafts, spreader grafts, and alar rim supporting grafts.

Several sources of grafting cartilage are readily available for these applications. The decision regarding the

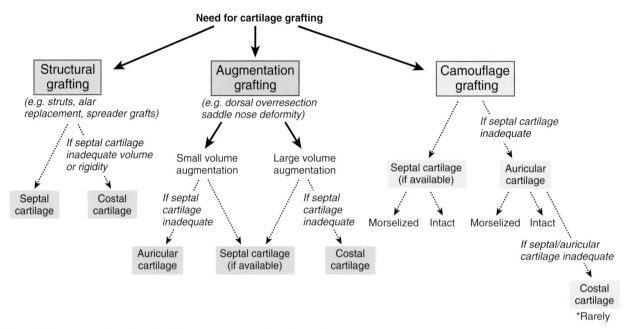

Figure 11-1 Decision-making algorithm for anatomic source of cartilage grafts.

source to be used is based on a number of variables including the presence or absence of donor cartilage related to prior surgery, volume of cartilage required, structural support requirements, desired contour of the grafted cartilage, graft rigidity, and donor site morbidity[10] (Figure 11-1).

SEPTAL CARTILAGE

When an adequate supply is available, the most desirable source of cartilage grafts is the nasal septum. As septoplasty is almost always performed concomitantly with rhinoplasty, there is no additional cartilage harvest morbidity. If used for nasal reconstructive purposes, the cartilage is within the field of reconstruction and easily accessible. Quadrangular cartilage tends to be flat and adequately rigid for structural support and can be scored, morselized, diced, or crushed if softer applications are desired. Grafts of various thicknesses can be harvested based on the grafting requirements.

Septal cartilage is most commonly harvested through a hemitransfixion or full transfixion incision as in a standard septoplasty. In external rhinoplasty, the cartilage can be harvested using an endonasal approach or from above through the medial crura. If there is a need for separation of the upper lateral cartilage from the dorsal septum, harvest from above is preferred. If the junction of the upper lateral cartilages with the dorsal septum is to remain intact, endonasal harvest is less destabilizing and requires less soft tissue dissection. Flap elevation is facilitated by

hydrodissecting the submucoperichondrial plane with local anesthesia (1% lidocaine with 1:100,000 epinephrine, 27-gauge 1¼-inch needle). Adequate dorsal and caudal septa (1.5 to 2.0 cm) must be preserved to prevent nasal collapse. If the amount of cartilage seems inadequate, it is better to seek an additional source rather than compromise nasal support (Figure 11-2).

Complications of septal cartilage harvest include compromise of dorsal or caudal support if adequate struts are not maintained, septal hematoma, septal perforation, and intranasal synechiae if raw mucosal surfaces are left in contact postoperative. Careful dissection of flaps, particularly in secondary cases, maintenance of adequate dorsal and caudal support, quilting sutures of 4-0 plain gut, and/or use of Silastic septal splints helps minimize these risks.

Disadvantages of septal cartilage are generally related to inadequate supply. Inadequate amount of cartilage may be harvested depending on the volume of cartilage required in primary rhinoplasty and the amount that can be safely removed without compromising the nasal support structure. The deficiency in septal cartilage is even greater in secondary procedures where the septum has been treated previously and there is an even greater need for rigidly supporting grafts. Some patients have anatomically inadequate available cartilage even if the septum has not been previously addressed. For instance, mesorrhine or platyrrhine noses more frequently present with larger than normal ratio of bony to cartilaginous septum. Thinner than average cartilage will also provide inadequate support in primary or secondary applications.

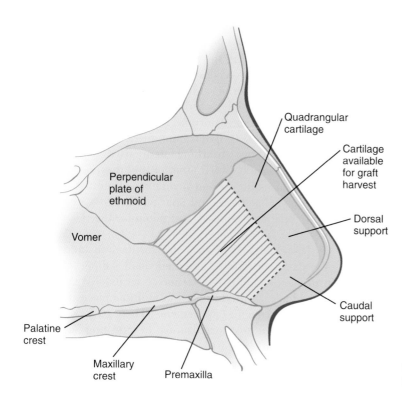

Figure 11-2 Nasal septal anatomy. The *shaded area* can be safely harvested for grafts.

AURICULAR CARTILAGE

When septal cartilage is inadequate in volume or rigidity, the next most common anatomic site for harvest of cartilage grafts is the ear.[8] Auricular cartilage is relatively easy to harvest with minimal donor site morbidity and little to no visible scarring or auricular deformity. Adequate volume of grafts is generally available and bilateral auricular cartilage can be harvested based on grafting requirements (Figure 11-3). The natural curvature of concha cymba and concha cavum reproduces the desired concavities or convexities of the nasal contour. Composite grafts can be taken with overlying skin as needed.

Auricular cartilage can be harvested from an anterior or posterior approach. In both approaches, the area that can be safely harvested is marked (Figure 11-4) and both the anterior and posterior aspects of the conchal bowl are infiltrated in a subperichondrial plane with 1% lidocaine with 1:100,000 epinephrine. Although it has been proposed that vasoconstriction with epinephrine is to be avoided in the ear, no ischemic events have been documented using this technique. Anterior harvest is performed through an incision along the inferior crus of the antihelix down toward the antitragus. This incision is well camouflaged if kept just anterior to the antihelix (on the conchal side). Dissection is carried out in a subperichondrial plane anteriorly. Maintenance of the crus of the helix helps prevent any deformity of the auricle post-operatively (Figure 11-5). Anterior harvest is somewhat faster and easier than the posterior approach but does carry the risk

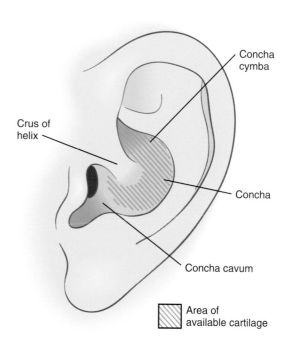

Figure 11-3 Auricular anatomy. The *shaded area* can be safely harvested without distorting the size or contour of the ear.

of a visible scar. Composite grafts of cartilage and skin are most frequently harvested from an anterior approach with an attempt made to match the desired curvature of the graft.

A posterior approach for auricular graft harvest is chosen in the majority of patients as the donor site scar

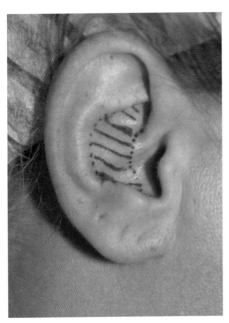

Figure 11-4 The *shaded area* of the conchal bowl can be safely harvested.

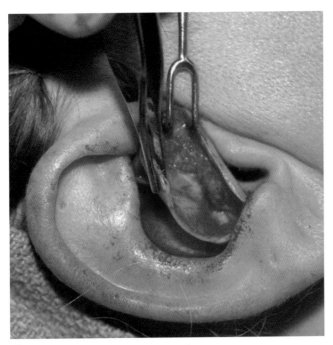

Figure 11-5 Anterior harvest approach.

visibility is further minimized. The ear is infiltrated as in the anterior approach and the incision is placed in the postauricular sulcus. In planning this incision, it is prudent to err 2 to 3 mm anteriorly up onto the posterior concha, leaving the resultant scar directly in the sulcus rather than onto the mastoid surface. Dissection is again subperichondrial and carried out to the edge of the conchal bowl. Introduction of a 27-gauge needle helps define the edge

of the conchal bowl beyond which dissection should not continue. Some surgeons outline this border preoperatively with a needle and methylene blue as would be done in an otoplasty procedure (Figure 11-6).

In both anterior and posterior harvest techniques, risks include visible scarring, auricular hematoma, and auricular contour deformity. Meticulous closure of the incision with 6-0 nylon minimizes scarring. Quilting sutures of 5-0 fast absorbing gut are used to obliterate the potential space between anterior and posterior perichondrial surfaces, to prevent hematoma. Limiting dissection to the conchal bowl and sparing the crus of the helix ensure adequate support and minimize the risk of deformation of the auricle.

Disadvantages of auricular cartilage include fragility of grafts, poor rigidity, and inadequate support, as well as insufficient length. Grafts may occasionally need to be stacked and sutured or used in multiple pieces to address volume or strength requirements. These grafts tend not to hold up well to morselization or crushing techniques. Fragmentation of cartilage and loss of form are common. Auricular cartilage in older patients tends to be brittle and fragments more easily.

COSTAL CARTILAGE

Costal cartilage is an excellent option if stronger support is required and in cases where septal and/or auricular cartilage grafts have been previously used. Rib grafts provide an almost unlimited supply of grafts in cases where a larger volume of cartilage grafts are required.[9,10] Costal cartilage is the most structurally supportive of all autologous cartilage grafting material. The grafts can be carved and shaped into various lengths, widths, and contours to replace or augment the cartilaginous and bony framework of the nose. Osteocartilaginous segments can be harvested if a bony component is required. Overlying perichondrium is frequently harvested and used as a camouflaging "blanket" over dorsum and tip in thin or compromised soft tissue (Figure 11-7).

Rib can be easily harvested by the rhinoplasty surgeon. Many techniques have been described either focusing on the fifth and sixth ribs or lower in the thorax on the eighth and ninth ribs. Our preference is to harvest segments of either the fifth or sixth rib through a well-camouflaged inframammary incision. This approach is used in male and female patients with minimal postoperative visibility. Careful dissection is required in patients who have had previous augmentation mammoplasty to avoid disruption of the implant. Rib harvest is always on the right side so as not to be confused with chest pain of a cardiac origin if the left side was used. Segments of the eighth or ninth ribs may be chosen if longer segments of cartilage or composite osteocartilaginous grafts are required.

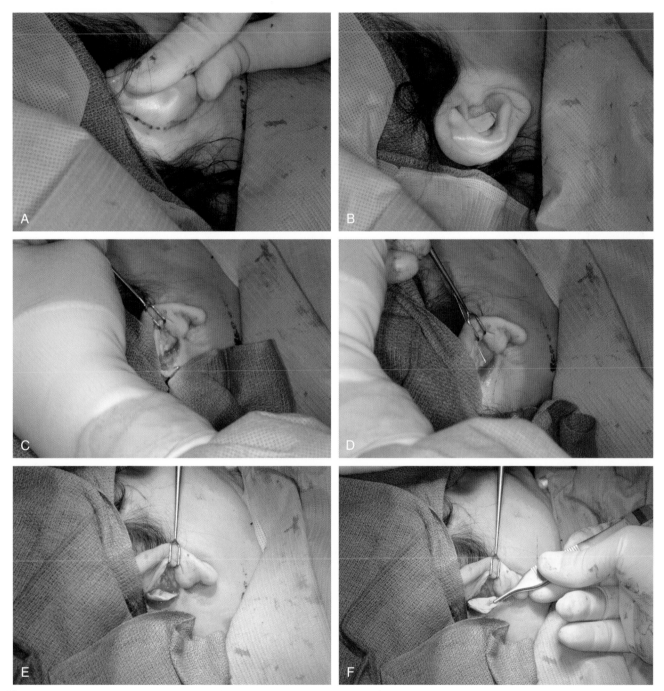

Figure 11-6 A, Postauricular harvest approach. **B,** Template measuring amount of cartilage required. **C,** Postauricular skin elevation. **D,** A 25-gauge needle can be passed to mark the anterior edge of the conchal bowl. **E,** Available cartilage for harvest. **F,** Templated amount of cartilage removed.

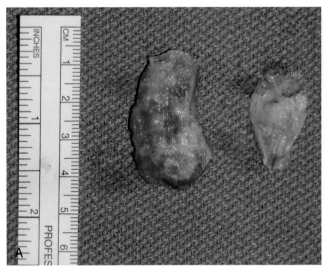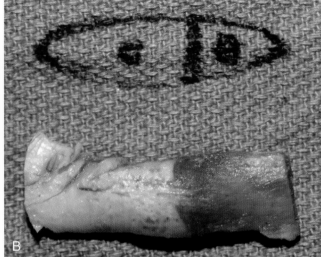

Figure 11-7 A, Harvested costal cartilage (*left*) and perichondrium (*right*). **B,** Osteocartilaginous rib graft with cartilaginous component (*left*) and bony component (*right*).

The skin is infiltrated with 1% lidocaine with 1:100,000 epinephrine. Upon encountering the extrathoracic musculature, every effort is made to not transect any fibers and instead to incise along and retract the fibers to expose the glistening rib below. This careful dissection significantly decreases postoperative pain and splinting, which can lead to atelectasis. Upon identifying the selected rib, the osteocartilaginous junction is easily identified. Dissection is carried out anteriorly to expose more of the cartilaginous component of the rib. If perichondrium is required, parallel incisions are made at the upper and lower edge of the rib. Extreme care must be taken not to drop off the edge of the cartilage thereby preventing injury to the neurovascular bundle or underlying pleura. The incisions are connected vertically just anterior to the osteocartilaginous junction. The perichondrium is elevated off of the cartilage and a perichondrial graft of appropriate length is harvested. A larger than required graft is often taken to account for shrinkage of the graft. The cartilage is now clearly visible. Based on the volume requirements, a decision is made whether to take a full-thickness segment of rib or to dissect a "chevron"-shaped segment from the central portion.

If a full-thickness segment harvest is required, dissection in a subperichondrial plane is performed with a combination of Freer and Doyen elevators. Upon ensuring that the underlying pleura has been safely dissected free of the undersurface of the rib, a segment can be harvested. The wound is carefully examined for any evidence of bleeding or violation of the pleura. The cavity is filled with saline and the anesthesiologist is asked to apply a large positive pressure to maximally inflate the lung. Presence of bubbles indicate a pleural rent, which should be identified and repaired. Upon identifying the pleural defect, a purse string suture of 3-0 Vicryl is placed around a red

rubber catheter. While applying suction, the red rubber catheter is slowly removed and the suture is cinched down while the anesthesiologist maintains positive pressure. A postoperative upright chest radiography should be performed.

More frequently, a "chevron"-shaped segment is harvested, providing adequate grafting material while leaving the rib contour intact and decreasing the risk of pleural injury and significantly minimizing postoperative pain. The absence of flail anterior and posterior segments of rib markedly reduces pain on inspiration in these patients. The technique begins with incising the rib cartilage along the superior and inferior borders beveling toward the center of the rib. Next an incision is made at the articulation of the bony and cartilaginous rib, and, last, an incision is made anteriorly connecting the horizontal limbs. The cartilage is dissected with a freer elevator maintaining a shelf of cartilage on the pleural aspect of the rib. The harvested cartilage is measured to assure adequacy of length and volume. The cavity is tested for air leaks as previously described (Figure 11-8).

Prior to closure, the area is infiltrated with 6 to 8 mL of 0.25% bupivacaine with 1:200,000 epinephrine. Closure is performed by obliterating the dead space with 3-0 vicryl and closing the skin edges with a 4-0 monocryl. The appearance of the scar postoperatively is minimal and well camouflaged in the inframammary crease (Figure 11-9).

A drawback of costal cartilage is the need for a distant secondary harvest site with risks of scarring, postoperative pain, and pneumothorax. Additionally, many patients express concern about having segments of rib(s) removed for nasal surgery. Candid discussion with prospective rib graft patients helps to allay many fears regarding the procedure. Careful harvesting techniques and

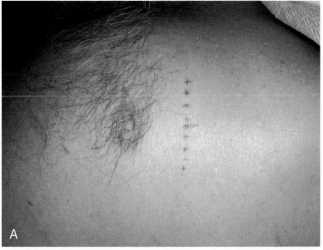

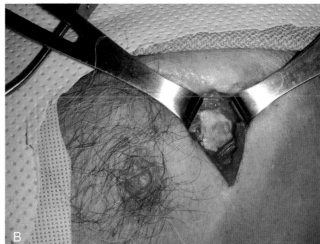

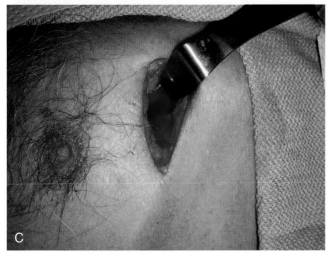

Figure 11-8 A, Planned incision for costal cartilage harvest. **B,** Adequate exposure with limited incision. **C,** Checking for air leak after removal of cartilage.

management of postoperative pain are crucial to this end. Other disadvantages of costal cartilage grafts include the potential for warping, resorption, visibility under thin or compromised soft tissue envelope, and difficulty in morselizing or crushing the grafts.

INDICATIONS FOR CARTILAGE GRAFTING

The application of grafts once harvested is limited only by the skill and creativity of the surgeon. Septal grafts alone can be used for support and augmentation (Figure 11-10). Auricular donor cartilage can be fashioned into planoconcave or planoconvex orientations to support or replace absent or deficient nasal structures (Figure 11-11). Often, in camouflaging applications, the harvested cartilage will be rendered more pliable and conforming by gently morselizing the cartilage with a morselizer or flattening contour irregularities with a Cottle cartilage crusher (Figure 11-12). Numerous grafts from multiple sources can be applied in both morselized and nonmorselized applications in situations requiring support,

and camouflage of nasal cartilage (Figure 11-13). Costal cartilage grafts provide an excellent source of autologous cartilage in revision rhinoplasty patients who lack septal or auricular cartilage. Individuals who require significant augmentation or rigid support are also best treated with use of costal grafting (Figure 11-14). The large volume of harvested cartilage can be fashioned into dorsal augmentation, alar replacement, batten, and columellar strut grafts (Figure 11-15).

CONCLUSION

Cartilage grafting is one of the most important tools in structural rhinoplasty and nasal reconstruction. There is an abundance of autologous cartilage with varying characteristics. Cartilage grafts are biocompatible and incorporate seamlessly when properly used in areas of adequate soft tissue coverage. Resorption is minimal even with large-volume grafts. Complications seen with

Text continued on page 157

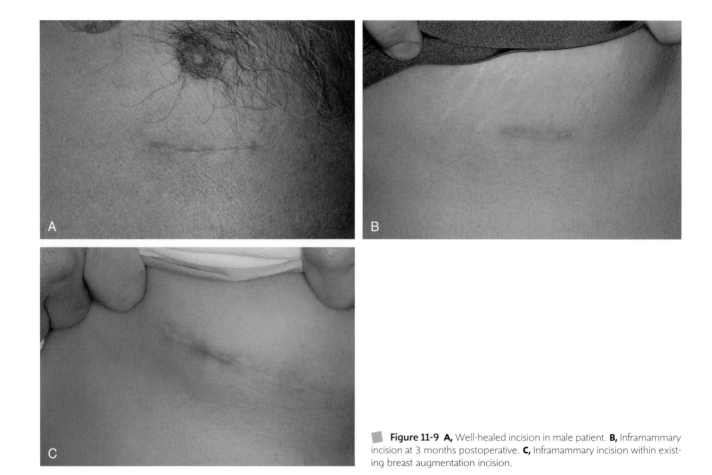

Figure 11-9 A, Well-healed incision in male patient. **B,** Inframammary incision at 3 months postoperative. **C,** Inframammary incision within existing breast augmentation incision.

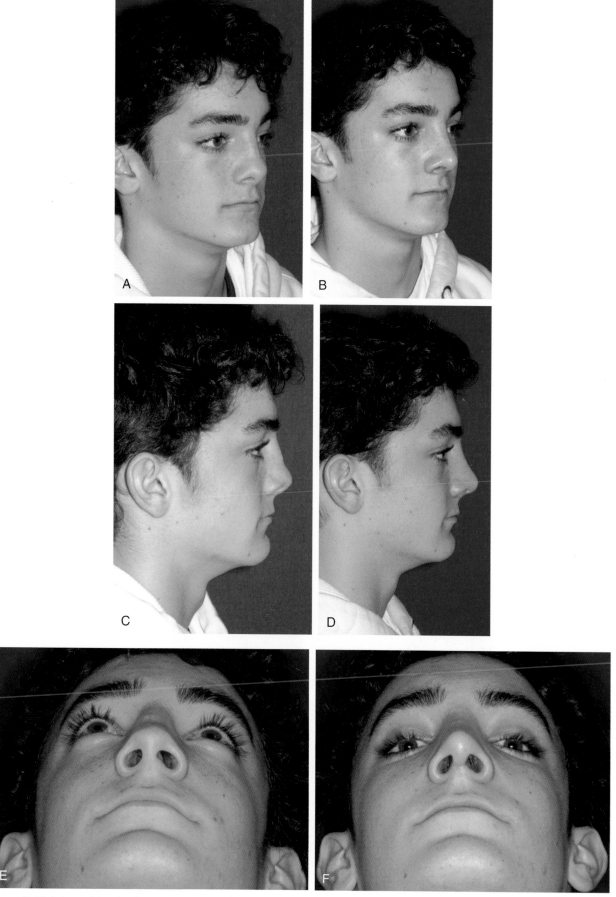

Figure 11-10 A, Loss of dorsal and tip support post nasal trauma. Preoperative oblique view. **B,** Postoperative oblique after septal cartilage dorsal onlay and tip support grafting. **C,** Preoperative lateral. **D,** Postoperative lateral. **E,** Preoperative base view. **F,** Postoperative base view.

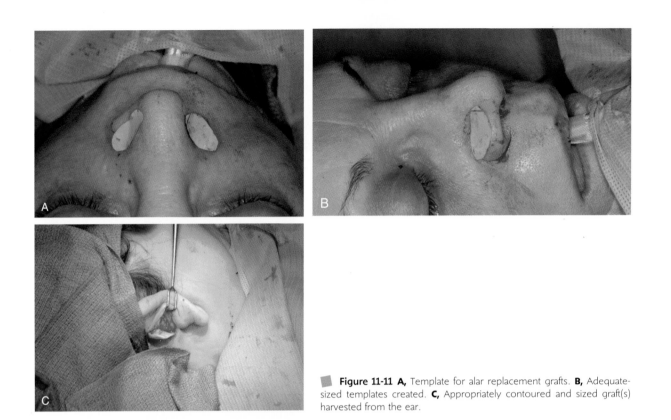

Figure 11-11 A, Template for alar replacement grafts. **B,** Adequate-sized templates created. **C,** Appropriately contoured and sized graft(s) harvested from the ear.

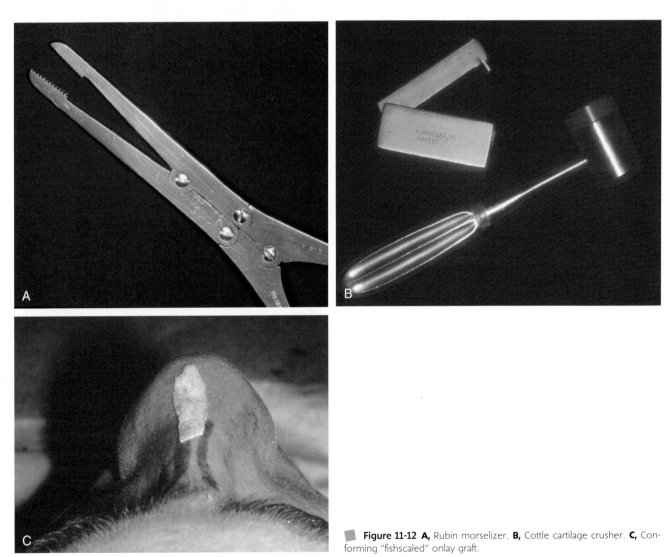

Figure 11-12 A, Rubin morselizer. **B,** Cottle cartilage crusher. **C,** Conforming "fishscaled" onlay graft.

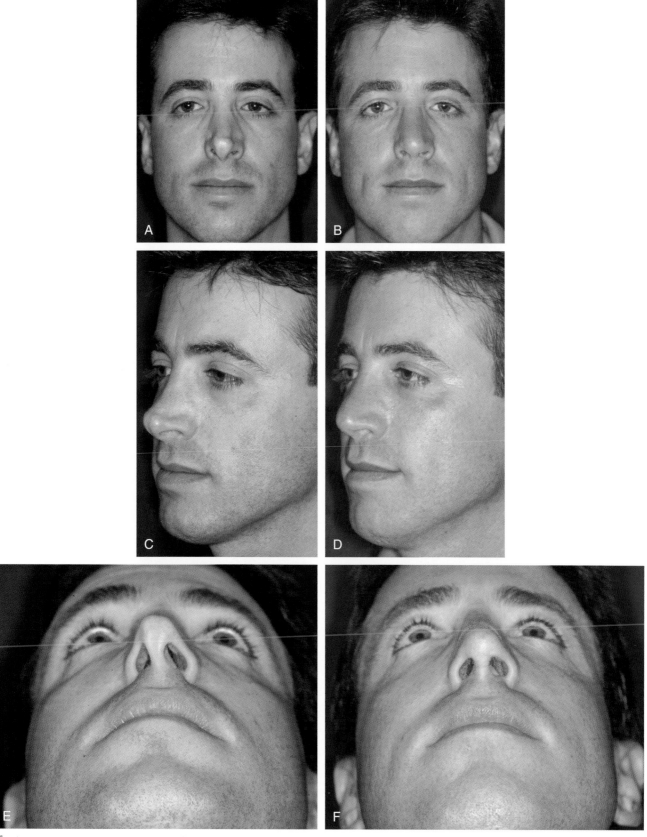

Figure 11-13 A, Contour abnormalities after three previous failed rhinoplasties. Preoperative frontal view. **B,** Postoperative frontal view after grafting with septal and auricular cartilage. Nonmorselized grafts used for support and morselized grafts used for camouflage. **C,** Preoperative oblique view. **D,** Postoperative oblique view. **E,** Preoperative base view. **F,** Postoperative base view.

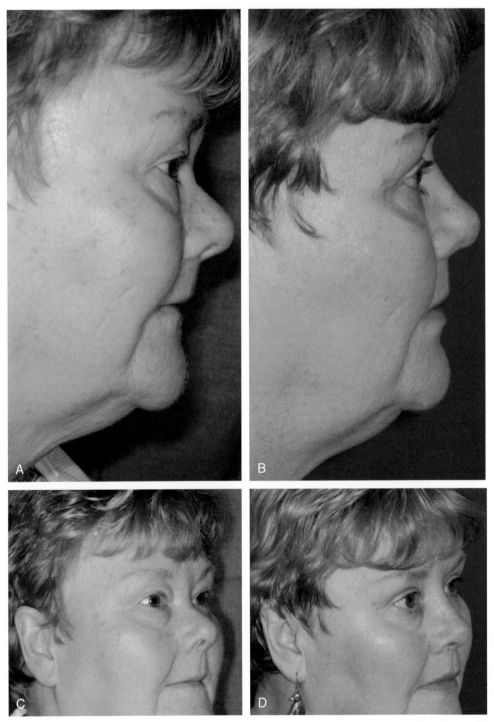

Figure 11-14 A, Traumatic loss of dorsal support. Preoperative lateral view. **B,** Postoperative lateral view after costal cartilage graft rhinoplasty. **C,** Preoperative oblique view. **D,** Postoperative oblique view.

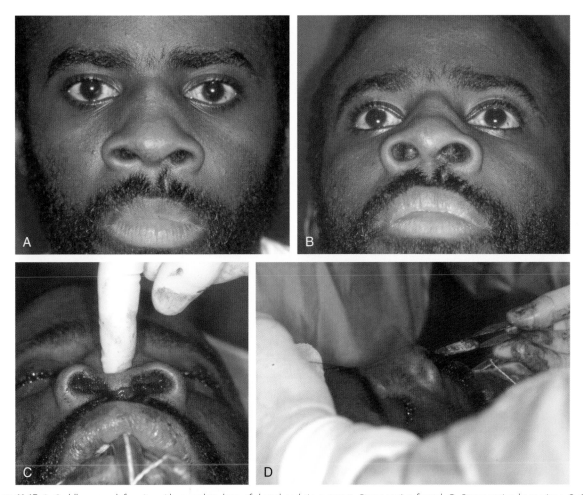

Figure 11-15 A, Saddle nose deformity with complete loss of dorsal and tip support. Preoperative frontal. **B,** Preoperative base view. **C,** Complete absence of tip support. **D,** Dorsal augmentation costal cartilage graft guided in with transcutaneous suture.

Continued

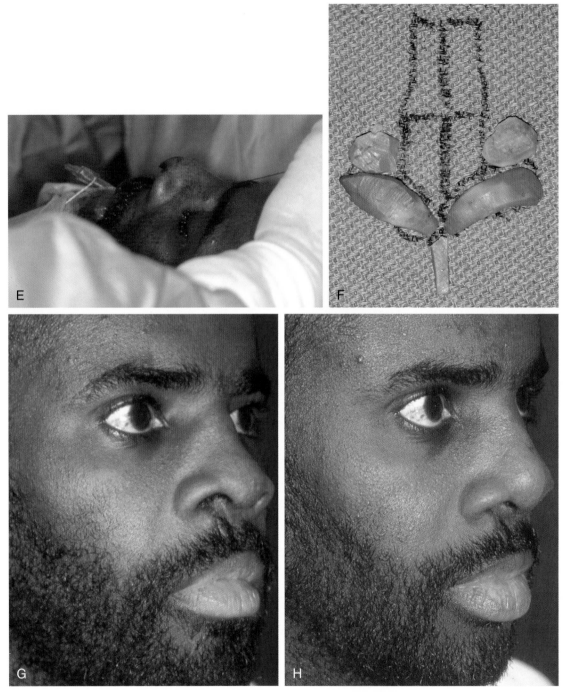

Figure 11-15, cont'd. E, Suture externalized and tied over a bolster. **F,** Numerous grafts fashioned from rib cartilage. **G,** Saddle nose deformity with absent tip and dorsal support. Preoperative oblique. **H,** Postoperative oblique after dorsal, alar replacement, batten, tip, and columellar strut grafts.

alloplastic material such as migration, extrusion, and chronic infection are rarely seen with autogenous tissue. Despite biomaterial research into alloplastic alternatives, it is unlikely a graft with the same reliability and safety profile will be available soon. With further research into bioengineering, plastic surgeons should look forward to the availability of "off-the-shelf" bioengineered cartilage with similar characteristic with regard to rigidity, resistance to resorption, ability to be carved, and host compatibility.[12]

REFERENCES

1. Berghaus A, Stetler K. Alloplastic materials in rhinoplasty. *Curr Opin Otolaryngol Head Neck Surg.* 2006;14(4): 270–277.

2. Acaturk S, Arslan E, Demirkan F, Unal S. An algorithm for deciding alternative grafting materials in secondary rhinoplasty. *J Plast Reconstr Aesthet Surg.* 2006;59(4): 409–416.

3. Romo 3rd T, Kwak ES. Nasal grafts and implants in revision rhinoplasty. *Fac Plast Surg Clin North Am.* 2006;14(4): 373–387.

4. Godin MS, Waldman SR, Johnson Jr CM. Nasal augmentation using Gore-Tex. A 10-year experience. *Arch Fac Plast Surg.* 1999;1(2):118–121.

5. Quatela VC, Jacono AA. Structural grafting in rhinoplasty. *Fac Plast Surg.* 2002;18(4):223–232.

6. Erol OO. The Turkish Delight: A pliable graft for rhinoplasty. *Plast Reconstr Surg.* 2000;105(6):2229–2241.

7. Daniel RK, Calvert JW. Diced cartilage grafts in rhinoplasty surgery. *Plast Reconstr Surg.* 2004;113(7):2156–2171.

8. Becker DG, Becker SS, Saad AA. Auricular cartilage in revision rhinoplasty. *Fac Plast Surg.* 2003;19(1):41–52.

9. Sherris DA, Kern EB. The versatile autogenous rib graft in septorhinoplasty. *Am J Rhinol.* 1998;12(3):221–227.

10. Defatta RJ, Williams 3rd EF. The decision process in choosing costal cartilage for use in revision rhinoplasty. *Fac Plast Surg.* 2008;24(3):365–371.

11. Cakmak O, Buyuklu F, Yilmaz Z, et al. Viability of cultured human nasal septum chondrocytes after crushing. *Arch Fac Plast Surg.* 2005;7(6):406–409.

12. Skodacek D, Brandau S, Deutschle T, et al. Growth factors and scaffold composition influence properties of tissue engineered human septal cartilage implants in a murine model. *Int J Immunopathol Pharmacol.* 2008;21(4):807–816.

The Middle Vault: Upper Lateral Cartilage Modifications

Kate Elizabeth McCarn • *Brian W. Downs* • *Ted A. Cook* • *Tom D. Wang*

The importance of the middle third of the nose has been increasingly recognized in recent years. Reductive rhinoplasty techniques performed without regard for the structural integrity of this region can cause structural and functional compromise. In this chapter, the anatomy, physiology, and pathologies in this important region will be described, followed by a discussion of the various techniques that are used to address the middle third, including hump reduction, spreader grafts, butterfly grafts, and batten grafts. Focus will be placed on preserving or augmenting the support in the middle vault so that pleasing functional and cosmetic results are maximized.

ANATOMY AND PHYSIOLOGY

The middle third of the nose is important both cosmetically and functionally. The middle nasal vault encompasses the region bounded superiorly by the rhinion, inferiorly by the cephalic border of the lower lateral cartilages, and laterally at the piriform aperture.[1] The soft tissue envelope is the thinnest over the dorsum of the middle third of the nose, making cartilaginous irregularities difficult to conceal and presenting a challenge to the surgeon, especially in thin-skinned patients. The mucosa lining the middle third of the nose is thin and tightly adherent to the upper lateral cartilage and cartilaginous septum.

The structural framework of the middle third of the nose consists of the cartilaginous septum and the upper lateral cartilages (Figure 12-1). Superiorly, the upper lateral cartilages fuse with the deep surface of the caudal edge of the nasal bones. Caudally, the upper lateral cartilage curves under and articulates with the lower lateral cartilages in the scroll region, which is considered to be a major tip support mechanism. Medially, the upper lateral cartilages fuse with the cartilaginous dorsum via dense fibrous attachments, while inferiorly the medial edge of the cartilage is often free. It is important to note that the cartilaginous septum widens to a T-like shape dorsally where it articulates with the upper lateral cartilages, forming a single unit that defines the dorsal subunit of the

nose. The lateral aspect of the upper lateral cartilage is adherent to fibrous tissue that approaches the piriform aperture and, if present, the sesamoid cartilages. Violation of the support for the upper lateral cartilages can cause cosmetic and functional problems, including nasal obstruction and the inverted-V deformity.

The internal nasal valve is an important functional anatomic unit. It is bounded medially by the septum, superiorly by the caudal edge of the upper lateral cartilages and fibrofatty tissue adjacent to the piriform aperture, and inferiorly by the anterior head of the inferior turbinate and nasal floor. It is the point of maximum narrowing of the airway and resistance to airflow on inspiration.[2] In Caucasians, the ideal angle between the upper lateral cartilage and the septum is 10 to 15 degrees. The valve measures between 55 and 83 mm².

EXAMINATION

A thorough examination of the middle third of the nose is critical for accurate diagnosis and surgical planning. The examination is straightforward and is best achieved in the office during the initial consultation. After a detailed history has established the patient's goals for surgical intervention, the nose is examined in a systematic fashion. With respect to the middle third of the nose, it is important to notice the character of the soft tissue envelope, the relation of the middle third to the patient's midline and the upper and lower thirds of the nose, the brow-tip aesthetic line, and the radix. The surface of the nose should be examined during quiet and deeper inspiration from a frontal and base view, looking for collapse of the internal or external nasal valves. The strength and integrity of the upper lateral cartilages and the character of the cartilaginous dorsum can be ascertained by palpation. Using a nasal speculum and headlight, all three components of the nasal valve (side wall, septum, and turbinate) should be examined. A cerumen curette can be used to identify precisely the site of nasal collapse. Targeted use of the curette provides more detailed information than the traditional Cottle maneuver. Finally, if there

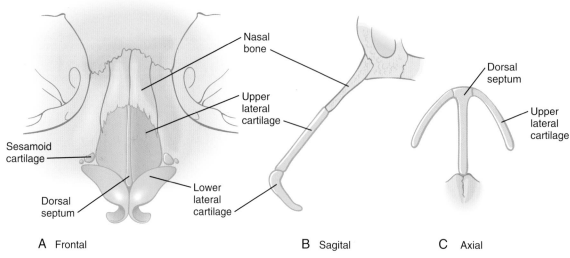

Figure 12-1 Middle nasal vault anatomy.

is any question of allergic or other mucosal disease, the nose can be sprayed with a topical vasoconstrictor and the examination repeated to determine whether further evaluation for allergic or other sinonasal pathology is warranted. Endoscopy can also be a useful tool in evaluating the internal nasal valve and in documenting valve collapse.

PROBLEMS OF THE MIDDLE THIRD

The middle third of the nose must be harmonious with the upper and lower thirds of the nose. The brow-tip aesthetic line should be unbroken, and the width between the brow-tip line should fall between the tip-defining points laterally and philtral columns medially. The most frequent request from cosmetic rhinoplasty patients is to take down a dorsal hump. While it is important to respect the patient's wishes, it is also critical that they are aware of the limitations posed by their anatomy and the consequences of overresection including narrowing of the dorsum and nasal obstruction.

Septorhinoplasty may cause collapse of the upper lateral cartilages or excessive narrowing of the dorsum. Destabilization of the upper lateral cartilages can result in cartilaginous collapse, causing the caudal contour of the nasal bones to become visible (the inverted-V deformity). Overly aggressive resection of the cartilaginous dorsum can cause a saddle nose deformity when the septum is lowered or separated from the nasal bones. A twisted or crooked middle third can result from septal deviation or fracture, trauma, or prior surgery.

Functional problems of the middle vault can be caused by a variety of pathologies. Those patients with

inherently short nasal bones, a thin soft tissue envelope, and weak cartilages are particularly susceptible to postoperative problems and therefore require careful planning at the time of surgery to maintain the integrity of this critical anatomic region.

Internal nasal valve obstruction can be static or dynamic. Static valve obstruction can be caused by a deviated dorsal septum, mucosal disease, or any other anatomic variation that blocks the valve. Dynamic valve collapse occurs when the strength of the upper lateral cartilages and soft tissue of the valve are unable to withstand the forces of inspiration (Figure 12-2). Even small changes in the radius of the valve can have an impact on nasal airflow as predicted by Poiseuille's law (proportional to the radius to the fourth power).

MATERIALS FOR USE IN THE MIDDLE THIRD

Grafting material used in the middle third falls into two broad categories: structural and camouflage. The ideal structural material in the middle third is biocompatible, strong enough to provide support, soft enough to achieve a natural feel, and able to be shaped or molded in order to obtain a smooth contour. Septal cartilage is readily available in the primary rhinoplasty patient. In patients undergoing revision rhinoplasty or those patients with insufficient septal cartilage, autologous costal cartilage is useful but is associated with donor site morbidity in a small number of patients. Alternatives include irradiated homologous costal cartilage,[3] calvarial bone, porous polyethylene (Medpor; Porex, Newnan, GA), and autologous conchal cartilage. Camouflage grafting materials include

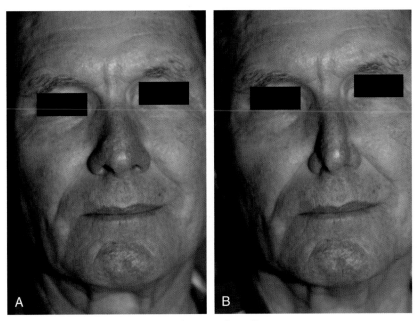

Figure 12-2 A, Patient at rest. **B,** With inspiration, demonstrating dynamic valve collapse.

GORE-TEX (Gore, Newark, DE), cartilage, fascia, and a wide variety of injectable fillers.

APPROACHES

The middle third of the nose is readily accessible via either the endonasal or external approach. Choice of approach is ultimately up to the surgeon and should be determined by the anatomy and the degree of exposure required based on the preoperative evaluation. The endonasal approach is useful for creating precise pockets for placement of grafts, and it has the advantage of minimizing edema and avoiding external scars. However, it affords less exposure than the external approach. If the endonasal approach is used and access to the dorsal septum is necessary (i.e., spreader grafts are going to be placed), a hemitransfixion incision will provide better access than a Killian incision. The external approach is useful in those cases, where, due to trauma or previous surgery, the anatomy is uncertain or in cases where modification of the tip or septum requires the exposure afforded by this approach. The main advantage of the external approach for the middle vault is that it allows for accurate visualization and precise positioning and securing of grafting materials. The proper approach is the one that allows the surgeon adequate visualization and the best control over the maneuvers that are being performed while minimizing scarring and edema.

Regardless of the approach, careful attention to technique is important. Of particular importance in the middle third is identifying the plane deep to the subnasal superficial musculoaponeurotic system (SMAS). Injection of local anesthetic can assist in this dissection. Mucosa and mucoperichondrium should be carefully dissected and left intact. Mucosal tears or cartilage exposure can lead to scarring, cosmetic deformity, and airway compromise.

TECHNIQUES

GENERAL

The sequence of maneuvers in rhinoplasty is a widely debated topic among surgeons and ultimately a matter of preference. One logical sequence, and the sequence used at our institution in those patients requiring an open structured approach, is to perform a standard external approach via a transcolumellar and bilateral marginal incisions. The soft tissue envelope is elevated, exposing the upper lateral cartilages, and then elevation is continued in a subperiosteal plane over the nasal bones. After adequate exposure is obtained, the septal cartilage is exposed starting at the anterior septal angle. Dissection continues dorsally to the junction of the upper lateral cartilages and the septum. The upper lateral cartilages are then sharply divided from the dorsal septum. The septum is addressed and is often a source of cartilage for spreader, tip, and onlay grafting. Care is taken to maintain the continuity of the mucoperichondrium of the septum and nasal lining and to leave behind a sufficient L-strut for nasal support. The resected cartilage is placed in saline for later use. Further modification of the middle vault is carried out after the osteotomies have been performed. Once the septum and bony pyramid have been addressed, any inherent deviation of the remaining middle third is corrected and structural grafting performed as needed. Tip work is done last so that the tip is harmonious with the upper two thirds of the nose

HUMP REDUCTION AND ONLAY GRAFTING

Taking down a dorsal hump is a common request of the rhinoplasty patient and can be performed via the endonasal or external approach. The cartilaginous dorsum can be resected using a 10-mm osteotome, taking the cartilage in continuity with the bony dorsum or via sharp dissection using a No. 15 scalpel or sharp dissecting scissors. Hall describes a modified Skoog dorsal reduction wherein the cartilaginous hump is taken in continuity with the bone, further resection is then carried out, the excised dorsum is sculpted and replaced, and the remaining upper lateral cartilages are suspended to the dorsal cartilaginous remnant.[4] The dorsal remnant essentially functions as a dorsal onlay spreader graft. Gassner et al.[5] describe the use of septal cartilage as a dorsal onlay graft that is sutured to the septum and upper lateral cartilages for reconstruction of the middle vault. In those patients who require narrowing of the dorsum and do not have nasal valve compromise, selective resection of the medial portion of the upper lateral cartilage can be performed such that the incision is beveled in order to leave more cartilage on the ventral surface (Figure 12-3). This bevel in the cartilage assists the cartilages in maintaining their convex confirmation rather than bowing in to form a C-shape that can pinch the middle third and narrow the nasal valve.[6]

Regardless of the technique used to take down the dorsum, care must be taken to preserve the mucoperichondrium at the angle of the upper lateral cartilage and dorsal septum. Maintaining this tissue improves support in this important area preventing collapse of the upper lateral cartilages.

SPREADER GRAFTS

Spreader grafts are the workhorse of middle nasal vault surgery. Many permutations of spreader grafts have arisen since its original description by Sheen[7] (Figure 12-4). The original spreader graft is a matchstick-shaped graft that is secured between the upper lateral cartilage and septum extending from the bony–cartilaginous junction to the anterior septal angle. The spreader graft has proved useful in correction of the twisted nose, where it can be used to help anchor the septum into a straighter configuration. They can be used in primary rhinoplasty to re-secure the upper lateral cartilages to the dorsal septum, helping to

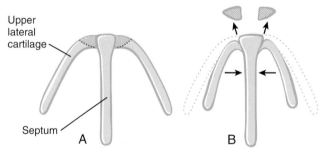

Upper
lateral
cartilage

Septum   A   B

Figure 12-3 Beveled resection of upper lateral cartilage to minimize narrowing of the nasal vault.

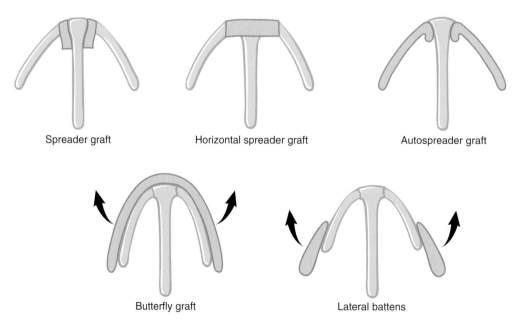

Spreader graft   Horizontal spreader graft   Autospreader graft

Butterfly graft   Lateral battens

Figure 12-4 Grafting in the middle third of the nose cross-sectional anatomy. **A,** Spreader grafts. **B,** Horizontal spreader grafts. **C,** Autospreader grafts. **D,** Butterfly graft. **E,** Lateral battens.

improve the structural integrity of the roof of the middle nasal vault and preventing postoperative collapse and inverted-V deformity. The use of spreader grafts has been described in functional rhinoplasty. It is useful in addressing static narrowing of the nasal valve, but most surgeons believe that it does little to address dynamic collapse unless combined with other techniques such as flaring sutures as described by Park.[8]

The spreader graft is most often fashioned from a straight piece of septal cartilage, although any straight piece of cartilage or other grafting material may be used. Spreaders can be placed via either the external or endonasal approach. When the endonasal approach is used, precise mucoperichondrial flaps are raised along the dorsal septum and the grafts placed within these pockets. The graft measures 1 to 4 mm in width and 3 to 6 mm deep, and the length should approximate the length of the upper lateral cartilages so that the graft extends from the osseocartilaginous junction to just past the anterior septal angle. Using the external approach, the graft is placed between the dorsal septum and upper lateral cartilages under direct visualization (Figure 12-5). It is important to position the graft so that the dorsal margin of the graft is flush with the dorsal septum and no contour irregularity is visible. PDS (polydiaxanone; Ethicon, Sommerville, NJ) suture is used to secure the grafts in place via a horizontal mattress suture through bilateral grafts and the dorsal septum. If necessary, a straight 27-gauge needle can be placed though-and-through to hold the grafts in position while suturing. Papel describes suturing the caudal edge of the upper lateral cartilage to the septum to provide traction and prevent buckling of the upper lateral cartilage.[9] Depending on the deformity that is being corrected, slightly wider grafts or stacked multiple grafts can be used unilaterally to achieve a more symmetric result or help maintain the crooked dorsal septum in a straighter configuration (Figure 12-6).

When spreader grafts are used in conjunction with flaring sutures, measurable improvements in the area of the nasal valve and nasal airflow are possible.[10] The flaring suture is a horizontal mattress suture extending across both upper lateral cartilages and supports the upper lateral cartilages. Critics of this technique site are concerned about the long-term stability of the suture.

The autospreader graft[11] can be used to restore support to the middle vault after hump reduction. The medial edge of the upper lateral cartilage is scored and folded in onto itself and suture secured (see Figure 12-4). This helps restore a convex configuration of the upper lateral cartilages, thus resisting collapse of the internal nasal valve. Figure 12-7 illustrates a case in which this technique was applied in a primary rhinoplasty patient.

The horizontal spreader graft is used in those circumstances where sufficient width cannot be achieved with a conventional spreader graft. It is a wide, flat piece of cartilage resting atop the dorsal septum and secured to both upper lateral cartilages. Securing this graft can be challenging but it can yield more significant improvements in the nasal airway and restore the width of the overresected dorsum (Figure 12-8).

Extended spreader grafts are used to achieve purposes beyond stabilization of the upper lateral cartilages, and they have use in lengthening the short nose, stabilizing an "open roof" of the nasal bones, and widening the pinched dorsum.[12] Caudal extension of the spreader graft can lengthen a foreshortened nose and counteract the forces of contraction and healing to maintain desired tip rotation. The graft is fashioned in the usual manner but with added length so that the tip is supported. If the graft extends much beyond the septal angle, it can push the domes laterally, producing a widened tip. In the upper third, spreader grafts can be extended superiorly between the septum and nasal bones to add width to the bony dorsum in the pinched nose.

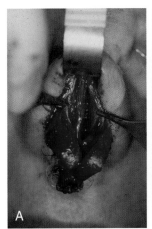
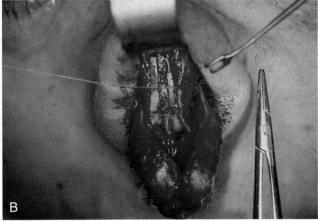

Figure 12-5 A, Intraoperative photo demonstrating the exposure and dissection used via the external approach to place spreader grafts. Note the upper lateral cartilages have been separated from the dorsal septum. **B,** Spreader grafts in situ.

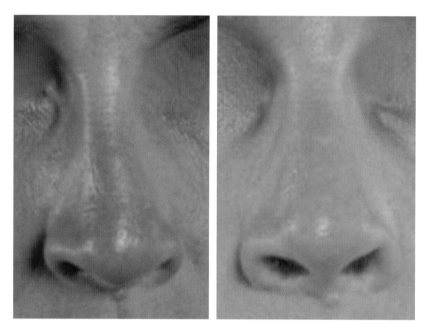

Right unilat spreader

Figure 12-6 A, Preoperative photo of patient with nasal asymmetry. **B,** After placement of a right-sided spreader graft.

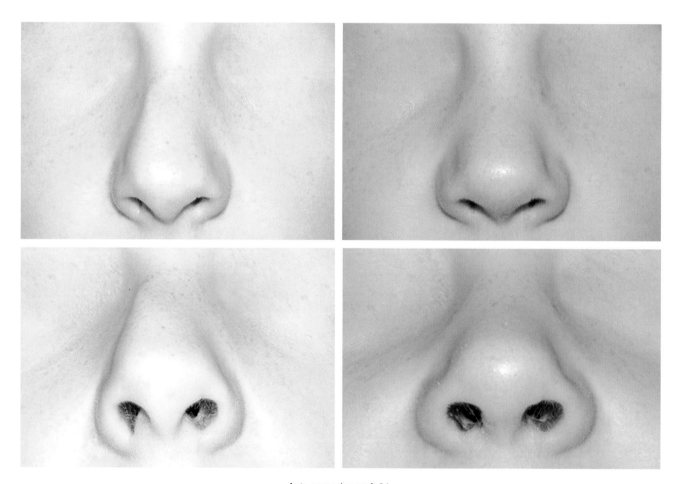

Auto spreader graft 01

Figure 12-7 *Upper left,* Preoperative frontal view. *Upper right,* After primary rhinoplasty with removal of the dorsal hump and use of the autospreader graft. *Lower left,* Preoperative base view. *Lower right,* Postoperative.

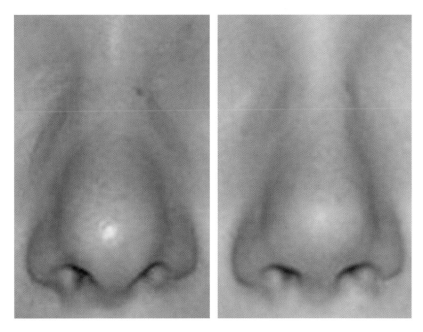

Horizontal spreader

Figure 12-8 *Left,* Preoperatively. *Right,* After placement of a horizontal spreader graft.

BUTTERFLY GRAFTS

The butterfly graft is a useful tool in treating collapse of the middle nasal vault.[2] It is an oval-shaped cartilage that is placed so that it lies on the dorsal surface of the upper lateral cartilages. It addresses both dynamic and static collapse by opening the angle between the upper lateral cartilages and the septum and providing support for weak upper lateral cartilages against the negative forces generated by inspiration.

Conchal cartilage is the ideal material for use as a butterfly graft. The graft is harvested via the anterior approach, elevating skin and perichondrium of the conchal bowl. A curved piece of cartilage measuring at least 3 cm in length by 1 cm in width is harvested, and the donor site closed using an absorbable suture, with a bolster placed to prevent hematoma accumulation. Donor site morbidity and deformity are generally minimal.

The graft is shaped so that any irregularities are minimized and the ends tapered to smooth the skin over the graft. The graft can be placed either by creation of a precise pocket via the endonasal approach or via the external approach. Care must be taken with the endonasal approach to create a pocket that will not allow shifting of the graft. Via the external approach, the graft may be sutured to the lower lateral cartilages with a permanent monofilament suture. Figure 12-9 illustrates the harvest and anatomic placement of a butterfly graft.

The butterfly graft gives patients seeking improvement in their nasal airway good results. The complaint that is sometimes encountered is that the graft broadens the dorsum and can cause some supratip fullness. Shaping and placing the graft appropriately and resecting some septal cartilage to create a bed for the graft can minimize these potential pitfalls, as can counseling the patient preoperatively regarding the objectives of the procedure. Figure 12-10 illustrates a case in which a butterfly graft was placed.

LATERAL BATTEN GRAFTS

In those patients with internal valve collapse due to a weak lateral nasal side wall, a cartilage graft in this area can be helpful and avoids the dorsal deformity that can sometimes result from a butterfly graft. This area is particularly prone to collapse in the aging patient and the patient with facial paralysis.

A batten graft measuring up to 1.5 × 1.5 cm is fashioned from either septal or conchal cartilage (Figure 12-11). The external or endonasal approach may be used, creating a lateral pocket that approaches and overlaps the piriform aperture. Care must be taken in ensuring hemostasis as this region is well vascularized. The graft is placed laterally over the lateral aspect of the upper lateral cartilage and within the dense fibrous tissue that approaches the piriform aperture (see Figure 12-4). The graft may be secured with an absorbable suture.

DORSAL GRAFTING

Grafting of the nasal dorsum falls into one of two categories: structural or camouflage. Beyond spreader grafts,

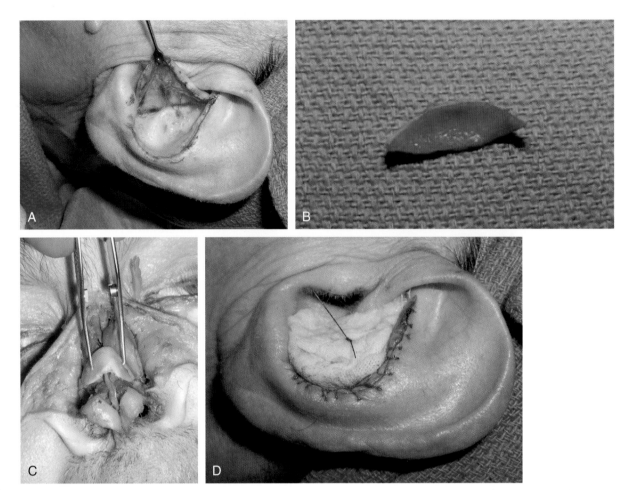

Figure 12-9 A, Harvest of conchal cartilage for use as a butterfly graft. **B,** Butterfly graft. **C,** Proper placement of the butterfly graft. **D,** Dressing for donor site.

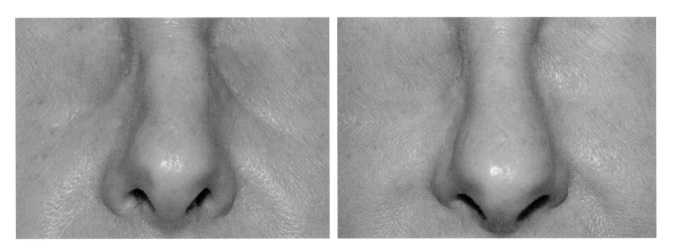

Butterfly graft 01

Figure 12-10 *Left,* This patient has undergone rhinoplasty and now presents with nasal airway obstruction. *Right,* After revision rhinoplasty with placement of butterfly graft.

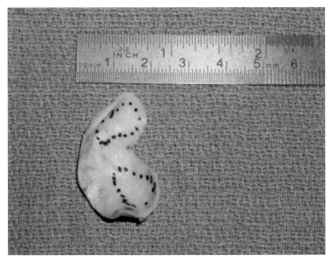

Figure 12-11 Harvested conchal cartilage with batten grafts outlined.

dorsal grafts can also be used to reconstruct the middle third of the nose in the patient with a severely injured, weak, or cartilage-depleted nose. Dorsal grafting material must be compatible with use in the middle third, keeping in mind that the thin skin overlying the dorsum here will readily reveal any contour irregularity. Autologous and irradiated rib are useful tools in dorsal grafting—the complication of warping can be minimized by using a central portion of cartilage and by soaking the cartilage in saline so as to reveal and address any deformity. Using irradiated rib can yield good results with minimal resorption[3] and minimizes the potential donor site morbidity associated with costal cartilage harvest. Stacked conchal or septal cartilage may be used but often is not available in those patients who truly need substantial dorsal grafting. Calvarial bone is strong but hard in comparison with cartilaginous grafts and can require rigid fixation techniques to secure.

In those patients who are unable or unwilling to undergo calvarial bone or costal cartilage harvest, porous polyethylene has also been used to graft the dorsum. Infection and extrusion are the main complications that may be encountered, but meticulous technique such as distancing the graft from the incision can be helpful in avoiding them. Extruding porous polyethylene dorsal grafts can be replaced with irradiated costal cartilage in a single stage.

Camouflage can become necessary in the management of the middle nasal vault, particularly in thin-skinned individuals requiring structural grafts. Morselized cartilage and fascia are useful biocompatible materials for this purpose. The 1-mm GORE-TEX sheets can be used for this purpose as well. The sheets may be stacked to provide additional thickness and achieve a stronger dorsal profile. A press can be used to crimp and taper the edges,

helping to blend the graft in with the surrounding tissue and minimize contour deformities. Finally, for slight contour irregularities in the postoperative patient, a wide variety of injectable fillers are available and, though none have U.S. Food and Drug Administration approval for use in the nose, their use for this purpose is growing.

CONCLUSION

The middle third of the nose is important both structurally and functionally; simple maneuvers such as taking down a dorsal hump can violate the integrity of this region. Providing support for the upper lateral cartilages is possible via a variety of methods and can prevent cosmetic deformity and nasal airway obstruction. The well-equipped surgeon will have a familiarity with a variety of techniques to achieve functionally and aesthetically pleasing results that will withstand the test of time.

REFERENCES

1. Tardy ME, Hendricks D, Alex J, Dayan SH. Surgical anatomy of the nose. In: Bailey B, ed. Head and neck surgery–Otolaryngology. 2nd ed. Philadelphia: Lippincott; 1998: 641–660.
2. Clark JM, Cook TA. The 'butterfly' graft in functional secondary rhinoplasty. *Laryngoscope.* 2002;112(11): 1917–1925.
3. Weber SM, Cook TA, Wang TD. Irradiated costal cartilage in augmentation rhinoplasty. *Oper Tech Otolaryngol.* 2007;18: 274–283.
4. Hall JA, Peters MD, Hilger PA. Modification of the Skoog dorsal reduction for preservation of the middle nasal vault. *Arch Fac Plast Surg.* 2004;6:105–110.
5. Gassner HG, Friedman O, Sherris DA, et al. An alternative method of middle vault reconstruction. *Arch Fac Plast Surg.* 2006;8:432–435.
6. Thomas JR, Prendiville S. Overly wide cartilaginous middle vault. *Fac Plast Surg Clin N Am.* 2004;12:107–110.
7. Sheen JH. Spreader graft: a method of reconstructing the roof of the middle nasal vault following rhinoplasty. *Plast Reconstr Surg.* 1986;73:230–239.
8. Park SS. The flaring suture to augment the repair of the dysfunctional nasal valve. *Plast Reconstr Surg.* 1998;101(4): 1120–1122.
9. Papel ID Management of the middle vault. In Papel ID, Frodel J, Holt GR, et al, eds. Facial plastic and reconstructive surgery. 2nd ed. New York: Thieme; 2002:407–414.
10. Schlosser RJ, Park SS. Surgery for the dysfunctional nasal valve: cadaveric analysis and clinical outcomes. *Arch Fac Plast Surg.* 1999;1:105–110.
11. Steve BH, Mead RA, Gonyon DL. Using the autospreader flap in primary rhinoplasty. *Plast Reconstr Surg.* 2007;119(6): 1897–1902.
12. Palacin JM, Bravo, FG, Zeky R, Schwarze H. Controlling nasal length with extended spreader grafts: A reliable technique in primary rhinoplasty. *Aesthet Plast Surg.* 2007;31:645–650.

CHAPTER THIRTEEN

The Mobile Tripod Technique: A Universal Approach to Nasal Tip Modification

Robert A. Glasgold • Alvin I. Glasgold • Sanjay P. Keni

One of the most important and difficult aspects of rhinoplasty surgery is creating a nicely shaped, natural-appearing nasal tip. This generally involves altering nasal tip definition, width, projection, and/or rotation. Nasal tip appearance is primarily determined by the shape and strength of the lower lateral cartilages (LLCs). In addition, the tip shape and position are affected by the relationship of the LLCs with adjacent support structures (i.e., septum and upper lateral cartilages [ULCs]) and the characteristics of the overlying skin envelope. Changing nasal tip appearance is usually accomplished by modifying the shape or configuration of the LLCs to create a new tip structure. Reshaping the cartilages requires both maneuvers to release the tip's support mechanisms creating a mobile structure, followed by reconstructive maneuvers to establish a cartilaginous foundation that will translate into a structurally sound and aesthetically pleasing appearance. Many techniques have been described to accomplish these changes.[1-4] The ideal technique for modifying the LLCs should be flexible enough to address a variety of issues, as well as provide predictable and lasting results. The central component of our preferred technique for modifying the nasal tip is vertical angle division of the LLCs to create a "mobile tripod."[5] This separates the lateral crura from the medial and intermediate crura, creating a structure that is more amenable to reshaping as seen in this patient (Figure 13-1).

A description of this technique, and an explanation of its rationale, must be prefaced with a description of the anatomy and relevant terminology. The LLCs consist of a lateral crus, a medial crus, and the variable presence of an intermediate crus between these two. The angle of the LLC is the junction of the medial (or intermediate) crura and lateral crura (Figure 13-2). The dome of the LLC is generally the most prominent portion of the lateral crus, and is located lateral to the angle. The major and minor tip support mechanisms have been reviewed previously in the text. Some of these structural relationships must be released in order to modify nasal tip shape, appearance, projection, and rotation.

Anderson's[6] tripod concept provides a simplified explanation of how alterations to the crural components of the LLCs change the external nasal appearance. This relies on conceptualizing the LLCs as a tripod in which the combined medial-intermediate crura comprise a single inferior limb and each lateral crura comprises the remaining two limbs (Figure 13-3). Altering any one limb of the tripod will affect the position of the lower third of the nose, whether through a change in its projection, rotation, or length. Practical implementation of these concepts may be more challenging as the intact crural arch resists many of the desired changes to the tripod. In the technique described in this chapter, vertical angle division is the centerpiece to developing a "mobile tripod" by removing the forces resisting alar restructuring.[5]

Three key steps isolate the limbs of the "mobile tripod" for subsequent manipulation: (1) releasing the membranous septal attachment between the medial crura and caudal septum; (2) vertical angle division, separating medial (and intermediate) crura from lateral crura; and (3) freeing the cephalic margin of the lateral crura from the ULCs. These steps allow for the individual limbs of the tripod to be modified and repositioned independent of one another. Having released structural supports to facilitate changes to the LLCs, an emphasis must be placed on reestablishing a solid structural foundation to provide a durable result.

The distinction between vertical angle division and traditional dome division technique cannot be emphasized enough. Dome division involves transecting the LLC at the domal portion of the lateral crura; similar to performing a lateral crural steal, with the medial post consisting of the medial, intermediate, and a portion of the lateral crus (Figure 13-4). The resulting tip structure is defined by the apex of the medial post with the lateral crura remnants collapsing to its side. The most common problems

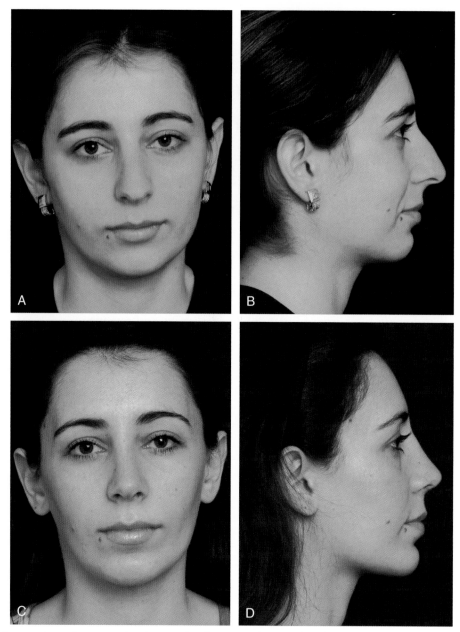

Figure 13-1 A–D, Preoperative and postoperative photographs of patient undergoing rhinoplasty using a vertical angle division to create nasal tip narrowing, definition, rotation, and deprojection.

associated with this technique were tent pole deformities, due to a narrow pointed medial post defining the tip, and alar collapse, due to inadequate support of the lateral crura remnant. In contrast, vertical angle division transects the LLC at the angle, the natural junction between medial-intermediate crura and lateral crura. The entire lateral crura remain intact. The tip structure is created by the contoured medial edge of the lateral crura overriding the slightly splayed medial-intermediate crural complex (Figure 13-5). This produces a more natural and attractive nasal tip appearance and avoids the problems associated with dome division.

TECHNIQUE

OVERVIEW

All cases are performed through an open/external rhinoplasty approach using an inverted-V columellar incision. A relatively consistent sequence of steps is adhered to in this technique, as outlined next.

- Skin flap elevation
- Separate medial crura and identify caudal septum
- Septal mucoperichondrial flap elevation

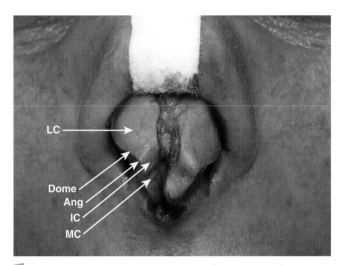

Figure 13-2 Intraoperative photograph demonstrating the components of the lower lateral cartilages: lateral crura (*LC*), intermediate crura (*ic*), medial crura (*MC*), angle (*Ang*), and dome.

- Septal shortening (as needed)
- Septal cartilage harvest
- Closure of septal mucosal flaps
- Elevate vestibular mucosa from under the angle
- Vertical angle division
- Medial crura sutured together
- Mucosal elevation under cephalic margin of lateral crura and separation of lateral crura from ULC (scroll)
- When additional rotation is needed — release and transaction of the lateral tail of the lateral crura
- Cephalic trim of lateral crura
- Graft creation (columella strut) from septal cartilage
- Placement and suture fixation of columella strut in an intracrural premaxillary pocket
- Medial (and intermediate) crural modification — height and shape
- Membranous septal sutures (as needed)
- Extended shield graft (if needed)
- Dorsal modifications

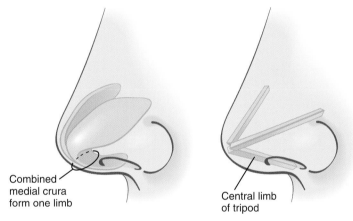

Figure 13-3 Illustration demonstrating lower lateral cartilages forming the nasal tripod. The combined medial crura form one limb and each lateral crura represents the remaining two tripod legs.

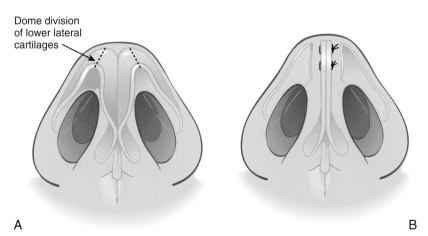

Figure 13-4 A, B, Schematic diagram demonstrating location of lower lateral cartilage transaction with classic dome division. The medial crural post forms the tip and the lateral crura collapse to its side.

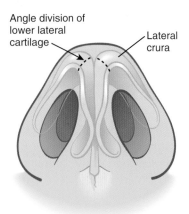
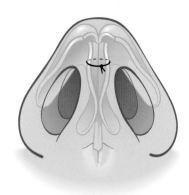

Angle division of
lower lateral
cartilage ⌐   Lateral
                          crura

Figure 13-5 Illustration demonstrating vertical angle division with the tip complex being formed by the lateral crura overriding the splayed apices of the medial crura.

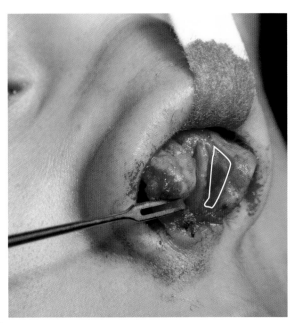

Figure 13-6 Anterior approach to septum. The medial crura are separated and the membranous septum is dissected through to expose the caudal septum. The membranous septum, separating the left lower lateral cartilage and the caudal septum, is indicated by the *white line*.

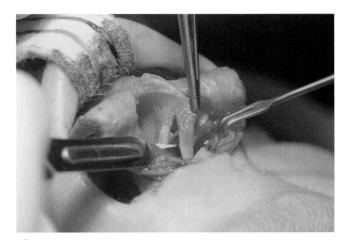

Figure 13-7 The medial crura are retracted to allow for shortening of the caudal septum with a No. 15 blade.

SEPTUM

The caudal septal cartilage is attached to the LLC through the membranous septum. By virtue of this relationship the caudal septum affects nasal tip projection, length, and rotation. The external anterior approach to harvesting septal cartilage requires separation of the medial crura and taking down the membranous septum (Figure 13-6). Releasing this attachment deprojects, shortens, and rotates the nasal tip. Even when these are not the primary goals for a particular patient, this release will also facilitate subsequent efforts to lengthen, counterotate, and/or project the nasal tip freely.

Following the takedown of the membranous septum and elevation of the septal mucosal flaps, caudal septal length is evaluated to determine the need for septal shortening (Figure 13-7). An excessively long septum may interfere with efforts to rotate or shorten the nasal tip impairing free mobilization of the LLC. Septal length is also assessed to ensure adequate room to place a columella strut graft without changing nasal length. After addressing caudal septal length, the septal cartilage is harvested and the mucoperichondrial flaps are sutured together using a quilting suture technique.

LOWER LATERAL CARTILAGES

The angle of the LLC is identified at the junction of the medial (or intermediate) and lateral crus (Figure 13-8). This angle varies in appearance: it can be a well-defined breakpoint or a more subtle and less-defined transition point between medial (or intermediate) and lateral crura.

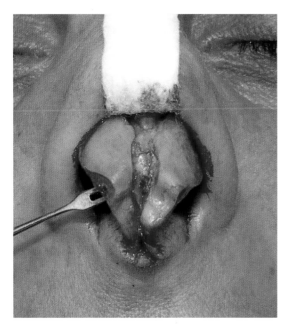

Figure 13-8 The angle of the lower lateral cartilage is identified at the junction of the medial (or intermediate) crus with the lateral crus. In this patient, the angle appears as a well-delineated crease.

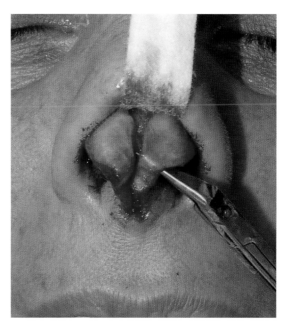

Figure 13-9 The vestibular mucosa is elevated from the undersurface of the angle prior to angle division.

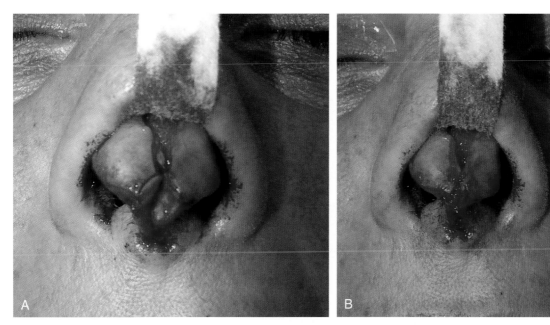

Figure 13-10 A, The right lower lateral cartilage angle has been transected; the left remains intact. **B,** Following transaction of the right and left angles, the medial (and intermediate) crura are sutured together.

The vestibular mucosa is elevated from the undersurface of the angle (Figure 13-9). Vertical angle division is performed with a Converse scissors without violating the underlying mucosa (Figure 13-10A, B). The medial (and intermediate) crura are sutured together below their apex using a 5-0 PDS reconstructing the single medial limb of the tripod (Figure 13-11). These two maneuvers narrow the tip by bringing together the medial (and intermediate) crura, which normally splay apart, and allowing the

domal portion of the lateral crura to medialize. Reducing the interdomal distance produces a more narrow and defined tip (Figure 13-12).

Once separated, the lateral and medial crura can be reshaped and manipulated independently of one another. This is especially helpful when addressing ala-columellar disproportions, particularly in the setting of excessive columellar show where the inherent shape of the LLCs create an unfavorable relationship of lateral to medial

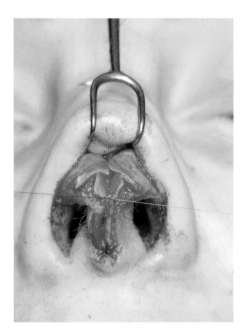

Figure 13-11 Following vertical angle division, the medial crura are sutured together below their apex. The visible overlap of the medial aspect of the lateral crura creates a supratip fullness, which is subsequently corrected during lateral crura modification.

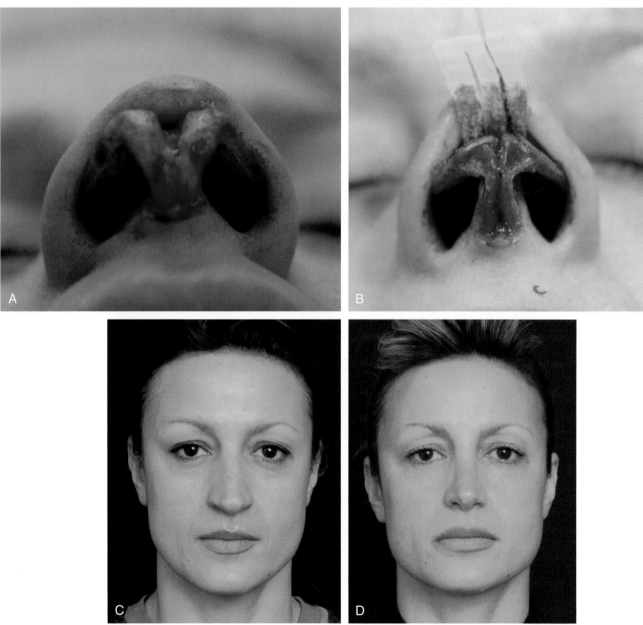

Figure 13-12 A, Intraoperative base view of a wide nasal tip after elevation of the nasal skin. B, Following vertical angle division and suturing of the medial crura. The lateral crura override the medial component. The tip structure is visibly narrowed. C, Preoperative photograph of the same patient. D, Postoperative photograph showing the tip narrowing and rotation that was obtained with vertical angle division.

crura.[7] After completing the vertical angle division, the lateral and medial crura can be effectively repositioned to reestablish an appropriate relation with less vertical separation of the lateral and medial crura (Figure 13-13).

Lateral Crura

The lateral crura are released by freeing their cephalic margin from the ULCs (Figure 13-14). The mucosa underlying the cephalic margin is elevated prior to dividing the LLC–ULC attachment (scroll). This allows for lateral crura freeing and trimming of the cephalic component, without violating the underlying mucosa (Figure 13-15).

Care is taken to preserve at least 7 mm of the lateral crura in vivo to prevent alar collapse. Following domal angle division and separation of the lateral crura from the ULC, the medial ends of the lateral crura may overlap and produce supratip fullness. Reduction of the cephalic portion of the lateral crura is done primarily in the medial two-thirds of the lateral crura to narrow the tip and reduce supratip fullness. Releasing the lateral crus–ULC attachment (scroll) facilitates lateral repositioning of the lateral crura, and thus nasal tip rotation. Additional rotation can be achieved, when necessary, by dissecting out and transecting the lateral most aspect of the lateral crura,

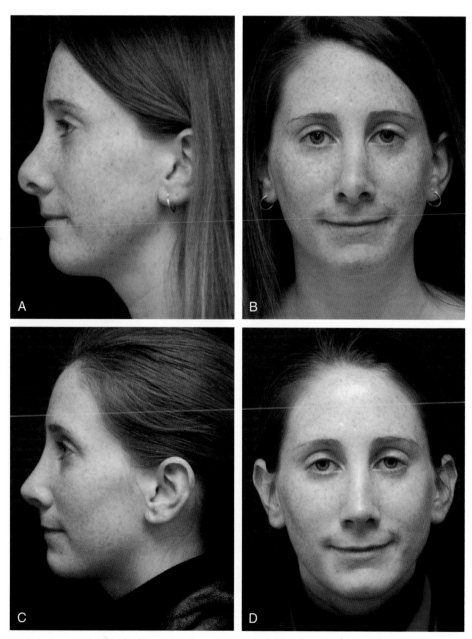

Figure 13-13 Preoperative photographs (**A, B**) of a patient who previously had rhinoplasty resulting in alar-columella disharmony and a blunted tip. Postoperative photographs (**C, D**) following revision rhinoplasty, the patient demonstrates correction of the alar-columella disharmony with vertical angle division.

where they abut the sesamoid cartilages (Figure 13-16). This lateral release allows the lateral crura to further migrate out toward the pyriform aperture.

Medial Crura

Having isolated and modified the lateral crura, attention is shifted to addressing the medial and intermediate crural complex. The medial crura are now relatively mobile, having been separated from the lateral crura and freed

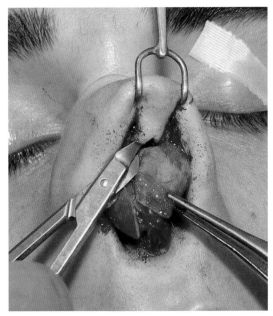

Figure 13-14 The cephalic border of the lateral crus is separated from the upper lateral cartilage.

from the caudal septum. Modifications to the medial crura are aimed toward modifying tip projection, rotation, and columellar position. Separating the medial from the lateral crura provides tremendous flexibility to alter nasal tip projection. In an overprojected nose, the apex of the medial crura can be reduced as much as needed for deprojection (Figure 13-17). Even in cases where deprojection is not needed, the apex of the medial–intermediate crural complex will generally need to be modified after angle division. Following vertical angle division, the cephalic portion of the apical (free) margin of the medial-intermediate crura will generally project higher than the caudal portion. Trimming the cephalic portion of the free apical edge of the intermediate crura is often necessary to prevent supratip fullness (Figure 13-18). Once the desired nasal projection has been established, a columella strut graft is sutured into place to prevent loss of tip projection during the healing process. When addressing an under-projected nose, a longer columella strut graft can be used to increase tip projection.

COLUMELLAR STRUT GRAFT

A columella strut graft is used in all patients, even when deprojecting the tip, to ensure maintenance of tip position (Figure 13-19). It is also useful for modifying the shape of the medial-intermediate crura complex. An overly curved medial-intermediate crura may lead to a hanging columella postoperatively. The columella strut graft can be used to straighten the medial–intermediate crural complex, as a means to address the alar–columella relationship. The columella strut graft is ideally carved out of

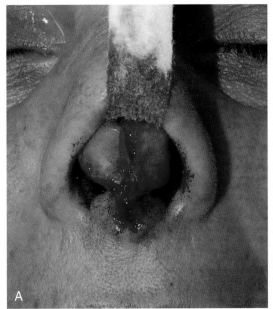
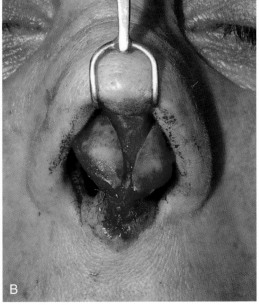

Figure 13-15 Before (**A**) and after (**B**) cephalic trim of the lateral crura. Reduction of the medial cephalic border narrows the tip and reduces supratip fullness.

a relatively strong strip of septal cartilage. It is approximately 2.5 cm long and 0.5 cm wide, tapering to a narrow base. An intercrural pocket is created between the feet of the medial crura staying anterior to the maxillary spine (Figure 13-20). The graft is placed with its narrow base into the pocket, then slid between the medial crura with its apex positioned immediately under the suture binding the medial crura together. The graft length is modified as needed to fit into the pocket. A longer graft can be used to increase projection. When using a longer columellar strut to increase projection, it is important to bear in mind that as the apex of the graft pushes against the medial crura suture, increased rotation of the nasal tip will be accomplished, thereby opening the nasolabial angle (Figure 13-21). Projection and rotation should be assessed before suture-fixating the graft. The skin is redraped and the tip height, narrowing, position, and rotation are reassessed.

MEMBRANOUS SEPTUM

During the process of LLC modification, emphasis is placed on reinforcing the anatomic supports that may have been weakened, in order to create a long-lasting and functional result. The columella strut graft, as described earlier, provides structural reinforcement of the medial crura and is used to maintain the newly established nasal tip projection and rotation. Another structure that often needs to be reinforced is the membranous septum. The open approach to the septum eliminates the space between the medial crura and caudal septum, leaving a potential space where the membranous septum had been. This allows the medial crura to drop back against the caudal septum, facilitating rotation, shortening, and deprojection (see Figure 13-6). The columella strut helps compensate for some of the loss of support from membranous septum take-down, but reestablishment of the membranous septum is generally needed to further modify nasal length and tip rotation. The membranous septum can be variably

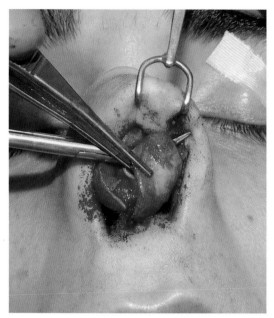

Figure 13-16 Additional tip rotation is facilitated by dissecting out and transecting the lateralmost aspect of the lateral crura. The scissor is positioned under the most lateral portion of the lateral crura.

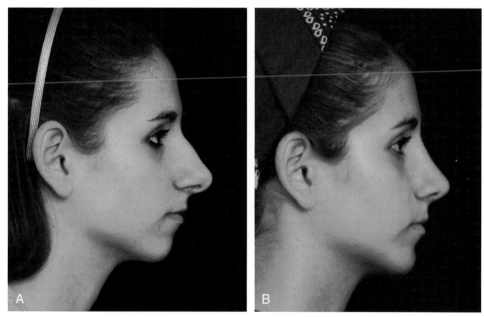

Figure 13-17 Preoperative (**A**) and postoperative (**B**) photographs demonstrating tip deprojection accomplished through vertical angle division followed by reduction of the medial crural height.

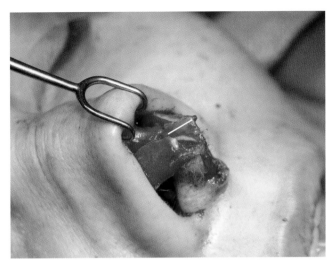

Figure 13-18 Fullness in the supratip is prevented by reducing the cephalic portion of the medial crural apex (cartilage reduction performed along *white line*).

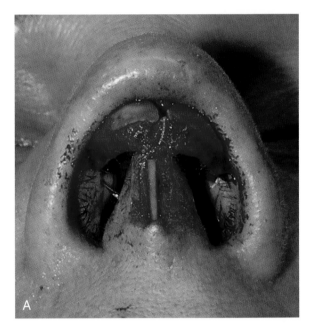

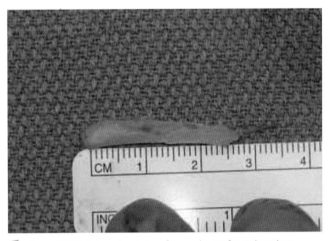

Figure 13-19 Columella strut graft carved out of septal cartilage.

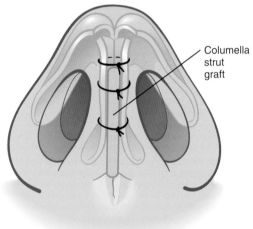

Columella strut graft

B

Figure 13-20 A, The columella strut is placed in an intracrural pocket with its base extending in front of the maxillary spine. **B,** Schematic showing the position of the columella strut and placement of sutures for fixation.

recreated depending on the changes that need to be made to the tip. Conceptually, the potential membranous septum can be envisioned as having a low, middle, and high component, each of which can be addressed independently. The membranous septum is reconstituted by placing a 4-0 chromic suture through the portion of the membranous septum that needs to be reestablished. The suture is placed through mucosa only. If the columella is retracting, a low and mid suture will lengthen these portions of the nose, bringing out the columella. If the tip is rotating too much and overshortened, a high membranous septal stitch will prevent its collapse in the cephalad direction, creating a longer, less rotated tip.

Having modified both the lateral and medial crura, a new tip structure has now been created. This new nasal

tip is formed by the medial ends of the lateral crura overriding the apical portion of the medial–intermediate crural complex. As the skin flap is pulled down, the lateral crura are pulled forward and medial into their final position overriding the apex of the medial crura, and the nasal tip is evaluated with the skin flap redraped (Figure 13-22). Based on evaluation of the tip, the need for further tip grafting is needed.

EXTENDED SHIELD GRAFT

In some cases, the above-mentioned steps may fall short of producing the desired tip definition, projection, narrowing, or overall appearance. This is more often seen in patients with thicker skin, for whom the tip structure is

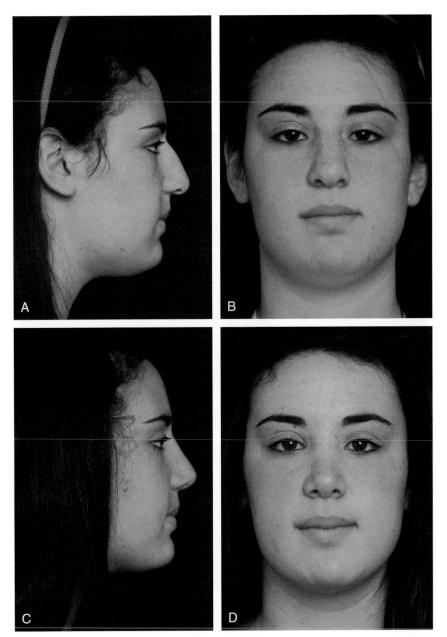

Figure 13-21 Preoperative (**A, B**) and postoperative (**C, D**) photographs demonstrating the effect of a strong columella strut after vertical angle division. The columella strut can rotate and project the tip, opening the nasolabial angle.

not adequately defined or narrowed, and for patients undergoing revision rhinoplasty procedures in whom the LLCs have been previously altered by either aggressive resection or reshaping, leaving an inadequate tip structure. In these instances, a new tip-defining structure needs to be created. An extended shield graft is an effective means for creating a more defined tip structure.[8,9] This graft is versatile and can be used to lengthen the nose, increase projection, narrow the tip, or even widen a pinched tip from prior surgery (Figure 13-23). The extended shield graft is a columella-lobular graft, with a shield shape at its lobular component. It is placed into a pocket in front of the medial crura and becomes the new

tip-defining structure (Figure 13-24). This relegates the medial aspect of the lateral crura (previously the tip-defining structure) as the new supratip structure. The extended shield graft is carved out of septal cartilage or, alternatively, conchal cartilage. The graft is approximately 2.5 cm in height and 10 mm in width at its apex, narrowing toward its base (Figure 13-25). The apical edges of the graft are thinned and beveled and the apical corners are blunted to better camouflage it under the tip skin. If the effect of the graft on tip shape and height is appropriate, it is then carefully sutured in place, taking care not to leave any exposed sharp edges that can later become visible. The skin envelope is then redraped and the effect

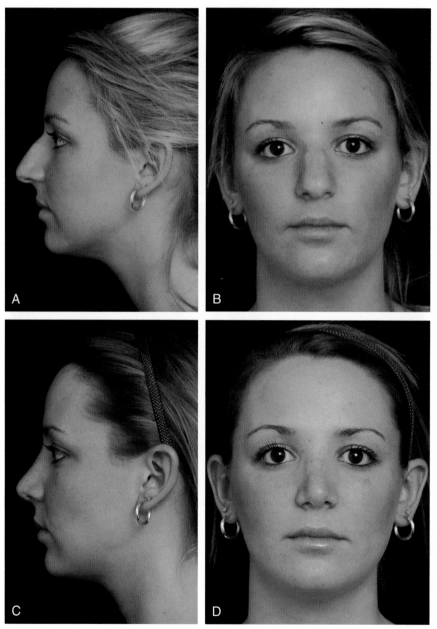

Figure 13-22 Preoperatively (**A, B**), this patient had an overprojected, wide, and ptotic tip. Rhinoplasty included vertical angle division, reduction of the cephalic margin of both the lateral crura and apex of the medial crura, and placement of a columellar strut graft. Postoperative (**C, D**) photographs demonstrate the ability to deproject, rotate, narrow, and improve tip definition with these techniques.

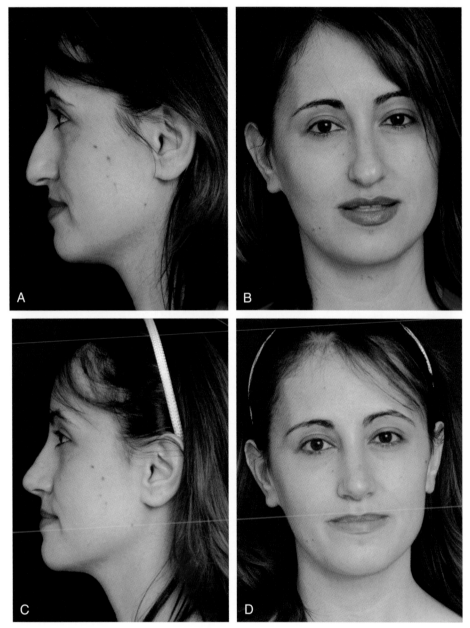

Figure 13-23 Preoperatively (**A, B**), this patient had a wide, poorly defined ptotic tip. Rhinoplasty, including vertical angle division, lower lateral cartilage cephalic trim, and columella strut placement were performed. An extended shield graft was needed to create appropriate tip definition (**C, D**) due to her relatively thick nasal skin.

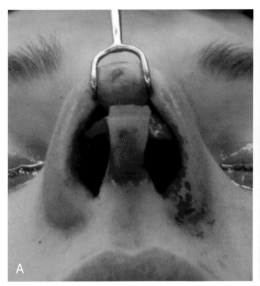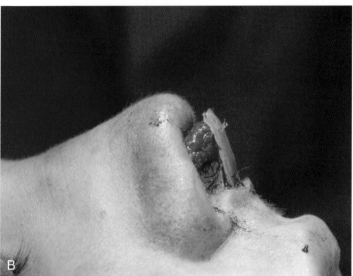

Figure 13-24 A, B, An extended shield graft is placed in a precrural pocket. The graft becomes the new tip and the lower lateral cartilages are now suptratip structure.

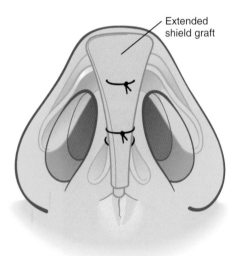

Extended shield graft

Figure 13-25 The extended shield graft is double suture-fixated to the medial crura and columella strut.

of the graft reassessed. Again, it is useful to place a suture to reapproximate the columella incision so as to accurately assess the result of the graft.

CONCLUSION

Vertical angle division is a useful technique for altering the LLCs to modify nasal tip appearance. Formation of a fully mobile tripod with this technique facilitates modification of each of the pods independently of one another.

In conjunction with structural cartilage grafts, this technique is applicable in all primary and revision rhinoplasties and has provided consistent long-term results.

REFERENCES

1. Toriumi DM. New concepts in nasal tip contouring. *Arch Fac Plast Surg.* 2006;8:156–185.
2. Adamson PA, McGraw-Wall BL, Morrow TA, et al. Vertical dome division in open rhinoplasty. An update on indications, techniques and results. *Arch Otolaryngol Head Neck Surg.* 1994;120:373–380.
3. Quatela VC, Slupchynskyj OS. Surgery of the nasal tip. *Fac Plast Surg.* 1997;13:253–268.
4. Kamer FM, Pieper PG. Nasal tip surgery: a 30-year experience. *Fac Plast Surg Clin North Am.* 2004;12:81–92.
5. Glasgold AI, Glasgold MJ, Rosenberg DB. The mobile tripod technique: the key to nasal tip refinement. *Fac Plast Surg Clin North Am.* 2000;8:487–502.
6. Anderson JR, Ries WR. Surgery of the nasal base: setting tip projection and location. In: Anderson JR, Ries WR, eds. *Rhinoplasty: emphasizing the external approach.* New York: Thieme; 1986:63–78.
7. Joseph EM, Glasgold AI. Anatomical considerations in the management of the hanging columella. *Arch Fac Plast Surg.* 2000;2:173–177.
8. Glasgold MJ, Glasgold AI. Tip grafts and their effects on tip position and contour. *Fac Plast Surg Clin North Am.* 1995;3:367–379.
9. Kridel RW, Soliemanzadeh P: Tip grafts in revision rhinoplasty. *Fac Plast Surg Clin North Am.* 2006;14:331–341.

CHAPTER FOURTEEN

Suturing Techniques to Refine the Nasal Tip

Ronald P. Gruber • Kenton Fong • Chia Chung

Controlling the shape of the nasal tip can be one of the most challenging problems rhinoplasty surgeons face in practice. Prior to the advent of suture techniques, the cartilages of the nose were largely controlled, by excision, crushing, and scoring. At the time, these methods were thought to be the easiest method to create a new nasal shape. Unfortunately, they all potentially damaged the cartilage and consequently often led to instability, collapse, contour irregularities, and a host of secondary problems including alar retraction, pinched tips, retracted alae, and external valve collapse.

In the late 1980s, Tardy et al.[1] used what is now called a transdomal suture to narrow the tip cartilages in a closed (endonasal) rhinoplasty, and soon Daniel[2,3] began using this technique in the open approach, which was described as the "dome-definition suture." Emphasizing the need for nondestructive methods of controlling cartilage shape, Tebbetts[4] provided a comprehensive approach to suture techniques, including his lateral crural spanning suture that reduced tip convexity and narrowed the overall width of the nasal tip. Since that time, a wide variety of suture techniques have been proposed to control the width and position of the tip and to reduce lateral crural bulbosity. Rohrich et al.[5] provided an algorithm for the boxy tip, and most recently, Guyuron et al.[6] used sutures to control the shape of the foot plates and reviewed the entire subject of suture techniques. Over the past decades, suture techniques have gradually come into vogue and now represent a quantum leap in the ability to control the shape of the nasal architectural framework. However, suture techniques should not be considered as an all-encompassing substitute for cartilage grafting. When there are major changes to be made in the nasal region, cartilage grafting may be necessary as an adjunct to suturing techniques. The choice of suture techniques chosen here represents the personal favorite of the authors.

FUNDAMENTAL PRINCIPLES FOR SUTURE-BASED MODIFICATIONS OF THE NASAL TIP

1. *Models facilitate sculpting*

   In planning what could be termed "suture tiplasty," it is important to have a structural shape and goal in mind (Figure 14-1). A generic tip would consist of the following: the lateral crus should be fairly flat (not convex or concave) and at least 5 to 6 mm wide. The tip cartilages resemble McDonald's arches. The actual domes are separated from one another at the cephalic end by about 3 mm. Each dome has an axis, and the two axes form the "angle of domal separation" approximating 70 to 90 degrees.[7] On lateral view, one will note that the angle formed by the medial/middle crus is anywhere from 15 to 30 degrees. The tip will commonly lie 6 to 8 mm above (anterior) to the dorsal septum. Commercially available anatomic models can aid the novice surgeon in sculpting the tip cartilages to these dimensions. As any commercial artist will tell you, copying is much easier than creating from memory.

2. *Cephalic resection of the lateral crus*

   Before implementing the suture techniques to control the shape of the nasal tip during a primary rhinoplasty, the cephalic component of the lateral crus is typically trimmed. Cephalic resection should result in a lateral crus that is never narrower than 6 mm wide (Figure 14-2). There are two reasons for carrying out this maneuver in this fashion: (1) the shape of the lateral crus can more precisely be controlled to reduce its convexity and (2) the integrity of the lateral crus (which effectively constitutes the external valve) is maintained. After the cephalic trim is performed, one can use suture techniques to reduce any remaining

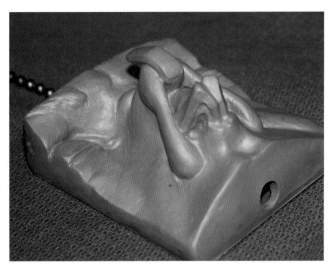

Figure 14-1 Anatomic model. The desired anatomical configuration of the tip cartilages are easier to sculpt with suture techniques if there is an anatomic model from which to copy.

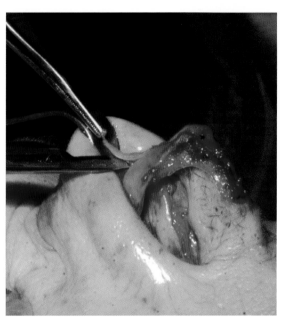

Figure 14-2 Cephalic trim of the lower lateral cartilage. Before beginning suture techniques on the nasal tip, a cephalic trim of the lateral crus is almost always needed in the primary rhinoplasty because there is almost always some tip bulbosity. At least 6 mm of lateral crus is maintained. This makes it easier to reshape and reposition the tip using suture techniques, preserving the integrity of the lower lateral cartilage both aesthetically and functionally.

convexity or concavity. Even if the lateral crus is cephalically oriented, as is commonly the case, the convexity of the entire lateral crus can and should be converted to a normal flat orientation with the aid of suturing techniques.

3. *Suture choice*

We have not found the suture type and size to be critically important factors. However, we routinely use 5-0 or 4-0 polydioxanone (PDS) sutures to control cartilage shape. We previously used nylon, but experience has demonstrated that the alar cartilage retains its new shape even after the PDS dissolves. Moreover, the potential problems of suture exposure in the nasal cavity are avoided given the dissolvable nature of the PDS suture. Suture color does not seem to be a critical issue either. Tapered needles are preferable because they are less likely to "cut through" the cartilage. However, cutting needles will work satisfactorily if round needles are not available.

4. *Intraoperative delayed suturing effect*

Cartilages will sometimes change their shape slightly after sutures are placed. This can be attributed to the local anesthetics diffusing through the soft tissues or to the gradual change of the shape of the cartilage over time.[8] Whatever the cause, it is helpful to plan to reassess the effect of the sutures that have been applied intraoperatively before completing the case. Minor warping changes can occur anywhere up to 45 minutes after a suture is placed in the cartilage. Fortunately, undesired changes are almost always reversible by removing and replacing the suture if the intended effect is not accomplished.

BASIC ALGORITHM (FOUR-SUTURE TECHNIQUE)

It is helpful to have a suture algorithm for the tip cartilages.[2,3,5,6,9] In the senior author's experience, four types of sutures[9] can control the entire tip shape in most cases (hemitransdomal, interdomal, lateral crural mattress, and columellar-septal). A few others are occasionally used.

HEMITRANSDOMAL SUTURE

Until recently, the senior author's first line and most commonly used suture was a transdomal suture to narrow the domal width. However, a modification of that technique developed by Tardy for the closed (endonasal) approach and further adapted by Daniel for the open (external) approach has become our first suture choice. The hemitransdomal suture is intended to narrow the cephalic end of the dome, thereby causing a small amount of eversion of the lateral crus and minimizing the chance of a collapsed marginal rim of the lateral crus.

The vestibular skin of the dome is infiltrated with local anesthesia to avoid needle penetration into the vestibular skin. A hemitransdomal suture (5-0 PDS) is then placed in the cephalic end of the dome. In essence, the cephalic end of the middle crus (*posterior or deep to the dome*) is pinched to the cephalic end of the lateral crus (*posterior or deep to* the dome) (Figure 14-3). The needle enters the cartilages parallel to the surface of the dome. The suture is usually located 2 to 3 mm below dome level. The lower the suture is placed from the dome, the more it tends to evert the lateral crus. Also, a more generous purchase into the cephalic dome will reduce the dome width. Typically, a short learning curve is involved before one corrects the dome with one attempt only.

Figures 14-4 and 14-5 demonstrate the effect of a hemitransdomal suture intraoperatively. Note that the cephalic part of the dome is narrowed but the caudal part of the dome is not narrowed much, if any. You can also notice that the caudal edge of the lateral crus is more everted, or at least not inverted, and that the caudal edge of the rim is not forced into concavity. A single hemi-transdomal suture is usually all that is required to reshape

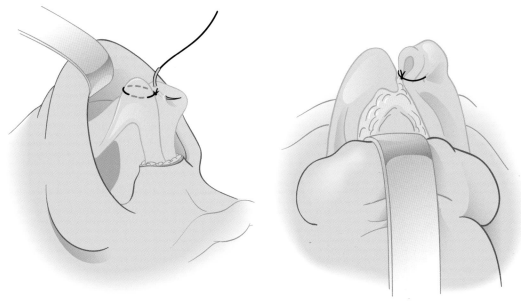

Figure 14-3 Schematic depiction of the hemitransdomal suture. The needle enters the cartilages parallel to the surface of the dome. The suture is usually placed 2 to 3 mm below the dome level. The lower the suture is placed from the dome, the more it tends to evert the lateral crus. Also, the larger the purchase of the cephalic dome, the more the dome width is reduced.

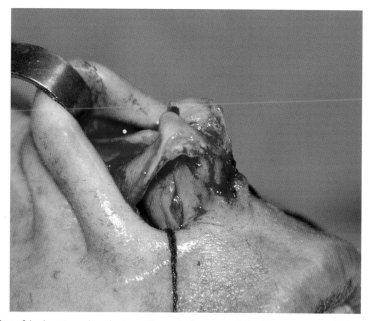

Figure 14-4 Intraoperative effect of the hemitransdomal suture. The cephalic aspect of the dome is narrowed. The caudal part of the dome is minimally narrowed if at all. Also note that the caudal border of the lateral crus is everted somewhat (or at least not inverted). Consequently, the caudal border of the rim is not forced to become concave.

the dome; however, some patients with a very broad or thick-walled dome may also require a transdomal suture as well.

The classic transdomal suture may inadvertently result in a pinched appearance that exhibits slight concavity of the alar rims. This suture may also unintentionally cause twisting of the lateral crus such that the alar rim is turned medially or inverted. Guyuron[6] and Daniel[2,3] suggested placing the transdomal suture at the cephalic end of the dome to minimize this side effect. Toriuimi[10] warned that tip sutures can displace the caudal margin of the

lateral crus well below the cephalic margin resulting in a pinched nasal tip. He suggested correcting this with the use of an alar rim graft. However, in our experience, eversion of the lateral crus often times cannot be achieved by just putting the transdomal suture at the cephalic end. Thus, the final result may on occasion still be a pinched nasal tip. One solution to this problem is to place the suture *posterior (deep)* to the very cephalic end of the dome and let it fully evert the lateral crus while narrowing the cephalic end of the dome.

TRANSDOMAL SUTURE (OCCASIONALLY USED)

When the transdomal suture is needed it is executed as follows (Figure 14-6): The vestibular skin of the undersurface of the dome is first infiltrated with local anesthesia to thicken that layer temporarily to prevent the needle from penetrating the underlying epithelial surface. Usually a 5-0 PDS (sometimes 4-0) mattress suture is applied such that the knot is on the medial side of the dome. To verify that the needle did not penetrate the vestibular skin, the needle is momentarily left sitting in the cartilage after taking a bite of it. The needle holder is then used to palpate the undersurface of the lateral crus for metal.

INTERDOMAL SUTURE

The second suture that is often, but not always, necessary is the *interdomal suture*[2-6,9,10] (Figures 14-7 and 14-8). Also known by other names, it is used when (1) asymmetry of the domal height is noted, (2) when a reduction

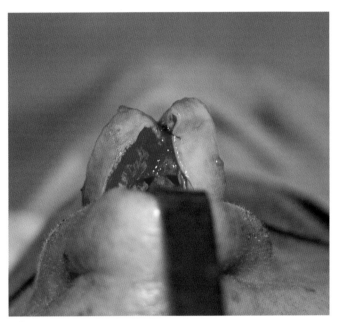

Figure 14-5 Hemitransdomal suture. View from head of bed.

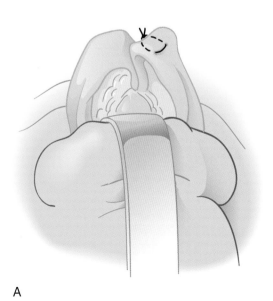

A

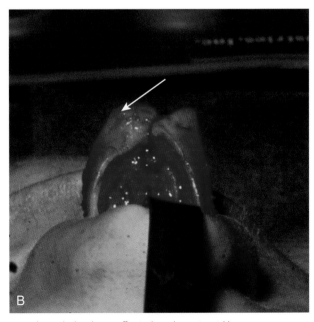

B

Figure 14-6 Transdomal (dome defining) suture. A horizontal mattress suture through the dome effectively reduces its width.

in interdomal width is desired, or (3) the domes feel weak or tend to splay apart easily when pressed upon with a finger. Symmetry and interdomal width are best appreciated from the head of the operating table. Asymmetry can be more noticeable following placement of transdomal sutures.

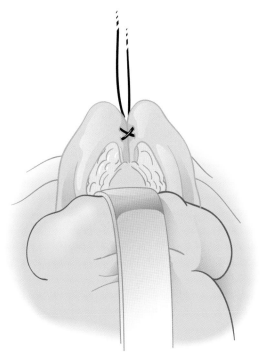

Figure 14-7 Schematic of interdomal suture. An interdomal suture provides symmetry and strength to the tip cartilages. It is applied by approximating the middle crura with a 5-0 PDS at a level that is about 3 to 4 mm posterior to the dome.

The interdomal suture is made by approximating the middle crura with a 5-0 PDS at a level that is about 3 to 4 mm posterior to the dome. It is important to select a suture location level that is far enough posterior to the domes so that there is a normal separation between the domes (approximately 3 mm) yet holds the middle crura together in symmetric fashion.

LATERAL CRURAL MATTRESS SUTURE

Horizontal mattress suture reduce and eliminate any cartilage convexity.[11] The lateral crural mattress suture (Figures 14-9 and 14-10) is useful to correct the broad or bulbous or ball and boxy tip.[9] The vestibular skin is hyperinfiltrated with local anesthesia just prior to inserting the lateral crural mattress suture. The lateral crus is grasped with Brown-Adson forceps at the apex of the convexity and a 5-0 PDS on a P-3 needle is inserted on one side of the forceps perpendicular to the direction of the lateral crus. The point of entry for the needle should stay on the caudal side of the lateral crus so that the knot ends up on that side (rather than the cephalic side where it is more likely to be palpable). A second purchase with the needle is made on the other side of the forceps approximately 6 mm away from the first pass. A slip knot is used to adjust tension on the suture until the lateral crus reaches the desired level of flatting.

If the spacing between each pass is too small, the convexity of the cartilage may not be sufficiently corrected. If the spacing is too wide, the convexity is corrected but the cartilage will tend to buckle and stability is lost. If the spacing is ideal, the convexity is largely eliminated and the lateral crus is approximately 30% stronger than

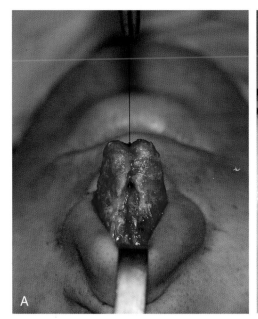
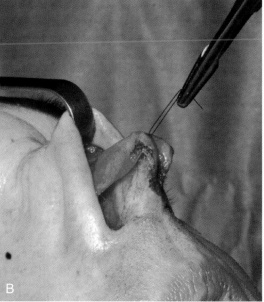

Figure 14-8 Intraoperative view of interdomal suture. View from the top of the head (**A**) and oblique view (**B**).

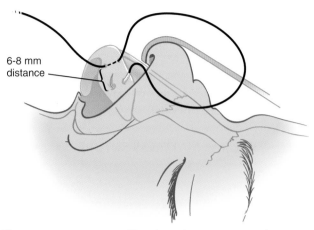

6-8 mm
distance

Figure 14-9 Schematic of lateral crural mattress suture placement. It consists of one or two horizontal mattress sutures applied to the most convex portion of the lateral crus following cephalic trim with the purpose of removing most of the unwanted convexity. The needle pass is perpendicular to the long axis of the lateral crus. A second pass is made 6 to 8 mm from the first one.

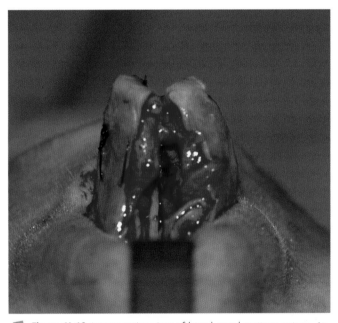

Figure 14-10 Intraoperative view of lateral crural mattress suture. As the knot is tied, the convexity tends to disappear. With further tightening of the suture, a small degree of concavity will result. A lateral crural mattress suture has the added benefit of applying a lateral vector, which tends to open the external valve slightly. This is particularly evident if one of the lateral crural mattress sutures is placed at the posterior end of the lateral crus.

it was before the suture was placed. If the convexity is not completely corrected (as occurs if the lateral crus is convex from one end to the other), a second mattress suture is placed adjacent to the first in order to correct convexity not corrected by the first suture. On occasion, a total of three such sutures are placed on a very convex and difficult to control lateral crus. Each suture provides additional strength to the cartilage.

Another advantage of the lateral crural mattress suture is its concurrent improvement in external valve function. As the mattress suture knot is tightened, the posterior aspect of the lateral crus tends to become more stable and is slightly lateralized. It does so by imposing a flaring vector force on the posterior aspect of the lateral crus. Thus, to a limited extent, the external valve is opened slightly and is stabilized. This is particularly noticeable for mattress sutures placed on the posterior aspect of the lateral crus.

COLUMELLA-SEPTAL SUTURE

There are four potential applications for this suture: (1) to reestablish tip support that may have been lost by a transfixion/intercartilaginous incision; (2) to provide a subtle degree of tip projection; (3) to help increase tip rotation, which can help address a hanging columella; and (4), in some selected instances, to help deproject the tip.

Before placing the columella-septal suture, it is helpful to determine the desired domal height in relation to the dorsal septum. Generally speaking the domes should lie 6 to 8 mm above the level of the dorsum. Thicker-skinned patients may require up to 10 mm, and thinner-skin patients less than 4 to 6 mm.

A 1-inch 27-gauge needle is used to impale the caudal septum between the middle crura. The hub of the needle is then clipped off, the skin is replaced over the alar cartilages (sutured with one stitch if needed), and the nasal profile is reexamined to evaluate if the desired degree of tip projection and rotation have been achieved. After satisfactory adjustments in height are made, the final suture is placed and the needle is then removed.

The suture is placed using a 4-0 PDS thrown between the leaves of the middle crura (Figures 14-11 to 14-13). The needle is then brought out into the transfixion space if there is one. If no transfixion incision has been made, the needle is passed between the medial crura. The needle is then passed through the septal cartilage usually at the level of the anterior septal angle. Then it is passed back between the middle crura.

Care is taken to prevent securing the suture too tightly, thereby creating an iatrogenic columellar retraction. After redraping the skin envelope, the tip is evaluated by observation and palpation aiming for a tip position projected just beyond the level of the dorsum. Slight firmness to palpation is desired to ensure adequate tip support. This will minimize the likelihood of a postoperative drop, tip counterrotation, or the development of a supratip deformity. The angle between the medial and middle crus (the columella/lobule angle) is evaluated. If columellar retraction exists, the suture is replaced. If a hanging columella is seen, the knot is secured until the desired angle and relation are accomplished.

In the case of an overprojected tip, the stabilizing needle is positioned posteriorly and the lower lateral cartilages are set back by securing them onto the posterior aspect of the caudal septum in order to decrease tip projection. This is one of the options available to deproject the nose.

INTERCRURAL SUTURE

At times, intercrural suture technique (Figure 14-14) can also be helpful during tiplasty.[12,13] This technique can reduce the width and flaring of the middle crura for nasal tips that exhibit widening at the level of the middle crus. Intercrural suture technqiue also helps create better symmetry. 5-0 PDS is typically used as a simple mattress suture that pulls the middle crura together but not too tightly.

CASE EXAMPLE

The patient shown in Figures 14-15 through 14-17 complained of a broad and bulbous tip. Physical findings confirmed a broad nasal tip, dorsal hump, broad nasal bones, and slightly long nose. At surgery, the following maneuvers were performed:

- Inverted-V columellar and marginal incisions
- Cephalic trim of lateral crus
- Hemitransdomal sutures
- Interdomal suture
- Columella-septal suture (to prevent tip drop)
- Lateral crural mattress sutures

The patient also underwent a dorsal hump reduction, osteotomies, and slight caudal shortening. At 13 months postoperatively, there is an improvement in tip bulbosity as shown.

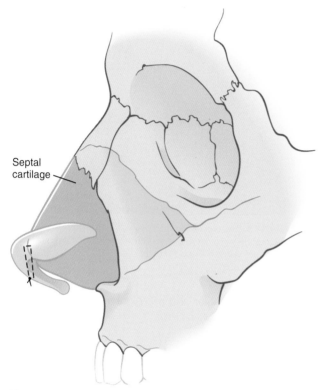

Septal cartilage

Figure 14-11 Schematic depiction of columella-septal suture.

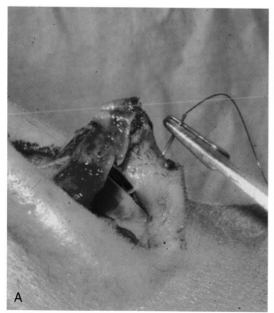
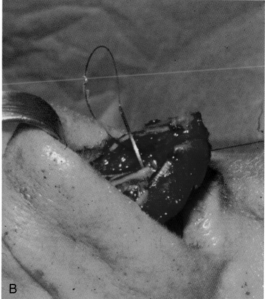

Figure 14-12 Columella-septal suture secures the tip complex to the caudal septum. A 4-0 PDS is passed between the leaves of the medial crura (**A**). The needle is then passed through the desired part of the caudal septum (anterior septal angle to increase projection and through the posterior septal angle to deproject the tip) (**B**).

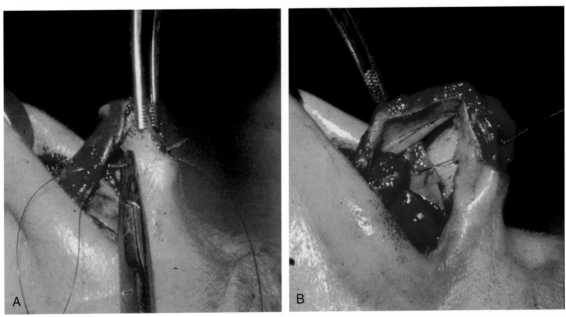

Figure 14-13 Columella-septal suture. The needle is passed back between the leaves of the medial crura from whence it came (**A**). The fibers between the medial crura are strong enough to provide a good support of the tip cartilages (**B**). Care must be taken not to overtighten the suture or it will cause columellar retraction. Placing a clamp between the tip cartilages and the caudal septum helps prevent that from happening.

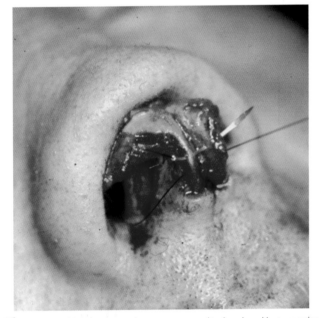

Figure 14-14 An intercrural suture may need to be placed between the caudal aspects of the middle or medial crura to reduce the flare, which can cause a wide columella. It can also help create symmetry.

CASE EXAMPLE

The patient in Figures 14-18 through 14-20 complained of a bulbous tip and preferred an endonasal approach. Physical findings confirmed a broad or bulbous tip. The patient also exhibited slightly broad nasal bones and a small dorsal hump. At surgery the following maneuvers were performed:

- Stair-step columellar and marginal incision
- Cephalic trim of lateral crus
- Transdomal sutures
- Interdomal suture
- Columella-septal suture
- Lateral crural mattress sutures

The patient also underwent a dorsal hump reduction and osteotomies. At 23 months after surgery, there is a significant improvement in tip bulbosity.

FOUR-SUTURE ALGORITHM IN ENDONASAL RHINOPLASTY

During endonasal rhinoplasty, a similar algorithm to external rhinoplasty can be used. The lower lateral cartilages are delivered onto the surgical field, one through each nostril via rim and intercartilaginous incisions. A hemitransdomal suture is then applied to one or both domes as needed (Figure 14-21). If any dome or tip asymmetry is detected externally and/or if the tip seems weak to palpation, both domes can be delivered through one nostril and an interdomal suture is applied.

If the delivered lateral crus exhibits convexity or if lateral crus convexity is seen externally, a lateral crural mattress suture is applied as in the open approach. If the tip can use slightly more projection or if it is weak upon palpation externally, a columellar-septal suture is applied. The columellar-septal suture is more technically challenging to perform through the endonasal approach than through the external approach. Marginal and transfixion

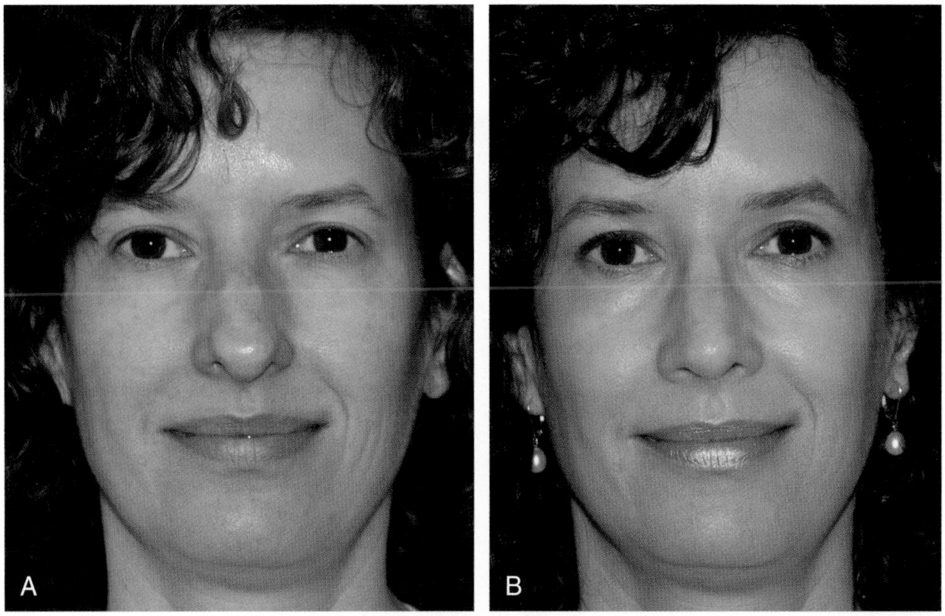

Figure 14-15 This patient presented with a broad tip and underwent a primary open rhinoplasty including the four-suture algorithm as well as hemi-transdomal suture. She also underwent a dorsal hump reduction, caudal shortening and osteotomies. **A,** Front view preoperatively. **B,** Front view postoperatively.

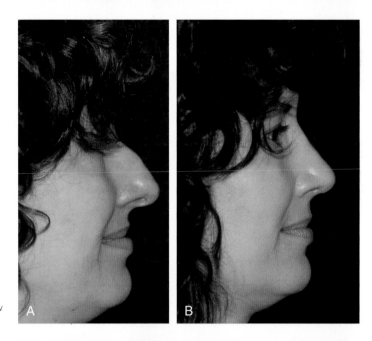

Figure 14-16 Same patient as in Figure 14-15. **A,** Lateral view preoperatively. **B,** Lateral view postoperatively.

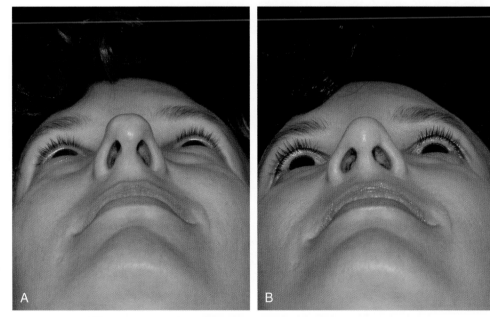

Figure 14-17 Same patient as in Figure 14-15. **A,** Base view preoperatively. **B,** Base view postoperatively.

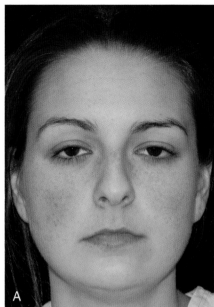
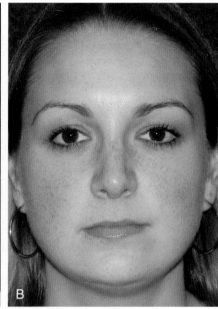

Figure **14-18** This patient presented with a broad tip and underwent a primary endonasal rhinoplasty including the four-suture algorithm, dorsal hump reduction, and osteotomies. **A,** Front view preoperatively. **B,** Front view postoperatively.

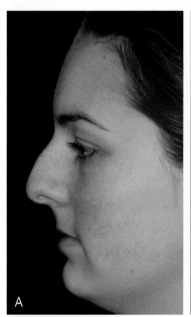
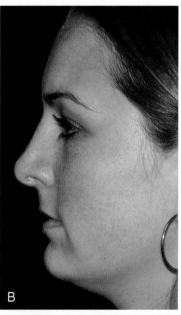

Figure **14-19** Same patient as in Figure 14-18. **A,** Lateral view preoperatively. **B,** Lateral view postoperatively.

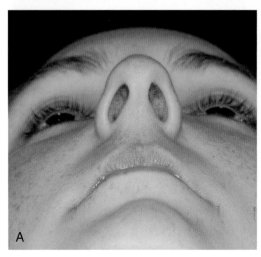
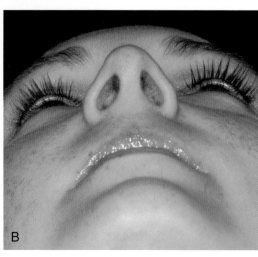

Figure **14-20** Same patient as in Figure 14-18. **A,** Base view preoperatively. **B,** Base view postoperatively.

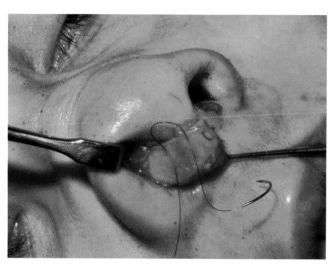

Figure 14-21 Hemitransdomal or transdomal suture being applied, taking advantage of the incisions carried out during a delivery technique.

incisions are in place for delivering the tip cartilages. The needle on a 4-0 PDS is passed between the medial crura and into the gap resulting from a transfixion incision. It is then passed through the anterior septal angle and brought back between the middle crura and back to the marginal incision area, where the knot is tied. The suture's resulting vector should have a slightly posterior to anterior orientation when it rotates and supports the tip cartilages.

FOUR-SUTURE ALGORITHM FOR SECONDARY RHINOPLASTY

As a general rule, the same algorithm described earlier is used during secondary external rhinoplasty. After the skin–soft tissue envelope is elevated, the existing dome is grasped with Brown-Adson forceps and a hemitransdomal suture is applied, followed if need be by an interdomal suture. The application of these two sets of sutures usually provides some strength and stability to the tip complex. More often than not, the lateral crus is found to be weak

and overresected. Consequently, a lateral crural mattress suture is usually not applicable. However, a columella-septal suture may be helpful to provide some additional tip projection and stability of the tip against the caudal septum. Ultimately, grafts are the building blocks for the secondary rhinoplasty. Thus, after executing the suture algorithm as described, the nose will commonly still require tip grafting.

REFERENCES

1. Tardy Jr ME, Patt BS, Walter MA. Transdomal suture refinement of the nasal tip: Long-term outcomes. *Fac Plast Surg*. 1993;9:275–284.
2. Daniel RK. Creating an aesthetic tip. *Plast Reconstr Surg*. 1987;80:775.
3. Daniel RK. Rhinoplasty: A simplified three-stitch, open tip suture technique. Part I: primary rhinoplasty. *Plast Reconstr Surg*. 1999;103:1491–1502.
4. Tebbetts JB. Shaping and positioning the nasal tip without structural disruption: a new, systematic approach. *Plast Reconstr Surg*. 1994;94:61–77.
5. Rohrich RJ, Adams Jr WP. The boxy nasal tip: Classification and management based on alar cartilage suturing techniques. *Plast Reconstr Surg*. 2001;107:1849–1863.
6. Guyuron B, Behmand RA. Nasal tip sutures, part II: The interplays. *Plast Reconstr Surg*. 2003;112:1130–1145.
7. Gruber RP. Discussion of "The boxy nasal tip: Classification and management based on alar cartilage suturing" by Rohrich, R.J. and Adams, W.P., Jr. *Plast Reconstr Surg*. 2001;107:1866–1868.
8. Harris S, Pan Y, Peterson R, et al. Cartilage warping: An experimental model. *Plast Reconstr Surg*. 1993;92:912–915.
9. Gruber RP, Friedman GD. Suture algorithm for the broad or bulbous nose. *Plast Reconstr Surg*. 2002;110:1752–1764.
10. Toriumi DM. New concepts in nasal tip contouring. *Arch Fac Plast Surg*. 2006;8:156.
11. Gruber RP, Nahai F, Bogdan MA, Friedman GD. Changing the convexity and concavity of nasal cartilages and cartilage grafts with horizontal mattress sutures: Part II. Clinical results. *Plast Reconstr Surg*. 2005;15:595–606.
12. Neu BR. Suture correction of nasal tip cartilage concavities. *Plast Reconstr Surg*. 1996;98:971–979.
13. Baker SR. Suture contouring of the nasal tip. *Arch Fac Plast Surg*. 2000;2:3442.

CHAPTER FIFTEEN

Rib Grafting Simplified

Kevin Brenner • Jay Calvert

The use of rib grafting in rhinoplasty has revolutionized the ability to treat complex nasal deformities. Its can be helpful for both primary nasal deformities (including posttraumatic, cocaine induced, and others), as well as secondary nasal deformities (including postoperative saddle deformities and otherwise graft-depleted patients).[1-4] Situations in which patients have had their septal cartilage or the majority of their conchal cartilage harvested during previous interventions leave few options for autogenous graft material. In addition, some primary nasal surgeries (i.e., patients with Binder syndrome) or other complex nasal reconstructions require the incorporation of structural grafting material using cartilage volumes that are not available even in the previously unoperated concha or septum. Although other autogenous material, homografts, and alloplastic materials are also available, they can be associated with potential complications including absorption, infection, and extrusion.[5,6] The lower likelihood of complications associated with costal cartilage grafts has popularized its use and made them the standard for complex nasal reconstruction despite the associated increased operative time and potential for donor site morbidity.

Many preeminent surgeons have described their successful use of rib grafts in reconstructive rhinoplasty.[7] Daniel[8] modernized the use of rib grafting.

Costal cartilage harvesting can be conceptualized as the natural progression and modification of the standard lateral and anterolateral thoracotomy exposures used during thoracic and cardiothoracic operations.[9] Currently, harvesting the fifth and sixth ribs through an inframammary incision is the most commonly used technique.[10] However, this approach is technically demanding, provides limited graft alternatives, and leaves a scar in an awkward location in male patients. The authors prefer a subcostal approach because of its ease of exposure, limited scarring, quick operative time (30 to 60 minutes), low morbidity, and great versatility of available graft material through the same incision. Furthermore, the subcostal approach is technically less demanding, making it an excellent choice for surgeons who are learning to incorporate costal grafting into their practice.

Costal cartilage harvesting is a safe technique, but the selected rib (or ribs) to be harvested will vary based on the specific grafting needs. Furthermore, rib anatomy will vary between individual patients. This chapter will discuss the technique of costal cartilage harvesting and will establish a practical approach toward rib selection based on individual grafting needs. Several rib graft harvesting techniques and choices are available, and each surgeon may develop a preferred algorithm to select one. The technique suggested here is meant to serve as a basic guide such that any surgeon can decide which approach best suits him or her.

EVALUATION OF THE PROBLEM

Describing the surgical decision-making process leading to the plan behind a complex nasal reconstruction is beyond the scope of this chapter. However, in the course of configuring an operative plan several factors must be incorporated. The plan begins with the defect to be addressed, which incisions need to be made to provide access to the surgical site, the operative maneuvers required to accomplish the desired modification, and, specifically with regard to rib cartilage harvesting, which grafts will need to be used. After having a clear idea of the grafts to be used, the surgeon can then select an appropriate donor site from which to harvest them, taking into account the quality and amount of cartilage necessary and available from each donor site (i.e., septum, conchae, or ribs). It is important to be clear about the intrinsic properties of cartilage and/or bone at each harvest site. The experience with harvesting and cutting cartilage grafts from different locations helps the surgeon to become familiar with the varying degrees of cartilage strength and consistency. The patient's age is important, as costal cartilage tends to ossify and become more brittle with advancing age. Marin et al.[10] have advocated preoperative computed tomography imaging for selected patients in order to assess for rib cartilage calcification.

As the surgeon selects the cartilage grafts necessary to perform the operation, the donor site morbidity associated with each site should be considered, operative reports from previous operations should be reviewed, and detailed physical examination of the septum and conchae will reveal if any residual cartilage remains to be harvested.

Secondary septal surgery is technically challenging and rarely produces an adequate amount of cartilage. Even if available in sufficient quantity, conchal cartilage often lacks the structural strength required to counteract the robust contractile forces resulting from cicatricial wound healing in a reoperated nose.

Once the decision to use costal cartilage has been made, the surgeon must next decide which rib or ribs will best serve the purposes for the planned operation (Figure 15-1). Factors integral to this decision include both the problem the surgeon is trying to solve with the cartilage graft and the patient's desires in terms of donor site morbidity. The most important questions the surgeon must ask are: What skin incision is required to obtain the necessary exposure to harvest the costal cartilage, and which rib or ribs will work best to carve the grafts? Of course this choice is both patient and problem dependent, but some guidelines to help make that decision will be outlined.

INFRAMAMMARY FOLD INCISION

This incision is useful in that it is cosmetically favorable for most women. We have found that some men find a breast scar unacceptable. It allows excellent access to the fifth, sixth, and sometimes even the seventh costal cartilage. Although it would seem that the risk of pneumothorax would be higher with this incision, this has not been found to be the case based on published studies.[10] The disadvantages to this approach include that it can be more technically difficult for the novice surgeon and the amount of cartilage harvested is typically less. Also, in patients who have previously undergone a breast augmentation procedure, there is a small yet distinct risk of damaging the existing implant. Nonetheless, this approach is popular and allows surgeons to accomplish the goal, and it rarely requires drain placement.

ABDOMINAL SKIN INCISION

The authors recommend the subcostal approach, as previously advocated by Sheen and Daniel, for multiple reasons (Figure 15-2).[8,11] The incision is generally no longer than 3 to 4 cm and is located well onto the abdomen, making it inconspicuous and unobtrusive. Second, the approach is safer, with a lower risk for pneumothorax since there is relatively more connective tissue in between the rib and the parietal pleura at this level. Third, and most important, the volume and variability of cartilage

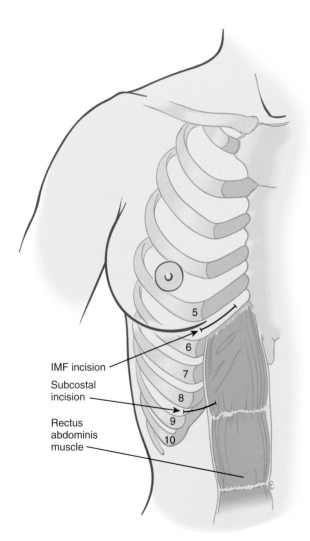

Figure 15-1 Inframammary fold and subcostal access incisions.

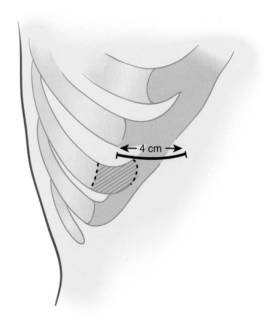

Figure 15-2 Subcostal incision closed with ninth rib cartilage and a portion of eighth rib cartilage.

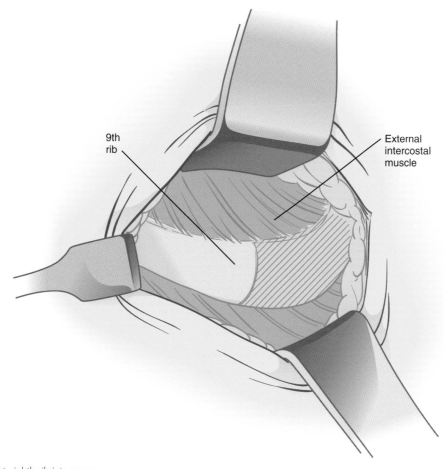

9th
rib

External
intercostal
muscle

Figure 15-3 Right eighth rib interspace.

available at this location are much greater than with the inframammary approach. Multiple ribs can be taken through the same incision, and in cases where osteochondral grafts are required, the incision simply needs to be shifted or extended to a more lateral position.

COSTOCHONDRAL GRAFT HARVEST

With the patient in the supine position, a 3- to 4-cm incision is designed over the junction between the floating ninth rib tip and the eighth rib above it (see Figures 15-1 and 15-2). The right rib cage is usually selected, particularly in older patients where postoperative chest pain could potentially mask cardiac-related pain. The incision is injected with 10 cc of lidocaine 1% with epinephrine 1:100,000 prior to preparation and draping, observing standard sterile technique. The incision is made and dissection is carried down through the external oblique muscle to identify the interspace between the eighth and ninth ribs (Figure 15-3). Commonly, the incision is carried deep at a point that is lateral to the lateral edge of the rectus abdominis muscle (Figure 15-4). Doing so allows

medial retraction (instead of division) of the rectus muscle and results in less postoperative pain and muscular denervation. For a ninth rib graft, the mobile, medial cartilaginous tip is identified and dissected in a retrograde and extraperichondrial fashion. Since it is a "floating rib," the extraperichondrial dissection is extremely quick with a total harvest time of less than 20 minutes in most cases. For the eighth rib, subperichondrial hydrodissection is performed using lidocaine 2-3 cc of 1% with epinephrine 1:100,000. Serial "H" incisions are carried out through the ventral perichondrium to allow a subperichondrial dissection. Frequently, these incisions must be carried both laterally and medially beyond the required amount of needed graft to facilitate dissection and prevent accidental tearing of the perichondrium. The costal arch is then freed with a periosteal elevator from the caudal aspect of the seventh rib (at the syncytium) and then dissected in a retrograde fashion to the bone–cartilage junction under direct vision. The bone–cartilage junction is easily identified both by a palpable ridge and by the very distinct color change from the white color of the cartilage to the reddish-gray color of the associated bone. This dissection is facilitated with a Doyen retractor (Figure 15-5),

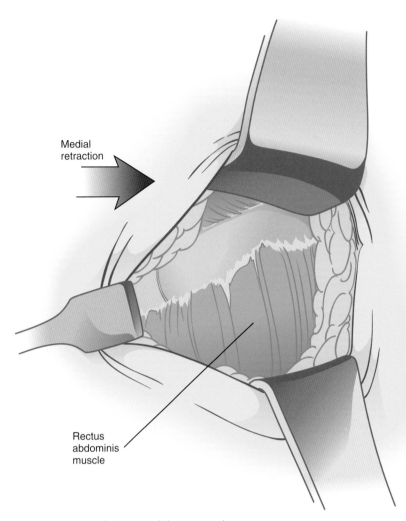

Medial
retraction

Rectus
abdominis
muscle

Figure 15-4 Dissection at lateral edge of the rectus abdominis muscle.

but caution must be heeded as tear of the intimately associated underlying pleura can occur if too much force is used. After the rib is transected under direct vision and removed (Figure 15-6), pleural integrity check is performed by filling the cavity with saline and having the anesthesia provider simulate a Valsalva maneuver. The wound is closed in different layers. Closure of the ventral perichondrium helps to splint the interspace and reduces postoperative pain. Closure of the external oblique fascia must be performed meticulously to help prevent the development of a postoperative hernia. Intramuscular and subcutaneous infiltration of 10 cc of bupivicaine 0.25% with Epinephrine during surgical closure greatly reduces immediate postoperative discomfort.

OSTEOCHONDRAL RIB GRAFT HARVEST

If a dorsal replacement graft is needed to support a severely shrunken skin envelope, a cantilevered bone–cartilage graft can be used. The patient is placed into the

lateral decubitus position on a bean-bag. The incision may need to be located slightly more laterally than for the graft using just cartilage. Dissection is carried through the subcutaneous tissue and external oblique muscle to identify the interspace between the ninth and tenth ribs. With adequate retraction, the osteocartilaginous junction of the ninth rib is identified. Hydrodissection using local anesthetic helps to facilitate subperiosteal retrograde dissection. The lateral portion (minimum 4 cm) of the osseous rib is first dissected with a Doyen elevator to allow for transection of the rib. Then an antegrade dissection is performed toward the medial cartilaginous portion along the same plane. Although quantity requirements will differ slightly between patients, a 4-cm cartilage segment for the columella and a minimum 5-cm osteocartilaginous segment for the dorsum frequently suffice for structural support. The ninth rib is usually sufficient to provide both a dorsal osteocartilaginous graft and a cartilaginous columellar strut. Should the rib stock be inadequate, harvesting the tenth rib can be accomplished through the same incision. The cartilaginous portion of the tenth rib is often

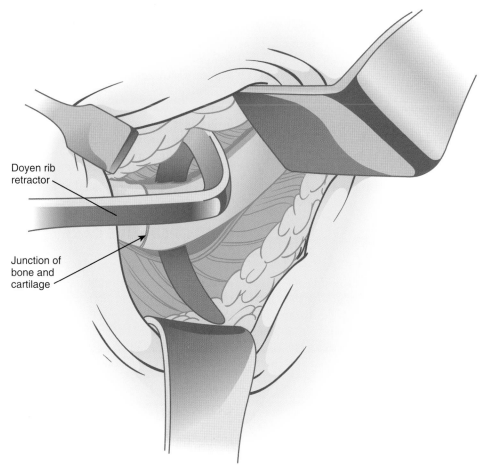

Figure 15-5 Doyen retractor facilitates rib dissection off of the posterior perichondrium.

Doyen rib
retractor

Junction of
bone and
cartilage

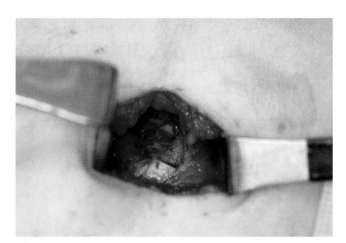

Figure 15-6 Posterior perichondrium with rib removed; ready for pleural integrity check.

short (less than 5 cm), which allows either a useable osteocartilaginous dorsal graft or a cartilaginous columellar strut. After checking for pleural integrity, layered closure starts by approximating the ventral perichondrium. Depending on the extent of dissection and the

individual's body habitus, a closed-suction drain may be placed prior to closure. Infiltration with 10 cc of Marcaine 0.25% with epinephrine is carried out into the wound for post-operative pain relief.

COMPLICATIONS

SEROMA AND HEMATOMA

Donor site seroma formation following rib graft harvest is unusual. In obese patients and in some patients requiring wide undermining, resulting in a larger than average dead space, it is prudent to place a closed suction drainage catheter. This allows efflux of any serous fluid and can be removed at the time of nasal splint and suture removal as long as the drainage output has decreased.

PLEURAL TEAR

If a pleural tear is identified intraoperatively, a purse-string suture closure is performed around a red-rubber suction catheter. The anesthesia provider produces and holds a Valsalva maneuver, while the surgeon simultaneously tightens the suture and removes the catheter. A careful layered soft tissue closure is then performed. If there is any question about the integrity of the repair, an additional intraoperative Valsalva maneuver can be performed.

A postoperative chest radiograph is not routinely performed following rib graft harvest. However, in cases of a pleural tear repair, it may be prudent to obtain an upright chest radiograph in the recovery room. Small residual pneumothoraces can then be treated with oxygen via nasal cannula overnight. Since these pleural tears are almost universally parietal (not visceral) in nature, treatment with thoracostomy tubes is not needed.

POSTOPERATIVE PAIN

Pain following rib graft harvest is expected after the procedure. One of the keys to reducing postoperative pain lies in the intraoperative sequence. Layered closure of the ventral perichondrium and periosteum helps reduce the intercostal space and splints together the adjacent ribs. Care should be taken not to encircle the caudally located intercostal neurovascular bundle, which will lead to postoperative neuropathic pain. Injection of bupivacaine solution prior to closure as described above helps reduce immediate postoperative pain, breaking up the pain cycle and reducing narcotic requirements for most patients. We have used indwelling pain pump catheters in the past. However, patients find these cumbersome and are not particularly useful for wounds requiring closed-suction drainage.

GRAFT FRACTURE

Costal graft fractures are uncommon, except for those exposed to significant trauma. In particular, rib grafts used for component reconstruction virtually never fracture.

INFECTION

Use of intraoperative and postoperative third-generation cephalosporin antibiotics is routine for patients undergoing nasal reconstruction with autologous rib grafting. Donor site infection is virtually nonexistent as long as sterile technique is followed meticulously. The incidence of postoperative graft infection is very low but is still a concern. The risk of infection increases significantly in patients with traumatized intranasal lining and in those with severely scarred nasal skin envelopes.

WARPING

Costal cartilage graft warping is a well-known risk and complication and has been well documented in the

literature.[12] While warping is possible with cantilevered grafts, the risk is significantly reduced and in fact is almost totally eliminated when rib cartilage is used in component reconstruction (with underlying structural support below and underlying camouflage grafting superficially) of the nose. In this way the major structural support is buried underneath a superficial concealing layer, such as diced cartilage wrapped in fascia. The authors do not use axial K-wires as a means of reducing or preventing graft warping. Attention to the carving process following a well-described protocol will minimize the likelihood of unpredictable warping.[13]

POSTOPERATIVE CARE

All operations are performed in an outpatient surgery center without an overnight stay. Pain is easily controlled using oral pain medications. Patients with low pain tolerance are recovered in a nurse-supervised facility to allow for supplemental injectable medications if necessary. Suture removal, dorsal cast, and Doyle intranasal splints are managed conventionally.

CONCLUSION

Costal grafts have dramatically improved the results of secondary and complex primary nasal surgery. We favor the subcostal approach in our practice because of its increased surgical exposure and the variable amount and composition of donor material. The cartilaginous portion of the ninth rib can provide a columellar strut, spreader grafts, and alar rim or tip grafts. If additional material is required, the eighth and tenth ribs can be harvested through the same incision. For severely scarred soft tissue envelopes requiring cantilevered support, the surgical dissection can be modified to include the bony component of ribs 9 or 10. In our experience, the subcostal approach has some advantages, including ease of harvesting, brevity, flexibility, and variability of donor tissue.

REFERENCES

1. Shubailat GF. Cantilever rib grafting in salvage rhinoplasty. *Aesthet Plast Surg.* 2003;27(4):281–285.
2. Cervelli V, Bottini DJ, Gentile P, et al. Reconstruction of the nasal dorsum with autologous rib cartilage. *Ann Plast Surg.* 2006;56(3):256–262.
3. Yilmaz M, Vayvada H, Menderes A, et al. Dorsal nasal augmentation with rib cartilage graft: long-term results and patient satisfaction. *J Craniofac Surg.* 2007;18(6): 1457–1462.
4. Gurley JM, Pilgram T, Perlyn CA, et al. Long-term outcome of autogenous rib graft nasal reconstruction. *Plast Reconstr Surg.* 2001;108(7):1895–1905; discussion 1906–1907.

5. Caccamese Jr R, Ruiz B, Costello J. Costochondral rib grafting. *Atlas Oral Maxillofac Surg Clin.* 2005;13(2):139–149.

6. Eppley BL. Donor site morbidity of rib graft harvesting in primary alveolar cleft bone grafting. *J Craniofac Surg.* 2005;16(2):335–338.

7. Cakmak O, Ergin T. The versatile autogenous costal cartilage graft in septorhinoplasty. *Arch Fac Plast Surg.* 2002;4(3): 172–176.

8. Daniel RK. Rhinoplasty and rib grafts: evolving a flexible operative technique. *Plast Reconstr Surg.* 1994;94(5):597– 609; discussion 610–611.

9. Smith C, Kron I. Hemothorax. In: Cameron J, ed. Current surgical therapy. 7th ed. St Louis: Mosby, 2001:762–765.

10. Marin VP, Landecker A, Gunter JP. Harvesting rib cartilage grafts for secondary rhinoplasty. *Plast Reconstr Surg.* 2008;121(4):1442–1448.

11. Sheen JH, Sheen AP. Aesthetic rhinoplasty. 2nd ed. St Louis: Quality Medical Publishing, 1998.

12. Gibson T, Davis WB. The distortion of autogenous cartilage grafts: its cause and prevention. *Br J Plast Surg.* 1958;11: 177.

13. Kim DW, Shah AR, Toriumi DM. Concentric and eccentric carved costal cartilage: A comparison of warping. *Arch Fac Plast Surg.* 2006;8(1):42–46.

CHAPTER SIXTEEN

Calvarial Bone Grafting in Rhinoplasty

Robin W. Lindsay • *Tessa A. Hadlock* • *Mack L. Cheney*

Calvarial bone grafting is an established method of cranio-facial reconstruction in facial plastic surgery. Konig[1] and Muller[2] were the first to describe autogenous calvarial bone grafting in 1890, advocating a combined osteocutaneous flap. Smith, Abramson, and Tessier[3-5] popularized the technique for modern craniofacial reconstruction. More recently, split calvarial bone grafts have been shown to be safe and effective grafts for nasal reconstruction[6,7] and a viable alternative to autogenous cartilage and alloplastic implants for dorsal nasal augmentation.[8,9]

Two groups of patients undergoing rhinoplasty and/or nasal reconstruction require materials to augment the nasal dorsum. The first group has saddle nose deformity, arising from traumatic, infectious, idiopathic, or iatrogenic conditions. The second group of patients has a congenitally platyrrhine nose, characterized by a low, wide dorsum, poor tip projection and definition, and an acute nasolabial angle.[10] In modern reconstruction of the nasal dorsum, an ideal implant provides structural support, long-lasting augmentation, limited mobility, and reasonable resistance to infection.

Four categories of facial implants are in use today: alloplastic materials, homografts, xenografts, and autografts. Alloplasts are implants made of chemically composed polymers. Homografts refer to grafts obtained from a donor of the same species and include irradiated and nonirradiated cartilage, bone, and soft tissue. Xenografts refer to materials obtained from different species and are not used in contemporary augmentation rhinoplasty. Autografts are materials harvested from the patient's own body and include bone, cartilage, and soft tissue grafts.[8,10]

ALLOPLASTS

Presently, the literature supports the use of both alloplastic and autogenous material for nasal reconstruction. Employing alloplastic materials shortens the length of an operation by eliminating the harvesting step, eliminates donor site morbidity, and can be easily tailored to conform to the defect. These materials are available in unlimited quantities and undergo minimal resorption.[10] However, there are several important disadvantages to their use that

have prompted many surgeons to avoid their use when possible. These disadvantages include foreign body reaction at the implant–tissue interface, a limited ability to withstand infection, and a tendency to migrate. These implants must be placed under highly sterile conditions, preferably in a bed of healthy, robust native tissue; tension over the implant and compromise to the vascular supply of the recipient bed must be avoided.[8]

HOMOGRAFTS

Homografts represent another option for nasal reconstruction, and irradiated costal cartilage has been advocated as the preferred graft for dorsal nasal reconstruction by some surgeons, especially for those with extruded nasal alloplastic implants.[11,12] Irradiated costal cartilage is harvested from cadavers that meet the same criteria required for organ donation (Venereal Disease Research Laboratory, hepatitis B, human immunodeficiency virus, tuberculosis, and slow virus testing).[8] After harvest, the graft is irradiated with 30,000 to 40,000 Gy of ionizing radiation to eradicate potential pathogens.[10] Benefits of homografts include their availability, low infection rates, minimal host immunogenic response, and decreased operative times.[8,10,11] The use of homografts is limited by their tendency to resorb, sometimes unpredictably; resorption rates as high as 80% have been reported at 2 years.[8,13] Symmetric contouring of the graft, placement in areas of low mobility (such as the nasal dorsum), and K-wire insertion are techniques that have been developed to decrease the rate of absorption.[8,14] Homologous rib is best reserved for the elderly, to decrease operative times and donor site morbidity.[8]

AUTOLOGOUS IMPLANTS

Given the shortcomings of allopasts and homografts, many nasal surgeons believe that the preferred type of implant for correction of saddle nose deformities or severe structural deficiencies is autogenous cartilage or bone.[7,8] Autologous tissue is favored for its biocompatibility, low rate of infection and extrusion, and limited inflammatory response. It also lacks the risk of disease transmission that is present in homologous implants. Despite the limited availability and donor site morbidity, autologous implants remain the standard to which all other implants are compared.

CARTILAGE

Cartilages is an extremely popular graft material for most rhinoplasty surgeons and can be harvested from the septum, concha, or rib. Septal and conchal cartilages do not provide sufficient material for repair of most saddle nose deformities or severe tip structural deficiencies. Rib is the only source of cartilage that provides the structural support required for major nasal reconstruction. A significant advantage of rib is that it is readily available, although moderate absorption rates and a tendency to warp have been reported.[11,13–16] Removal of the perichondrium, accompanied by symmetric carving using the central core of cartilage for dorsal augmentation, is one technique described to reduce warping.[8] Internal fixation of the graft with a K-wire can also potentially reduce warping and decrease delayed graft malposition.[14] Donor site morbidities include the possibility of pneumothorax, a likelihood of postoperative pain, temporary atelectasis, potential chest wall deformity, and a visible scar. In older patients, ossification of the cartilage can make carving and shaping of costal cartilage difficult.

BONE

Autologous bone is rigid, provides excellent support, and can be contoured with an otologic drill to create the desired contour. For nasal reconstruction, osseous rib and iliac crest are common sources of endochondral bone, while calvarium is the most common source of membranous bone. Osseous rib has an unpredictable pattern and amount of absorption, with an inherent tendency to distort its shape over time. The iliac crest yields plentiful bone, which can be fashioned to fit a variety of defects, similar to calvarial grafts. However, absorption has been problematic, and donor site issues, including pain and walking impairment, have been substantial.[17,18]

CALVARIAL BONE

Calvarial bone offers advantages for nasal reconstruction based on its membranous origin. Experimental evidence suggests that graft volume is more consistently maintained in bone of membranous origin than from endochondral bone grafts.[7,19–24] When compared morphologically to endochondral bone, membranous bone demonstrates a thicker cortical plate, a smaller endocortical cancellous area, and stronger intracortical struts.[18]

Clinical advantages to calvarial bone grafting include decreased donor site pain, a hidden donor site, proximity of the donor site to the surgical field, and excellent graft shape.[6,7,19] An additional benefit of calvarial bone is its ability to establish a bony union, decreasing the risk of displacement. Calvarial bone can also be used safely in patients with infection, destructive infectious processes, and noninfectious inflammatory diseases.

ANATOMIC CONSIDERATIONS IN CALVARIAL BONE GRAFTING

The calvarium is composed of single frontal and occipital bones, along with paired parietal and temporal bones (Figure 16-1). The sagittal, coronal, lambdoid, and squamosal sutures separate these bones. There are three distinct layers in the adult human skull: the outer cortical layer, the middle spongy cancellous layer (also termed the diploic layer), and the inner cortical layer. The goal of the split calvarial bone technique is to harvest only the outer cortical layer (Figure 16-2). The dura adheres very closely to the undersurface of the inner calvarial layer, making it susceptible to tearing if the inner calvarium is inadvertently violated. The undersurface of the inner cortex is imprinted with numerous concavities formed by the underlying intracranial vasculature. The venous sagittal sinus is located in the midline and is approximately 1 to 1.5 cm wide. The temporal line represents the superior attachment of the temporal muscle, and both the outer cortical and the middle diploic layers are unacceptably thin lateral to this landmark. Moreover, the area above the temporal line possesses a natural curvature that mimics the nasal dorsum. Midline calvarial bone grafts place the sagittal sinus at risk, so bone within 2 cm of the midline should be left undisturbed.[19] The bone also becomes thin in the area of the sutures (Figure 16-3).[19] The parietal bone has been consistently noted to have the thickest bone.[23] Bone is thicker in males than in females by 1 or 2 mm.[3,6] With these anatomic areas in mind, the safest area to harvest a split calvarial bone graft is on the parietal bone between the temporal line, the sagittal sinus, and suture lines.

METHODS AND SURGICAL TECHNIQUES

The patient's hair is not shaved but instead is parted and coated with bacitracin ointment. The donor site and the recipient are prepped with povidone-iodine or alcohol and infiltrated with lidocaine (Xylocaine) with epinephrine (1:100,000) to promote hemostasis. Consideration should be given to using the nondominant side of the scalp, to

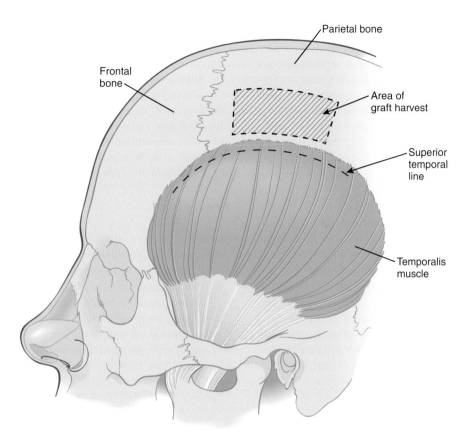

Figure 16-1 Typical donor site for harvesting the calvarial bone graft. Site should be superior to the superior temporal line and should not involve the central calvarium to avoid exposure of the sagittal sinus.

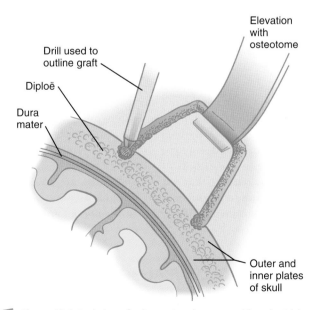

Figure 16-2 Technique for harvesting the outer table calvarial bone graft. The outer table troughs are created to the level of the diploic layers. Using Tessier osteotomies, the graft is elevated from the inner table of the calvarium.

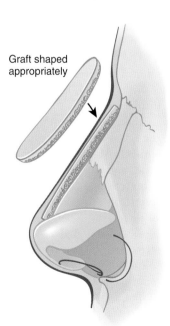

Figure 16-3 The bone graft is fashioned into a fusiform shape and introduced into the nasal pocket after rasping the nasal bones.

protect the dominant motor cortex in the event of a neurologic complication. A sagittal temporoparietal incision is made over the superior temporal line. An incision positioned medial to the superior temporal line risks exposure if male pattern baldness develops, and an incision placed laterally risks hematoma from dissection around the temporalis muscle and cerebrospinal fluid leak from calvarial dissection in the thinner bone of this region. After the incision is made to the level of the calvarium, the pericranium is elevated medially and laterally. Using an otologic cutting drill, a 1.5 × 4.5-cm graft is outlined, with the longest dimension in the sagittal plane. A trough is created around the graft with the cutting burr. The diploic level is identified when spongy bone and bleeding are encountered. The margins of the trough are beveled to facilitate the positioning of the osteotomes. The osteotomes are positioned in a plane tangential to the skull to prevent dural injury (Figure 16-4). A series of sequentially larger curved osteotomes are used circumferentially to separate the outer table calvarium from the inner table through the diploic layer. If dura is exposed during elevation, the margins should be burnished with a diamond drill. Typically, no further measures are necessary. The donor site defect can be obliterated by filling with methyl methacrylate, although this may occasionally lead to a pain syndrome, and also harbors all of the usual risks of a foreign body. The defect when left untreated is frequently imperceptible, given its location under hairbearing scalp, and most patients are not bothered by the slight palpable depression in that zone. The wound is closed in a single layer over a suction drain, and a head wrap is placed. The calvarial bone graft is then brought to a separate sterile field and irrigated copiously with a bacitracin-containing solution. At this point, the bone graft normally measures approximately 1.0 × 3.5 cm. An otologic drill is used to carve a fusiform shape to match the nasal defect. The graft is fashioned slightly wider caudally if correction of the internal nasal valve is required. The undersurface of the graft is hollowed along its central axis to prevent displacement.

Prior to or simultaneously with the harvest of the calvarial bone, the nasal dorsum is exposed via a closed or open nasal approach. Most frequently, a transcolumellar incision is made, and the nasal flap is raised off the cartilaginous and bony framework of the nose. The periosteum is elevated from the nasal bones, facilitating assessment of the defect and helping to determine the volume of bone to be harvested. The nasal bones are freshened with a rotating burr or a rasp to provide good contact with the diploic layer of the calvarial graft. With the open nasal approach, this step is performed under direct vision. The sculpted calvarial bone is placed under the nasal soft tissue envelope, and the columellar incision is closed with 6-0 nylon sutures. The vestibular incisions are closed with 5-0 chromic suture to ensure that the graft is isolated from the nasal cavity.[1,2,19,25]

IMPORTANT TECHNIQUE ISSUES

There are a few important technical points that tend to improve graft survival. Theoretically, graft survival improves by limiting the interval between bone graft harvest and implantation to less than 45 minutes and by avoiding bone temperatures above 42°C.[26] To avoid thermal injury to the bone graft, copious irrigation should be used while harvesting and contouring the bone graft.[7]

Additionally, the position of the bone graft as it bridges the upper two thirds of the nasal dorsum is of utmost importance. The bone graft should not project beyond the caudal margin of the upper lateral cartilages and the anterior septal angle. Using this principle, the nasal lower third will maintain its natural flexibility. If the graft does extend beyond this point, the nasal tip will become frozen and unnatural in appearance and feel.

Dead space between the nasal bones and the bone graft must be avoided. The diploic layer of the bone graft must interface directly and securely with the nasal bones. Proper preparation of the nasal bones with the cutting burr and careful sculpting of the graft so that irregular areas of contact are eliminated both ensure optimal interfacing. This technique promotes early fusion between the diploic layer and the bony nasal pyramid and eliminates the need for additional stabilizing measures such as plates, screws, or wires. Dead space between the cartilaginous framework of the middle one third of the nasal pyramid and the bone graft is acceptable and may be beneficial in selected cases.

A tight soft tissue pocket reduces the risk of graft migration and has a positive effect on the internal nasal valve. A tight subperiosteal pocket enables the surgeon to place the bone graft along the nasal dorsum with external casting alone.[7,27-30] Many surgeons do fixate the graft with wires, screws, or microscrews[8,25,31,32] based on experimental data supporting that fixation is necessary to maintain graft position and reduce the risk of resorption.[33] However, even groups using fixation have shown that mobile grafts have not decreased in size and that grafts were solidly fused to the underlying bone between 14 and 21 days.[25] Radiographic postoperative studies have demonstrated capacity for bone to bone healing with calvarial bone grafts.[7,27] In addition, experimental studies have shown that when bone grafts are placed in an area of limited motion, rigid fixation offers no advantage over placement of the graft in a compact soft-tissue envelope.[29,30]

EFFECTS OF CALVARIAL BONE GRAFTING ON FUNCTION

The mechanism by which a calvarial bone graft influences the internal nasal valve is by displacing the upper lateral cartilages laterally. Two factors influence the

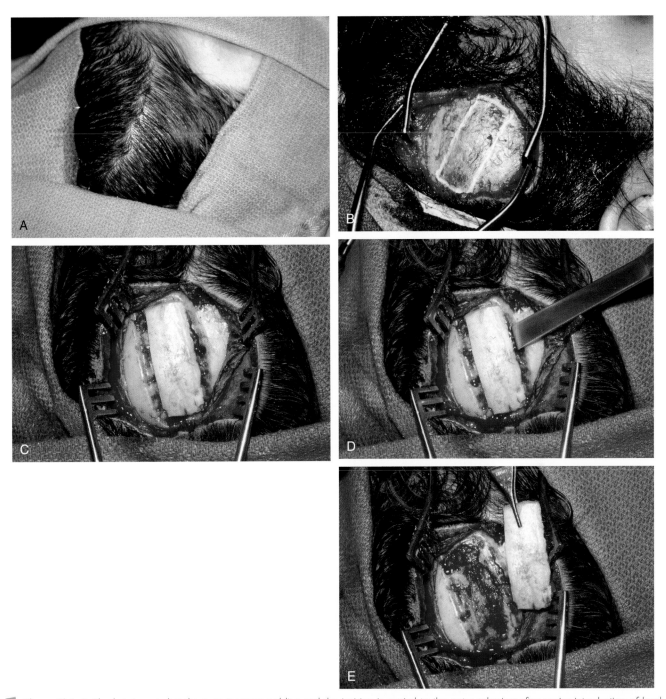

Figure 16-4 A, The hair is parted at the superior temporal line and the incision is carried to the outer calvarium after copius introduction of local anesthesia with epinephrine. **B,** Using an otologic drill with a cutting bit, an outline of the outer calvarium is performed. The average dimension is 3 centimeters by 1.5 centimeters. **C,** Troughs are created to the mid-diploic layer of the calvarium with attention to flattening the shoulder of the troughs so the osteotomies can easily be introduced. **D,** Using Tessier osteotomes, the bone graft is removed from the inner calvarium. Hemostatis is obtained with bone wax. **E,** Appearance of the bone graft after harvest and prior to creating a fusiform shape.

amount of lateralization that can be achieved. First, increasing the width of the bone graft, especially caudally, increases lateral displacement of the upper lateral cartilages from the nasal septum. Second, maintaining the attachments of the upper lateral cartilages to the overlying soft tissue when dissecting the soft-tissue pocket widens the internal nasal valve when the graft is placed (Figure 16-5).

COMPLICATIONS OF CALVARIAL BONE GRAFTING

DONOR SITE

Donor site complications include hematoma/seroma (1% to 8.3%), infection (1% to 2%), alopecia (2.8%), loss of sensation (2.8%), and dural tears (<1%).[6,7,19,27] However,

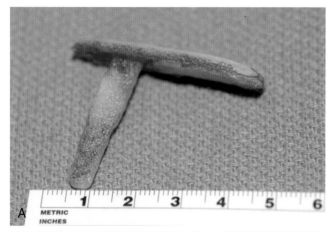

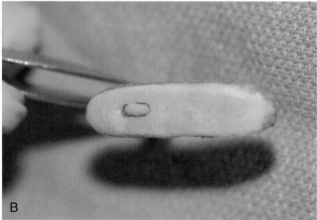

Figure 16-5 A, B: Additional structural support may be incorporated into the bone graft by using a tongue in groove technique to introduce a columellar strut into the dorsal bone graft.

in a series by Kline and Wolfe of 586 cranial bone harvests, no neurologic complications were reported.[34] Superior sagittal sinus laceration has been reported; however, it occurs extremely infrequently and can be avoided by being familiar with the surgical technique.[35]

MANAGEMENT OF DONOR SITE COMPLICATIONS

In case of dural exposure, the surgeon has several options. In most cases, the area of exposed dura is small and no attempt at osseous closure is needed. Bone dust may be placed in this defect or, if the defect is large (>2 cm), another split calvarial graft may be needed to repair the defect.[36]

In the case of a dural tear, it is important to visualize the laceration completely by removing additional bone. The dura is then carefully elevated and the brain examined for injury. If no injury exists, the dura is repaired with a 4-0 silk suture. If injury is suspected, there should be a low threshold for neurosurgical consultation.[19]

RECIPIENT SITE

Recipient site complications have been reported in the literature and include resorption, overcorrection, mobility, infection, graft exposure, graft fracture, and displacement of the graft.[6,7,37] In the series of 35 nasal reconstruction patients by Cheney and Gliklich, there was one case that was thought to be overcorrected, but no cases of graft displacement, mobility, extrusion, or significant resorption, and in the series of 87 calvarial bone graft patients by Emerick et al., one patient had a postoperative infection and three grafts became mobile (Figures 16-6 and 16-7).[7,27]

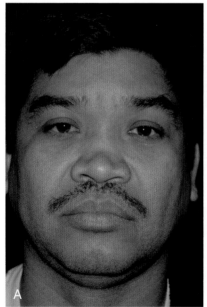

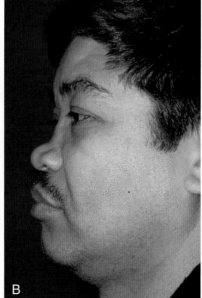

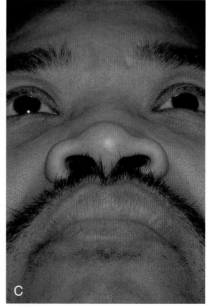

Figure 16-6 A–C: Preoperative photographs of a patient who suffered severe nasal collapse secondary to extensive nasal infection as a child.

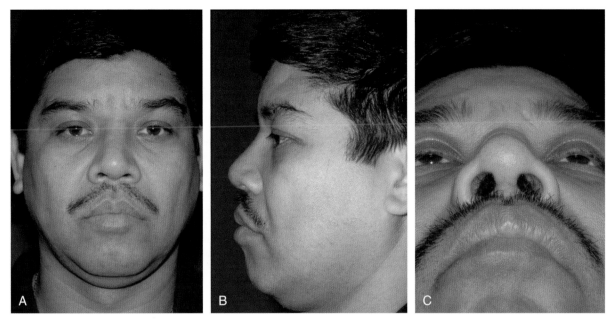

Figure 16-7 A–C: Postoperative result at 1 year after utilizing a calvarial bone graft with an integrated columellar strut for dorsal restoration.

CONCLUSIONS

Calvarial bone is an excellent source of grafting material for saddle nose deformities and congenitally platyrrhine noses. It provides structural support, long-lasting augmentation, limited mobility, and resistance to infection. These properties allow surgeons to utilize the graft in patients with destructive infectious processes and noninfectious inflammatory diseases. However, a detailed knowledge of the local anatomy and surgical technique is required to perform the operation safely.

REFERENCES

1. Konig F. Der knocheme Erstz grosser Schadelfekte. *Zentralbl Chir.* 1890;17:497–501.
2. Muller W. Zur Frage der temporaren Schadeldefekten an Stelle der Trepanation. *Zentralbl Chir.* 1890;17:65–66.
3. Tessier P. Autogenous bone grafts taken from the calvarium for facial and cranial applications. *Clin Plast Surg.* 1982;9: 531–538.
4. Tessier P. Aesthetic aspects of bone grafting to the face. *Clin Plast Surg.* 1981;8:279–301.
5. Sheen JH, Sheen, AP. *Aesthetic Rhinoplasty,* 2nd ed. St. Louis: Mosby; 1987; pp. 383–402.
6. Jackson IT, Choi HY, Clay R, et al. Long-term follow-up of cranial bone graft in dorsal nasal augmentation. *Plast Reconstr Surg.* 1998;102:1869–1873.
7. Cheney ML, Gliklich RE. The use of calvarial bone in nasal reconstruction. *Arch Otolaryngol Head Neck Surg.* 1995;121: 643–648.
8. Lovice DB, Mingrone MD, Toriumi DM. Grafts amd implants in rhinoplasty and nasal reconstruction. *Otolaryngol Clin North Am.* 1999;32:113–141.
9. Romo 3rd T, Jablonski RD. Nasal reconstruction using split calvarial grafts. *Otolaryngol Head Neck Surg.* 1992;107: 622–630.
10. Romo 3rd T, Pearson JM. Nasal implants. *Fac Plast Surg Clin North Am.* 2008;16:123–132, vi.
11. Clark JM, Cook TA. Immediate reconstruction of extruded alloplastic nasal implants with irradiated homograft costal cartilage. *Laryngoscope.* 2002;112:968–974.
12. Kridel RW, Konior RJ. Irradiated cartilage grafts in the nose. A preliminary report. *Arch Otolaryngol Head Neck Surg.* 1993;119:24–30; discussion 30–31.
13. Congdon D, Sherris DA, Specks U, et al. Long-term follow-up of repair of external nasal deformities in patients with Wegener's granulomatosis. *Laryngoscope.* 2002;112:731–737.
14. Gunter JP, Clark CP, Friedman RM. Internal stabilization of autogenous rib cartilage grafts in rhinoplasty: a barrier to cartilage warping. *Plast Reconstr Surg.* 1997;100:161–169.
15. Adams Jr WP, Rohrich RJ, Gunter JP, et al. The rate of warping in irradiated and nonirradiated homograft rib cartilage: a controlled comparison and clinical implications. *Plast Reconstr Surg.* 1999;103:265–270.
16. Strauch B, Wallach SG. Reconstruction with irradiated homograft costal cartilage. *Plast Reconstr Surg.* 2003; 111:2405–2411; discussion 12–13.
17. Silber JS, Anderson DG, Daffner SD, et al. Donor site morbidity after anterior iliac crest bone harvest for single-level anterior cervical discectomy and fusion. *Spine.* 2003;28:134–139.
18. Hardesty RA, Marsh JL. Craniofacial onlay bone grafting: a prospective evaluation of graft morphology, orientation, and embryonic origin. *Plast Reconstr Surg.* 1990;85:5–14; discussion 15.
19. Frodel Jr JL, Marentette LJ, Quatela VC, et al. Calvarial bone graft harvest. Techniques, considerations, and morbidity. *Arch Otolaryngol Head Neck Surg.* 1993;119:17–23.
20. Chen NT, Glowacki J, Bucky LP, et al. The roles of revascularization and resorption on endurance of craniofacial

onlay bone grafts in the rabbit. *Plast Reconstr Surg.* 1994;93:714–722; discussion 723–724.

21. Zins JE, Whitaker LA. Membranous versus endochondral bone: implications for craniofacial reconstruction. *Plast Reconstr Surg.* 1983;72:778–785.

22. Smith JD, Abramson M. Membranous vs endochondral bone autografts. *Arch Otolaryngol.* 1974;99:203–205.

23. Pensler J, McCarthy JG. The calvarial donor site: an anatomic study in cadavers. *Plast Reconstr Surg.* 1985;75:648–651.

24. Hunter D, Baker S, Sobol SM. Split calvarial grafts in maxillofacial reconstruction. *Otolaryngol Head Neck Surg.* 1990;102:345–350.

25. Jackson IT, Smith J, Mixter RC. Nasal bone grafting using split skull grafts. *Ann Plast Surg.* 1983;11:533–540.

26. Young VL, Schuster RH, Harris LW. Intracerebral hematoma complicating split calvarial bone-graft harvesting. *Plast Reconstr Surg.* 1990;86:763–765.

27. Emerick KS, Hadlock, TA, Cheney, ML. Nasofacial reconstruction with calvarial bone grafts in compromised defects. *Laryngoscope.* 2008;118(9):1534-1538.

28. Albreksson T. *Scand J Plast Reconstr Sur.* 1980;14:1–12.

29. Fry H. Cartilage and cartilage grafts: the basic properties of the tissue and the components responsible for them. *Plast Reconstr Surg.* 1967;40:526–539.

30. Lin KY, Bartlett SP, Yaremchuk MJ, et al. The effect of rigid fixation on the survival of onlay bone grafts: an experimental study. *Plast Reconstr Surg.* 1990;86:449–456.

31. Staffel G, Shockley W. Nasal implants. *Otolaryngol Clin North Am.* 1995;28:295–308.

32. Sullivan PK, Varma M, Rozzelle AA. Optimizing bone-graft nasal reconstruction: a study of nasal bone shape and thickness. *Plast Reconstr Surg.* 1996;97:327–335; discussion 36–37.

33. Phillips JH, Rahn BA. Fixation effects on membranous and endochondral onlay bone-graft resorption. *Plast Reconstr Surg.* 1988;82:872–877.

34. Kline Jr RM, Wolfe SA. Complications associated with the harvesting of cranial bone grafts. *Plast Reconstr Surg.* 1995;95:5–13; discussion 14–20.

35. Cannella DM, Hopkins LN. Superior sagittal sinus laceration complicating an autogenous calvarial bone graft harvest: report of a case. *J Oral Maxillofac Surg.* 1990;48:741–743.

36. Sammartino G, Marenzi G, Colella G, et al. Autogenous calvarial bone graft harvest: intraoperational complications. *J Craniofac Surg.* 2005;16:312–319.

37. Sheen JH. The ideal dorsal graft: a continuing quest. *Plast Reconstr Surg.* 1998;102:2490–2493.

CHAPTER SEVENTEEN

Mandibular Implants

William A. Kennedy III • Babak Azizzadeh • William J. Binder

Over the past two decades, great improvements have been made in the design of facial implants. Facial implants are able to enhance facial contour and provide permanent volumetric replacement. Facial implants can be used in many anatomic regions of the face, including the cheek, midface, nose, and mandible. Here we discuss the application of implants for the correction of profile imbalance as well as the rejuvenation of the lower third of the face. Mandibular augmentation is perhaps the simplest and most powerful aesthetic procedure available to the surgeon. Mentoplasty can create a stronger mandibular profile and improve the appearance of the nose by making it appear smaller and less imposing. In addition, augmentation of the prejowl sulcus and the mandibular angle can help enhance the effects of rhytidectomy by creating a sharper cervicofacial angle. Successful surgical results will be determined by the proper technique. The goals of mandibular augmentation are to reconstruct facial contour deformities or deficiencies with a high degree of predictability.

GENERAL CONSIDERATIONS

INDICATIONS FOR MANDIBULAR AUGMENTATION

The primary indications for mandibular augmentation include:

1. Stand-alone procedure for mandibular augmentation
2. Adjunctive procedure to rhinoplasty with an emphasis on profileplasty
3. Adjunctive procedure to rhytidectomy, which is often essential for patients with microgenia and/or prominent prejowl erosion

The key to mandibular augmentation lies in the restoration of anterior projection and/or expansion of lateral contour. In the aging process, the anterior mandible may develop flattening of the soft tissue button of the chin and form a deepening of the prejowl sulcus.

Augmentation of the bony mandible occurs over one of three zonal areas (Figure 17-1). The first zone is the central chin area, which extends from the mentum to mental foramen (Zone 1). The midlateral zone is defined by a line extending from the mental formen posteriorly to the oblique line of the horizontal body of the mandible (Zone 2). The third and last zone of the premandibular space ecompasses the posterior half of the horizontal body, including the angle of the mandible and the first 2 to 4 cm of the ascending ramus (Zone 3).

Augmenting a recessed central chin area is a key componenet of profileoplasty which can additionally improve the aesthetic outcome of rhinoplasty. The projection of the chin directly affects the illusory projection of the nose in an inverse relationship. The traditional chin implants, placed only within the central area (Zone 1) without lateral extension into the midlateral zones (Zone 2) often created suboptimal results (Figures 17-2 to 17-4). These early implants, unidimensionally designed and with a single vector, were often bulky and nonanatomic. This often resulted in a round chin protuberance, which can appear abnormal and unattractive. Similarly, a smaller implant, placed centrally had a greater tendency to shift or rotate than a larger more extended implant.

Most of these early problems were corrected with the design of the extended mandibular implants that occupied Zones 1 and 2. Placement of an implant that extends into at least two zones (central chin and midlateral) also results in a natural widening of the anterior jawline as well as an increased vertical dimension of the lower third of the face (Figure 17-5).

Augmentation of the posterior-lateral zone widens the jaw to produce a stronger posterior jawline contour. This can be achieved using a mandibular angle implant to augment the posterior lateral zone of the mandible (the posterior half of the horizontal body including the angle of the mandible and the first 2 cm to 4 cm of the ascending ramus).

Mentoplasty can also have a powerful impact in facial rejuvenation in addressing the structural elements of the jaw and neck. The prejowl and prejowl–chin implants can be used as stand-alone procedure or serve a complementary role to liposuction and rhytidectomy (Figures 17-6

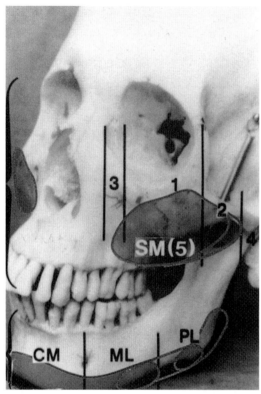

Figure 17-1 The mandible can be anatomically divided into three zones. The first zone extends from the mentum to mental foramen (CM-Zone 1). The midlateral zone is defined by a line extending from the mental formen posteriorly to the oblique line of the horizontal body of the mandible (ML-Zone 2). The third and last zone of the premandibular space ecompasses the posterior half of the horizontal body, including the angle of the mandible and the first 2 to 4 cm of the ascending ramus (PL-Zone 3). (From Binder W, Schoenrock L, eds. Facial contouring and alloplastic implants. Philadelphia: WB Saunders, 1994, Facial Plastic Surgery Clinics of North America.)

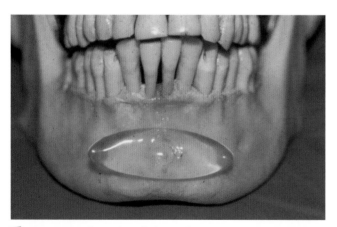

Figure 17-2 The traditional chin implants, as depicted in this photograph, were placed only wthin the central area (Zone 1) without lateral extension into the midlateral zones. These early implants were unidimensionally-designed utilizing a single vector.

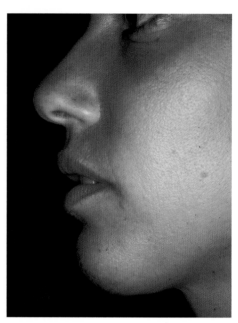

Figure 17-3 Traditional central implants placed in Zone 1 often created suboptimal results. This often gave the appearance of an abnormal and unattractive round chin protuberance.

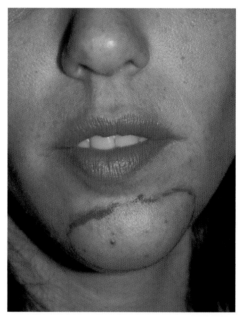

Figure 17-4 A smaller implant, placed centrally had a greater tendency to shift or rotate than a larger more extended implant.

to 17-8). Causative factors leading to the aging and ptotic face include loss of volume or atrophy of soft tissue and skin elasticity overlying Zones 1 and 2 of the mandible. Over the lower third of the face, this is seen as a loss of a straight jaw line and the development of jowling, prejowl

sulcus, and/or marionette lines (skin crease that extends from the oral commissure to the mandible). The marionette lines emerge due to the attachment of the depressor labii inferiorus muscle and depressor angulii oris to the inferior mandible.[1] These attachments create a point resistance by which drooping skin is caught producing a

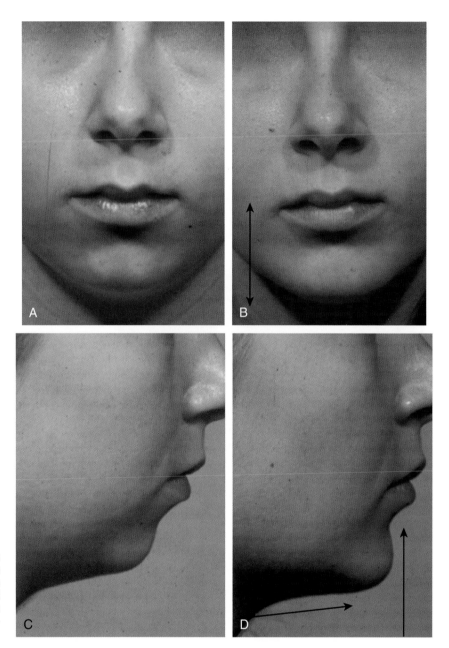

Figure 17-5 Placement of an implant that extends into at least 2 zones (central chin & midlateral) results in a natural widening of the anterior jawline as well as increasing the vertical dimenstion to the lower third of the face. **A, C** Pre-op; **B, D** Post-op photo after chin augmentation. The implant resides "low" on the mandible preserving a normal labiomental sulcus.

"hammock"-like bulge of skin. By removing these attachments, the skin is allowed to fall more naturally and the marionette lines are reduced or softened.

Careful evaluation leads to realization that an area of volume deficiency exists anterior to the jowl called the prejowl sulcus. The prejowl sulcus is a specific area anterior to the jowl exhibiting a marked dropoff in soft tissue volume and bony mandibular projection. The sulcus or depression can occur from several factors such as a deficiency of bone, congenitally narrow mandible, or aggregation of soft tissue around the mandibular ligament that contributes to the jowl. The skin overlying the prejowl sulcus is also significantly thinner than the skin lateral or medial to this location. As the aging process advances, the anterior mandibular groove deepens, which further accentuates the jowls.

Treatment of mandibular jowling and creation of a smooth mandibular line primarily require rhytidectomy, which repositions and tightens the soft tissue along the lower third of the face. Rhytidectomy alone, however, may not completely address the prejowl sulcus. Therefore, a secondary procedure that directly addresses this defect using a prejowl implant is required. A series of prejowl and chin implants have been designed for this use. The implants used in conjunction with facelift surgery increase its ability to create a smooth and straight jaw line.

IMPLANT CHARACTERISTICS

The ideal implant material for bony manidibular augmentation should be inert, easily shaped, conformable yet able to maintain its desired shape over the long term (Figure 17-9). The implant should be easily customized and modified for the needs of the patient while not compromising the integrity of the implant. Implant immobilization is partly related to the degree of encapsulation. All implants have some level of encapsulation.[6] Implants made from silicone elastomer have a high degree of encapsulation, while implants made from polytetrafluoroethylene (ePTFE; W.L. Gore & Asssociates, Inc., Flagstaff, AZ) encapsulate to a lesser degree yet provide some fixation

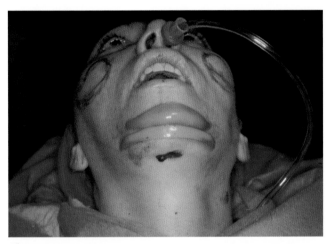

Figure 17-6 The prejowl and prejowl–chin implants along with other procedures such as liposuction and rhytidectomy address the structural elements of the lower face and the manifestations of aging.

with minimal tissue ingrowth.[6] Each implant material causes unique tissue–implant interactions. Ideal tissue–implant interaction will not cause significant tissue ingrowth and permanent fixation of the implant. As with any implantable material, ease of removal and replacement is essential to the quality of any implant, whether it be a breast implant or cardiac pacemaker. In aesthetic surgery, it is particularly important if the patient desires further change.[7]

The shape of the implant should also have tapered edges to ensure a smooth transition from implant to bony foundation. In newer generations of silicone implants, design efforts are focused on making the undersurface of the implant more malleable. Greater conformation to the irregular bony surfaces of the mandible prevents the formation of dead space and thereby reduces the movement and migration.[8]

IMPLANT COMPOSITION

BIOMATERIALS

Polymetric Materials

In use since the 1950s, silicone has proved to be a safe and effective implant material. Silicone is polymerized dimethylsiloxane and can take the form of a gel, solid, or liquid depending on the degree cross-linking and polymerization. The gel form of silicone has the potential to leak, but the most recent studies finds no cause-and-effect relationship between silicone and the development of lupus, scleroderma, or other autoimmune diseases.[9–11]

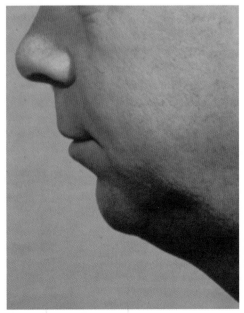
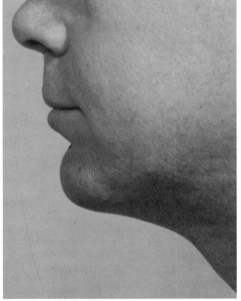

Figure 17-7 A, Pre-op; **B,** Post-op after chin augmentation and submental liposuction.

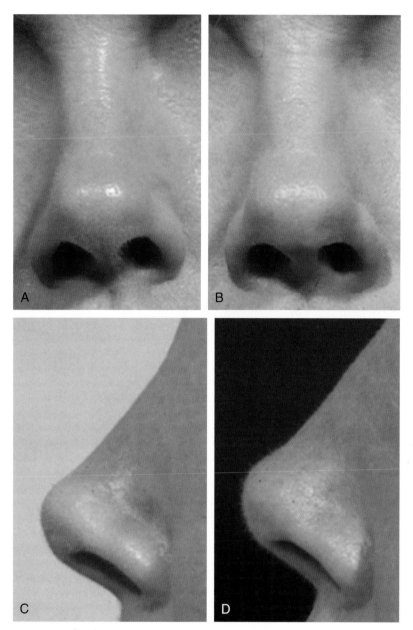

Figure 17-8 A, C, Pre-op; **B, D,** Post-op after chin augmentation.

Solid silicone has a higher degree of inertness than gel silicone with no evidence of toxicity or allergic reactions.[12] Tissue reaction to solid silicone consists of the formation of a fibrous capsule around the implant but without tissue ingrowth. Capsular contraction and secondary implant deformity are rare and occur secondary to an implant that is placed improperly at a superficial plane. Seroma formation or inflammatory tissue reaction usually occurs as a result of implant mobility.

Polymethacrylate (Acrylic) Polymers

These can be supplied as a powdered material or preformed. The powder is mixed at the time of surgery to form a hard material. Due to its rigidity, placement of larger implants through relatively smaller openings can be difficult and even impossible. Preformed implants also lack the ability to conform to the vagaries of underlying bone.

Polyethylene

In the porous form, also known as MEDPOR (Porex Surgical, Inc., Newnan, GA), polyethylene can be developed to take on a variety of forms and consistencies. It elicits minimal amounts of inflammatory cell reaction. The material is rigid and thus difficult to mold to fit the underlying bony foundation. The porosity of the implant allows for significant tissue ingrowth and tissue stability, but as a drawback the biomaterial is therefore difficult to remove.

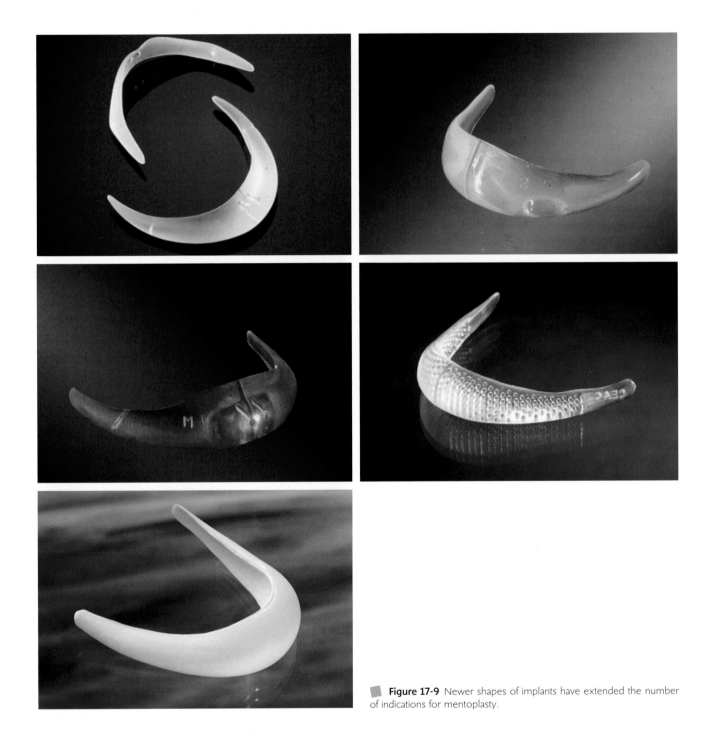

Figure 17-9 Newer shapes of implants have extended the number of indications for mentoplasty.

Polytetrafluoroethylene

Formerly marketed under the brand name of Proplast, this group of materials is no longer marketed in the United States secondary to its complications with temporomandibular joint use. Under high mechanical stress, this implant often broke down and elicited intense inflammatory reaction, thick capsule formation, and extrusion

Expanded Polytetrafluoroethylene (ePTFE)

Originally produced for cardiovascular applications, this material has the benefit of producing minimal tissue ingrowth, capsule formation and inflammatory reaction. Given its limited tissue ingrowth, ePTFE is ideally suited for subcutaneous tissue augmentation where ease in secondary modification or removal may be desired.

Mesh Polymers.

The mesh polymers include Marlex (Chevron Phillips Chemical Company, The Woodlands, TX), Dacron (Unify, Inc., Greensboro, NC), and Madrilène (Ethicon, Cincinnati, OH). They have similar advantages of being able to be folded, sutured, and shaped with ease. Unfavorable characteristics include ingrowth of fibrous tissue. Supramid (Resorba Wundversorgung, Nurnberg, Germany) is a polyamide mesh derivative of nylon that is unstable in vivo. It elicits a mild foreign body reaction and over time causes implant degradation and resorption.[13]

METALS

Metals consist mainly of stainless steel, vitallium, gold, and titanium. Gold and titanium are commonly used for upper eyelids for facial reanimation. Titanium has become the metal of choice for long-term implantation. It has high biocompatibility and a low corrosive index and is primarily used in craniofacial reconstruction.

CALCIUM PHOSPHATE

Calcium phosphate or hydroxyapatite is not an osteoconducive material but does provide a substrate into which bone can be deposited.[14] The granule form of hydroxyapatite has been shown useful for augmentation of the alveolar ridge in oral surgery and as an interposition graft in mandibular osteotomies, although it has been shown to have little value in facial augmentation. This is due to the product's brittleness, difficult contouring, and inability to mold to bony surface irregularities.

AUTOGRAFTS, HOMOGRAFTS, AND XENOGRAFTS

Autografts are available as autogenous bone, cartilage, and fat and are limited by donor site morbidity and availability. Both autograft and processed homograft cartilage are additionally limited by eventual resorption and fibrosis.[15]

TISSUE-ENGINEERED BIOCOMPATIBLE IMPLANTS (TEBIS)

TEBIs offer the advantage of minimal donor site morbidly, precise three-dimensional design, long-term effects, and reduced operative time. Although still in the developmental stage, the technique involves the seeding of cells in a suspension that provides a three-dimensional structure that promotes matrix formation. The three-dimensional structure anchors the cell and permits nutrition, and gas exchange provides for the ultimate formation of a new gelatinous tissue in the precise shape desired.[16] Several tissue-engineered implants have previously been used for joint articular cartilage, tracheal rings, and auricular cartilage.[17] The field of tissue engineering has advanced in recent years in parallel with advances in material science, tissue culture, and transplantation, and its usefulness in creating contoured facial implants is currently under evaluation.

SURGICAL PROCEDURE

PREOPERATIVE CONSIDERATIONS

Controlling the size, shape, and position of the implant is important in determining the overall final outcome. Examination and evaluation of the patient's mandible as well as the overlying soft tissue are paramount to appropriately selecting the necessary and anatomically correct implant.

Evaluation of a person's lower face centers on the mandible. The lower border of the mandible defines the jaw line and should be a smooth and consist straight line extending from the midline of the chin to the angle of the mandible.

In general, profileplasty has always emphasized an endpoint whereby the chin should project to the level of the vermillion border based on the Gonzalez-Ulloa vertical line (perpendicular from the Frankfort horizontal). However, it is extremely important to differentiate between males and females when trying to define goals and endpoints of size (Figures 17-10 and 17-11). Females generally require less projection anteriorly than male patients. It is also most important to assess the entire mandible including the need for lateral augmentation, particularly within the prejowl area. Augmentation of the chin with implants such as a small anterior button-type implant can have the unwanted effect of actually increasing the jowls and accentuating the prejowl sulcus.

The location of the mental foramen must be determined preoperatively (Figure 17-12). The area of the mental nerve marks the point of maximal resorption of the alveolar process. Edentulous patients often exhibit excessive thinning in the region. However, resorption of the jaw, particularly associated with the edentulous patient, is primarily from the superior alveolar ridge downward. The area below the mental nerve remains relatively stable in dimension. It should also be noted whether the patient has had previous dental implants, posts, or plates that may influence the positioning of the implants, as well as history of fractures or other mandibular trauma.

CHOICE OF IMPLANTS

Choosing the correct mandibular implant is crucial to achieving a good outcome. There are many designs of extended mandibular implants that are available for

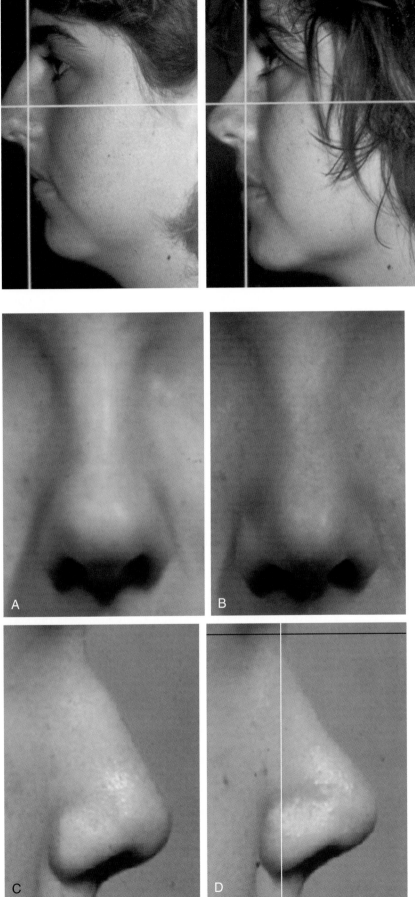

Figure 17-10 In general, profileplasty has always emphasized an endpoint whereby the chin should project to the level of the vermillion border based on the Gonzalez-Ulloa vertical line. However, it is important to differentiate between males and females when trying to define goals and endpoints of size. These pre- and post-operative photos demonstrate that the old definitions of profileplasty are not necessarily desirable in females.

"More subtle in females"
(slightly **less** than G-U profileplasty line)

Figure 17-11 A, C; Pre-op; **B, D;** Post-op after mandibular augmentation and rhinoplasty. Females generally require less projection anteriorly than male patients. It is also most important to assess the entire mandible including the need for lateral augmentation particularly within the prejowl area.

patients who require both anterior augmentation of the chin and a softening of the prejowl sulcus. They are available in multiple sizes and serve to augment both the chin and jaw line.

Injectable soft tissue fillers, such as hyaluronic acids, calcium hydroxyapatite, and collagen, offer a temporary option for improving the jaw line aesthetics in minor circumstances. Fillers, however, as opposed to implants, lack the ability to provide significant dimensional contour change of the bony skeleton or a major degree of permanent volume enhancement.

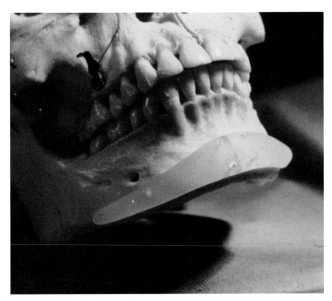

Figure 17-12 Extended anatomical implants are placed just inferior to the mental foramen.

SURGICAL TECHNIQUE

On the day prior to surgery, patients are typically started on broad-spectrum antibiotics for a total of 7 days. Intraoperatively, intravenous antibiotics and dexamethasone are given. Prior to surgery, the patient is placed in the upright position and the precise area to be augmented is outlined with a marking pen. At this time, final decisions are made to anticipate implant size, shape, and position.

Chin implants can be placed through either an intraoral or external approach. The intraoral route provides the obvious advantage of leaving no external scars (Figure 17-13). The entry wound is a transverse incision through the mucosa anterior to the incisors at the level of the gingival-buccal border. The mentalis muscle is divided vertically in the midline raphe to avoid transaction of the muscle belly or detachment from the bone. The midline incision provides for adequate access to the inferior edge of the mandible and prevents potential weakness from transsection of the mentalis muscle.

The external approach utilizes a 1- to 1.5-cm incision in the submental crease, located approximately 2 to 3 cm below the level of the inferior edge of the mandible (Figure 17-14). The advantages of the external route include avoidance of intraoral bacteria, direct access to the inferior mandibular bone, limited retraction of the mental nerve, and ease of fixation of the implant to the periosteum at the inferior border of the mandibular. We prefer the external approach since it avoids disinsertion of the mentalis muscle. The external approach will keep the attachment of the superior-most portions of periosteum to the area below the labial mental sulcus. This is extremely important in preventing the implant from being

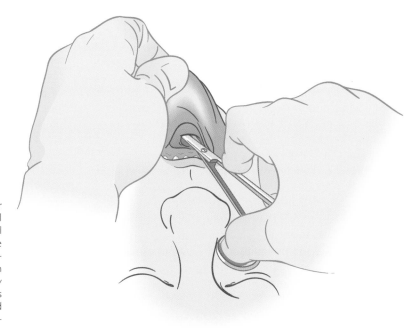

Figure 17-13 Chin implants can be placed either through an intraoral or external approach. The intraoral route provides the obvious advantage of leaving no external scars. The entry wound is a transverse incision through the mucosa anterior to the incisors at the level of the gingival-buccal border. The mentalis muscle is divided vertically in the midline raphe to avoid transaction of the muscle belly or detachment from the bone. The midline incision provides for adequate access to the inferior edge of the mandible and prevents potential weakness from transection of the mentalis muscle.

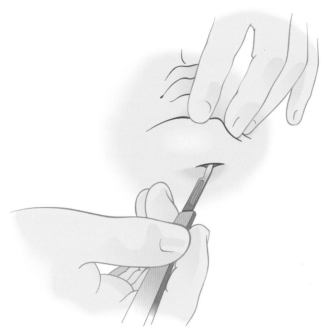

Figure 17-14 The external approach utilizes a 1–1.5 cm incision in the submental crease, located approximately 2–3 cm below the level of the inferior edge of the mandible. The advantages of the external route include avoidance of intraoral bacteria, direct access to the inferior mandibular bone, limited retraction of the mental nerve and ease of fixation of the implant to the periosteum at the inferior border of the mandibular.

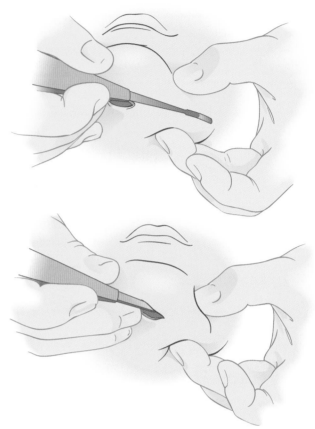

Figure 17-15 During the periosteal dissection, the mental nerves should be avoided by compressing the tissues around the mental foramen with the opposite hand. This helps to direct the elevator away from the nerve and along the inferior border of the mandible.

positioned in an undesirable superior location, which would have the potential of reducing the vertical dimension and natural contour of the labiomental sulcus (Figure 17-9). To ensure the same critical positioning via an intraoral approach would require the use of a permanent screw fixation system. In addition, the external approach provides a more direct route of access for dissection along the inferior mandible, which reduces the risk of injury to the mental nerve.

Whatever route of insertion is chosen, there are five golden rules that will help ensure safe and successful mandibular enhancement:

1. Stay on bone through the subperiosteal approach. This ensures a firm and secure attachment to the bony skeleton for the implant.
2. Elevate the soft tissues gently.
3. Ensure the dissection space is slightly larger than the implant.
4. Avoid the mental nerves by compressing the tissues around the mental foramen with the opposite hand. This helps to direct the elevator away from the nerve and along the inferior border of the mandible (Figure 17-15).
5. Maintain a dry operative field to ensure accurate visualization, precise dissection, and proper implant placement and to prevent postoperative hematoma or seroma.

THE EXTERNAL APPROACH

The incision is initially made through the subcutaneous tissue. From this point, either scissors or cautery is used to carry the incision down to the level of the mandibular periosteum. With a small two-prong or Parkes retractor, the periosteum is incised and the elevator is inserted; subperiosteal dissection is carried over Zone 1, making sure to leave a cuff of soft tissue at the superior edge of the pocket (see Figure 17-10). There are some who leave the periosteum attached anteriorly and continue laterally in a subperiosteal plane, believing that there is less bone resorption if the implant resides in a supraperiosteal plane. However, there is potential for implant mobility if it is placed in the supraperiosteal plane. Bone resorption does occur with all implants; however, it has not been considered to be clinically significant.[18]

At this point, the pocket is further developed laterally to access Zone 2. The most important part of accessing the lateral component of the mandible via the anterior approach is to appreciate the areas of condensations of fibrous tissue similar to a ligamentous attachment. These ligamentous attachments at the level of the periosteum are identified just lateral to the midline of the mentum and transected bluntly with its periosteal elevators. This enables an easy plane of dissection directed posteriorly along the most inferior border of the mandible. This avoids inadvertent misdirection of the elevator and potential injury to the mental nerve.

Using a Joseph or 3- or 4-mm periosteal elevator, a subperiosteal tunnel is then created along the inferior mandibular border that extends 6 to 7 cm laterally. The length of this lateral tunnel is confirmed with a flexible malleable retractor. It is important during the dissection that adequate length of the tunnel and dissection inferior to the mental nerve is achieved. Elevation onto the nerve or compression of the nerve can lead to injury and resultant hypoesthesia, bleeding, or malposition of the implant.

Once the pocket has been created, sizing of the implant is undertaken with sets of blue "Sizers" (Figure 17-16). Once the shape and size of the intended implant are assessed, the smaller and larger sizes are purposely inserted into the pocket and also assessed for size and shape to validate the choice of the implant. The average projection needed for the central portion of the chin in men is between 6 and 9 mm, and in women, it is between 4 to 7 mm. Occasionally, in patients with severe microgenia, implants with 10 to 12 mm of projection are necessary to create a normal profile and broad jaw line.

The authors find that an end result representing a square shape to the anterior chin is desirable in males. Men usually desire and can accept a larger and more square appearance to the mandible. In the majority of cases in females, particularly when larger implants are required to achieve the desired level of anterior projection, it becomes necessary to modify the extended implant to achieve a rounder anterior shape to the chin (see Figure 17-16). The areas of the implant that represent the position over the anterior-lateral areas of the chin are identified and reduced in projection to ensure a rounder appearance to the chin (Figure 17-17). Asymmetry is compensated for in similar fashion by reducing specific areas over the external surface of the implants.

The pocket is then irrigated with antibiotic solution. The implant is then removed from antibiotic solution and inserted into the lateral portion of the pocket on one side and then folded upon itself whereby the contralateral portion of the implant is inserted into the other side of the pocket (Figure 17-18). Care is taken to place the implant inferior to the mental nerve and positioned so it is not buckled or folded onto itself. It is important to extend the pocket beyond the extent of the implant. The pocket closes down rapidly, so there is no worry of a pocket being made too large. Displacement or infolding of an implant is usually secondary to a pocket that is too small with the surrounding soft tissue impinging on a particular area of the implant.

The implant is then palpated externally to check for symmetry and to ensure the implant does not extend beyond the inferior border, especially the lateral tip. Once the position is confirmed, the anterior edge of the implant

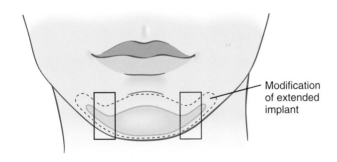

Modification of extended implant

Figure 17-16 In the majority of cases in females, particularly when larger implants are required to achieve the desired level of anterior projection, it becomes necessary to modify the extended implant to achieve a rounder anterior shape to the chin. This will often prevent a "square" chin from occurring in females.

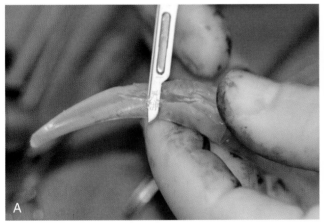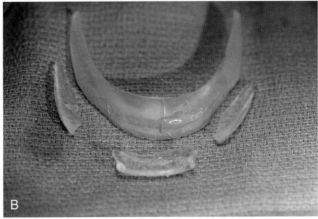

Figure 17-17 A, B, The areas of the implant that represents the position over the anterior-lateral areas of the chin are identified and reduced in projection to ensure a rounder appearance to the chin.

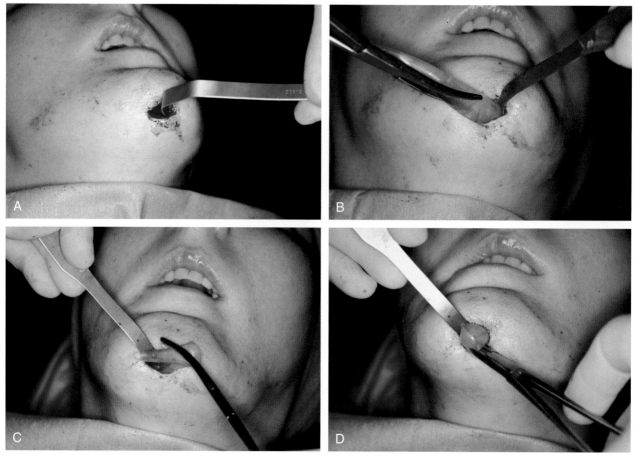

Figure 17-18 A-D, The implant is inserted into the lateral portion of the pocket on one side and then folded upon itself whereby the contralateral portion of the implant is inserted into the other side of the pocket.

is secured to the periosteum with two sutures of 4-0 clear nylon or 5-0 Prolene. The wound is again irrigated and closed in two layers with a deep subcutaneous suture and skin closure.

COMPLICATIONS

Complications with mandibular implants are rare. Most common among them is unilateral hypoesthesia or paresthesia of the lower lip or chin. Reports of incidence range from approximately 8% to 35%.[2,3] A reduced complication rate has been attributed to direct visualization of the lateral subperiosteal dissection tunnel using a headlight and ribbon retractor that does not stretch the mental nerve. If hypoesthesia manifests, it lasts approximately 1 to 2 weeks. Dysesthesia is rare and usually unilateral and can be caused by the malposition of the implant impinging on the mental nerve. All implant material induces the formation of fibroconnective tissue, which encapsulates the implant and acts as a barrier between the host and the implant.[4,5] Therefore, infection rates and displacement of the implant are rare. Rates of infection can be further reduced by care in the handling of the implant, soaking the implant in antibiotic solution, meticulous hemostasis,

antibiotic irrigation of the subperiosteal tunnels, and perioperative antibiotics. Rates of displacement can be reduced with tacking sutures attaching the implant to the periosteum.

Mobility of the implant is enhanced if dissection of the tunnel is carried below and inferior to the mandible and should therefore be avoided. One should also be cognizant that preoperative asymmetries in the patient's mandible will be present postoperatively and should be pointed out to the patient preoperatively.[18]

ANGLE OF THE MANDIBLE IMPLANTS

Access to the angle of the mandible is achieved through a 2- to 3-cm mucosal incision at the retromolar trigone. This gives direct access to the angle of the mandible. Dissection is then performed on the bone and beneath the masseter muscle to elevate the periosteum upward along the ramus and anteriorly along the body of the mandible. A curved (90-degree) dissector is used to elevate the periosteum around the posterior angle and ramus of the mandible. This permits accurate placement of the angle implants that are designed to enhance the posterior border of the ascending ramus and thus angle definition. These implants are then secured with titanium screws. No screws are needed if custom implants such as three-dimensional Accuscan are used.

CONCLUSION

Chin augmentation is an extremely important tool in aesthetic surgery. When assessing facial form, it is imperative to apply a three-dimensional approach to facial contouring so that the correct implant can be chosen for achieving the optimum result. Identifying components related to facial size, form, dimension, and factors of aging are all important in determining the correct implant shape and size to optimize the results in mandibular contouring.

REFERENCES

1. Anderson J. *Grants Atlas of anatomy.* 7th ed. Baltimore, MD: Williams & Wilkins, 1978:7–17.
2. Mittleman H. The anatomy of the aging mandible and its importance to facelift surgery. *Fac Plast Surg Clin North Am.* 1994;2(3):301–309.
3. Cortez EA. Extended pre-jowl implants enhance lower face. *Cosmet Surg Times.* 2004;14.
4. Anderson JM, Miller KM. Biomaterial biocompatibility and the macrophage. *Biomaterials.* 1984;5:5
5. Ziats NP, Miller KM, Anderson JM. In vitro and in vivo interactions of cells with biomaterials. *Biomaterials.* 1988;9:5.
6. Binder WJ, Azizzadeh B, Tobia GW, eds. Aesthetic facial implants. In: *Facial Plastic and Reconstructive Surgery,* 3rd edition, New York: Thieme Medical Publisher; 2009.
7. Broadbent TR, Mathews VI. Artistic relationships in surface anatomy of the face. Application to reconstructive surgery. *Plast Reconstr Surg.* 1957;20:1.
8. Belinfante LS, Mitchell DI. Use of alloplastic material in the canine fossa-zygomatic area to improve facial esthetics. *J Oral Surg.* 1977;35:121.
9. Binder W, Schoenrock L, eds. *Facial contouring and alloplastic implants.* Philadelphia: WB Saunders, 1994, Facial Plastic Surgery Clinics of North America.
10. Gabriel SE, O'Fallon WM, Kurland LT, et al. Risk of connective-tissue diseases and other disorders after breast implantation. *N Engl J Med.* 1994;330:1697.
11. Park AJ, Black RJ, Sarhadi NS, Chetty U, Watson ACH. Silicone gel-filled breast implants and connective tissue diseases. *Plast Reconstr Surg.* 1998;101:261.
12. Park JB, Lakes RS. Polymeric materials. In: *Biomaterials: An Introduction.* New York: Plenum; 1994:164.
13. Brown BI, Neel III HB, Kern EB. Implants of Supramid, Proplast, Plasticpore, and Silastic. *Arch Otolaryngol Head Neck Surg.* 1979;105:605.
14. Alexander H. Calcium-based ceramics and composites in bone reconstruction. *CRC Crit Rev Biocompat.* 1987;4:43.
15. Salyer KE, Hall CD. Porous hydroxyapatite as an onlay bone graft substitute in maxillofacial surgery. *Plast Reconstruc Surg.* 1989; 84:236.
16. Rodriguez A, Vacanti CA. Characteristics of cartilage engineered from human pediatric auricular cartilage. *Plast Reconstr Surg.* 1999;103:1111.
17. Langer R, Vunjak G, Freed L, et al. Tissue engineering: Biomedical applications. *Tissue Eng.* 1995;1:151.
18. Terino EO. Complications of chin and malar augmentation. In: Peck G, ed. *Complications and problems in aesthetic plastic surgery.* New York: Gower Medical; 1991.

CHAPTER EIGHTEEN

Alloplasts in Nasal Surgery

Anthony P. Sclafani

Few concepts in rhinoplasty engender as much discussion and conflict as the use of alloplasts in the nose. Clear divisions within the specialty have developed, with some surgeons using alloplastic implants liberally while others staunchly maintaining that alloplasts should never be used in rhinoplasty. Central to this dichotomy is the risk versus benefit analysis and the thresholds one sets as acceptable. Should an alloplast ever be used in cosmetic or reconstructive rhinoplasty? Does sparing the patient an additional incision and operative site with additional risks (including potential intracranial or thoracic penetration) and donor site morbidity outweigh a small but finite risk of implant material extrusion or infection? Can an alloplast effectively simulate the tissue characteristics (such as bulk, shape, texture, and stability) it is designed to replace? Unfortunately, it is often the patients who most need significant bulk and/or structural support, due to prior surgery, trauma, or inflammatory disease, who may be the worst candidates for alloplastic augmentation. Significant scarring or a thinned, devascularized skin–soft tissue envelope may lead to poor implant integration, skin erosion, and breakdown, as well as implant mobility and/or exposure. This chapter will review the benefits and risks of alloplastic nasal augmentation and will discuss the use of implants in the nose in the context of implant biocompatibility and as related to wound healing.

HISTORY

At its most basic level, rhinoplasty is an alteration in the form and function of the nose by removal, modification, or augmentation of existing nasal structures. Historically, nasal mutilation was inflicted with the intention of leaving a visible marker of a degraded social status for thieves, adulterers, and military or political prisoners. The syphilis epidemic in Western Europe in the sixteenth and seventeenth centuries caused a significant number of saddle nose deformities and left victims with conspicuous sequelae of sexual promiscuity. Military wounds also left victims with nasal deformities requiring treatment.

The simplest form of augmentation is the prosthesis. Justinian II ("Rhinotmesis"), a Byzantine emperor whose nose was amputated after he was deposed (nasal and facial deformities precluded individuals from ruling), wore a nasal prosthesis when he reclaimed his throne. Tycho Brahe, the Danish astronomer, wore a silver prosthesis to camouflage a nasal deformity.

Soft tissue reconstruction of the nose with forehead or cheek skin flaps dates from as early as the sixth century BC in India, and forearm pedicled flap repair was well known in Italy prior to Tagiacozzi's publication in the sixteenth century. These early surgical interventions in the preanesthetic era were intended to replace large amounts of nasal volume and skin coverage. More focused reconstruction of nasal deformities—in particular, the saddle nose deformity—began in earnest in the late nineteenth to early twentieth centuries, as modern anesthetic techniques and antisepsis were introduced. While subtler than the earlier treatment of more dramatic nasal amputations, the repair of these injuries was primarily aimed at restoration of nasal volume and skin coverage. Some of the materials used, including stones from the Black Sea, duck breastbone, pearls, and ivory, may seem inexact and perhaps more than a little odd, but the deformities being treated were severe and even modest improvements were appreciated. At best, the materials may have been well-tolerated foreign bodies with fibrous encapsulation, but it seems obvious they were chosen more for their physical qualities than for their biocompatibility.

The development of synthetic polymers in the mid to late twentieth century led to the greatest increase in the use of nasal implants. In particular, solid silicone implants were introduced and are still in use today. These were designed primarily for dorsal augmentation but some later designs incorporated struts for columellar and tip support. These implants are fairly well tolerated, but implant infections and extrusions have been reported and will be discussed later in this chapter. Other implants have also been developed over the past two decades for isolated columellar support, premaxillary augmentation, and nasal valve support; their use will also be covered in this chapter.

ANATOMY

Five main areas can typically be considered for alloplastic nasal augmentation: the dorsum, premaxilla, nasal valve, ala, and columella. Additionally, some implants will include aspects designed to augment the nasal tip. Congenitally shallow nasal dorsal profiles often seen in Asian and African American patients are amenable to dorsal onlay implants. In patients with limited or weak tip projection and support, a single-piece implant can be used to both augment dorsal height and to provide tip support. A retruse premaxilla can be augmented with an implant to restore proper balance to the lower third of the nose. Recently, new implants have been introduced to modify/support the internal nasal valve without adding excessive bulk. Implants can be added to the nasal ala to correct alar contour, while implants placed in the columella can aid in augmenting tip projection, altering tip rotation or reshaping the columella itself. In general, space-occupying implants are better tolerated than those that provide structural support; there are exceptions to this rule, and factors such as the health and vascularity of the local soft tissues, implant stabilization, and the physical and chemical characteristics of the implant itself will also have a significant impact on implant success.

ALTERNATIVES

Traditional teaching of rhinoplasty techniques dictates the use of autologous materials whenever possible. Autologous septal, conchal, and costal cartilage are the most commonly used material for nasal grafting. They are readily harvestable, have minimal donor site morbidity, can generally provide sufficient volume of cartilage, are relatively easy to carve, and provide fairly predictable results. Alternatively, outer table calvarial or iliac crest bone grafts can be used, but due to their rigidity, they are only practical for dorsal onlay (and columellar support) grafts. Temporalis fascia can be used to soften graft edges but provides neither volume augmentation nor support. Erol and colleagues[1,2] described the use of the "Turkish Delight" graft: minced cartilage is mixed with autologous blood and wrapped in oxidized cellulose. The subsequent fibrotic response provides bulk augmentation for the nasal dorsum but cannot be used in structural settings.

Homografts, such as irradiated rib cartilage (IRC), can be considered as an alternative if autologous tissue is unavailable or insufficient or the patient refuses a second surgical incision. IRC is harvested from human cadavers and processed to reduce the potential for infection transmission or immunologic host rejection. It has been in use for over 20 years and the literature is mixed as to the ultimate fate of irradiated cartilage. Schuller et al.[3] initially described good results using IRC. However, subsequent long-term follow-up in these cases is mixed with preservation of volumization but loss of tip support reported when IRC is used. Considerable warping can also occur over time.[4-6]

Another homograft, acellular dermal matrix (ADC; LifeCell Corp., Branchburg, NJ), has been used as a dorsal onlay implant, either alone or in combination with autologous cartilage. ADC provides a three-dimensional collagen scaffold for host tissue ingrowth and fibrosis and can be used to provide subtle volume augmentation (especially in the radix). It can also be used to camouflage irregularities of the dorsum or from other cartilage grafts. At best, only a portion of the volume of ADC will persist long term.[7]

Finally, temporary injectable fillers such as hyaluronic acids and calcium hydroxylapatite have been described for nasal contouring.[8,9] These are generally simple and effective but temporary solutions, and the long-term safety of permanent filler material in this area is unclear.

IMPLANT BIOCOMPATIBILITY

The body's biologic response to an alloplast is dependent on factors related to both host and implant. The chemical composition, surface electrical charge, surface texture, and porosity all contribute to the specific response that occurs around an alloplastic implant. Simply put, a nasal implant is a rather large subcutaneous or submuscular foreign body. Following implantation, the implant is coated with host proteins such as fibrin, fibronectin, and other proteins that become partially denatured on contact with the implant. These proteins are essential for the subsequent host inflammatory response. The severity, cellular activity, and longevity of this response are determined in large part by the qualities of the implant. Neutrophils and monocytes migrate to the implant surface. When the initial inflammatory response subsides, the neutrophilic content decreases, giving way to macrophage increase and accumulation of giant cells, fibroblasts, and some lymphocytes around the material. A fibrotic response ultimately results, with a capsule of fibrosis around the implant; any fragments, left behind in the manufacturing of the implant, related to surgical technique, or formed as a result of implant degradation in situ, will promote additional inflammatory reactions around each particle of material. Some early implants no longer in use today were found to undergo degradation and released new fragments into the surrounding tissues; a vibrant secondary foreign body response developed and persisted around the implant causing significant collateral damage. By contrast, the three most commonly used solid nasal alloplasts today (expanded polytetrafluoroetheylene [e-PTFE], porous high density polyethylene [PHDPE], and silicone) are associated with quite different early responses, which represent different points on a common spectrum. These implants have been designed to avoid particulate degradation.

SILICONE

Silicone nasal implants are nonporous and smooth surfaced. The inert nature of the polymer generally is associated with a thin fibrous capsule with quiescent fibroblasts and rare giant cells. There is no tissue ingrowth making removal simple but predisposing the implant to infection (from early contamination or late bacteremia) and instability within the implant pocket. As there is no rigid fixation of the implant, the micromotion of the implant can cause a synovial reaction within the implant.

e-PTFE

e-PTFE is a soft and pliable microporous material. The most commonly used e-PTFE was produced by W.L. Gore & Associates but the manufacturer has ceased production. Currently, a preformed composite e-PTFE/silicone implant is available (Implantech Associates, Inc., Ventura, CA). These implants have a solid silicone core with a bonded e-PTFE coating. The e-PTFE acts as a cushion between the firm silicone core and the soft tissue envelope, and the porous surface of the e-PTFE allows limited tissue ingrowth into the periphery of the implant. This ingrowth effectively binds the implant to the surrounding tissue and seals it from the outside environment, eliminating dead space and potential micromotion, while the silicone core can provide structural support. The surrounding capsule is composed of a few thin layers of collagen and relatively quiescent fibroblasts.

PHDPE

PHDPE (MEDPOR; Stryker Corp., Kalamazoo, MI) is a rigid implant with pores averaging 150 microns in size. These larger pores promote a more vibrant fibrovascular soft tissue ingrowth than e-PTFE, and ultimately the implant, which is 50% porous, is completely ingrown by host tissue. This provides a dense attachment to the surrounding soft tissue and assists with implant fixation. Porous implants have been shown to be more susceptible to early infections (prior to soft tissue invasion of the implant) but more resistant to late infections (because of the protective effect of host tissue invasion and integration of the implant) compared to solid implants.

SPECIAL CONSIDERATIONS

A careful assessment of surgical needs for which the implants will be used to address is critical in choosing the correct implant. Each area is examined to assess the patient's surgical requirements. Is dorsal augmentation necessary, and if so, to what degree? If the dorsum is to be augmented, is tip projection required as well? Does the alar base or the columella need additional volume? The

answers to these questions will help select the most appropriate implant.

In assessing patients preoperatively, standard functional and aesthetic rhinologic evaluation should be performed. Specific aesthetic and structural needs should be identified. The intended volume augmentation should be assessed, as should the anticipated amount and quality of autogenous cartilage available. In general, autogenous cartilage is better tolerated and more forgiving in the nose (especially in revision and posttraumatic cases), and should be considered as a "first-line" choice. If septal and/or conchal cartilage is insufficient for the patient's needs, costal cartilage and calvarial bone grafts are considered. Patient preference and the potential associated morbidity of these autografts make consideration of alloplasts reasonable. Both short- and long-term risks and benefits should be fully discussed with the patient. The decision to use an alloplastic implant is made jointly.

A major factor affecting the success of nasal alloplasts is the integrity of the skin–soft tissue envelope beneath which the implant is placed. The overlying tissues must be sufficiently thick and healthy to withstand contact with and pressure from a solid implant. Patients with exceptionally thin skin may be more prone to skin compromise when an alloplast is used; likewise, the multi-revised rhinoplasty patient or patients with known vascular compromise will have an increased risk of implant/soft tissue complications due to diminished vascularity. Patients with septal perforation are also at an increased risk of complications because of diminished local tissue vascularity secondary to prior surgery or trauma. Additionally, chronic nasal crusting of the perforation edges may allow transient bacterial seeding of the local tissues. When an alloplast is present, this can lead to chronic inflammation or infection around the implant. When present, septal perforation should be closed if an alloplast is used, and if there is any uncertainty as to the anticipated success of the perforation repair, placement of the alloplast should be deferred. Tobacco use, while always a hindrance to wound healing, is especially problematic in the postoperative period after placement of a nasal implant; success of the alloplast is dependent on proper healing of the soft tissue pocket surrounding the implant, especially in the early postoperative period.

SPECIFIC ALLOPLASTS

Silicone

Silicone refers to a family of polymers of the compound dimethysiloxane ($[(CH_3)_2SiO_2]_x$). Silicone implants have been used extensively for dorsal augmentation and enhancement of tip projection, while single L-shaped silicone implants can be used for both purposes. As silicone is nonporous and is surrounded by a fibrous capsule, stability of the implant depends primarily on creation of a precisely positioned and sized pocket, one that allows neither implant movement nor excessive pressure against the overlying soft tissue. The implant should be placed directly over the nasal bone periosteum from the nasal root to just above the anterior septal angle. If an L-shaped implant is chosen, the vertical strut portion is placed in between the medial crura of the lower lateral cartilages and rests anterior to the anterior nasal spine. These implants can be placed via an external approach, but creation of a discrete implant pocket may be more effective via an endonasal approach. All incisions should be closed meticulously so as to establish a distinct and separate cavity from the external environment.

PHDPE

PHDPE implants are made of a highly porous material that facilitates fibrous ingrowth. The standard nasal dorsal implant should rest directly over the nasal bones from the nasal root to rest over the cartilaginous dorsum. In patients with reasonable tip support and form, the implant can be used without the nasal tip portion; however, in patients with thick nasal tip skin or those with limited nasal tip architecture, the nasal dorsum/nasal tip implant can be used. In general, the soft tissue fibrosis that occurs

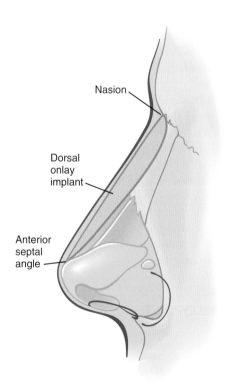

Nasion

Dorsal onlay implant

Anterior septal angle

Figure 18-1 A dorsal nasal implant provides bulk augmentation of the nasal dorsum. To ensure a smooth, continuous dorsal line, the implant is placed so as to overlay the nasal bones and dorsal septum, ending at the anterior septal angle. Piecemeal dorsal augmentation is generally discouraged to avoid irregularities.

postoperatively coapts the nasal tip skin to the nasal tip portion of the implant yielding an acceptable form. A thin PHDPE sheet (0.85 or 1.5 mm thick) can be cut into an ovoid or rectangle shape, for use as an alar batten or a columellar strut, respectively.

Because of the rough surface of the PHDPE, these implants do not slide easily into position and will catch on the surrounding soft tissue. A wider dissection pocket than required for a silicone implant must be created; this is especially true for columellar and dorsal placement. A useful trick is to wrap the implant in its sterile plastic liner prior to placement; this will allow the implant to slide into position more easily. Once properly positioned, the wrapper can be advanced out, leaving the implant in the desired location. Stabilization of dorsal PHDPE implants is not mandatory, although this can be performed with a monocortical titanium screw placed through the implant into the nasal bone. This is recommended when premaxillary implants are placed. Implants at other sites can be secured much in the same was as cartilage grafts, although effective soft tissue apposition to the implant is essential for long-term success.

e-PTFE

e-PTFE implants are porous materials that also promote soft tissue ingrowth. The pore size in e-PTFE is notably smaller than in PHDPE, which limits the fibrous ingrowth of the implant to the outer few tenths of a millimeter. e-PTFE does not result in a well-developed capsule. This degree of ingrowth stabilizes the implant and isolates its interior from bacteria, while allowing for relatively simple implant removal when necessary. e-PTFE alone, however, is soft and flexible and cannot be used to provide structural support. Numerous studies have been published documenting the safety and efficacy of e-PTFE implants.[10-12]

Recently, preformed e-PTFE nasal implants have become unavailable, and e-PTFE–coated dorsal as well as dorsal/columellar silicone implants have been introduced. (Implantech Associates, Inc, Ventura, CA). These implants are covered by a thin layer of e-PTFE bonded to a silicone core. The e-PTFE integrates the implant with surrounding soft tissues and serves as a cushion between the overlying skin and soft tissues and the firmer silicone, while the central silicone portion of the implant maintains a consistent shape and structure. In theory, these implants should perform as well as standard e-PTFE implants; however, e-PTFE implants were never used to provide structural support, and in this setting these implants may behave similarly to all-silicone implants. Care should be taken to avoid applying excessive pressure of the implant against the skin.

Again, the implant is placed into the dissected pocket, sliding easily into position. e-PTFE/silicone implants require a relatively precise pocket; alternatively, the edge can be sutured to the surrounding soft tissue to maintain implant position.

SPECIAL MANEUVERS AND TECHNICAL PEARLS

GENERAL CONSIDERATIONS

It is essential to ensure that no fragments of material are unintentionally implanted. All implants should be sterilely rinsed prior to use. Prior to placement, all implants should be soaked in an appropriate antibiotic solution, and any small particles remaining from carving should be rinsed off the implant prior to placement.

To facilitate antibiotic diffusion into porous implants, the implant should be placed in a 20-mL syringe filled with an antibiotic solution; all air should be expelled from the syringe. With a gloved finger over the tip of the syringe, the plunger is pulled back creating a vacuum; air bubbles can be seen emerging from the implant pores, being replaced by the antibiotic solution.

Implants should be placed in the smallest dissection pocket possible, to limit the potential for early implant migration. Adequate fixation with titanium screws or sutures is essential. Implants should be kept as far away as possible from suture lines, and excessive soft tissue pressure against the implant should be avoided. PHDPE implants can be heated in sterile hot water and bent to the most appropriate shape; they are then held in this shape while they cool and subsequently will hold this shape. Consideration should be given to the use of autologous platelet/fibrin gel (Selphyl®, Aesthetic Factors, Inc., Wayne, NJ) to enhance and accelerate wound healing. Postoperatively, the nose should be taped appropriately to limit edema and obliterate any dead space in the area surrounding the implant.

DORSAL ONLAY AND COMBINED ONLAY-STRUT IMPLANTS

Dorsal onlay implants are the simplest implants to use. They should rest symmetrically over the nasal dorsum from the nasal root to the anterior septal angle (see Figure 18-1). While these implants can be placed endonasally, an external approach is preferred to reduce the potential for contamination with nasal bacteria. The rough surface of PHDPE implants prevents sliding along the dorsum into position, so the nasal soft tissues need to be adequately elevated to allow the implant to be inserted into the pocket before it is allowed to contact the surrounding soft tissues. As discussed previously, this requires dissection of a more ample pocket than other implant materials. However, the rough surface generally stabilizes the implant well and generally precludes the need for rigid fixation. Implants made of smoother materials, such as

e-PTFE and silicone, will slide into smaller pockets more easily; fibrovascular tissue ingrowth into both PHDPE and e-PTFE occurs fairly rapidly, further stabilizing these implants. Silicone becomes encapsulated by fibrous tissue, and excessive motion of the implant will promote a thicker capsule and greater inflammation.

Combined onlay-strut implants are placed similarly, except that the additional strut portion rests between the medial crura (see Figure 18-2). Care should be taken to ensure that the domes rest at a higher point than the angle of the L-strut and cushion the overlying skin from the implant. Also, a thick nasal tip skin is preferred when using this type of implant; scarred or thinned nasal tip soft tissues, as often seen in revision rhinoplasty, increase the risk of implant exposure and extrusion.

NASAL VALVE IMPLANTS

Two types of nasal valve implants are available. Individual pieces of thin PHDPE can be used in a fashion similar to cartilage in reconstructing the internal nasal valve as an alar batten spanning from the pyriform aperture to the dorsal septum to stabilize and reinforce a flail internal nasal valve (Figure 18-3). A more recent addition is a combined e-PTFE–coated titanium "butterfly" shape (Monarch Adjustable Implant, Hanson Medical Inc.,

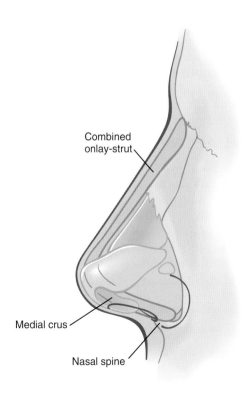

Figure 18-2 An "L-strut"-type implant can be used to augment the dorsum and simultaneously provide tip support. The dorsal segment rests on the bony and cartilaginous dorsum, while the caudal strut portion is sutured in between the medial crura and rests over the nasal spine.

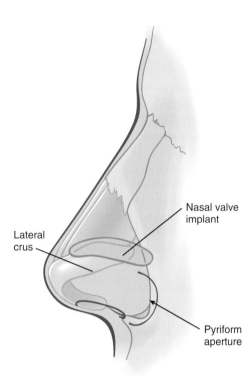

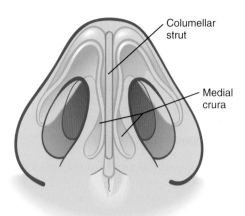

Figure 18-4 In cases of isolated weakness or inadequacy of the medial limb of the nasal tripod, a semirigid implant can be sutured in between the medial crura and used to strengthen columellar support.

Figure 18-3 Semirigid implants, if thin enough, can be used to reinforce and strengthen the area of the internal nasal valve. Nonelastic implants should span from the nasal septum to the pyriform aperture; in cases of prior resection of lateral crura when the remnant crura are weak or collapsed, the cartilage can be sutured and suspended directly to the implant.

Kingston, WA), which spans over the nasal dorsum and is designed to "spring open" and enlarge the nasal valve area.[13,14] The PHDPE implant is placed and secured through an external approach, while the Monarch implant requires a direct dorsal incision.

COLUMELLAR STRUT IMPLANTS

Silicone implants are not recommended for use as isolated columellar struts due to the high incidence (over 50% in some reports) of extrusion when used in this location.[15] PHDPE, though, is generally well tolerated and can add strength and support to the medial limb of the nasal tip tripod. However, great care must be taken to preserve some soft tissue between the nasal spine and the columellar implant above. It is also essential to completely bury the implant between the medial crura, ensuring complete soft tissue coverage (Figure 18-4). The medial crura can be sutured onto the implant, increasing tip support and projection.

PREMAXILLARY IMPLANTS

Patients with medial maxillary and/or premaxillary deficiency can be augmented with preformed PHDPE implants.[16] These are best placed at the pyriform rim

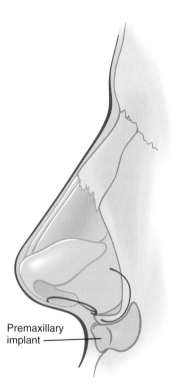

Figure 18-5 Limited maxillary and premaxillary retrusion can be treated with a peri-alar premaxillary implant placed via a transoral approach.

through a sublabial approach and should be secured in place with titanium screws (Figure 18-5). In cases of mild premaxillary retrusion, small particulate implants of PHDPE (2- to 3-mm pieces) can be placed directly through the columellar incision.

RADIX AND RIM IMPLANTS

Radix and rim implants are more technically challenging to place. In patients with isolated nasal root deficiency, a small implant can be placed to create a smooth dorsal

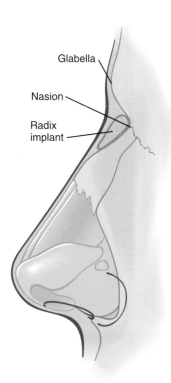

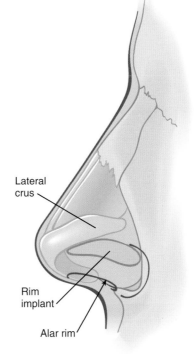

Figure 18-6 An isolated deep nasal root can be augmented with an implant placed at the deepest point of the root. Care should be taken to place the implant in a deep pocket and to avoid extension beyond the sides of the nose.

Figure 18-7 A retracted alar rim can be repaired by placing an implant between the skin of the rim and the caudal end of the lateral crura. Extreme caution should be used in these cases to avoid excessive skin tension and possible implant extrusion.

profile. Any implant placed in this location should be feathered at its edges to blend in smoothly with the nasal sidewalls as well as the caudal and dorsal contours of the radix (Figure 18-6).

An alar rim implant can be placed caudal to the lateral crus to correct a retracted ala (Figure 18-7). An implant here should be used with great caution, as these tissues often are scarred and exposure/extrusion of the implant is not uncommon. Generally, sufficient amounts of autologous cartilage can be found for these areas and are preferred to any type of alloplastic implant.

COMPLICATIONS

One must discuss the issue of complications of nasal implants in the proper perspective. Most rhinoplasties in which alloplasts are used fall into one of the following categories: major revision rhinoplasty, major trauma, congenital deformity, or need for large volume augmentation. These situations entail a high degree of complexity and are associated with higher complication rates. In light of this, a 3% to 6% removal rate of alloplasts[17] can be considered acceptable. A thoughtful appreciation of the biologic events that occur around the implant after surgery not only explains this risk but suggests rational management options as well. As described earlier, silicone is

encapsulated postoperatively by fibrous tissue, e-PTFE is invaded peripherally, and PHDPE is ultimately completely invaded by the patient's fibrovascular tissue. Thus, infection or exposure almost certainly dooms a silicone implant at any point in time. In contrast, after an initial critical healing period and soft tissue ingrowth, PHDPE and e-PTFE implants are less likely to become infected, as the patient's immune response has access to sites of bacterial seeding.[18]

Indeed, in cases of late experimental exposure, PHDPE implants have healed by secondary intention and have (after debridement) supported full-thickness skin grafts.[19] After fibrovascular tissue has developed around the implant surface over the first few weeks, any signs of infection around the implant should be treated aggressively with prolonged antibiotic treatment using both a quinolone and a macrolide antibiotic. Bacterial colonization of a synthetic surface can be extremely difficult to treat. Mucopolysaccharides secreted by the pathogenic bacteria can form a protective covering for the bacterial colonies, making antibiotic penetration and eradication of infection slow and difficult. Antibiotic coverage should be continued for at least 4 to 6 weeks, to ensure full penetration and elimination of any biofilm, which may have developed at the implant surface.

Because of the stabilization of the implant by the patient's fibrous response around the implant, extrusion

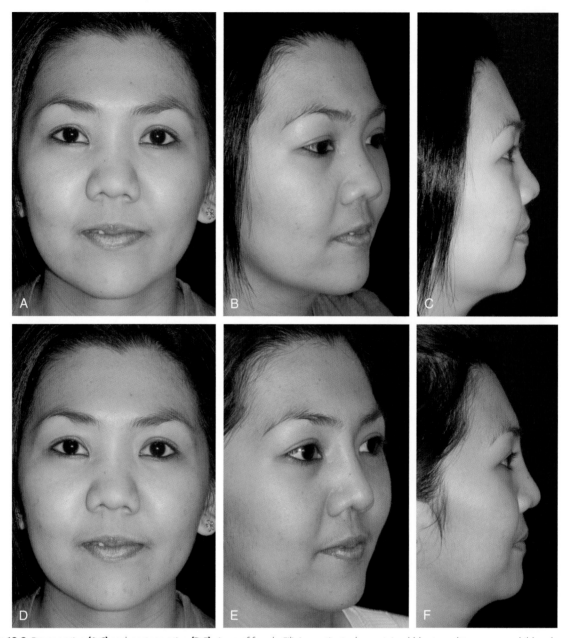

Figure 18-8 Preoperative **(A-C)** and postoperative **(D-F)** views of female Filipino patient who sustained blunt nasal trauma as a child and matured with an underprojected nasal tip and dorsum. Reconstruction required septal cartilage for spreader, columellar strut, and shield grafting, while an e-PTFE–coated silicone dorsal implant was used to provide dorsal augmentation.

of e-PTFE and PHDPE implants is uncommon. However, silicone implants, once exposed, generally extrude or require removal. Careful attention to technique, maintenance of healthy soft tissues around the implant, avoidance of wound tension, and placement of the implant distant from any suture lines are essential to the successful use of any nasal implants but especially those made from silicone.

Undercorrection or overcorrection of the nasal dorsum is due to an error in judgment. While most nasal dorsal implants come in a variety of sizes, implants may require tailoring to suit the patient's needs by shaving the implant to a desired size. This can generally be done with a No.

10 or 15 blade. It is essential that all implant edges are feathered, and that the implants are rinsed to remove any adherent loose particles, as these will increase the risk of foreign body granulomatous response around the implant. Any changes to the nasal tip should be made first, so that the amount of dorsal augmentation can suit the tip projection.

Should overcorrection be noted postoperatively, the implant can be removed, trimmed down or replaced with a smaller implant more easily in the case of silicone implants. On the other hand, the fibrovascular tissue ingrowth into PHDPE and e-PTFE implants that helps stabilize these implants makes implant removal more difficult. In removing these implants, the surgeon should dissect down directly against the implant, leaving as much fibrous tissue on the overlying flap. In densely adherent areas, hydrodissection by injecting 1 to 2 mL of local anesthetic directly onto the implant surface can aid in dissecting the implant from the surrounding tissues.

CONCLUSIONS

Autologous tissue is the preferred material for nasal reconstruction. However, in carefully selected patients, with specific indications and in discrete locations, thoughtfully chosen alloplasts can be successfully used in rhinoplasty (Figure 18-8).

REFERENCES

1. Erol OO. The Turkish Delight: A pliable graft for rhinoplasty. *Plast Reconstr Surg.* 2000;105:2229–2241.
2. Velidedoeglu H, Demir Z, Sahin U, et al. Block and Surgicel-wrapped diced solvent-preserved costal cartilage homograft application for nasal augmentation. *Plast Reconstr Surg.* 2005;115:2081–2093.
3. Schuller DE, Bardach J, Krause CJ. Irradiated homologous costal cartilage for facial contour restoration. *Arch Otolaryngol.* 1977;103:1–15.
4. Welling DB, Maves MD, Schuller DE, Bardach J. Irradiated homologous cartilage grafts. Long-term results. *Arch Otolaryngol Head Neck Surg.* 1988;114(3):291–295.
5. Burke AJ, Wang TD, Cook TA. Irradiated homograft rib cartilage in facial reconstruction. *Arch Fac Plast Surg.* 2004;6(5):334–341.
6. Kridel RW, Konior RJ. Irradiated cartilage grafts in the nose. *Arch Otolaryngol Head Neck Surg.* 1993;119:24–31.
7. Sclafani AP, Romo 3rd T, Jacono AA, et al. Evaluation of acellular dermal graft (AlloDerm) sheet for soft tissue augmentation: A 1-year follow-up of clinical observations and histological findings. *Arch Fac Plast Surg.* 2001;3(2):101–103.
8. Stupak HD, Moulthrop TH, Wheatley P, et al. Calcium hydroxylapatite gel (Radiesse) injection for the correction of postrhinoplasty contour deficiencies and asymmetries. *Arch Fac Plast Surg.* 2007;9(2):130–136.
9. de Lacerda DA, Zancanaro P. Filler rhinoplasty. *Dermatol Surg.* 2007;33(Suppl 2):S207–S212.
10. Queen TA, Palmer FR. Gore-Tex for nasal augmentation: A recent series and a review of the literature. *Ann Otol Rhinol Laryngol.* 1995;104:850–852.
11. Godin MS, Waldman SR, Johnson Jr CM. Nasal augmentation using Gore-Tex. A 10-year experience. *Arch Fac Plast Surg.* 1999;1(2):118–121.
12. Conrad K, Torgerson CS, Gillman GS. Applications of Gore-Tex implants in rhinoplasty reexamined after 17 years. *Arch Fac Plast Surg.* 2008;10(4):224–231.
13. Hurbis CG. An adjustable, butterfly-design, titanium–expanded polytetrafluoroethylene implant for nasal valve dysfunction. *Arch Fac Plast Surg.* 2006;8:98–104.
14. Hurbis CG. A follow-up study of the monarch adjustable implant for correction of nasal valve dysfunction. *Arch Fac Plast Surg.* 2008;10:142–143.
15. Milward TM. The fate of Silastic and Vitathrene nasal implants. *Br J Plast Surg.* 1972;25:276–278.
16. Pessa JE, Peterson ML, Thompson JW, et al. Pyriform augmentation as an ancillary procedure in facial rejuvenation surgery. *Plast Reconstr Surg.* 1999;103:683–686.
17. Peled ZM, Warren AG, Johnston P, Yaremchuk MJ. The use of alloplastic materials in rhinoplasty surgery: A meta analysis. *Plast Reconstr Surg.* 2008;121:85e–92e.
18. Sclafani AP, Thomas JR, Cox AJ, Cooper MH. Clinical and histologic response of subcutaneous expanded polytetrafluoroethylene (Gore-Tex) and porous high density polyethylene (MEDPOR) implants to acute and early infection. *Arch Otolaryngol Head Neck Surg.* 1997;123:328–336.
19. Sclafani AP, Romo T, Silver L. Clinical and histologic behavior of exposed porous high-density polyethylene implants. *Plast Reconstr Surg.* 1997;99:41–50.

CHAPTER NINETEEN

Correction of the Pinched Nasal Tip Deformity

Santdeep H. Paun • Gilbert Nolst Trenité

The "pinched nasal tip" is a deformity caused primarily by collapse of the lateral crura of the lower lateral cartilages. Such collapse may be congenital due to inherent hypoplasia, weakening, or malposition of the cartilaginous support but is often secondary to acquired, commonly iatrogenic, causes. The resultant pinching effect gives an unaesthetic appearance characterized by an alar groove, which extends to the alar rim, causing shadowing between the tip and alar lobules. Such shadows give rise to a ball-shaped tip, and the basal view exhibits a typical pinched appearance. At its worst, it can lead to severe knuckling and bossae formation in the nasal dome region with resultant nasal obstruction by impedance of the airflow on inspiration.[1-3] Correction of the functional and aesthetic components to this problem is achieved with restoration of the alar cartilaginous strength and structure and requires appropriate, ideally autogenous, grafting material. This chapter describes the relevant anatomical basis for the deformity, causes and prevention of iatrogenic problems, and techniques for correction.

ANATOMY OF THE NASAL VESTIBULE

The ideal aesthetic of the basal view of the nasal tip is that of an equilateral triangle. The lateral crura should have an outward convexity of the posterior alar rims and gentle rounding in the dome region; specifically there should be no pinching of the lateral alar walls. Various factors, including thickness of the overlying skin, musculature (dilators), and strength and position of the lower lateral cartilages, can directly influence the tip shape and dynamics.

The caudal margin of the lateral crus should ideally lie in a horizontal plane such that it lies just inferior to the cephalic margin. If the cartilage is angulated such that there is a significant superior to inferior relationship between the cephalic and caudal margins, this may predispose to loss of support in the lateral alar region and consequent pinched tip deformity[4] (Figures 19-1 and 19-2).

Inherent or postoperative weakness in the lateral crus can cause the anterior and midportion of the tip to collapse. Posterolaterally, there is thick alar soft tissue and skin, so fewer problems are encountered.

CAUSES OF DEFORMITY

Weakness of the lateral cartilaginous support leads to the nostril rim contracting inwards under the weight of the thick alar skin and soft tissue envelope. Inspiration may exacerbate this collapse. The basal view exhibits a typical appearance resembling a teat on a baby's bottle[5] (Figure 19-3).

CONGENITAL

Congenitally weak lower lateral cartilages predispose to this deformity. The lateral nasal rim is typically convex and its most severe form can buckle in so dramatically so as to restrict the nasal airway even in the resting state.

ACQUIRED/IATROGENIC

By far the most common cause for this deformity is iatrogenic weakening of the lower lateral cartilages due to overresection of the cephalic edge of the lower lateral cartilages with subsequent weakening of the intact rim strip. The useful edict of leaving behind more cartilage than that resected should always be remembered although the authors recommend an absolute minimum of 6-mm cartilaginous support but leaving more may be favorable.

Knuckling of the lower lateral cartilages in the domal area forms "bossae" (Figure 19-4).

The inexperienced rhinoplasty surgeon may not be aware of the triad of thin skin, strong alar cartilages, and bifidity of the tip, which together predispose to their formation when there is an excess cephalic strip reduction and inadequate narrowing of the domes.[6] Postoperative scar contracture in this area causes the deformity.

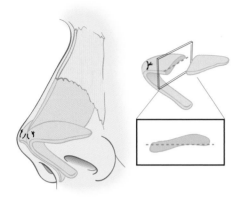

Figure 19-1 The caudal aspect of the lateral crus is situated ideally in the horizontal plane with the cephalic margin just superior to it.

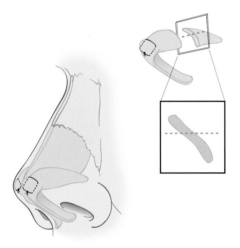

Figure 19-2 With a more vertical orientation of the lateral crus, the alar lobule is weaker and may further be weakened by cephalic rim excision, predisposing to a pinched tip appearance.

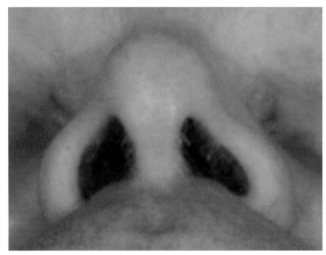

Figure 19-3 Typical "baby bottle teat" appearance of the pinched nasal tip.

Controversy surrounds the predisposition of vertical dome division techniques to formation of the pinched tip and bossae, and distinguished authors have both suggested[7] and refuted[8] this possibility.

Overzealous cephalic strip resection can further lead to alar retraction due to the visoring effect caused by contraction as healing occurs. If vestibular mucosa is not preserved, this complication, too, can contribute to contracture and promote further retraction.

Aggressive domal suturing with its resultant alteration in tip orientation and dynamics can cause notching in the dome region predisposing to a pinched tip effect. Ensuring the suture is not tied overtightly such that significant pinching of the domes occurs should reduce the risk of this.[9]

Other more unusual causes of this deformity include collapse of the alar cartilaginous region following inflammatory conditions (see Fig. 19-5) such as Wegener's granulomatosis, but this may also occur following cocaine abuse.

ASSESSMENT

A complete and discerning history regarding the perceived cosmetic problem and function, any prior procedures, and accurate chronologic detailing of postoperative changes is important when considering revision surgery. As ever, copies of a detailed prior operative report are helpful but rarely available for the revision rhinoplasty surgeon. Overall, it is vital to ensure that the patient's concerns and expectations are elucidated early in the consultation. Dissatisfaction expressed by the patient should be specific rather than general and should be perceived as realistic and true by the evaluating specialist.

The surgery is best not performed if the patient's expectations are thought to be unrealistic. When in doubt, sensitive counseling of the patient and referral for psychiatric review is always prudent, and surgery is deferred pending this.[10]

Diagnosis of the underlying anatomic deformity is essential prior to embarking upon a surgical plan. Inspection and palpation of the integrity of lower lateral support are equally important. It may not be possible to assess whether there is an intact strip of the lower lateral cartilage, and prior operative notes may be helpful in this regard.

Specific assessment for analysis of the pinched nasal tip includes analysis of functional obstruction. It is important to check whether there is alar collapse on inspiration, but in its absence, valve collapse cannot be excluded. Assessment with the Cottle maneuver is often advocated but can be nonspecific[11] and lateralizing the alar cartilage with a probe or cotton tip applicator may be a better evaluator.

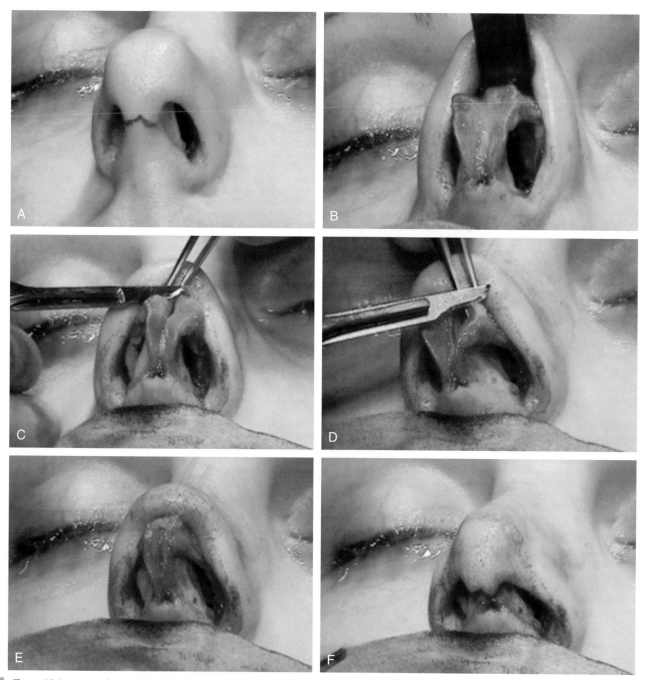

Figure 19-4 A, B, Tip bossae. Knuckling occurs due to inherent strength of the lower lateral cartilage, excessive cephalic reduction, and inadequate narrowing of the nasal domes. **C, D,** Bossae are excised by trimming and gentle scoring of the knuckled cartilages. **E,** Suture reconstitution of the domes. **F,** Intraoperative tip configuration after bossae correction.

OPERATIVE TECHNIQUES

ENDONASAL APPROACH

Correction of the pinched tip deformity can be achieved in a variety of ways. For a minor deformity, an endonasal approach may prove adequate for placement of supporting grafts in primary surgery or to correct prior overzealous tip suturing.[5] Marginal incisions may allow delivery of the lower lateral cartilages that can be repositioned and modified as required. Small specific pockets can also allow batten grafts to be inserted to correct concavities caused by weakness of the cartilage. An isolated aesthetic deformity caused by inherent concavity of the lateral crus may be corrected by complete mobilization of the lower lateral cartilage from the vestibular skin. An incision is then made just lateral to the domal area and the lateral crus flipped over such that the concavity now becomes a

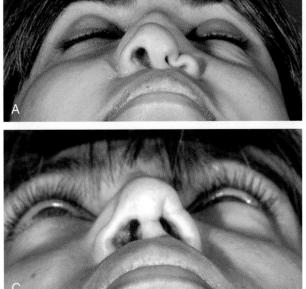

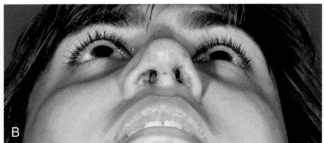

Figure 19-5 A, Preoperative view of inflammatory nasal deformity with complete bilateral vestibular stenosis. **B,** Early and **C,** late postoperative views after reconstruction using rib cartilage, composite auricular cartilage grafting, application of topical mitomycin C and medium term use of a custom made vestibular stent.

convexity. The rotated, reconstructed crus is then sutured to the medial segment. Figure 19-6 outlines such a reconstruction, albeit performed via an external approach.

EXTERNAL APPROACH

It is our preference to employ the external approach for most revision cases. This allows accurate evaluation of the orientation, integrity, and strength of the alar cartilages.

CARTILAGINOUS AUGMENTATION

Restoration of cartilaginous support is paramount with this deformity. The firmness and straightness of septal cartilage may be advantages for alar batten and lateral crural strut grafting, but auricular cartilage can be carved to shape very well even if it is a little weaker. Rib cartilage may be the preferred option in severe postinflammatory contraction and in the presence of multiple other grafting needs. Other nonautogenous material is generally not advocated by the authors.[5,12]

ALAR BATTEN GRAFTS

Alar batten grafts are fashioned from curved auricular or septal cartilage and placed to support the alar rim. A precise pocket is created, and the graft is placed from laterally over the pyriform aperture to the area of maximal collapse. The graft may need to extend to the caudal lateral crus. A more anatomically placed such graft extending along the weakened lateral crus to the pyriform aperture is termed a *lateral crural graft* (Figure 19-7). The convex side of the graft is placed laterally to help correct the pinch deformity. It is important to maintain as

much skin and soft tissue cover to reduce the risk of the graft showing postoperatively. If inserted into a specific "hand in glove" manner, fixation may not need to be necessary, particularly if performed via an endonasal approach. When an open approach is preferred, the grafts can be suture fixated to the lateral crus.

When using tip or shield grafts, particularly when they project 3 mm beyond the domes, a pinched type appearance may be created. Lateral crural grafts and alar rim grafts placed into a pocket along the caudal margin of the marginal incision can help to recreate the gentle curve to the nasal tip contour.[4]

LATERAL CRURAL STRUT GRAFTS

Lateral crural strut grafts are placed in a pocket between the lateral crus and vestibular skin such that they extend laterally to the pyriform aperture (Figure 19-8). They are not to be confused with lateral crural grafts, which are positioned between the external skin and lateral crus (see section on alar batten). While they essentially have the same function as alar battens, they have the advantage of causing less visible distortion externally in thin-skinned patients. Such grafts are also useful in providing support when cephalically malpositioned lateral crura are repositioned caudally in patients with a "parenthesis"-type tip deformity.[13]

Careful dissection is required between the vestibular skin and lateral crus, making this technically more difficult than alar battens. Care has to be taken to avoid the graft protruding into the airway.

Dome suturing is used to narrow the domal angle but may also cause significant concavity or occasionally convexity of the lateral crus in the process. If such deformity

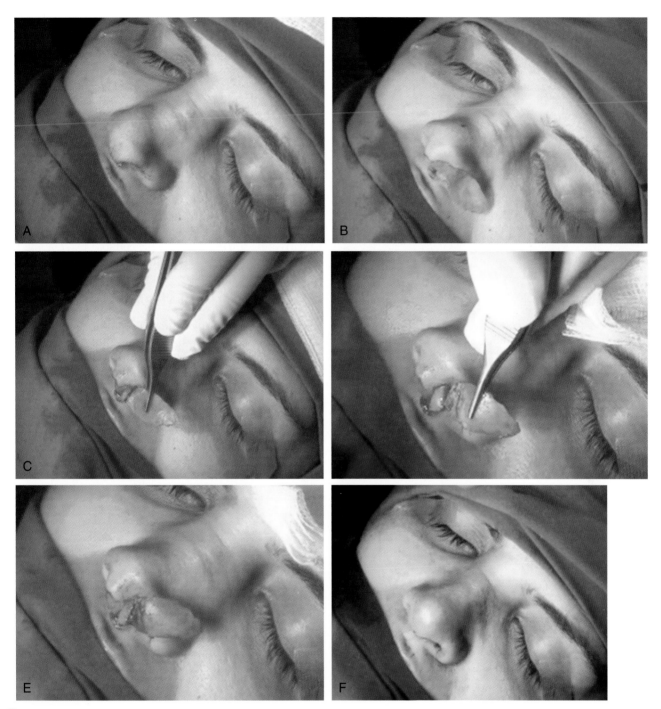

Figure 19-6 Diagram to illustrate the technique of "flipping" of a concave lateral crus to produce a favorable convexity of the alar lobule. **A,** Significant concavity of the lateral crus causing a pinched, collapsed effect. **B, C,** The lateral crus is fully mobilized from vestibular skin and then marked and divided in domal area. **D, E,** The lateral crus segment is "flipped" over and reconstituted with permanent sutures. **F,** A natural convexity to the lateral crus is restored.

cannot be resolved by repositioning of the sutures, lateral crural strut grafts can effectively flatten this area, giving rise to an aesthetic contour.[4]

ALAR RIM GRAFTS

Alar rim grafts are fashioned from thin, soft cartilage. They are approximately 2 to 3 mm wide. A pocket is created between the external skin and vestibular skin

along the caudal margin of the marginal incision along the alar rim border (Figures 19-9 and 10). Care is taken to remain as close to the vestibular skin as possible to avoid any risk of puncture through the alar skin and to reduce potential postoperative visibility of the graft. The medial-most border of the graft is particularly prone to such visibility and is thus camouflaged by crushing the cartilage in that region. The grafts are suture-fixated to the regional soft tissue. Alar rim grafts act to support and elevate the alar margin. They can also be used to displace the alar margin inferiorly, which may be helpful where there is an alar–columellar disproportion. They usefully reduce any pinching deformity following dome suturing by eradicating any significant visible transition between the domal area and the alar lobule.[14,15]

ALAR SPREADER GRAFTS

When an overresected rim of cartilage is found to be causing the pinching effect, a bar-type graft can be placed horizontally in the space between the remnants to correct the collapse. Such an "alar spreader graft" acts to lateralize the concavities[16] (Figure 19-11). Pockets are dissected between the vestibular skin and alar cartilage at the area of maximal collapse. A preferred septal cartilage graft is fashioned to sit into the created pockets and trimmed to a length such that the concavity in the alar cartilages becomes a gentle convexity. The cartilage is then sutured with an absorbable suture to the lateral crura to ensure stability. The skin–soft tissue envelope is replaced, and it is ensured that there is no evidence of nostril flaring necessitating trimming of the graft. A triangular or butterfly-shaped graft can be inserted instead of a single bar. The graft is partially incised in the midline to give a lateralizing spring effect. This may have the additional benefit of correcting internal nasal valve collapse by splaying the upper lateral cartilages laterally.[17]

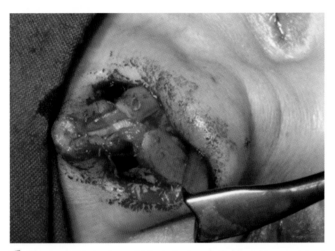

Figure 19-7 Lateral crural (alar batten) grafts fashioned to reconstruct alar collapse following prior dome division of the lower lateral cartilages.

REORIENTATION OF LATERAL CRURA

Ideal orientation of the caudal margin of the lateral crus should be in a horizontal plane such that it lies just inferior to the cephalic margin. A loss of support in the lateral alar region may be predicted if there is a significant superior-to-inferior relationship between the cephalic and caudal margins and subsequent pinching anticipated. A cephalically positioned lateral crus may also give rise to lack of support laterally in the alar lobule with fullness cephalically giving rise to the "parenthesis deformity" of the nasal tip.[18] Reorientation of the cartilage into a more caudally placed ideal form can be achieved by dissecting

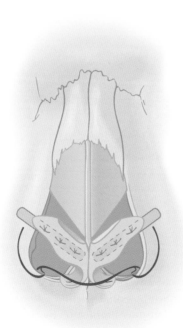

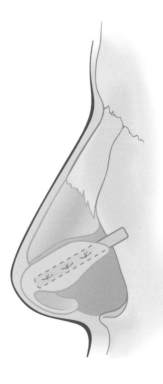

Figure 19-8 Lateral crural strut grafts.

the lateral crus fully from the vestibular skin. A lateral crural strut is attached to the freed edge to provide structural support. This extends laterally to the pyriform aperture. An appropriately fashioned caudally placed pocket is created to hold the lateral crus with attached strut in position. The resulting position should be at near to 45 degrees to the midline. This deals with the laterally based pinching effect and gives significant lateral support to this area.

TREATMENT OF NASAL BOSSAE

Nasal tip bossae are often associated with other postoperative problems, including alar collapse. Clearly, cartilaginous augmentation procedures as described here may be required in addition to the specific correction of the bossae. Treatment options include trimming or complete

resection of the domal knuckling with suture reconstruction of the lower lateral cartilages. If resection is required, it should be conservative to avoid significant deprojection of the tip. Isolated bossae deformities may be corrected through a small marginal incision with careful undermining to separate the knuckled cartilages from the underlying vestibular skin, which should be preserved intact wherever possible. More significant deformities are better visualized and managed via an external approach. Approximation of the domes with sutures is important to prevent recurrent postoperative splaying of the nasal domes predisposing to further bossae formation. A crushed or bruised cartilaginous tip graft may usefully camouflage any minor underlying irregularity remaining after the domal area has been reconstituted[5] (Figures 19-4, 19-12, and 19-13).

SUMMARY

The pinched nasal tip deformity is an unaesthetic consequence of weakness in the lateral alar region. Such weakness may be congenital but is often iatrogenic, most commonly due to excessive cephalic reduction of the lateral crus in primary rhinoplasty surgery. Other causes may include the lack of recognition of the pinching effect of dome suturing that may lead to concavity of the lateral crus. Similar unaesthetic changes may occur after insertion of a protruding shield or tip graft, which gives the effect of a transition between the tip dome lobule and the alar lobule. Cephalically positioned lateral crura give rise to bulkiness in the tip region, but the absence of more laterally based support of the alar lobules can cause a pinching effect leading to the "parenthesis"-type deformity of the nasal tip. Similarly, malpositioned lateral crura such that the caudal edge does not lie just inferior to the cephalic edge may predispose to pinching.

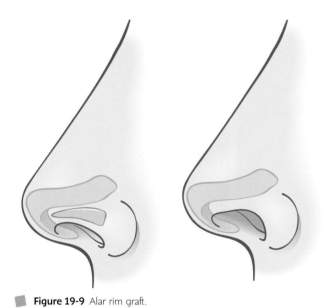

Figure 19-9 Alar rim graft.

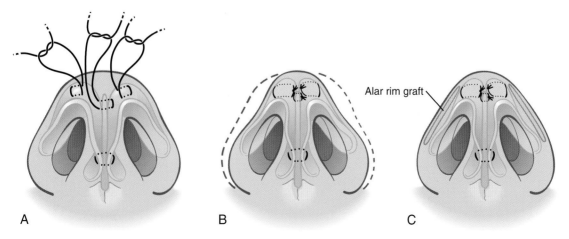

Figure 19-10 A pinched tip can result from overly suture techniques. In this example, the issue is remedied with alar rim grafts.

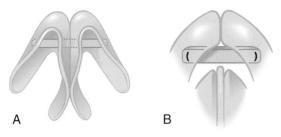

Figure 19-11 Alar spreader grafts are placed to lateralize collapse of the alar cartilages.

Grafting techniques as described here act to flatten the lateral crural region and add stability and support to this area, thus addressing both functional and aesthetic concerns with this deformity. The curved nature of conchal cartilage lends itself well to such grafting but can be a little weak at times. Gently scored septal cartilage to encourage curving may be better from a structural, functional point of view. As with all grafting procedures, there is a risk of postoperative visibility and care has to be taken to ensure pockets created for graft insertion are deep enough within the skin–soft tissue envelope and that such grafts are feathered and crushed appropriately.

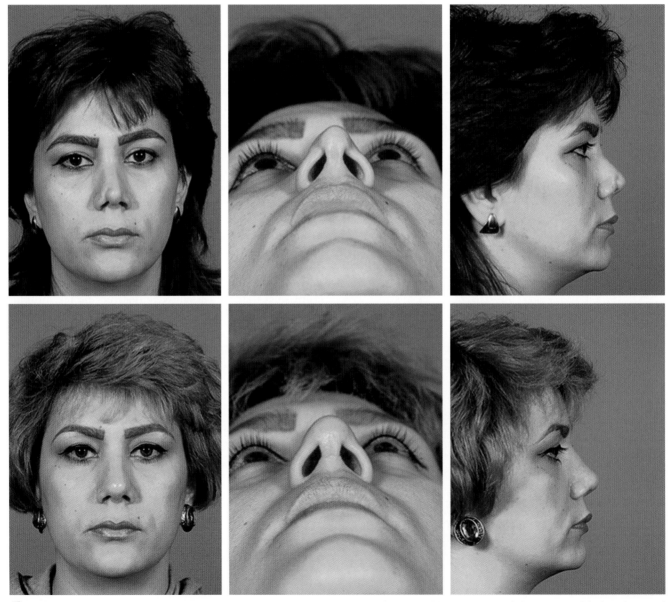

Figure 19-12 Pre and post operative views of a revision rhinoplasty to correct for bossae caused by excessive cephalic resection of the lateral crus and surrounding soft tissue with scar contracture.

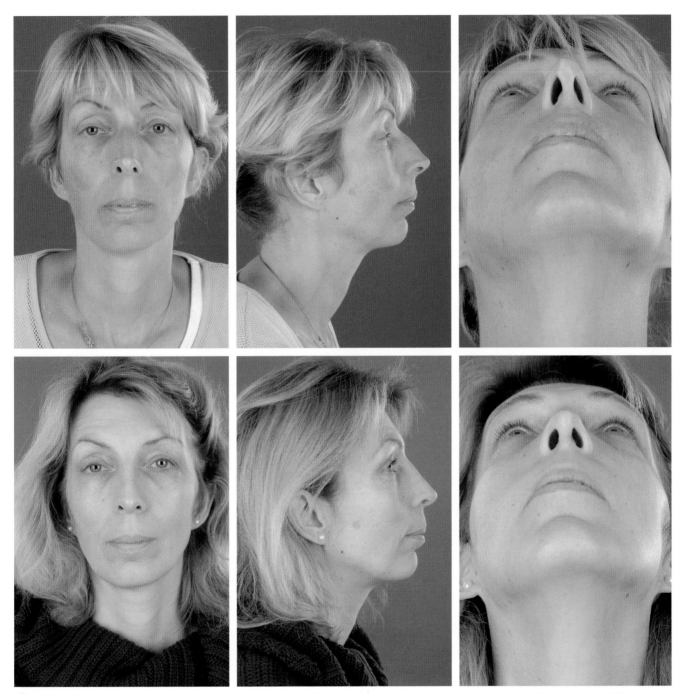

Figure 19-13 Deformities of dorsum and nasal tip improved with hump reduction, osteotomies, tip deprojection, and improvement of the irregular bossae type deformity.

REFERENCES

1. DesPrez JD, Kiehn CL. Valvular obstruction of the nasal airway. *Plast Reconstr Surg.* 1975;56(3):307–313.
2. Cottle MH. The structure and function of the nasal vestibule. *AMA Arch Otolaryngol.* 1955;62(2):173–181.
3. Haight JS, Cole P. The site and function of the nasal valve. *Laryngoscope.* 1983;93(1):49–55.
4. Toriumi DM, Checcone MA. New concepts in nasal tip contouring. *Fac Plast Surg Clin North Am.* 2009;17(1):55–90, vi.
5. Paun SH, Nolst Trenite GJ. Revision rhinoplasty: an overview of deformities and techniques. *Fac Plast Surg.* 2008;24(3):271–287.
6. Nolst Trenite G, ed. *Rhinoplasty: a practical guide to functional and aesthetic surgery of the nose.* 3rd ed. Amsterdam: Kugler Publications; 2008.
7. Kamer FM, ed. *Revision rhinoplasty.* Philadelphia: JB Lippincott; 1998.
8. Gillman GS, Simons RL, Lee DJ. Nasal tip bossae in rhinoplasty. Etiology, predisposing factors, and management techniques. *Arch Fac Plast Surg.* 1999;1(2):83–89.
9. Nolst Trenite GJ, Paun, S. External rhinoplasty. In: Watkinson J, ed. *Scott Brown's Otolaryngology.* 7th ed. London: Arnold; 2008.
10. Vuyk HD, Zijlker TD. Psychosocial aspects of patient counseling and selection: a surgeon's perspective. *Fac Plast Surg.* 1995;11(2):55–60.
11. Constantian MB. The incompetent external nasal valve: pathophysiology and treatment in primary and secondary rhinoplasty. *Plast Reconstr Surg.* 1994;93(5):919–931; discussion 32–33.
12. Nolst Trenite GJ. Grafts in nasal surgery. In: Nolst Trenite GJ, ed. *A practical guide to aesthetic surgery of the nose.* 3rd ed. Amsterdam: Kugler Publications; 2005:49–67.
13. Gunter JP, Friedman RM. Lateral crural strut graft: technique and clinical applications in rhinoplasty. *Plast Reconstr Surg.* 1997;99(4):943–952; discussion 53–55.
14. Toriumi DM. Structure approach in rhinoplasty. *Fac Plast Surg Clin North Am.* 2005;13(1):93–113.
15. Rohrich RJ, Raniere J Jr, Ha RY. The alar contour graft: correction and prevention of alar rim deformities in rhinoplasty. *Plast Reconstr Surg.* 2002;109(7):2495–2505; discussion 506–508.
16. Gunter JP, Rohrich RJ. Correction of the pinched nasal tip with alar spreader grafts. *Plast Reconstr Surg.* 1992;90(5):821–829.
17. Clark JM, Cook TA. The "butterfly" graft in functional secondary rhinoplasty. *Laryngoscope.* 2002;112(11):1917–1925.
18. Sheen JH, Sheen AP. Aesthetic rhinoplasty. 2nd ed. St Louis: CV Mosby; 1987.

CHAPTER TWENTY

Postrhinoplasty Nasal Lobule Deformities: Open Approach

Peter A. Adamson • Jason A. Litner • Peyman Solieman

Older reduction tip rhinoplasty techniques are effective in altering tip contour and definition, yet they depend on aggressive cartilage resection, morselization, and sacrifice of tip supports to achieve these goals. Weakening of the crura in this manner, when subjected to long-term forces of contracture, may lead to tip distortion and commonly seen postrhinoplasty deformities. Beginning in the 1980s, advancements in understanding of nasal tip anatomy and dynamics allowed for technical innovations in tip alteration that emphasize more conservative handling of the tip while better preserving structural support and functional integrity.[1-6] Despite these developments, the incidence of revision rhinoplasty remains considerable. Kamer,[7] in a 1981 review, reported rates of revision rhinoplasty in the range of 8% to 15%, while more recent reports place the incidence closer to 5% in the hands of experienced surgeons.[8,9] The senior author (P.A.A.) previously reported[10] a 6% revision rate in a cohort of his patients. The general decline in revision rates has been attributed in part to increasing acceptance and employment of open rhinoplasty approaches[11] but may also be due to better public understanding of the need to choose experienced rhinoplasty surgeons when undergoing this procedure.

Residual and iatrogenic aesthetic deformities are the primary indications for revision; however, a functional deficit coexists in roughly two-thirds of patients.[12,13] While the authors' experience reflects a higher revision rate for mid-vault abnormalities, several studies spanning five decades suggest tip deformities are the leading reason for revision surgery.[8,13-15] Failures of philosophy and ability to accurately diagnose and properly implement techniques during the primary procedure account for the patterns of deformities seen. Even when accurate diagnosis is possible, the capacity to execute surgical goals may be diminished in revision surgery for several reasons: (1) tip anatomy is typically distorted, (2) tip supports are often compromised, necessitating augmentation procedures, (3) aesthetic goals are sometimes supplanted by functional needs, and (4) the skin envelope is often scarred and inelastic, rendering redrapage unpredictable and less forgiving.[10]

This chapter will discuss the most frequently seen postrhinoplasty lobule deformities and summarize indications and techniques for their correction.

ANATOMY AND NASAL TIP DYNAMICS

The techniques available for manipulation of the nasal tip are widely known. Yet, the challenge is in knowing when to apply specific techniques to achieve the appropriate correction. Another way of looking at this is that the surgeon must have both a clear aesthetic understanding of the surgical goals as well as the technical expertise to recognize which procedures will achieve them.

In the revision scenario it is especially important to have a clear conceptual framework with which to create a surgical plan. The Tripod Concept, first advanced by Jack Anderson, M.D.,[16] is widely taught in training programs and still represents a useful algorithm for nasal tip reduction. However, the Tripod Concept was conceived at a time when reduction tip rhinoplasty using a closed technique was the norm. Thus, it does not provide for understanding of techniques for achieving greater projection or for better understanding of the need for tip stabilization in open cases. In addition, the Tripod Concept predates the further characterization of the intermediate crura, and so it does not address the effects of alteration of this structure to achieve refinement of the lobule.

A contemporary model of nasal tip dynamics, termed the M-arch model,[17,18] has been proposed in an effort to expand on the Tripod Concept (Figure 20-1). This model views the lower lateral cartilages as paired parabolic cartilaginous arches having their vertices at the tip-defining points. The most significant determinants of tip-alteration are the overall length of the arch and the specific site of the alteration (Figure 20-2). Shortening the arch in close proximity to the vertex will have a greater effect on deprojection (such as a vertical lobule division), while shortening *by the same amount* farther from the tip-defining point will have a greater influence on rotation (such as a lateral crural overlay technique). Furthermore, shortening

245

Peter A. Adamson · Jason A. Litner · Peyman Solieman

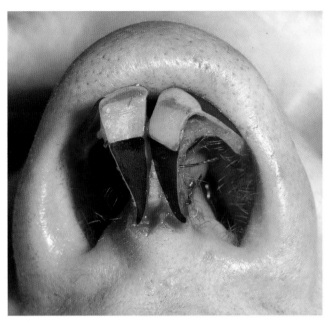

Figure 20-1 The anatomy of the tripod arch seen from the basal view. The central segment of the M-arch is termed the domal arch or lobular arch and comprises the intermediate crus and the most medial aspect of the lateral crus.

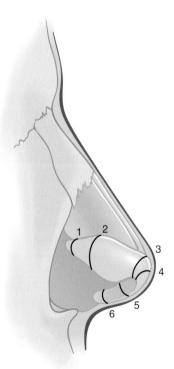

Figure 20-2 The various locations that have been described as sites to divide the lower lateral cartilages: (*1*) hinge area, (*2*) lateral crural flap, (*3*) Goldman maneuver, (*4*) vertical lobule division, (*5*) Lipsett maneuver, and (*6*) medial crural feet.

of the arch lateral to the tip-defining point serves to deproject, rotate, and shorten the nose, whereas shortening medial to this point will deproject, counterrotate, and lengthen the nose.

The same principles may be applied to understanding of the relative effects of arch-lengthening maneuvers such as suture or tip-grafting techniques. Suture techniques such as the lateral crural steal[5] effectively increase the vertical arch segment by borrowing length from the more horizontal segment just lateral to the tip-defining point. Lobular grafts, on the other hand, achieve improvements in projection by adding *apparent* length or vertical height to the M-arch. In our practice, columellar struts are routinely used to stabilize the length and strength of the medial crura and thereby uphold the nasal tip projection without, in and of themselves, actually increasing arch length.

The M-arch model allows for application of specific arch-altering maneuvers to achieve simultaneous predictable changes in nasal length, projection, rotation, and tip definition. Division at the medial crural feet will generate tip deprojection and some counterrotation and may be used to diminish excessive flaring of the medial crural footplates if the soft tissue attachments between the footplates have been released. Division in the mid-medial crus may be used to adjust columellar asymmetries, in addition to providing counterrotation and deprojection. Division at the angle or junction of the medial and intermediate crus will yield primarily tip deprojection and vertical shortening and may also diminish a hanging infratip lobule. Division within the intermediate crus or at the dome will deproject the tip and engender greater acuity of the domal arch, thus producing lobular refinement. Asymmetric division in this region may be used to improve lobule symmetry with sutures concealed within the infratip. Division in the mid-lateral crus, known as a lateral crural overlay, represents the most powerful maneuver for obtaining rotation along with deprojection. Finally, division at the hinge area will achieve mild tip deprojection and rotation. This setback technique is preferred when lobular contour is acceptable; however, this is rarely the circumstance in revision tip surgery. Furthermore, occasionally it can lead to crural in-flaring and obstruction within the vestibule, so we avoid this maneuver if possible. In our practice, the vertical lobule division and lateral crural overlay are the workhorse techniques for obtaining the desired alterations in major nasal parameters.

Vertical arch manipulations represent extraordinarily powerful techniques for achieving predictable changes in lobular contour. In fact, it is the experience of the authors that such techniques are the only reliable method for accomplishing meaningful modification of tip projection and rotation. Maneuvers that do not cause real or apparent changes in arch length cannot, therefore, achieve real or apparent changes in tip projection. By example, traditional methods for achieving changes in projection or rotation, such as full transfixion incisions, resection of the nasal spine, shortening of the caudal septum, and cephalic crural excision, among others, are not dependable options and most often are conducive to postrhinoplasty tip destabilization and pollybeak deformity.

ETIOLOGY OF POSTRHINOPLASTY TIP DEFORMITIES

Postrhinoplasty tip deformities can be categorized as those caused by either undertreatment or overresection of preexisting abnormalities.[19,20] Persistent primary deformities comprise aesthetic problems that were not adequately treated during the primary procedure. These may be attributed to an oversight in diagnosis or failure to properly account for postoperative soft tissue healing. Common deformities include (1) a persistently overprojected or underprojected nasal tip, (2) a counterrotated or ptotic tip, (3) a wide, boxy, bulbous or asymmetric tip, (4) a discordant alar–columellar relationship, and (5) a broad or flared alar base.

By contrast, aggressive reductive efforts at primary surgery may give rise to the spectrum of overresected nasal tip deformities. Examples of these abnormalities include (1) an underprojected, collapsed tip, often in combination with a pollybeak deformity, (2) an overrotated tip, leading to a shortened nasal appearance, (3) an excessively narrowed, pinched tip, (4) alar-columellar contour irregularities caused by bossae formation, alar retraction or a hanging columella, or grafts that have become visible or palpable, (5) an aggressively narrowed alar base, and (6) external soft tissue irregularities caused by excessive soft tissue thinning or unsatisfactory scar formation. Associated functional consequences may typically include external valve collapse, caudal septal instability, and vestibular stenosis.

INDICATIONS FOR SURGERY

The desirable revision tip rhinoplasty candidate has a clearly defined and realistic complaint. One must remember that the degree of subjective concern that a patient experiences bears no direct relationship to the objective severity of the defect.[21] Thus, reasonable distress over a minor deformity is not, as such, a contraindication to surgery. Equally important, the defect must be technically treatable in the surgeon's hands. The quality of cutaneous health and vascularity should be used as the yardstick to measure technical suitability rather than the absolute number of prior surgeries. A patient with a real, definable complaint and a history of four prior rhinoplasties may be a reasonable revision candidate, whereas a patient having had only one prior procedure may be a poor candidate in the presence of severe scarring or vascular compromise.

A sound rapport must be developed with the prospective patient, one that will weather potential postoperative problems. The patient must be medically fit and psychologically prepared for yet another surgery. He or she must clearly understand and accept the likely range of outcomes, the limitations, and risks of surgery. In our own practice, we apply the above selection criteria stringently before embarking on revision surgery.[22,23]

SURGICAL TECHNIQUES

ADVANTAGES OF THE OPEN APPROACH

While technical preferences vary from surgeon to surgeon, most experienced revision rhinoplasty surgeons today prefer the open approach for revision tip surgery because of the undistorted exposure it affords.[11] We believe that open rhinoplasty is the approach of choice for both primary and revision cases unless an equivalent improvement can be obtained with a closed approach. This is seldom the case in our estimation. It is our perception that closed revision rhinoplasty approaches more often result in common postrhinoplasty deformities such as persistent overprojection, underrotation, tip asymmetry, contour deformities from graft distortion and migration, and soft tissue irregularities owing to a compromised plane of dissection, as well as bossae and pinched tip formation resulting from overly aggressive resection. The open approach offers distinct, well-described advantages in the form of more precise dissection, careful exposure and diagnosis of complex deformities, accurate measurement of proposed tip-altering maneuvers, and suture stabilization of both native cartilage as well as grafts. The avoidance of vestibular incisions near the internal nasal valve will also decrease the likelihood of incipient valve obstruction or vestibular stenosis postoperatively, which is more common following revision rhinoplasty.

Our preferred incision is the midcolumellar, inverted gull-wing design. If planned and closed carefully, this incision rarely, if ever, is cause for scar revision. If open rhinoplasty was performed previously, we will incise through the existing scar unless it is unfavorable, in which case it is revised. We routinely elevate the columellar flap following this incision, while the marginal incisions are made during scissor dissection over the domes and lateral crura. This permits more accurate identification of the crural margins. Occasionally, severe scarring may necessitate first making the marginal incisions, followed by retrograde dissection over the domes. We elevate as much as possible in the supraperichondrial plane, thereby maintaining scarred soft tissue on the flap. This helps to preserve flap vascularity and to prevent "buttonholing," and it better delineates the residual extent of the alar cartilages. At times, one may find that infiltration of the scar tissue with local anesthetic can aid in hydrodissection.

Extreme care must be exercised in multiple revision cases since thick scar tissue often complicates the dissection. Those surgeons who routinely perform revision rhinoplasty need not be told of how difficult this dissection can be. Alar cartilage remnants may be abnormally thin, tenuous, and easily penetrated by an excessively deep dissection. In fact, scar tissue is sometimes the only tip support remaining in the severely deformed tip. Similarly, the subdermal plane may be filled with scar, predisposing to dermal ischemia with an overly shallow dissection. The safest initial approach in the heavily scarred patient may be to leave a rind of scar tissue on the crura. This can be further painstakingly dissected and excess scar tissue may be discarded or saved for soft tissue augmentation elsewhere. To compensate for the thick, inelastic skin that is often encountered in a revision case, it is necessary to undermine the soft tissue envelope widely to encourage favorable redrapage. Once the tip and dorsum have been adequately exposed, precise corrective maneuvers may be undertaken.

VERTICAL ARCH DIVISION

Prior to any division, the cartilage is extensively released from vestibular skin in the surrounding region to allow for cartilage advancement. The location for arch division is chosen in accordance with the desired alterations in tip dynamics. The cut ends of cartilage are then overlapped from 2 mm up to 6 mm in some cases and are secured with 6-0 nylon mattress sutures. Two buried sutures are placed in every case, the first to set the length of overlap, and the second to set the longitudinal axis of the neoarch. Alternatively, 4-0 Vicryl sutures may be used in the lateral crus to fixate the cartilage segments through the underlying vestibular skin. This is sometimes preferred since it may be technically challenging to bury sutures in this location. Overlapping suture fixation is a critical component of this technique in order to avert inflaring or collapse of the arch upon contraction of the skin–soft tissue envelope. In general, the cartilage segment closest to the tip-defining point represents the overlying segment when overlapped (Figure 20-3).

CARTILAGE GRAFTING TECHNIQUES

Columellar Strut

Once fundamental tip parameters have been set, attention is then directed toward reconstructing the nasal tip from its base upward. This begins in nearly all instances with placement of a strong cartilaginous columellar strut. Septal cartilage is preferred to conchal cartilage, if available. A strut provides enduring support for the medial crura and acts as a secure foundation for further lobule grafting. While it will not inherently procure increased projection, we believe that a strut is essential to sustain the rotation and projection achieved with other maneuvers.[24] The strut is best positioned directly on the maxillary spine, if present, and assiduously secured to the medial crura by two horizontal mattress sutures via long Keith needles. To provide a reliable foundation for the strut, the maxillary spine may be assiduously flattened with a rongeur, although it should never be excised. The strut is encased in a pocket by an anterior suture placed through the strut and medial crura and a posterior suture placed through the membranous septum just cephalic to it. Placing just one suture through the strut minimizes the risk of its fracture. These sutures set medial crural symmetry at the base, in both vertical and craniocaudal dimensions. Columellar widening is prevented by dissection of intercrural ligaments and scar, which are either preserved as a soft tissue columellar flap or free graft within the premaxillary space, or are discarded when nasolabial augmentation is undesirable.

Nasolabial Angle Augmentation Grafts

When further nasolabial augmentation is desired, we find cartilaginous nasolabial grafts to be very efficacious. These can be exploited to improve a posterior columellar retraction or to increase apparent tip rotation. One or more cartilaginous wafers are shaped and positioned within a deep pocket in the premaxillary space (Figure 20-4). The authors prefer to secure these first to each other and then either through the premaxillary skin or to the caudal margins of the medial crura via peripheral sutures. Conchal cartilage works well for this purpose.

Lobule Grafts

As a consequence of overresection, many postrhinoplasty nasal tips appear overrotated and underprojected, giving the nose a foreshortened appearance. Such situations call for lobular grafts that, depending on their precise placement, may secure greater lobule projection, definition, counterrotation, lengthening, and camouflage of remaining asymmetries. It is not uncommon for the authors to use multiple grafts in revision tips; however, the fewest necessary grafts should be used. In thick-skinned or severely scarred tips, tiered grafts may often be necessary to obtain any amount of tip definition. The authors do not follow a defined formula for tip grafting but rather individualize the configurations to each patient. The main goal is to reconstruct the ideal aesthetic lobule utilizing whatever surgical techniques are necessary. In most instances, a shield-type[25] infratip lobule graft, possibly supported by one or two domal onlay grafts, will achieve the desired lengthening and/or projection (Figure 20-5). Increased projection or counterrotation can be selectively favored by rotating the axis of the graft upon the underlying lobule. Grafts are generally secured to the lobule by

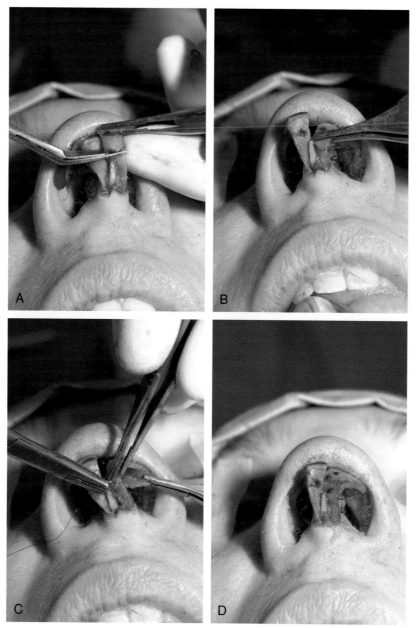

Figure 20-3 Intraoperative photos demonstrating vertical lobule division. **A,** Intended point of division is marked at the junction of the medial and intermediate crus. **B,** Overlap of the divided cartilage segments. **C,** Suture stabilization with two horizontal mattress sutures. **D,** Final view showing the degree of deprojection achieved.

peripherally placed 6-0 nylon sutures after the tip has already been set and appropriate interdomal and intercrural sutures have been positioned. Careful feathering of the graft edges is crucial, especially in thin-skinned individuals. When the columella also requires augmentation, an extended infratip graft is usually placed to span the columella as a batten. This is also fixated with transfixion sutures of 6-0 nylon. Supratip deficiencies, occurring from unbalanced resection of the anterior septal angle, may also be addressed by grafting techniques. These may be camouflaged by placement of a supratip onlay cartilage graft. Alternatively, a dorsal septal extension graft may be

placed to bridge the gap between the residual dorsal septal remnant and the columellar strut. Occasionally, a unilateral supratip depression may be resolved by apt positioning of a caudally situated spreader graft.

Lateral Crural Grafts

Lateral crural grafts may be used as support or contour grafts. In cases of severe alar deficiency and associated external valve collapse resulting from overresection, a lateral crural graft is best designed as a batten spanning from the dome to the hinge area over the pyriform margin. This is usually placed in an onlay fashion in order to

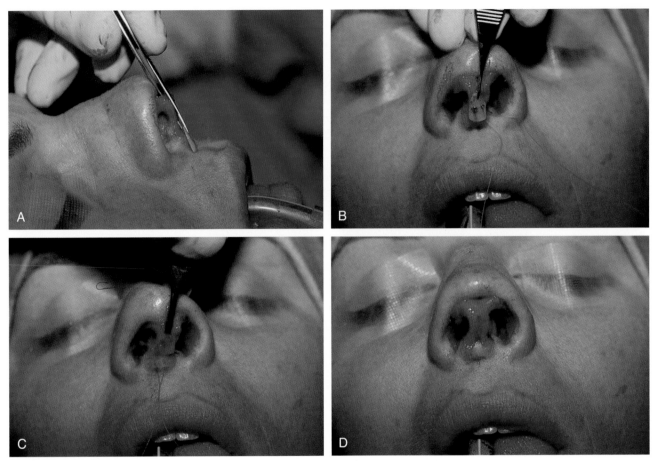

Figure 20-4 Intraoperative photographs demonstrating nasolabial angle augmentation (NLA) grafting. **A,** Lateral view of the location of the NLA graft. **B,** Horizontal mattress suture placement through the graft. **C,** Sutures being drawn through the premaxillary skin. **D,** Final view showing nasolabial augmentation achieved.

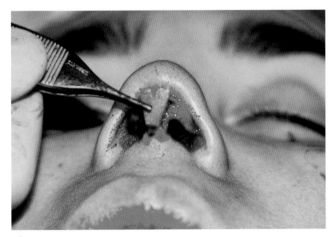

Figure 20-5 Intraoperative photograph demonstrating an infratip lobule graft.

impart reinforcement and to enhance alar contour. A native lateral crus that has adequate width, but requires support and contour, such as for a concavity, is amenable to placement of an alar strut graft. This is formulated as a cartilaginous slab designed to provide an inversion of

convexity. It is best positioned deep to the concave surface in an underlay fashion (Figure 20-6). While very effective, care must be taken in appropriate placement of this strut. Ideally, it should be located cephalically near the scroll region so as to enhance support in this area and to reduce potential valve collapse. Placement too close to the marginal incision will increase the chances for postoperative palpability and potential narrowing of the vestibular inlet. Otherwise, patients will tend to complain of a palpable lump within the vestibule.

SUTURING TECHNIQUES

Suture techniques provide invaluable versatility in revision tip surgery to help alter the length and contour of the M-arch either independently or as an adjunct to other maneuvers. The greatest applicability occurs in situations requiring increased projection, rotation, and lobular narrowing or refinement. Most surgeons are familiar with various intradomal and interdomal suturing techniques (Figure 20-7). The authors' preferred suture protocol consists of the use of single-dome unit mattress sutures to individually narrow each domal arch as needed and a

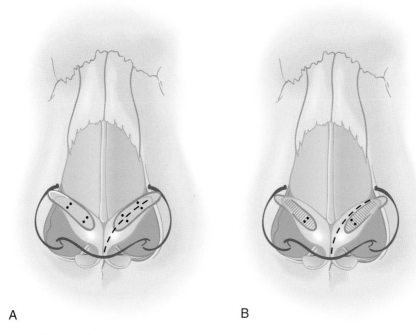

A   B

Figure 20-6 Lateral crural grafts. **A,** Overlay alar batten grafts. **B,** Underlay alar strut grafts.

double-dome unit mattress suture to conjointly medialize the domal arches. Lobular "bunching" mattress sutures located more cephalically near the scroll region may also aid in decreasing supratip fullness though overnarrowing should be avoided. For this reason, the authors rarely make use of this type of suture for fear of creating a postoperatively pinched tip. Moderately increased projection may be acquired with the lateral crural steal technique.[5] A very powerful technique that the authors use regularly is an intermediate crural horizontal mattress suture. Transfixion of the caudal margins of the intermediate crura is accomplished along a vertical axis. Depending on its exact placement, this suture may be exploited to strengthen the medial crural–strut complex, to set the intercrural and alar-columellar angles, to narrow the infratip columella, and to diminish a hanging infratip. These techniques are applied in a graduated fashion to achieve the ideal outcome. Great precision is attainable through precise suture adjustment; 5-0 and 6-0 nylon sutures are generally preferred, with the knots always buried.

SOFT TISSUE TECHNIQUES

Resection of undesired soft tissue can be accomplished guardedly and meticulously in the revision tip via the open approach, especially in the lobular and lateral supratip areas. This tissue can first be hydrodissected with local anesthetic to create a bleb of scar tissue that may then be

safely resected. This tissue may be discarded or reserved for volume filling of the nasolabial angle or for contour grafting elsewhere in the nose. When the tip has been significantly deprojected, it may be advisable to excise 1 to 2 mm of the distal columellar flap to reduce the chances of skin redundancy imparting a hanging columella effect. Conversely, in cases of substantially increased projection, it may be necessary to develop an inferiorly based advancement flap of the columellar skin to allow for a tension-free closure. In very thin-skinned noses, soft tissue may be placed over lobule grafts to camouflage their firmness, and especially their perimeters.

ALAR BASE NARROWING

Patients in need of alar base narrowing postrevision are those having undergone significant tip deprojection causing alar flaring. Lobules that have been substantially narrowed may also benefit from basal narrowing in an effort to maintain a balanced, harmonious nasal appearance. The desired amount of resection of the internal (nostril circumference) and external (basal width) circumference is measured and marked within the sill. Identical or asymmetric excisions may be performed. A cut-back incision is made just above the alar-facial groove to allow advancement-rotation of the alar flap. Alar wall flaring may be treated simultaneously by excision of a tissue wedge in this location. The incision is closed with simple, well-everted 6-0 nylon sutures.

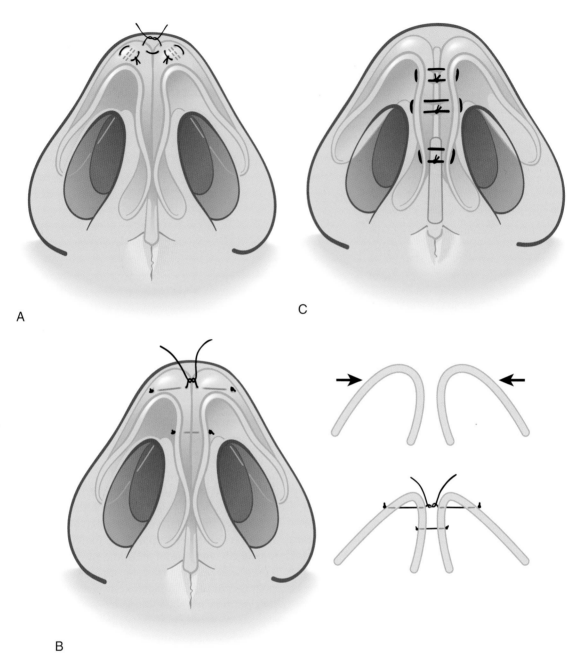

Figure 20-7 Intercrural suture techniques. **A,** Single-dome unit and intradomal sutures. **B,** Double dome unit. **C,** Intercrural horizontal mattress sutures.

APPLICATION OF THE M-ARCH MODEL TO SPECIFIC POSTRHINOPLASTY LOBULE DEFORMITIES

Revision tip surgery often requires a combination of reduction and augmentation techniques. Reduction maneuvers are used in the modification of persistent primary deformities. Conservation is the order of the day where these techniques are used. Deformities caused by overresection, on the other hand, will necessitate augmentation techniques.

THE PINCHED LOBULE

A pinched lobule may be encountered for several reasons in the revision nose. More often than not, this outcome is the result of overzealous cephalic resection of the lateral crura (Figure 20-8). In this case, poor lateral crural support leads to postoperative in-flaring and apparent pinching of the lobule. For this reason, the authors prefer to preserve at least 8 mm of lateral crural width, at its widest point, whenever a cephalic margin resection is performed and especially in the setting of a scarred or

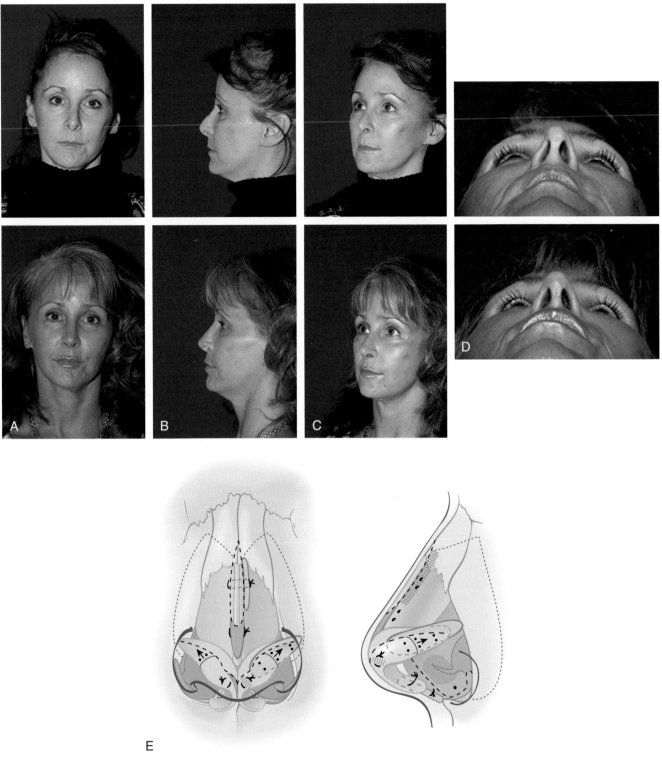

Figure 20-8 A postrhinoplasty pinched lobule secondary to overresection. Preoperative and postoperative (**A**) frontal, (**B**) lateral, (**C**) oblique, and (**D**) basal views. Schematic (**E**) showing tip correction with a right extended alar batten graft, left domal onlay graft, infratip lobule graft, columellar strut, interdomal spacer graft, and bilateral rim grafts.

thickened soft tissue envelope. In the revision setting, restoration of lateral crural support often entails lateral alar grafting in the form of alar batten grafts for severe overresection and alar strut grafts for moderate in-flare and/or support.

Another common cause for a pinched lobule is over-aggressive suture techniques. While single-dome unit, double-dome unit, and other suture maneuvers provide near-infinite possibilities for tip contouring, they can also be applied excessively. Our experience has been that tip narrowing suture effects are increased by temporal contracture of the skin envelope. So, every attempt should be made in the primary setting to preserve a normal or greater than normal alar–columellar relationship. We prefer to maintain a 90-degree intercrural angle of divergence to create an attractive diamond-shaped, two-point light reflex at the tip-defining lines. Risks of a pinched lobule and uni-tip deformity are elevated with an overly snug double-dome suture or supratip bunching suture, especially in the setting of weak cartilage.[6] Fortunately, the great advantage of suture techniques is their reversibility, so these unwanted effects are easily remedied in the revision case.

Poorly designed grafts may be at fault as well in giving the appearance of a pinched lobule. A too prominent columellar strut may abnormally fill the natural interalar groove and may even give an unnatural "tent pole" effect if it becomes the most projecting point within the infratip lobule. This seems to occur more frequently after a strut has been placed in an intercrural pocket via a closed approach without adequate stabilization. A shield-type tip graft[25] that is too narrow by design or that is placed too cephalically and too projected in relation to the natural domes may give rise to the undesired effect of a pinched appearance. This scenario owes to the fact that the graft itself overtakes the function of single-handedly creating the lobular contour without appropriately merging with the lateral alar contour. This effect can be corrected or prevented by fastidious attention to blending and "feathering" of the graft edges. We also find that stabilization of the crura behind the graft and peripheral location of multiple fixation sutures helps to ensure that the graft and intermediate crura appear as a single unit. Placement of a vertical notch at the midpoint of a tip graft may also preserve normal tip bifidity. When more projection is desired, use of a CAP graft (Cartilage Augmentation and Projection graft) similar to Peck's originally described onlay tip graft[26] can be advantageous. The graft is designed as a rectangular block of customizable thickness that is commonly secured immediately behind and cephalic to the shield graft. In this way, the graft acts as both a buttress to support caudal projection of the shield graft and a spacer to create a natural supralobular transition in contour. As with suture problems, pinched lobules as a result of poor graft technique may be repaired by graft alteration or replacement as necessary.

The final basis for a postrhinoplasty pinched lobule is utilization of inadvisable methods for cartilaginous arch division. Pinched lobules have been noted by the authors in patients having previous Goldman-type lateral crural division procedures[27] due to in-flare of the "floating" lateral crural remnants. While proponents of these techniques point to tip stability in their practice experiences, it has been our observation that the Goldman maneuver, and its derivatives such as the "hockey stick" excision, may place the lobule at risk for long-term instability and

deformity after many years in some patients. This occurs because the natural elastic spring of the cartilaginous arch is forfeited by interruption of its continuity. It is our contention that any arch division technique must be accompanied by reconstruction of the arch by suture overlap of the cut elements. We do not advise resection of intervening cut cartilage when undertaking arch division. Rather, the overlapped cut segments are always secured by two-point fixation. In this fashion, arch continuity is upheld and, in fact, the tip will be sturdier than it was prior to any intervention. In secondary rhinoplasty, deformities owing to in-flare of cut arch segments may be reconstructed by suture overlap as they would in the primary setting. It may be necessary to "buy back" lost projection by use of a tip graft.

THE BROAD, UNDEFINED LOBULE

Rarely, a widened lobule may persist after primary rhinoplasty because excess lateral crural width went undertreated. This is unusual, however, because most rhinoplasties incorporate cephalic margin resection in the hopes that this maneuver will decrease supratip fullness. The problem lies in the fact that nondelivery approaches to closed rhinoplasty render suture treatment of the lobule more difficult. As a result, many surgeons rely too heavily on cephalic margin resection to overcompensate for undercorrection of a broad interdomal angle. Horizontal cephalic cartilage excision, as opposed to vertical division, may achieve some small measure of lobule refinement and rotation but may rather, in excess, promote alar retraction and in-flaring, as mentioned. While excessive cephalic margin resection is not intrinsically a significant inducement to tip rotation, this maneuver will allow for excessive rotation and shortening of the nose by alternate techniques. When a persistently broad lobule is encountered, it should be treated as in the primary setting by suture techniques. Scoring of the lower lateral cartilage can be very effective in narrowing a broad domal arch, flattening a biconvex arch, and creating a new tip-defining point, although caution must be exercised so as not to noticeably weaken the arch.

A far more frequent cause for a broadened postrhinoplasty lobule is the presence of excessive soft tissue thickening. This is especially common in the thick-skinned individual or in those undergoing multiple procedures (Figure 20-9). When the lobule is overaggressively deprojected or thinned, intervening accumulation of scar tissue within the dead space can undermine the intended gains. At times, in the revision setting, the surgeon is confronted with scar tissue that makes the dissection nearly impossible in the face of cartilage that is weakened (Figure 20-10). In these cases, the surgeon is advised to sculpt the cartilage–scar tissue block into the gross shape of a normal tip. A semblance of tip refinement can then be achieved by camouflage of the scar tissue block with a tip graft.

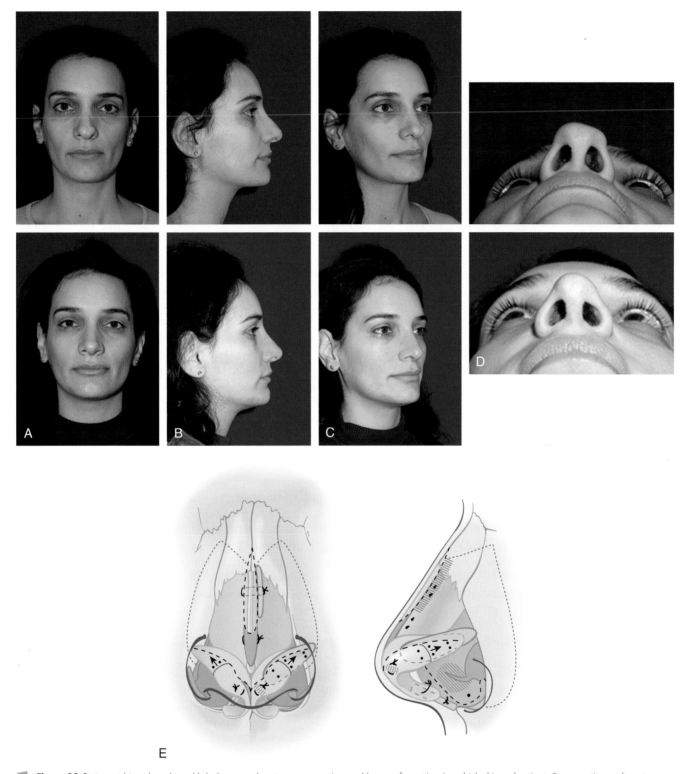

Figure 20-9 A postrhinoplasty broad lobule secondary to overresection and bossae formation in a thick-skinned patient. Preoperative and postoperative (**A**) frontal, (**B**) lateral, (**C**) oblique, and (**D**) basal views. Schematic (**E**) showing tip correction with a left underlay alar strut graft, columellar strut, bilateral lateral crural overlay, single-dome unit sutures, and soft tissue thinning.

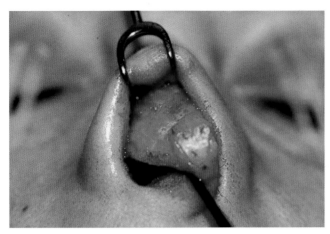

Figure 20-10 Dissection of a heavily scarred tip.

Occasionally, excessive scar in the scroll region may also need to be cautiously excised to achieve greater narrowing of the lateral supratip regions. It goes without saying that functional needs should not be undercut in the pursuit of aesthetic enhancement in these scenarios. It is especially important in the revision patient with thick, scarred, and inelastic skin to understand the need for augmentation and projection to achieve any measure of lobule refinement. In thin-skinned patients, scar contraction following aggressive cephalic lower lateral cartilage resection can lead to the triad deformity of thin skin, knuckling, and intercrural bifidity.

THE BICONVEX LOBULE

A biconvex lobule is the term applied to a persistent deformity in which the domal arch contour exhibits an exaggerated natural convexity in both the longitudinal and horizontal axes (Figure 20-11). This finding disposes the M-arch to an abrupt "drop-off" lateral to the natural highlight at the dome region.[28] Externally, this can manifest in the appearance of a deep and anteriorly displaced alar groove. This deformity has been identified by some as resulting from cephalically malpositioned lateral crura.[29] The authors are of the opinion that a distorted, bowl-shaped lateral crural contour more readily accounts for this observation. Reversal of this concavity may be favorably obtained by use of alar grafts or arch division techniques. When rotation and deprojection are also desired, a lateral crural overlay technique can be very effective in achieving all of these objectives with one maneuver. In some cases, vertical lobule division will decrease the length of the domal arch and achieve the desired refinement. When the lateral crura are of adequate form and projection, alar strut grafts may be placed in an underlay fashion to increase crural support and straightening without affecting contour. In the setting of severely attenuated or asymmetric crura, larger alar batten grafts

may be placed in an overlay fashion to simultaneously enhance both form and function.

THE ASYMMETRIC LOBULE

An asymmetric postrhinoplasty lobular deformity usually results from unrecognized buckling of the domal arch secondary to trauma, unequal lower lateral cartilage excision, or scar contracture forces acting on the medial or lateral crura that cause the tip to twist.[30] The surgical maneuvers that contribute to bossae formation and tip asymmetry are those that fail to produce or secure symmetric domal cartilages, those that promote separation of the domes, and those that excessively thin the horizontal width of the lateral crura by aggressive cephalic margin resection.[31] To avoid the sequelae of tip bossae or asymmetry, a surgeon must always reconstitute the domes symmetrically, reinforce weak cartilage, and avoid excessive cartilage excisions.

As a general rule, the simplest and fewest possible techniques should be applied to achieve the desired outcome (Figure 20-12). In the asymmetric lobule, it may be possible to achieve normal symmetry by application of asymmetric suture techniques such as unilateral or asymmetric single-dome unit sutures. Once adequate symmetry has been obtained, the authors prefer to set the tip complex with a double-dome unit suture and an intercrural horizontal mattress suture within the intermediate crus. This suture is a very powerful way to simultaneously achieve appropriate intercrural height, angulation, symmetry, and support. Alternatively, when lobular contour is asymmetric owing to attenuated or distorted arch segments, vertical division within the domal arch segment may be used to simultaneously correct arch length and asymmetry in addition to irregularities of the lobular–columellar relationship such as a hanging infratip. Unilateral or asymmetric cartilaginous arch divisions or combinations of various maneuvers may be exploited in a graduated fashion and customized to each patient's particular anatomy. An elongated columellar strut extending upward between the intermediate crura can sometimes add the required support and enhance symmetry. Finally, grafts may be used to conceal any remaining asymmetries that prove too problematic to correct by other means.

SUMMARY

Increasing acceptance and utilization of the open rhinoplasty approach have provided for far greater diagnostic and therapeutic exactitude in the management of post-rhinoplasty lobule deformities. While the techniques depicted here are powerful and dependable, the experienced surgeon should not feel confined by this armamentarium. The authors frequently find themselves exploring novel variations in technique to uniquely tailor the

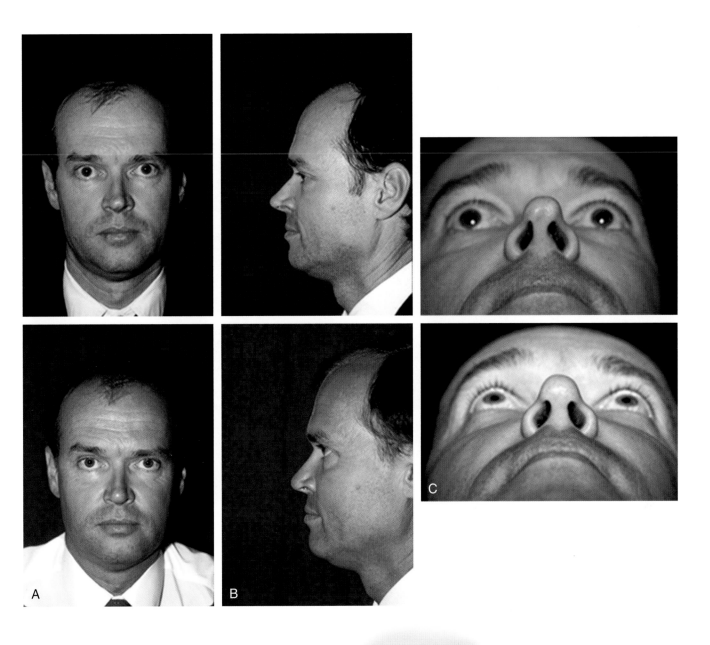

Figure 20-11 Treatment of a persistent primary biconvex lobule. Preoperative and postoperative (**A**) frontal, (**B**) lateral, and (**C**) basal views. Schematic (**D**) showing tip correction with bilateral onlay lateral crural grafts, a columellar strut, bilateral vertical lobule division, and division of the medial crural footplates.

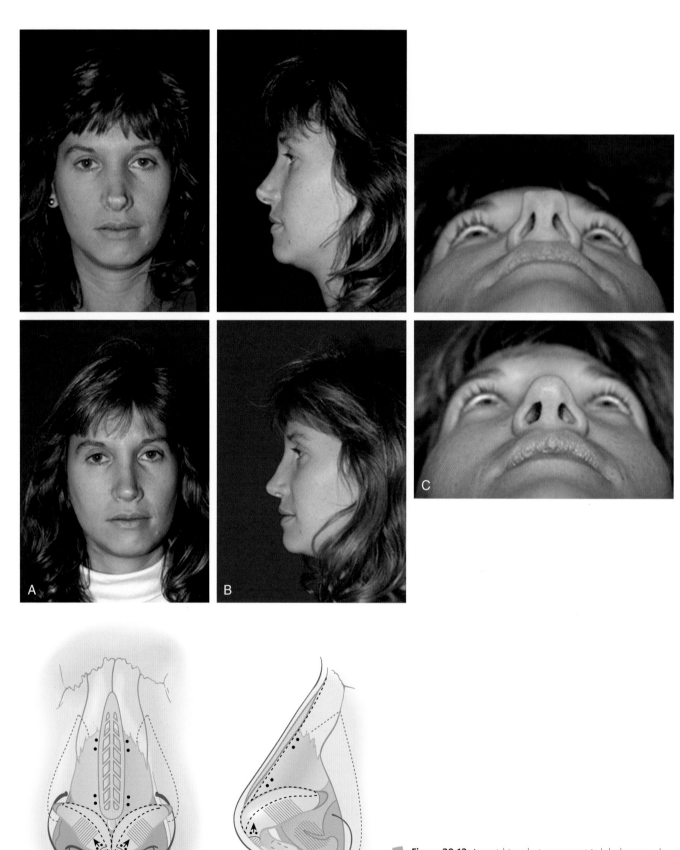

Figure 20-12 A postrhinoplasty asymmetric lobule secondary to overresection and bossae formation. Preoperative and postoperative (**A**) frontal, (**B**) lateral, and (**C**) basal views. Schematic (**D**) showing tip correction with a columellar strut, bilateral vertical lobule division, hinge setback, and lateral crural scoring to create inversion of convexity.

operation to the individual problems encountered. In this way, the revision tip rhinoplasty can accomplish meaningful improvements in structural and functional support in addition to harmonious restoration of lobular contour, definition, and refinement.

REFERENCES

1. McCullough EG, English JL. A new twist in nasal tip surgery: An alternative to the Goldman tip for the wide or bulbous lobule. *Arch Otolaryngol.* 1985;111(8):524–529.
2. Daniel RK. Rhinoplasty: Creating an aesthetic tip. A preliminary report. *Plast Reconstr Surg.* 1987;80:775–783.
3. Johnson CM, Toriumi DM. *Open structure rhinoplasty.* Philadelphia: WB Saunders; 1990.
4. Tardy ME, Cheng E. Transdomal suture refinement of the nasal tip. *Fac Plast Surg.* 1987;4:317–326.
5. Kridel RWH, Konior RJ, Shumrick KA, et al. Advances in nasal tip surgery: The lateral crural steal. *Arch Otolaryngol.* 1989;115:1206–1212.
6. Tebbetts JB. Shaping and positioning the nasal tip without structural disruption: A new, systematic approach. *Plast Reconstr Surg.* 1994;94:61–77.
7. Kamer FN, McQuown SA. Revision rhinoplasty: Analysis and treatment. *Arch Otolaryngol Head Neck Surg.* 1988;114:257.
8. Parkes ML, Kanodia R, Machida BK. Revision rhinoplasty: An analysis of aesthetic deformities. *Arch Otolaryngol Head Neck Surg.* 1992;118(7):695–701.
9. Perkins SW. The evolution of the combined use of endonasal and external columellar approaches to rhinoplasty. *Facial Plast Surg Clin North Am.* 2004;12(1):35–50.
10. Adamson PA. The failed rhinoplasty. In: Gates GA, ed. *Current therapy in otolaryngology–head and neck surgery.* 4th ed. Toronto, Ontario: BC Decker; 1990:137–144.
11. Adamson PA, Galli SK. Rhinoplasty approaches: current state of the art. *Arch Fac Plast Surg.* 2005;7(1):32–37.
12. Foda HM. Rhinoplasty for the multiply revised nose. *Am J Otolaryngol.* 2005;26(1):28–34.
13. Vuyk HD, Watts SJ, Vindayak B. Revision rhinoplasty: Review of deformities, aetiology, and treatment strategies. *Clin Otolaryngol.* 2000;25:476–481.
14. O'Connor GB, McGregor MW. Secondary rhinoplasties: Their cause and prevention. *Plast Reconstr Surg.* 1955;26: 404–410.
15. Nicoll FV. Secondary rhinoplasty of the nasal tip and columella. *Scand J Plast Reconstr Surg.* 1986;20:67–73.
16. Anderson JR. New approach to rhinoplasty. *Arch Otolaryngol.* 1971;93:284–291.
17. Adamson PA, Litner JA, Dahiya R. The M-arch model: A new concept of nasal tip dynamics. *Arch Fac Plast Surg.* 2006: 16–25.
18. Adamson PA, Litner JA. Applications of the M-arch model in nasal tip refinement. *Fac Plast Surg.* 2006;22(1):42–48.
19. Bagal AA, Adamson PA. Revision rhinoplasty. *Fac Plast Surg.* 2002;18(4):233–244.
20. Perkins SW, Tardy ME. External columellar incisional approach to revision of the lower third of the nose. *Fac Plast Surg Clin North Am.* 1993;1:79–98.
21. Goin JM, Goin MK. *Changing the body: Psychological effects of plastic surgery.* Baltimore, MD: Williams & Wilkins; 1981
22. Adamson PA, Strecker HD. Patient selection. *Aesthet Plast Surg.* 2002;26(Suppl 1):11.
23. Adamson PA, Kraus WM. Management of patient dissatisfaction with cosmetic surgery. *Fac Plast Surg.* 1995; 11(2):99–104.
24. Adamson PA. Nasal tip surgery in open rhinoplasty. *Fac Plast Surg Clin North Am.* 1993;1:39–52.
25. Sheen JH. Tip graft: a 20-year retrospective. *Plast Reconstr Surg.* 1993;91(1):48–63.
26. Peck GC. The onlay graft for nasal tip projection. *Plast Reconstr Surg.* 1983;71(1):27–39.
27. Goldman IB. The importance of medial crura in nasal tip reconstruction. *Arch Otolaryngol.* 1957; 65:143.
28. Toriumi DM. New concepts in nasal tip contouring. *Arch Fac Plast Surg.* 2006;8(3):156–185.
29. Constantian MB. The boxy nasal tip, the ball tip, and alar cartilage malposition: variations on a theme: A study in 200 consecutive primary and secondary rhinoplasty patients. *Plast Reconstr Surg.* 2005;116(1):268–281.
30. Kridel RWH, Yoon PJ, Koch RJ. Prevention and correction of nasal tip bossae in rhinoplasty. *Arch Fac Plast Surg.* 2003;5: 416–422.
31. Kridel RWH, Soliemanzadeh P. Tip grafts in revision rhinoplasty. *Fac Plast Surg Clin N Am.* 2006;14:331–341.

CHAPTER TWENTY-ONE

The Management of Alar–Columellar Disproportion

Russell W. H. Kridel • Robert J. Chiu • Anand D. Patel

Often unappreciated in rhinoplasty is the alar–columellar complex. Patients may present with a preexisting hanging or retracted columella or abnormal alar rim or columellar shape and configuration. In the patient with a preoperative normal relationship, certain surgical maneuvers, made to affect other desired changes elsewhere in the nose, may leave the patient with an unattractive alar–columellar complex after surgery. Alterations that are made to the lower third of the nose must take into account the relationship between the nostril border and ala to the columella. A seemingly attractive nose may be aesthetically displeasing if the alar–columellar relationship is not refined and proportional. Compared to other aspects of rhinoplasty, relatively little attention is devoted to the proper diagnosis and treatment of alar–columellar disproportion. To address this, it is paramount to discern the etiology of the alar–columellar disproportion, which requires a full understanding of the relevant nasal anatomy and commonly used rhinoplasty techniques that can alter it.

THE IDEAL ALAR–COLUMELLAR RELATIONSHIP AND THE AGING NOSE

Normal columellar show is classically defined as between 2 and 4 mm of visible columella below the alar margin on profile view[1] (Figure 21-1). However, this definition fails to differentiate between relative positions of the ala and the columella. Tardy qualitatively described the ideal appearance of the ala and columella on frontal view as a gentle "gull-in-flight" configuration where the columella represents the body of the gull and the alar margin represents the wings of the gull.[2] On profile view, the alar margin resembles a gentle S-shaped configuration. Gunter quantified the alar–columellar relationship by drawing horizontal lines through the tip-defining point, the alar rim, and the columellar–alar–facial junction.[3] This divided alar–columellar disproportion into six categories, depending on if whether the position of the ala or columella (or both) were contributing to the problem. Perhaps an all-encompassing method of analysis is to consider all the factors that contribute to a pleasing alar–columellar

relationship: width of columellar show, long axis of the nostril, shape of the nostril, shape of the alar margin, presence of a double break in the columella, length of the upper lip, columella-to-lip ratio, columella-labial angle, and the configuration of the lateral crus. With respect to the nostril shape, an oval shape is desirable.

The anatomic components (Figure 21-2) that determine the position and shape of the columella include the cartilaginous caudal septum, membranous septum, and intermediate and medial crus of the lower lateral cartilages. Their contributions may vary. Typically, the caudal-cephalic dimension of the medial crus is 4 mm,[4] which we refer to as the medial crural width. The position and shape of the ala are established by the width and orientation of the lateral crus of the lower lateral cartilages and the insertion and resilience of the fibroadipose component of the nasal ala.

Aging has a significant effect on these structures. Weakening of fibroelastic attachments in the scroll region as well as suspensory ligaments between the medial crura lead to tip ptosis, divergence of the medial crural footplates, and subsequent lengthening of the membranous septum. Also, with aging there is bone recession in the premaxillary region. In sum, these changes give the appearance of narrowing of the nasolabial angle and shortening of the columella, with a hanging columella anteriorly and a retraction posteriorly.[5–7]

Alteration of the tip rotation and projection in this case, in concert with adjunctive procedures, may itself correct the hanging columella defect. Numerous methods have been developed that define the ideal proportions and angles of the nose and nasal tip projection.[1,8–12] An approach to create an ideal alar–columellar relationship can only be undertaken after the desired tip projection and rotation are set.

THE HANGING COLUMELLA DEFORMITY

The hanging columella deformity is a common cause of alar–columellar disproportion. A retracted ala or alar notching can give the appearance of a hanging columella and must be differentiated, because the etiology and surgical repair are different. The anatomic configurations that make up the hanging columella deformity include overdevelopment of the caudal septal cartilage, which pushes down the medial crura, and/or the redundant membranous septum (Figure 21-3). Additionally, the medial and intermediate crura can be too wide,

excessively curved and convex, or vertically inclined. The long medial crus, with an excessive C-shaped curvature, has been cited as a prominent cause of the hanging columella deformity.[13] Adamson cited a broad vestibular vault and ptosis of the medial crura as additional causes.[14] In the senior author's experience, a large nasal spine is rarely the etiology because it is usually the septum that projects more forward and caudally than ever does the spine.

A hanging columella can result from previous rhinoplasty. Loss of tip projection and rotation causes loss of tip support and relative redundancy of the columella with apparent columellar show. Forward or caudal placement of a columellar strut or caudal septal extension graft can be the culprit. Suturing together previously bifid and lateralized medial crura can make the columella more caudally prominent. A tip graft that is too thick or a plumping graft that is too large can create the same problem.

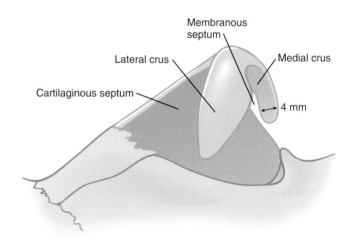

Figure 21-2 The anatomic components that help determine the position and shape of the columella. (© 2009 Russell W. H. Kridel, MD; used with permission.)

Figure 21-1 Normal columellar show is defined as 2 to 4 mm.

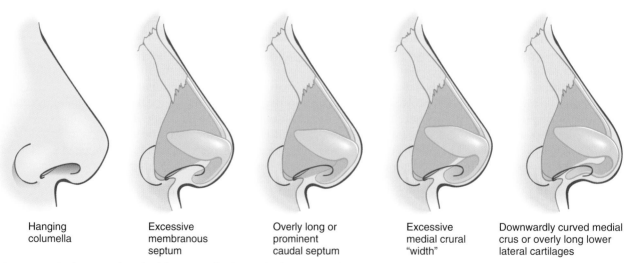

| Hanging columella | Excessive membranous septum | Overly long or prominent caudal septum | Excessive medial crural "width" | Downwardly curved medial crus or overly long lower lateral cartilages |

Figure 21-3 The hanging columella deformity can be the result of excess membranous septum, prominent caudal septum, excessively wide medial and intermediate crus, downwardly curved medial crus, or overly long lower lateral cartilages (LLCs). (From Kridel RWH, Chiu RJ. Alar columellar disproportion. Facial Plastic Surgery Clinics November 2006; used with permission.)

Treatment of the hanging columella deformity is based on the underlying etiology. Previous descriptions of surgical repairs have been separated into indirect and direct.[13,15] The direct repairs involve resection of the caudal margin of the medial crura, whereas the indirect repairs involve trimming the caudal septum or the membranous septum. In the senior author's experience, the tongue-in-groove (TIG) technique is very effective in correcting the hanging columella deformity in many cases, including defects caused by long, convex medial and intermediate crura, vertical inclination of the intermediate crura, or overdevelopment of the caudal quadrangular cartilage.[16] The TIG technique does not burn any bridges. In brief, mucoperichondrial flaps are developed on both sides of the caudal septum, a pocket is developed between the medial crura, and the caudal septum is positioned into the developed pocket. After assessment of the appropriate relationship, excess membranous septum is trimmed bilaterally on the septal (cephalic) side of the incision, allowing for the greatest excision in the area where the columella hangs the most. After closure of the transfixion incision, septocolumellar sutures are used to add strength or to affect change in the tip height. In select cases where the hanging columella defect still exists after the TIG procedure due to an overdeveloped caudal quadrangular cartilage, conservative excision of the caudal end of the cartilaginous septum is carried out. In contrast to some authors who have found a frequent need to reduce the maxillary spine,[17,18] the senior author rarely finds the need to trim the nasal spine to correct the hanging columella defect. Occasionally, the medial crura may be too caudally projecting, and conservative trimming of the caudal edge of the medial crura is performed and the medial crura are sutured together. In the treatment of excessively curved and long medial crura, division of the alar cartilages at the angle of the medial and lateral crura has been advocated with placement of a columellar strut to restore strength and tip support.[13,19] When the lower lateral cartilages are too long and are overdeveloped, a lateral crural overlay (LCO) can be used to shorten the lateral crura and rotate the tip, in concert with a TIG procedure to correct the hanging columella deformity by setting the medial crura back over the septum.[20] Last, in revision cases where previous graft placement is the causative factor for the hanging columella defect, the offending graft, whether it is a tip graft, columellar strut, or caudal septal extension graft, is removed, replaced, or trimmed.

TREATMENT ALGORITHM FOR THE HANGING COLUMELLA

Algorithms in rhinoplasty can only be guidelines since patients and noses are different and each treatment must be individualized. However, algorithms can help organize an approach to the problem. An algorithm has been developed to manage the hanging columella deformity in a systematic approach (Figure 21-4).[21] Once alar–columellar disproportion has been identified, the presence of a hanging columella is assessed. If a hanging columella is not present, the surgeon is directed to the diagnosis and treatment of alar retraction or notching with grafting. The next step is the palpation of the caudal septum at the columella to determine any contribution to the problem. At this point, the treatment algorithm diverges. If the caudal septum is normal, the surgical procedure to correct the hanging columella defect begins by performing a TIG procedure. Most cases of hanging columella with a normal caudal septum position will be resolved by a TIG procedure with trimming of the membranous septum. Conversely, if there is significant caudal septal excess, the caudal septum is trimmed first, followed by a TIG procedure. After reevaluation for persistent hanging columella, further conservative trim of the caudal septum may be performed, making sure to preserve an adequate caudal septal strut when septoplasty is also performed. If the hanging columella deformity persists, a TIG procedure involving medial crural setback on the caudal septum is considered and performed. Consideration is also given to the occasional presence of a prominent maxillary spine, with attendant reduction. We then proceed with external rhinoplasty to identify additional causes for any residual persistent hanging columella. Any cartilage grafts previously placed that are contributing to a hanging columella, including a columellar strut graft, tip graft, caudal septal replacement graft, caudal septal extension graft, or columellar batten grafts, are removed. If a hanging columella is still present, trimming of the caudal medial crura is performed, and consideration is given to a medial crural overlay (MCO) technique[22] in cases of long intermediate or convex intermediate crura, or an LCO technique in cases of excessively long lower lateral cartilages.

THE RETRACTED ALA

A retracted ala is usually encountered after previous rhinoplasty, but it can be secondary to a previously unrecognized disproportion. Familial variants contributing to a retracted ala include a highly arched alar lobule margin with high insertion into the cheek laterally or a plunging nasal tip with high-arched ala.[2] Vertically oriented lower lateral cartilages may significantly contribute to bilateral retracted alae.

More often, the retracted ala is due to aggressive excisional surgery or as a result of normal scar contracture from prior surgery. The cephalic trim of the lower lateral cartilage is a commonly used technique in rhinoplasty to refine and narrow the tip and to cause rotation of the tip via scar contracture at the scroll area. The degree of scar contracture is difficult to predict, and varying amounts of cephalic trim of the lateral crus can cause the alar margin

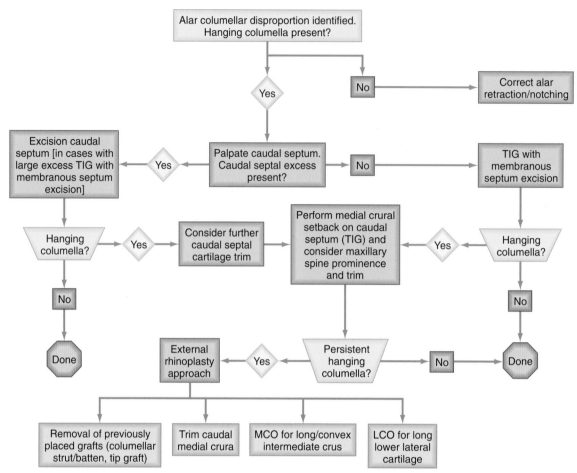

Figure 21-4 Treatment algorithm for managing the hanging columella deformity. (From Kridel RWH, Chiu RJ. Alar columellar disproportion. Facial Plastic Surgery Clinics November 2006; used with permission.)

to retract and result in alar–columellar disproportion. Other excisional techniques that can predispose to this condition include excision of the lateral-cephalic portion of lateral crura and vertical interruption of the lower lateral cartilages. Often specific to the closed rhinoplasty approach and causing a more difficult situation is the possibility that the vestibular skin under the lower or upper lateral cartilages was inadvertently trimmed via an intercartilaginous, intracartilaginous, or transcartilaginous incision, which, coupled with a cephalic trim, can predispose to alar retraction. Additionally, a tightened lateral crural spanning suture may be yet another iatrogenic cause for alar retraction, which can be relieved with removal and repositioning.[23] And, in the open technique, a tightened closure of the marginal incision may also predispose to such retraction.

In treating the retracted or notched ala, management depends first on the identification of any tissue deficiency. In cases of mild retraction with no tissue deficiency, the lateral crus can be detached after wide undermining of the scroll area, followed by repositioning of the lateral crus more inferiorly. A vertically oriented lower lateral

cartilage can be repositioned inferiorly in this manner. If tip rotation is needed as well, the Boccieri modification of the Kridel LCO technique is an excellent way to address this problem.[24] In the senior author's experience, double-dome sutures can solidify the position of the lower lateral cartilages and counteract the tendency for retraction, especially when the domes are brought together with a caudal rotation of the lower lateral cartilages. Retraction with high insertion of the lateral crus can also be treated with alar base resection and repositioning.[25] Alar rim grafts can be used to treat mild to moderately retracted alae or as a preventive measure to counteract floppy alae or potential future scar contracture with later retraction. Alar rim grafts can be placed through a closed or open technique via a precise pocket created in the alar rim (Figure 21-5). A properly sized graft is fashioned to fit the exact pocket, and the medial aspect is sewn to the alar rim soft tissue so as to prevent migration of the alar rim graft. If an alar base excision is to be carried out additionally, the rim graft may be inserted through that incision from lateral to medial. Alternatively, an alar batten onlay graft with an extension in the alar rim can be used

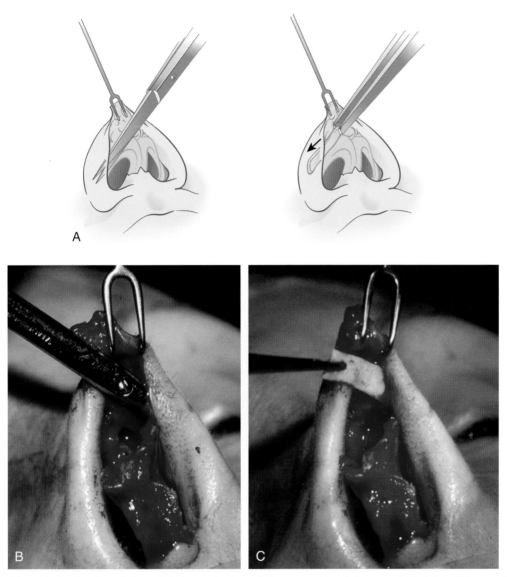

Figure 21-5 A, Schematic showing the technique of placing an alar rim graft via an open rhinoplasty approach. **B, C,** Actual intraoperative views showing the technique of placing an alar rim graft via an open rhinoplasty approach. (From Kridel RWH, Chiu RJ. Alar columellar disproportion. Facial Plastic Surgery Clinics November 2006; used with permission.)

effectively to treat a retracted ala. For the nose with a pinched nasal tip, an alar spreader graft can effectively treat the tip as well as the alar retraction.[26]

In many revision cases, however, retraction is accompanied by scar contracture and lack of mobile tissue to reposition the ala more caudally. In these cases, extra tissue must be obtained to "push" the alar rim inferiorly. The mainstay for management is the composite auricular skin–cartilage graft. The auricular skin and cartilage are harvested as a composite graft from an anterior approach, using a well-camouflaged incision (Figure 21-6). The composite auricular graft may be placed along the cephalic edge of the lateral crura, or scroll area, and can be sutured into the intercartilaginous incision through an endonasal approach (Figure 21-7). Alternatively, in the open technique, it may be sutured directly to the caudal edge of the lower lateral cartilage on the vestibular side (Figure 21-8). These composite grafts have a high take rate and are often necessary to correct a severely retracted or notched ala. One needs to allow for shrinkage of the grafts, but sometimes it is later necessary months down the line to intranasally trim any remaining bulk; however, it is preferable to overcorrect initially than to remain shy of the necessary correction. Alternatively, Guyuron has described using an internal lining V-Y advancement to lower the alar rim, in combination with structural cartilage reconstruction for any missing lateral crus.[27] For very severe alar retraction, reconstruction using a cutaneous alar rotation flap and autogenous cartilage batten grafts was described.[28]

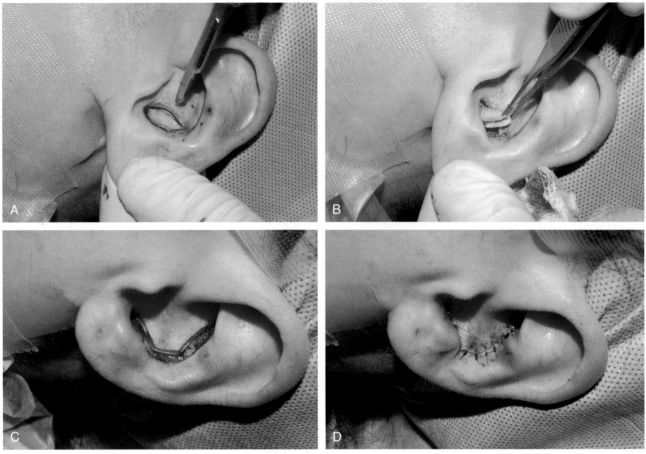

Figure 21-6 A, Harvest of free auricular composite grafts from both the concha cymba and concha cava. **B,** Conchal cartilage is taken with anterior conchal skin. **C,** The harvest leaves a symmetric defect. **D,** Closure is possible without auricular deformity. (© 2009 Russell W. H. Kridel, MD; used with permission.)

THE HANGING COLUMELLA COMBINED WITH A RETRACTED ALA

Often in revision rhinoplasty, the surgeon encounters concurrently the presence of a hanging columella defect with a retracted ala. In these cases, it is essential to arrive at the correct diagnosis and assess the relative contributions of each deformity. Only then can the correct techniques be selected to achieve an aesthetically pleasing alar–columellar relationship. Once again, attention is given to the shape of the nostril, the tip rotation, the presence of alar notching, the strength and volume of the lower lateral cartilages, the shape of the alar margin, the size of the quadrangular cartilage, and the relationship of the tip and columella to the upper lip. Excessive nostril show with a ptotic tip, rounding of the caudal nostril margin, short upper lip, long lateral crus, and relatively strong lateral crus with no apparent notching are all suggestive of a hanging columella etiology. Conversely, the presence of alar notching, weak lateral crura, retraction of the alar margin, and

excessive curve to the alar rim margin are suggestive of alar retraction as the etiology for excessive columellar show. In revision rhinoplasty, significant contributions from both the hanging columella defect and alar retraction commonly result in very significant amounts of columellar show. Failure to address the hanging columella in the original surgery, coupled with overly aggressive excisional techniques of the lateral crus, can result in this predicament. In these cases, the hanging columella defect is usually addressed first using the TIG technique, trimming of the membranous septum, and possible trimming of the caudal cartilaginous septum. After addressing the hanging columella, the surgeon can better assess the severity of the alar retraction and the amount of correction needed to achieve a columellar show less than 3 mm. The mainstay of treating severe retraction is the composite auricular cartilage graft, but in some cases, alar rim grafts can also be effective. Using a full armamentarium of techniques available to address the hanging columella and alar retraction, one can achieve an aesthetically pleasing columellar relationship, even in cases of severe alar–columellar disproportion (see Case Examples 5 and 6).

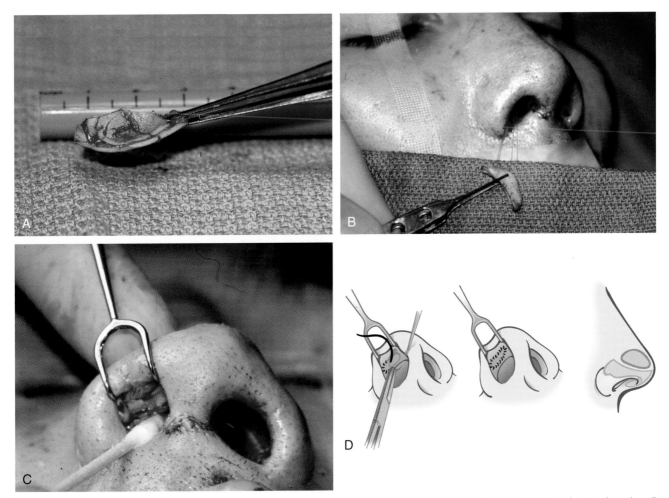

Figure 21-7 A composite cartilage graft can be placed in the scroll area to "push" the alar rim inferiorly. (From Kridel RWH, Chiu RJ. Alar columellar disproportion. Facial Plastic Surgery Clinics November 2006; used with permission.)

THE HANGING ALA

The hanging ala, or alar hooding, is a relatively more uncommon diagnosis and can represent a normal anatomic variant previously unrecognized. A prominent ala, including excessive alar flare, can contribute to a hanging ala. In correcting alar flare, improper insetting of the ala after alar wedge resection can cause a hanging ala deformity. Other causes of the hanging ala include improperly placed grafts along the alar rim. Simple repositioning of the ala with a deep stitch via a lateral alar-facial incision, as one might make for alar wedge reduction, may often solve the problem. The hanging ala also can be corrected by directly removing an ellipse of the alar rim or extra alar lining and underlying subcutaneous tissue.[3,29] Alternatively, techniques that promote alar retraction, including cephalic trim, can in this case help correct a hanging ala.

THE RETRACTED COLUMELLA

A retracted columella, in comparison, is commonly seen in primary or secondary rhinoplasty or posttraumatically. Etiologies unrelated to previous nasal surgery include normal anatomic variation and congenital causes. Patients with cleft lip and palate deformity can present with columellar retraction, secondary to an underdeveloped premaxilla. In addition, numerous processes that erode the cartilaginous septum or cause septal perforation may cause a columella to be retracted. A variety of rhinoplasty techniques can induce the columella to retract. Excessive resection of the caudal septum or medial crura causes columellar retraction, especially in the long term. Excessive resection of membranous septum, without cartilage manipulation, can result in the same predicament. The TIG maneuver is an effective technique to reposition a hanging columella.[16] However, excessive setback of the

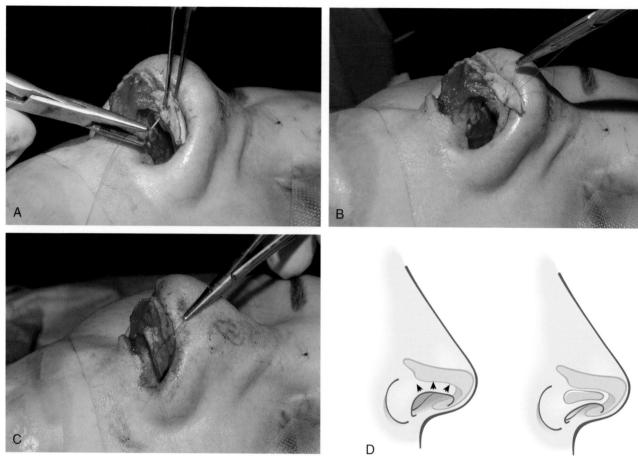

Figure 21-8 A composite auricular cartilage graft is placed on the caudal edge of the lower lateral cartilage to treat the retracted/notched ala.

medial crus on the caudal septum can cause columellar retraction. Failure to stabilize the medial crural relationship to the caudal septum can lead to columellar retraction onto the caudal septum.

Treatment of the retracted columella in revision rhinoplasty also depends on identifying the causative factor for the defect. In cases where the diagnosis of retracted columella was missed in the initial surgery and where it represents a natural anatomic variant, one can place a columellar batten graft or place a cartilage or crushed cartilage onlay in the columella. Where additional strength of tip support is also desired, an extended tip graft with a caudal component can be used to correct the retracted columella. Alternatively, a columellar strut can be fashioned to extend caudally beyond the caudal border of the medial crura (Figure 21-9). The columellar strut should be fashioned so that the most caudal extent of the strut is positioned in the area of greatest retraction. In cases where the caudal septum is weak or missing, a septal extension graft or a caudal septal replacement graft[30] can help improve tip support and correct the retracted columella (Figure 21-10). A plumping graft will specifically augment retraction near the columellar-lip angle (see Case Example 3). If the etiology is an improperly positioned medial crura

onto the caudal septum, the surgeon needs to reposition the medial crura through bilateral elevation of septal mucoperichondrial flaps to free up the membranous septum and then use suture techniques to recreate the fibrous attachments between the medial crura and the septum. Finally, cases of columellar retraction secondary to a large septal perforation repair may require cartilage augmentation of the columella.

PREVENTION OF IATROGENIC ALAR–COLUMELLAR DISPROPORTION

A thorough understanding of the ideal alar–columellar relationship and the surgical maneuvers that can modify it is of paramount importance in the prevention of iatrogenic alterations. Clearly, overly aggressive resections should be avoided, but even then, alar–columellar disproportions may result from normal scar contracture, as well as from the vagaries of wound healing that are beyond the control of a properly executed rhinoplasty. This is particularly true in revision cases.

Prevention of columellar show relies on the careful use of grafts used in the nasal tip or columella or for septal

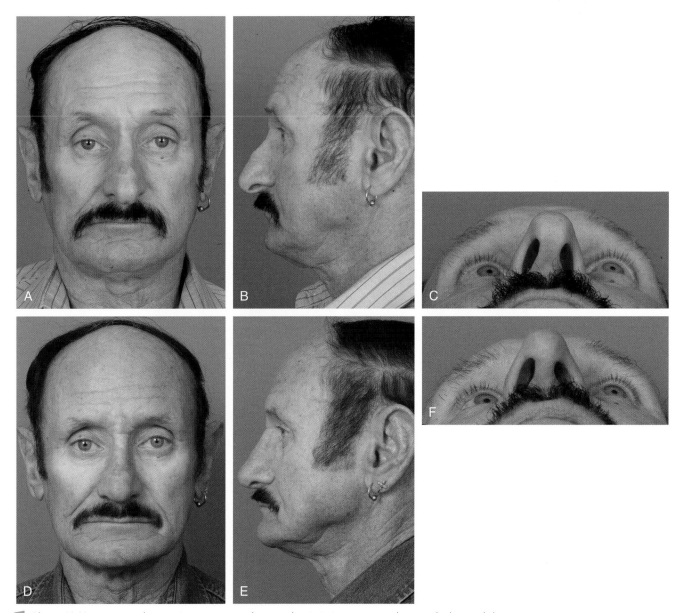

Figure 21-11 Case example 1. **A–C,** Preoperative photographs. **D–F,** Postoperative photographs (8 months).

curved, which produced a hanging columella anteriorly. The MCO and a localized resection of membranous septum helped to address this problem. A columellar strut was placed to maintain support to this region. A premaxillary cartilage graft was placed to address the posterior columellar retraction.

CASE EXAMPLE 4

A 37-year-old woman presents with a history of unsatisfactory primary rhinoplasty 18 years earlier, as well as subsequent nasal trauma in an automobile accident. She desires improved nasal breathing, a shorter nasal tip, and smaller nose overall with less show of her nostrils. The patient also had concerns about having a protrusive chin.

On examination, the patient has a deviated nasal septum; irregular dorsal hump; underrotated, overprojected tip with asymmetries; hanging columella with wide medial crura; and alar retraction (Figure 21-14).

Plan

· Septoplasty
· Dorsal reduction
· Trim membranous septum and medial crura with TIG
· Dome sutures
· Alar rim grafts

Here, mild hanging of the columella coupled with alar retraction is causing significant columellar show. The cause for the hanging columella, in this case, is not excess caudal septum. A slight trim of the wide medial crura and

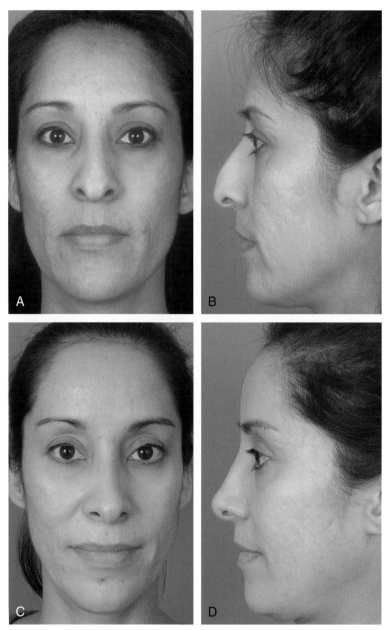

Figure 21-12 Case example 2. **A, B,** Preoperative photographs. **C, D,** Postoperative photographs (2 years).

membranous septum and the placement of alar rim grafts are relatively conservative maneuvers that additively create a substantial effect on columellar show. The patient also underwent placement of a chin implant.

CASE EXAMPLE 5

A 38-year-old woman who previously underwent rhinoplasty 22 years earlier, and had a satisfactory result, has noticed increasing droop and asymmetry of her nasal tip with more show of her nostrils over the past decade. On examination, she has a ptotic, overprojected tip; hanging

columella, composed of cartilaginous and membranous septum; and severe alar retraction (Figure 21-15).

Plan
- Dome truncation and binding sutures
- Trim of membranous and cartilaginous septum with TIG technique
- Alar batten grafts

This patient's severe alar retraction was likely a result of overly aggressive cephalic trim of the lower lateral cartilages. Here, alar rim grafts would not be sufficient, and instead, alar batten grafts were secured to the lateral crus

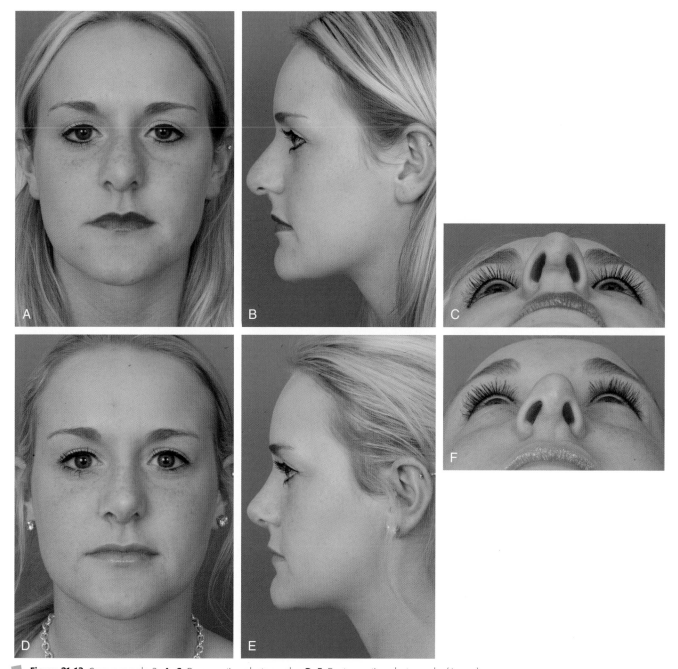

Figure 21-13 Case example 3. **A–C,** Preoperative photographs. **D–F,** Postoperative photographs (1 year).

remnants. The hanging columella required a conservative excision of caudal septal cartilage and membrane with a TIG maneuver.

CASE EXAMPLE 6

A 28-year-old woman presents with a history of nasal trauma during childhood and primary septorhinoplasty 4 years earlier, with resection of nearly all the cartilaginous septum, dorsal reduction, and some tip work through an external approach using rim incisions. She is concerned with a "scooped-out" appearance to her nasal dorsum, her unrefined nasal tip, and increased nostril show. On examination, we find an overresected nasal dorsum; boxy tip; hanging columella; and alar retraction. The patient has very little residual septal cartilage (Figure 21-16).

Plan

- Dorsal augmentation with irradiated rib cartilage
- Trim of membranous and cartilaginous septum with TIG technique

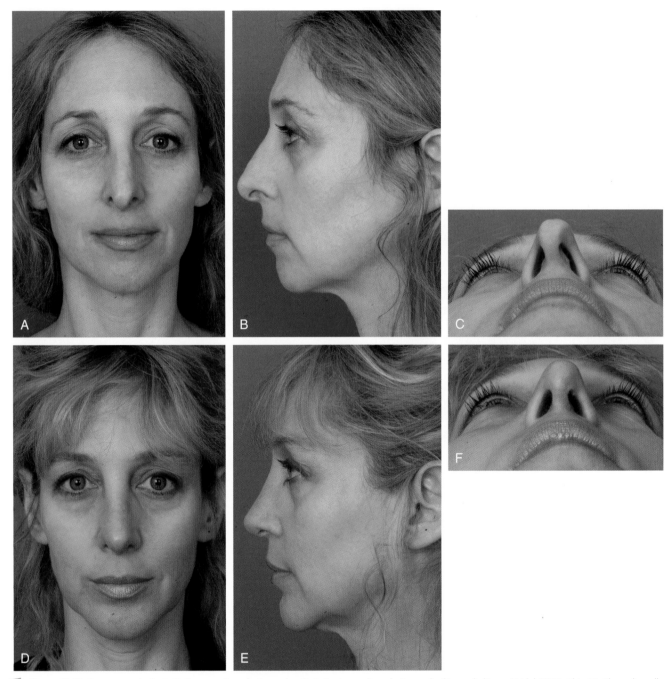

Figure 21-14 Case example 4. **A–C,** Preoperative photographs. **D–F,** Postoperative photographs (1 year). (From Kridel RWH, Chiu RJ. Alar columellar disproportion. Facial Plastic Surgery Clinics November 2006; used with permission.)

- Dome binding sutures
- Alar grafting with composite auricular tissue

Here the rotation and projection of the tip do not need to be altered much, and so will not affect the alar–columellar relationship. The hanging columella was addressed with a conservative trim of caudal cartilaginous and membranous septum. Overresection of cephalic lower lateral cartilages coupled with alar rim incisions likely contributed to this patient's alar retraction. New tissue needed to be

recruited to the area via an auricular composite graft, which was sutured to the caudal edge of the residual lower lateral cartilages.

CONCLUSION

The problem of alar–columellar disproportion in rhinoplasty presents a challenge to all surgeons. It is very important to proceed only after careful analysis of the

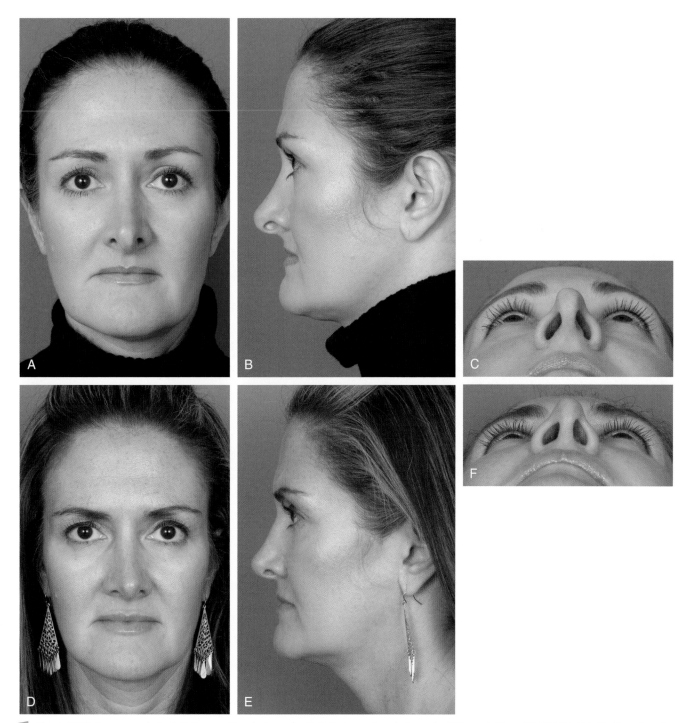

Figure 21-15 Case example 5. **A–C,** Preoperative photographs. **D–F,** Postoperative photographs (1½ years). (From Kridel RWH, Chiu RJ. Alar columellar disproportion. Facial Plastic Surgery Clinics November 2006; used with permission.)

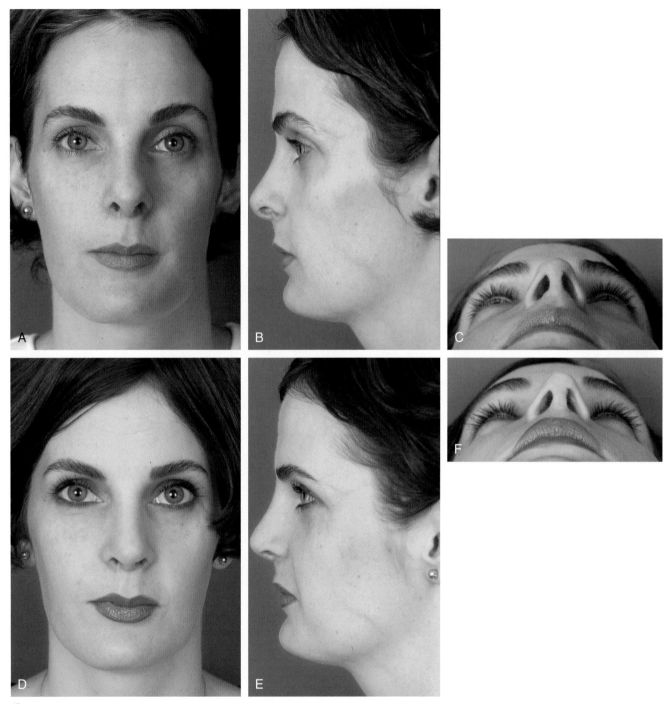

Figure 21-16 Case example 6. **A–C,** Preoperative photographs. **D–F,** Postoperative photographs (8 months).

defect and correct diagnosis of the problem. The surgeon then can choose among the myriad of approaches the particular techniques that will achieve the desired relationship between the alar margin and columella and create an aesthetically pleasing result. Keys to prevention are a heightened sensitivity to the maneuvers and mishaps that may lead to alar–columellar disproportion.

REFERENCES

1. Powell NP, Humphries B. *Proportions of the aesthetic face.* New York: Thieme-Stratton; 1984:8.
2. Tardy ME, Genack SH, Murrell GL. Aesthetic correction of alar columellar disproportion. *Fac Plast Surg Clin N Am.* 1995;3:395–406.

3. Gunter JP, Rohrich RJ, Friedman RM. Classification and correction of alar columellar discrepancies in rhinoplasty. *Plast Reconstr Surg.* 1996;97:643–648.

4. Bernstein L. Aesthetics in rhinoplasty. *Otolaryngol Clin North Am.* 1975;8:705–715.

5. Guyuron B. The aging nose. *Dermatol Clin.* 1997;15(4): 659–664.

6. Romo T 3rd, Soliemanzadeh P, Litner JA, Sclafani AP. Rhinoplasty in the aging nose. *Fac Plast Surg.* 2003;19(4): 309–315.

7. Stupak HD, Johnson CM Jr. Rhinoplasty for the aging nose. *Ear Nose Throat J.* 2006;85(3):154–155.

8. Crumley RL. Aesthetics and surgery of the nasal base. *Fac Plast Surg.* 1988;5:135–142.

9. Crumley RL, Lanser M. Quantitative analysis of nasal tip projection. *Laryngoscope.* 1988;98:202–208.

10. Simons RL. Nasal tip projection, ptosis, and supratip thickening. *ENT.* 1982;61:452–455.

11. Goode RL. Personal communication, 1983.

12. Kridel RWH, Konior RJ. Controlled nasal tip rotation via the lateral crural overlay technique. *Arch Otolaryngol Head Neck Surg.* 1991;117:411–415.

13. Joseph EM, Glasgold AI. Anatomical considerations in the management of the hanging columella. *Arch Fac Plast Surg.* 2000;2:173–177.

14. Adamson PA, Tropper GJ, McGraw BL. The hanging columella. *J Otolaryngol.* 1990;19:319–323.

15. Armstrong DP. Aggressive management of the hanging columella. *Plast Reconstr Surg.* 1980;65:513–516.

16. Kridel RWH, Scott BA, Foda HM. The tongue-in-groove technique in septorhinoplasty. *Arch Fac Plast Surg.* 1999;1: 246–256.

17. Davis RE. Diagnosis and surgical management of the caudal excess nasal deformity. *Arch Fac Plast Surg.* 2005;7:124–134.

18. Honrado CP, Pearlman SJ. Surgical treatment of the nasolabial angle in balanced rhinoplasty. *Arch Fac Plast Surg.* 2003;5:338–344.

19. Adamson PA. Commentary: Anatomical considerations in the management of the hanging columella. *Arch Fac Plast Surg.* 2000;2:178–179.

20. Kridel RWH, Konior RJ. The underprojected tip. In: Krause C, Mangat D, Pastorek N, eds. *Aesthetic facial surgery.* Philadelphia: Lippincott Williams & Wilkins; 1991:191–228.

21. Kridel RWH, Chiu RJ. Management of alar columellar disproportion. *Fac Plast Surg Clin North Am* 2006;4:313–329.

22. Soliemanzadeh P, Kridel RW. Nasal tip overprojection: Algorithm of surgical deprojection techniques and introduction of medial crural overlay. *Arch Fac Plast Surg.* 2005;7(6):374–380.

23. Baker SR. Suture contouring of the nasal tip. *Arch Fac Plast Surg.* 2000;2:34–42.

24. Boccieri A, Raimondi G. The lateral crural stairstep technique: A modification of the Kridel lateral crural overlay technique. *Arch Fac Plast Surg.* 2008;10(1):56–64.

25. Guyuron B. Alar base abnormalities. Classification and correction. *Clin Plast Surg.* 1996;2:263–270.

26. Gunter JP, Rohrich RJ. Correction of the pinched nasal tip with alar spreader grafts. *Plast Reconstr Surg.* 1992;90(5): 821–829.

27. Guyuron B. Alar rim deformities. *Plast Reconstr Surg.* 2001; 107:856–863.

28. Jung DH, Kwak ES, Kim HS. Correction of severe alar retraction with use of a cutaneous alar rotation flap. *Plast Reconstr Surg.* 2009;123(3):1088–1095.

29. Meyer R. Residual deformities of the ala. In: Secondary rhinoplasty. 2nd ed. Berlin: Springer-Verlag; 2002:295–318.

30. Kridel RWH, Lunde K. Nasal septal reconstruction, review and update. *Fac Plast Surg Clin North Am.* 1999;7:105–113.

31. Kridel RW, Konior RJ, Shumrick KA, Wright WK. Advances in nasal tip surgery. The lateral crural steal. *Arch Arch Otolaryngol Head Neck Surg.* 1989;115(10):1206–1212.

CHAPTER TWENTY-TWO

Evaluation and Correction of the Crooked Nose

Michael J. Brenner • Peter A. Hilger

GENERAL CONSIDERATIONS

The crooked nose is neither a single entity nor a specific description. Crooked noses represent a spectrum of nasal deformities, most commonly of traumatic origin, that are associated with a deviated or irregular appearance to the nose. For the casual onlooker, the crooked nose may be unsettling because of its disharmony with the rest of the face, much like a picture frame that sits askew on a wall. In common usage, "crooked" connotes not only a lack of straightness but also traits of dishonesty or unsavory character, as contrasted to the forthright person who is "playing it straight." The term "crooked nose" is thus apt because it not only captures the distinctive external appearance of a misaligned, deviated nose but also suggests the potential for social stigmatization. The surgeon should thus be attentive to not only the anatomic characteristics of the crooked nose but also the potential effects of this deformity on the patient's self-image.

Correction of the crooked nose remains a notoriously difficult challenge for the rhinoplasty surgeon. The complex interplay of functional and aesthetic considerations is coupled with the predilection of this deformity for gradual recurrence, often despite initially successful surgical treatment. The contracture forces of scar formation combined with cartilage thickening and deformation may resist definitive correction. Cartilage's elastic memory, the progressive formation of adhesions, and the collapse of a weakened septum are all contributory factors. An understanding of the relevant anatomy and pathogenesis of the deformity informs the surgical approach. This chapter covers the etiology, analysis, and surgical correction of the crooked nose.

ANATOMY OF THE CROOKED NOSE

The anatomy of the crooked nose is best understood relative to the constituent components of the osseocartilaginous framework. The upper third of the nose comprises the bony pyramid with its paired nasal bones and ascending processes of the maxillae. Bone thickness tapers along the nasal bones' caudal aspect. The lower two thirds of the nose are cartilaginous, including the nasal septum, the paired upper lateral cartilages, and the alar cartilages. The cartilage of the septum is relatively wide along the floor of the nose, flattens in the midportion, and is thickest near the dorsum, adjacent to the takeoff of the upper lateral cartilages.

Crooked noses exhibit greater diversity in their patterns of deformity than do isolated bony fractures. This heterogeneity is a reflection of the ability of cartilage to not only fracture but also twist, bend, and remodel in response to injury. The nasal septum behaves much like the rudder of a boat that both acutely and chronically guides the direction of the external nose, lending credence to the surgical maxim, "Where the septum goes, so goes the nose." Traumatic injury may cause angulation, telescoping, stepoffs, flattening, or splaying of the framework of the nose. The entire nasal pyramid may be deviated to one side, or a canted bony pyramid may be at an angle with the mid vault or lower third of the nose.

CLASSIFICATION OF THE CROOKED NOSE

The common patterns of crooked or deviated noses are the C-, S-, and I-type deformities shown in Figure 22-1. The C-shaped deformity usually begins cephalad at the nasal dorsum, proceeds posteroinferiorly through the perpendicular plate of the ethmoid, and then extends into the cartilaginous septum. The S-shaped deformity is characterized by a serpentine twisting of the external nose, usually with corresponding septal deviation. The I-shaped deformity corresponds to a deviation of the entire nasal pyramid. The nose is considered truly deviated if it departs from the midline position, with or without curvature. These deformities are associated with varying degrees of nasal obstruction.

Not all crooked noses fit neatly into this classification scheme. Prior rhinoplasty, pathologic disease processes, and saddling may all produce unpredictable patterns of asymmetry. Some noses that appear crooked do not have a true deviation. For example, when a laterally directed

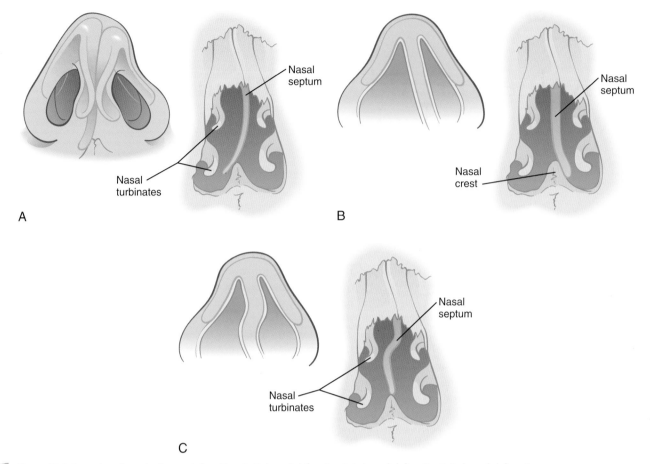

Figure 22-1 Examples of crooked nose deformities. **A,** C-shaped deformity. **B,** I-shaped deformity. **C,** S-shaped deformity.

force causes unilateral collapse of a nasal bone, the resulting concavity makes the nose appear deviated to the opposite side. Unilateral infracture of the bony pyramid side wall is often not associated with displacement of the septum. This infracture injury has a more favorable long-term prognosis with surgery and requires less extensive reconstruction than does a true deviation.

ETIOLOGY AND PATHOGENESIS OF THE CROOKED NOSE

TRAUMATIC CAUSES

The nasal bones are the most commonly fractured bones in the face, and nasal injury is the most common cause of the crooked nose. True deviation is indicative of a high energy injury and requires greater force than an isolated nasal bone depression or fracture. Usually a significant frontal vector is required for deviation to occur. With trauma, the nasal septum is often fractured or displaced from the maxillary crest. Because the nasal framework becomes more ossified and brittle with age, younger patients tend to have larger fracture segments than older

patients, who are more prone to nasal bone comminution. As a general rule, nasal trauma associated with septal fracture requires extensive reconstruction and is unlikely to be adequately treated with closed reduction. The surgeon should also consider psychological repercussions of the incident; such factors may influence the patient's readiness to undergo an elective surgical intervention.

The crooked nose deformity may reflect either the acute outcome of a traumatic episode or a remote injury that has been compounded by years of scarring and soft tissue contracture. The cartilaginous septum is the primary shock absorber of the nose, with lesser contributions from the upper lateral cartilages, alar cartilages, and bony components. Patients with untreated or inadequately reduced nasal fractures may develop a crooked nose gradually, with surface irregularities and asymmetries becoming more conspicuous with the passage of years. Cartilage has a low metabolic rate and frequently heals with scar formation. In cases of remote trauma, the patients may recount a worsening of the deformity with time, often associated with progressive nasal airway obstruction due to disruption of nasal support mechanisms. Repetitive fractures may cause profound structural deficiency, and comminution often will induce aberrant growth.

Many patients with a crooked nose do not remember the inciting traumatic injury. The patient with a severely twisted nose and without history of antecedent trauma is likely to have sustained a childhood injury that was overlooked. Relatively minor cartilage trauma may lead to dramatic deformation over time with chondrocyte growth. The pediatric nose lacks a well-developed bridge and is capable of absorbing substantial energy without showing irregularity until later in life. Children's noses are mostly cartilaginous and are susceptible to injuries that produce progressive deformation over subsequent years of growth. In some cases, septal subluxation or fracture may have occurred during birth. Forceps delivery and breach delivery are risk factors, although the head is also subjected to powerful compressive forces during normal passage through the birth canal. Such early deformities may first become evident during adolescence, as shown in Figure 22-2.

IATROGENIC CAUSES

Prior nasal surgery is an important cause of the crooked nose. Asymmetric or incomplete osteotomies often result in deviation and step-off deformities of the upper third of

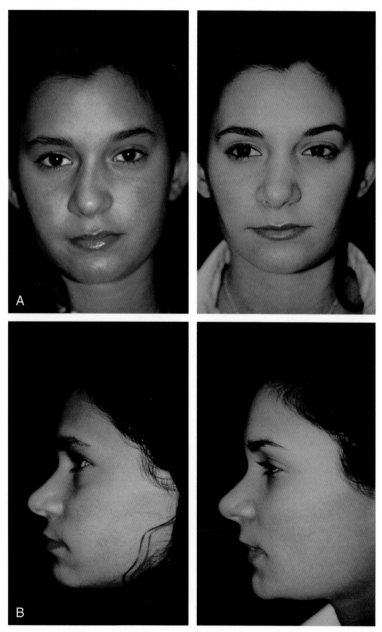

Figure 22-2 Patient with no history of antecedent nasal trauma. The patient developed progressive nasal deformity during adolescence. Examination demonstrated facial asymmetry with maxillary midline shifted to the right and nasal framework twisted and canted to the right, as well as a broad nasal tip. A shim spreader graft was created by drilling holes through a bone graft derived from the perpendicular plate of ethmoid. Medial and lateral osteotomies were performed to restore the nose to midline, and a dorsal onlay crushed cartilage graft was placed.

the nose. With green-stick fractures, the bony vault may be subject to residual memory and deviating forces from scarring. Alternatively, if adequate osteotomies are performed but the underlying septal deformity is not addressed, the nasal pyramid will often regress to its original, deviated position. Removal of a dorsal hump in the nose with a straight dorsum and a caudal deviation may unmask an underlying deformity that was not previously visible. Closed reduction of a nasal fracture may result in persistence or creation of a crooked nose if the fracture is not adequately reduced.

Reduction rhinoplasty deserves special consideration due to its potential for creating severe asymmetries that usually become apparent years after surgery. Resection of the nasal osseocartilaginous framework disrupts nasal support mechanisms, often with insidious destabilizing effects. Over the course of years, the contractile forces of scar formation, gravity, and aging conspire to warp and collapse the attenuated nasal scaffold. Such distortions may require major reconstruction years later to address progressive disfigurement and impairment of nasal function. Most rhinoplasty techniques have effects in adjacent zones of the nose during healing. Thus, unexpected deviations often occur from manipulations elsewhere, for example mid vault narrowing and upper lateral cartilage collapse occurring after dorsal hump reduction.

DISEASES INVOLVING THE SEPTUM AND INTERNAL NOSE

Several relatively rare pathologic processes may lead to a crooked nose. The surgeon should inquire about symptoms of nasal obstruction and history of epistaxis, allergy, and systemic disease. Autoimmune or immunologically mediated diseases may cause resorption of bony or cartilaginous nasal structures. Granulomatous disease, such as Wegener's granulomatosis or sarcoidosis, and collagen vascular/connective tissue disorders are important diagnostic considerations, particularly in patients with nasal septal perforation or saddling. A history of inhalant abuse, such as cocaine, oxymetazoline, nasal steroids, or NeoSynephrine use, should be considered in cases of mucosal atrophy, ulceration, or nasal perforation. The surgeon should also be alert to infectious etiologies such as tuberculosis, syphilis, and HIV infection. Sinonasal polyposis or neoplastic disease may also induce remodeling and/or splaying of nasal framework.

EVALUATION

PHYSICAL EXAMINATION AND NASAL ANALYSIS

The physical examination begins with an assessment of overall facial symmetry to ensure that all nasal pathology is viewed in relation to facial asymmetries. Many patients are unaware of asymmetry of the facial bones or soft tissues that may influence the perceived straightness of the nose. One of the defining features of the crooked nose is disruption of the brow–nasal tip aesthetic line, a line that runs from the medial brow to the ipsilateral nasal tip defining point. Identification of a break in this contour line helps localize the site of fracture or deformity that will require correction. Visual inspection and palpation are complementary in the nasal analysis.

The bony pyramid, nasal mid vault, and lower third of the nose are then systematically evaluated. The bony pyramid may be canted or have palpable surface irregularities. Angulation is often present at the transition of the upper and lower two thirds of the nose. Careful examination of the mid vault region will differentiate true deviation from isolated unilateral collapse of a nasal bone and/ or upper lateral cartilage. The nasal tip is assessed for asymmetry, deviation, presence of bossae, and alar retraction. Poor recoil of the tip to gentle finger pressure is indicative of compromised tip support. The anterior septal angle is palpated for its location and orientation. Basal view demonstrates caudal septal deviation and subluxation of the caudal septum off the maxillary crest. The anterior nasal spine serves as an anchoring point for the septum. Malposition of the septum due to prior trauma or surgery will alter nasal alignment and is best appreciated upon inspection of the nasal base.

Internal nasal examination is crucial from both a functional and aesthetic standpoint because septal deformity is the primary driver of the external appearance of the crooked nose. The nose should be examined both before and after constriction of the nasal mucosa to visualize potential sites of obstruction. The nasal lining will provide clues as to the extent of scarring and inflammation. Septal fractures, spurs, deviations, and other deformities are noted. The attachment of the upper lateral cartilage to the septum should create an angle of at least 10 to 15 degrees to avoid internal nasal valve collapse. The Cottle maneuver, performed by retracting the cheek soft tissues laterally, decreases the nasal obstruction from internal nasal valve collapse. Dynamic alar collapse with inspiration indicates external nasal valve collapse. Recurvature of the lower lateral cartilage into the nasal airway makes an often unrecognized contribution to airway narrowing and is an impending source of deformity following tip surgery. Turbinate hypertrophy may require a reduction or submucosal resection.

Photography is necessary in all patients with crooked nose, including those with purported interest in the relief of nasal obstruction only. Photography allows for precise recording of deformities and for computer imaging during patient consultation. In addition to the standard 7 rhinoplasty views (frontal, base, bilateral three-quarters, bilateral side, and lateral smiling views), the authors find it helpful to include a helicopter or sky view from above the nose highlighting any twisted configuration. Analysis of the patient followed by review of photographs taken in these views will assist the surgeon to determine whether camouflaging, structural reorientation, or both are needed.

SELECTION OF SURGICAL APPROACH

The decision to undertake anatomic reconstruction (structural reorientation) versus masking of the deformity (camouflage) will dictate the surgical approach. Camouflage techniques will best preserve existing structural support but fail to introduce new support and often involve some compromise in the aesthetic outcome. In contrast, structural reorientation can achieve excellent contour and can correct airway obstruction but does so at the expense of more extensive surgery and the potential risk for collapse if support mechanisms are not reconstituted. In performing nasal analysis, the surgeon should differentiate between the intrinsic forces and extrinsic forces that contribute to the nasal deformity. Intrinsic forces are due to aberrant growth and development of the cartilaginous septum. Extrinsic forces result from deviation of the nasal pyramid. Extrinsic forces are transmitted to the nasal septum through attachments to the nasal bones, the upper and lower cartilages, the vomer and perpendicular plate, and the maxillary crest.[1] For more severe deformities, especially those with airway compromises, we often use a combination of structural realignment and camouflage of residual minor deformities.

When nasal airway obstruction is present or when there is concern for impending nasal airway compromise, a structural reorientation approach is preferred. This approach involves release and deconstruction followed by rebuilding of structural elements of the osseocartilaginous skeleton. In such cases, an open rhinoplasty approach is advised. Camouflaging methods, which create the illusion of correction without actual manipulation of the deviated framework, do not influence nasal airway patency. In the absence of nasal obstructive complaints, camouflage alone may be adequate for correcting limited deformities. Camouflage techniques, when used in isolation, are usually conducive to an endonasal approach. It should be kept in mind that this method may only partially correct the crooked appearance and grafts may become visible in patients with thin skin. In some cases, it is desirable to use both techniques, as shown in Figure 22-3.

The Role of Closed Reduction

Closed reduction is best reserved for simple nasal fractures resulting from lateral forces. With such injuries, the nose may appear deviated but the actual deformity is usually limited to a single depressed bone fragment of the nasal side wall. The ipsilateral upper lateral cartilage may also be pulled medially. The casual observer will often erroneously perceive the nasal dorsum to being deflected to the opposite side. With either closed reduction or rhinoplasty, this type of injury carries a favorable prognosis. Closed

reduction should be performed within 24 hours of the injury, prior to the onset of edema, or at 10 to 21 days, by which time soft tissue edema has resolved. For unilateral nasal bone fracture, the Boies elevator usually suffices to restore the bone to its native position. Closed reduction is also useful in the neonatal period, when a difficult delivery is associated with a displaced septum and can be reduced with blunt forceps.

Unfortunately, the aesthetic outcomes following closed reduction are frequently unsatisfactory for the deviated or crooked nose. Closed reduction has limited precision in realigning bony and cartilaginous structures that are askew, telescoping, or markedly displaced. Walsham and Asch forceps are designed to reduce the displaced septum and impacted nasal bones, respectively. However, revision rates after closed reduction are unacceptably high when significant septal pathology is present.[2] Another drawback is the possibility of mucosal crushing injuries, synechia formation, and septal hematoma. In general, closed reduction can be unsatisfying for traumatic deformities that have bony comminution, extensive cartilaginous injury, or septal fracture.

If one chooses to perform a closed reduction, assessment of postreduction fragment stability is essential. Most fractures are, in fact, comminuted injuries that tend to collapse readily with minimal pressure. In adults, we often wait 10 to 21 days following their injuries when the fragments start to get "sticky." In this early phase of healing, the fragments are more stable. In addition, we will often support unstable fragments with a section of compressed cellulose sponge that can be wedged beneath the mucosal surface of the bone and anchored with absorbable sutures. The sutures are passed through the dorsal fracture fragments and nasal skin and then taped to the dorsum. These splints eliminate the need for traditional nasal packing and are removed within 5 to 7 days.

External Approach to the Crooked Nose

Much debate has centered on the indications for use of external versus endonasal approaches in rhinoplasty. In the authors' opinion, the preferred surgical approach is the one that confers the highest likelihood of a successful and durable surgical outcome. The literature confirms that the columellar scar from the external approach is a concern in less than 1% of patients. This figure is quite small compared to the overall published revision rates for rhinoplasty. Therefore, we use the external approach whenever improved exposure and precise graft placement can provide a meaningful advantage. These two criteria are met in the majority of patients with crooked noses.

The external approach affords the surgeon unparalleled exposure for counteracting the intrinsic and extrinsic forces responsible for cartilaginous septal deviation. Release of diffuse scar tissue, realignment of collapsed or twisted lateral cartilages, and repair of septal deviations involving the dorsal or caudal septum are all cumbersome

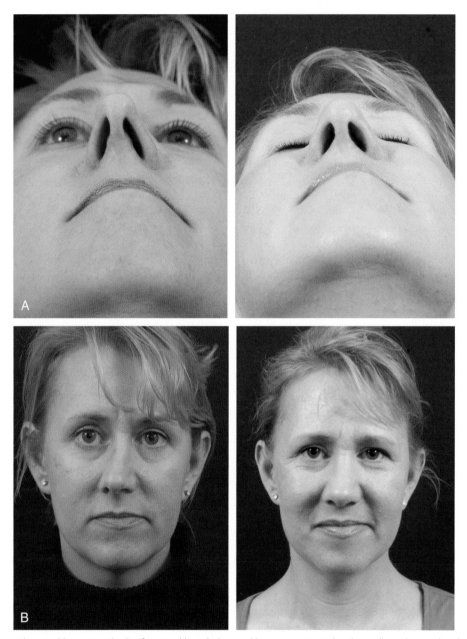

Figure 22-3 Patient with canted lower two thirds of nose. Although the nasal bones are situated in the midline, the nasal mid vault and lower third of the nose are deviated to the patient's right. Intraoperative assessment confirmed deviation at the bony–cartilaginous junction. An external rhinoplasty approach with division of the upper lateral cartilages afforded excellent exposure of the structural deformity. A combination of anatomic realignment with structural grafting and camouflage techniques were required to restore nasal function and achieve an aesthetic result.

through intranasal incisions. Using the external approach, the surgeon can expose the septum from the dorsum to the maxillary crest and from the caudal margin back to the anterior face of the sphenoid. As a result, structural reorientation involving graft placement under direct visualization and precise suture fixation is possible. In our experience, placement of spreader grafts after dividing the upper lateral cartilages through an external approach results in far more predictable results than endonasal placement. In addition, the lower third of the nose is seen in broad relief and easily manipulated, providing the best

opportunity for achieving symmetry in the deviated or twisted nasal tip.

Endonasal Approach to the Crooked Nose

The endonasal approach is useful for a more limited subset of crooked noses. One of the most significant advantages of this approach is that is allows for precise pocket preparation for camouflage grafts. In addition, this approach decreases operative time, avoids a columellar incision, may decrease postoperative edema, and obviates the need to reconstitute the structural elements disrupted by the open approach. An intercartilaginous incision allows for camouflage techniques in the middle third of the nose, as well as conservative hump reduction and osteotomies, provided the nasal airway remains widely patent. Grafts are placed immediately above perichondrium or deep to periosteum to minimize the risk of visible or palpable grafts. Although the delivery approach has proven very useful in refinement of the bulbous nasal tip, correction of tip asymmetries is less reliable endonasally.

SELECTION OF GRAFT MATERIAL

Septal cartilage is the grafting material of choice because of its versatility, ease of harvest, and minimal donor site morbidity. When adequate septal cartilage is not available, usually auricular cartilage or costal cartilage may be used. Autologous tissues have long track records of success and are associated with low risks of infection, extrusion, and resorption. Conchal cartilage is best for alar batten grafts and for filling small dorsal concavities, whereas costal cartilage is often necessary for correction of a saddle deformity or when previous surgery has reduced other grafting options. Crushing cartilage significantly improves camouflage and malleability but may predispose to resorption if chondrocyte viability is impaired by excessive trauma. We rarely use calvarial or other bone grafts due to the favorable attributes of cartilage, which include its natural feel and facile harvest, carving, and fixation. Acellular dermal matrix may be used selectively for camouflage of minor irregularities, although we prefer autologous fascia, perichondrium, or fibroconnective tissue for this purpose.

When costal cartilage is required, we prefer to use the "floater" tenth rib as a dorsal onlay graft. Harvesting from this site decreases pain, carving time and risks of flail chest and pneumothorax. Harvesting additional cartilage from other ribs may be necessary if additional grafting material is needed. The floater rib has less curvature than attached ribs and contains both bone and cartilage, thus mimicking the structural elements to be replaced. The bony portion of the graft is cantilevered on the rasped bony foundation of the upper third of the nose to promote a bony union. If cartilage is harvested from the seventh or eighth ribs, the grafts should be taken from the center of a relatively straight cartilage segment to decrease risk of warping.

Dorsal costal cartilage grafts serve to provide sufficient structure to recreate a straight dorsal line and simultaneously camouflage and modify irregularities. Costal cartilage dorsal grafts are not immune to distortion during or after surgery, and a few pearls may decrease the risk of warping. Carving the graft symmetrically by trimming from both lateral edges and placing a Kirschner wire in the middle of the graft has been recommended. We routinely place the dorsal graft along the entire dorsum, from the radix to the supratip to avoid distortion that can occur if a graft ends at the rhinion. In the uncommon case where a patient is unwilling or unable to undergo costal cartilage harvest, homologous irradiated rib graft is useful. It is readily carved and compares favorably with the commercially available alloplastic implants.

Numerous fixation techniques have been used to secure dorsal grafts. Our preferred method is to suture the caudal portions of the graft to the dorsal edges of the upper lateral cartilages, as in an onlay spreader graft and anchor the cephalic end to the bony dorsum with one or two percutaneous Kirschner wires that are removed in 3 weeks as a minor office procedure that rarely requires even local anesthesia. Lag screw fixation, although preferred by some, has been unsatisfactory for use due to the tendency for the screw to extrude long term.

TECHNICAL ASPECTS OF SURGERY

Common steps in surgery of the crooked nose include exposure of the nasal deformity, release of septal attachments, hump reduction (often performed in an asymmetric manner), straightening of the bony pyramid, and correction of the deformity with structural and/or camouflage grafting. While various algorithms for treatment of the crooked nose have been proposed,[1,3] the complexity and variability of the crooked nose render most such approaches of more theoretical than practical value. Ultimately, sound nasal analysis will dictate the sequence of steps. Discussion of technical aspects of crooked nose surgery begins with consideration of the crooked nasal septum, which plays a pivotal role in pathogenesis of the crooked nose deformity. A detailed discussion on management of the upper, middle, and lower third of the nose follows. Several instructive case studies are detailed in the accompanying case examples shown in Figures 22-4 and 22-5.

Care must be taken during the surgical exposure to preserve cartilaginous elements amid the disrupted, scarred tissue planes. These characteristics necessitate meticulous dissection during elevation of the skin–soft tissue envelope in a sub–superficial musculoaponeurotic system (SMAS) plane. Release of adhesions and structural attachments optimizes exposure and relieves distortional forces.

SEPTAL DEFORMITY IN THE CROOKED NOSE

The septum is the crux of the nasal osseocartilaginous framework. Because the crooked nose is driven by a crooked septum, failure to correct an underlying dorsal or caudal septal deformity will inevitably result in migration of the nose back to a crooked configuration. If the bony and cartilaginous skeletons are shifted in opposite

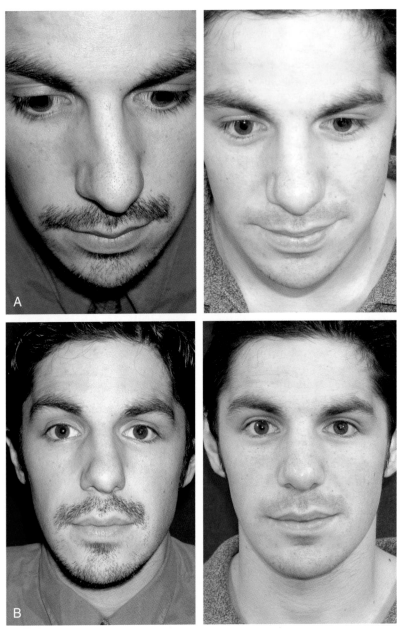

Figure 22-4 Crooked nose with I-shaped deformity. This patient had a history of nasal trauma 5 years earlier and complained of a crooked nose and a fixed nasal obstruction, more severe on the right side. The osseocartilaginous vault is deviated to the patient's left. Sky view emphasizes the preoperative deviation to the patient's left. Surgical management included medial and lateral osteotomies, unilateral spreader graft to right to correct for asymmetric collapse, and use of a crushed cartilage graft to camouflage depression of the right nasal mid vault.

directions, addressing the deviation of the nasal bones alone may actually worsen the septal component. Attachments between the nasal septum and other nasal framework transmit distortions of the septum to the external nose (Table 22-1). The septal perichondrium has significant tensile strength, so dissection deep to this layer prevents tearing and perforation. In contrast, dissection between the mucosa and perichondrium is associated with decreased flap viability, bleeding, and tears. When the correct plane of cleavage is identified with a Cottle elevator, the subsequent flap dissection proceeds easily, such

that gentle sweeping with a Frazier suction is sufficient to elevate the flap off the nasal septum.

An area requiring special attention during elevation of mucoperichondrial flaps is the intersection of the nasal septum with the vomerine-maxillary groove. At this location, the septal perichondrium, maxillary periosteum, and vomerine crest form a line of dense adhesions that must be released. This adhesion is sometimes referred to as a conflicting line (Figure 22-6). We prefer to elevate inferior and superior tunnels separately and then use a hockey stick–shaped dissector to lyse these fibrous attachments.

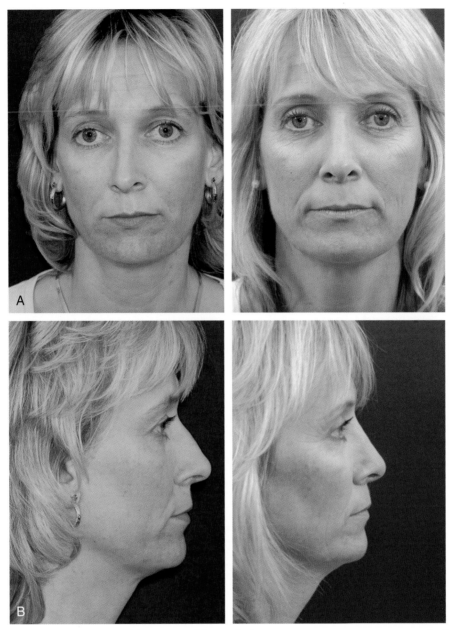

Figure 22-5 Crooked nose and thin skin. Successful correction of the crooked nose requires extra precision in patients that have thin nasal skin. In this patient, dorsal hump reduction and medial and lateral osteotomies were followed by spreader grafts, alar rim grafting, and onlay crushed cartilage grafting. Grafts that are placed immediately under the skin–soft tissue envelope are poorly concealed in patients with thin skin; thus, precise anatomic realignment was necessary.

This approach avoids violation of the intranasal mucosa and unintended scarring. If the caudal anterior septum is subluxed off the maxillary crest, a "swinging door"–type approach may be used, wherein a small triangular wedge of caudal septum near the posterior septal angle is judiciously trimmed to bring the septum back into the midline position.[4,5] The septal base is then secured with suture to the periosteum of the maxillary crest periosteum (Figure 22-7). Dissection then proceeds posteriorly and superiorly to free the mucoperichondrium under the upper lateral cartilages.

Deviated portions of the quadrangular cartilage may then be addressed using a variety of techniques. Scoring, crosshatching, gentle crushing, and morselization of septal cartilage may be adequate to improve mild deviations when used in conjunction with Mustarde-type mattress stitches. Deviated cartilage may also be resected with preservation of a 1.5-cm dorsal and caudal L-shaped strut that spans from the rhinion to the posterior septal angle. Failure to preserve this L-shaped strut predisposes to saddle nose deformity, columellar retraction, and tip ptosis. Some authors have gone so far as to describe this

Table 22-1 Septal Deformity and Corresponding External Deformity

Septal Deformity	Corresponding External Deformity
Dorsal septal deviation	Asymmetric upper lateral cartilages or mid vault collapse
Caudal septal subluxation	Medial crura and columella displacement into nasal airway
Anterior septal angle distortion	Twisting of cartilaginous domes and nasal tip asymmetry
Posterior septal angle deflection	Columellar base asymmetry and medial footplate malposition

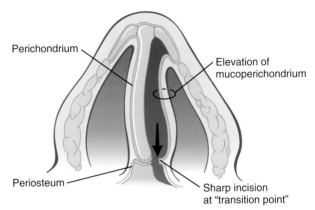

Figure 22-6 Lysis of the "conflicting line" during septoplasty. After the superior mucoperichondrial and inferior mucoperiosteal tunnels have been elevated, the fused connective tissue (conflicting line) between the vomerine maxillary crest and cartilaginous septum is divided sharply to avoid inadvertent fenestration of the flap during this portion of the dissection.

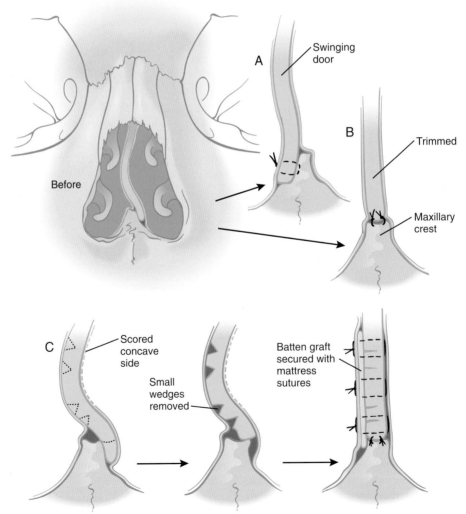

Figure 22-7 Correction of caudal septal deflection with a "swinging door" technique. The initial septal deformity (*left*) may be corrected through a variety of techniques depending on severity of the deformity. For minor distortions, it may suffice to swing the caudal septum to the opposite side. Alternatively, the caudal septum may be conservatively trimmed and placed back on maxillary crest. For more severe cases, it may be necessary to incise, score, or trim the septum and then stabilize the septum with septal batten or shim spreader grafts.

crucial L-shaped strut as "sacrosanct,"[6] with the caveat that this L-shaped strut can be removed and reconstructed. When performing the septoplasty through an open approach, the supporting attachments of the L-shaped strut are disrupted and must be reconstituted with a columellar strut or other structural support.

When the caudal and dorsal septal components are both severely deviated, it may be necessary to perform an extracorporeal septoplasty, in which the septum is removed and replaced after being rotated 180 degrees. This technique exploits the tendency of the posterior septum to be closer to the midline position than the anterior septum. Whenever possible, a small strut of cartilage in the keystone area is preserved as a fixation point for the reimplanted septum. Disruption of this area increases the risk of irregularity over the rhinion, which has thin skin and may show notching. In cases where the septum does not provide adequate salvageable grafting material, the deformed septum may be removed and the L-shaped strut replaced with a strut made from costal cartilage.

After completion of the septoplasty, bilateral mucoperichondrial flaps are secured over the nasal septum with a quilting mattress stitch. An often overlooked technical pearl is elevation of the lower third of the nose during flap resuspension. This maneuver is performed by having an assistant apply steady traction to a suture that has been passed through the domes of the alar cartilages. Doing so ensures smooth redraping of the flap, which otherwise falls and bunches at the caudal portion of the septum. While neglect of this detail seldom has immediate repercussions, over time the contractile forces acting on the distorted nasal lining will predispose to nasal collapse as the lining pulls against the newly reconstructed framework.

When the septum tends to warp we may place a vomer or perpendicular plate of the ethmoid "shim spreader graft." With this technique, a bony graft measuring $2\frac{1}{2} \times 1\frac{1}{2}$ cm is harvested. Multiple 1-mm holes are then drilled through it. The graft is then secured to the concave side of the septum flush with the dorsal edge. Suture fixation of the graft to the septum allows the graft to function as a rigid, permanent intranasal stent.

UPPER THIRD/BONY PYRAMID OF THE CROOKED NOSE

Overview

Deformity of the bony nasal pyramid is often a major component of the crooked dorsum. A severely deviated bony dorsum may be addressed early in the operation to provide a stable foundation for the lower two thirds of the nose. The surgeon should perform osteotomies only after careful analysis of the dimensions of each side of the nasal pyramid. Various permutations of medial, intermediate, and lateral osteotomies, illustrated in Figure 22-8, are

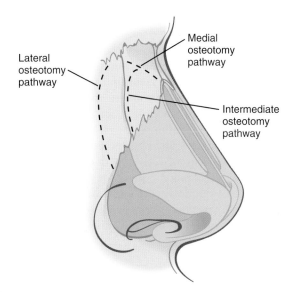

Figure 22-8 Medial, lateral, and intermediate osteotomies. The medial osteotomy preferably fades laterally as it proceeds cephalad, and it is not always necessary if a hump reduction is performed. Intermediate osteotomies are used selectively due to risk of comminution. Intermediate osteotomies must be performed prior to lateral osteotomies. The lateral osteotomy is usually performed in a high–low–high pathway through the ascending process of the maxilla.

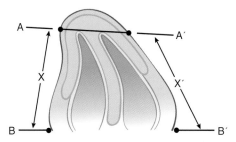

Figure 22-9 Angled hump reduction. In the case of a deviated nose, an angled hump reduction with preservation of mucoperichondrium is necessary to achieve nasal sidewalls of equal length. Removal of the hump in a beveled manner equalizes the lateral walls such that the distance "X" from point A to point B (right side) is equal to the distance "X'" from point A' to B' (left side). After hump reduction, the nose is restored to the midline with septoplasty and osteotomy.

used depending on the specific deformity present. Rarely, repositioning of the bony vault will achieve simultaneous correction of lower two thirds of the nose by virtue of attachments of the upper lateral cartilages to the displaced nasal bones, although a septal deformity must not been overlooked.

Dorsal Hump Reduction

In the crooked nose, it is common for the posterior portion of the septum to be straighter than the dorsum. As a result, dorsal hump reduction alone may markedly diminish the extent of deformity. When performing resection of a dorsal hump, the Rubin osteotome is advanced at an incline that will preserve equal height on either side of the nose. As shown in Figure 22-9, his technique prevents overresection of the more vertical component. If a dorsal hump reduction is deferred until after the septoplasty, particular care is taken to ensure that an adequate septal L-shaped strut remains, lest the hump reduction have the unintended consequence of compromising dorsal support. This error will undermine reconstructive efforts and predispose to saddle nose deformity. In the patient with a reasonably straight dorsum, short nasal bones, and long upper lateral cartilages, the resected dorsal hump may be sculpted and repositioned on the dorsum as an onlay graft, thereby obviating the need for osteotomies.[7] This useful approach simultaneously achieves reduction of the dorsal hump, correction of the open roof deformity, preservation of the middle vault, and restoration of natural dorsal contour.

Osteotomies

Osteotomies are inherently destabilizing, and foremost consideration must be given to avoiding unintended complications when undertaking these maneuvers. One of the most common errors is inadequate preservation of maxillary periosteum. As shown in Figure 22-10, the periosteum maintains the integrity of the nose after medial and lateral osteotomies. It protects from nasal collapse and comminution. Precise use of a sharp osteotome minimizes periosteal shearing and postoperative edema. When performing sliding (continuous) endonasal osteotomies, use of a smaller osteotome or directing the guard downward minimizes trauma. Interrupted percutaneous osteotomies

are often used. "Inside-out" osteotomies can prove extremely helpful in minimizing periosteal injury if multiple osteotomies are necessary. With this method, postage stamp–type perforations of the nasal bone are created endonasally, and the intervening bone bridges are fractured with minimal periosteal disruption.[8,9] This approach is ideal for correction of traumatic medial displacement of a nasal bone. An alternative approach involves accessing the pyriform aperture through a sublabial approach just over the canine fossa. The risk of comminution of the nasal side wall is greatest when medial, intermediate, and lateral osteotomies are performed.

Medial osteotomies are performed prior to lateral osteotomies in order not to destabilize the nasal pyramid. Medial osteotomies are directed obliquely at approximately 25 degrees off midline and fade laterally along their course. This path avoids the "rocker deformity" in which the osteotomy is inadvertently carried into the frontal bone resulting in a mobile fragment that rocks in the cephalocaudal dimension (percutaneous osteotomy across the nasal bridge will correct this deformity). Medial osteotomies may be unnecessary if an open roof deformity results from dorsal hump reduction or when the nasal bones are symmetric and the deviated pyramid can be corrected with lateral osteotomies alone. Incomplete osteotomies are to be avoided, as these "green-stick" fractures may predispose to bony irregularities and unpredictable healing. The intermediate osteotomy is useful for restoring a collapsed lateral wall to a neutral position or reducing the outward bowing of an overly convex lateral wall. Intermediate osteotomies are performed after medial osteotomies to avoid performing osteotomy on mobile bone segments.

Lateral osteotomies are most commonly performed in a high–low–high pattern. This particular trajectory confers several advantages for most patients:

1. Initiating the osteotomy high on the pyriform aperture avoids disruption of the inferior turbinate and preserves nasal airway patency by maintaining a ledge of bone at Webster's triangle (the base of the pyriform aperture).
2. Proceeding low along the mid-dorsum achieves aesthetic narrowing of the ascending process of the maxilla and masks the osteotomy site beneath the thicker soft tissues in the nasofacial sulcus.
3. Returning to a high position prevents excessive narrowing of the root of the nose.

When the nasal base is broad, the osteotomy may be performed in a low–low–high path, so long as this can be performed without impairing the airway. A unilateral osteotomy is especially useful in the midline nose with a convex side wall. This convexity may create the illusion of deviation where none exists; therefore, a unilateral osteotomy corrects the perceived irregularity.

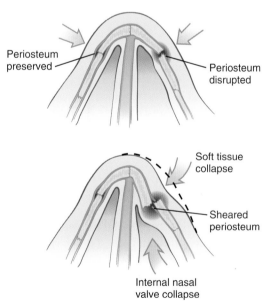

Figure 22-10 Demonstration of the importance of preservation of periosteum. The periosteum is crucial in maintaining support and preventing nasal collapse after osteotomies. On the left side, the periosteum has been kept in continuity allowing for aesthetic narrowing with preservation of structural support. On the right side, the periosteum has been inadvertently sheared during osteotomy. As a result, there is soft tissue collapse and compromise of nasal airway patency due to telescoping of the bones and excessive medial displacement of the anterior bony framework.

MIDDLE THIRD OF THE CROOKED NOSE

Straightening the crooked middle third of the nose involves treatment of complex functional and aesthetic deformities. Usually, an underlying septal deviation is present. Unfortunately, the commonly used techniques of septal scoring, partial resection, shaving, crushing, and cross-hatching all weaken the cartilage. In addition, the patency of the mid vault is often compromised by collapse or depression in the crooked nose. Preexisting nasal airway problem may be further exacerbated by osteotomies that narrow the mid vault region. For these reasons, spreader grafts or broad sandwiching stent grafts play a major role in reconstruction of the crooked mid vault.

Spreader grafts, originally described by Sheen,[10] stent the airway open while also addressing the aesthetic problems of a pinched or twisted middle third of the nose and open roof deformity. These grafts are secured in a submucoperichondrial plane, flanking the septum. They embrace the L-shaped septal strut to restore rigidity to otherwise flaccid septal cartilage. These grafts also increase the angle of the internal valve angle, improve airway patency, and maintain a straight dorsum. Although septal cartilage is preferred, ethmoid bone, other autologous cartilage, or an alloplastic implant may be used. Recently, there has been interest in extended spreader grafts made from high density porous polyethylene (MEDPOR). This alloplast allows fibrous ingrowth and resists resorption, thereby stabilizing the upper lateral cartilages and straightening the septum. Although experience is limited, these rigid grafts can provide mid vault and tip support.

A number of variations on spreader grafts have found application in treatment of the asymmetric mid vault associated with the crooked nose. A planoconvex spreader graft, which is flat on one side and rounded or beveled on the other surface, may be placed in between the upper lateral cartilage and septum. The flat side of the graft faces outward such that the convex surface of the graft fills the concavity created by curvature of the dorsal septum.[11] A side wall spreading suture can be used to elevate a depressed upper lateral cartilage. The triangular spreader graft, unilateral spreading graft, or asymmetric spreaders are refinements of the classic spreader technique. Alternatively, a septal extension graft secured to the convex surface of the septum may be paired with a spreader graft on the contralateral concave side. To camouflage mild deviations, a concave region of the dorsal septum may be augmented with crushed cartilage and the contralateral convexity shaved.

Suture-based techniques are useful adjuncts to structural grafting and camouflaging defects of the nasal middle vault. For example, a differential suturing technique may be applied to the upper lateral cartilages and spreader graft–septum complex. As a general rule, we do not rely on sutures for permanent fixation; instead, sutures are used to align raw surfaces in a particular configuration during the acute phase of healing. Scar formation provides permanent stabilization. Side wall spreading/flaring sutures are a type of mattress suture that elevate a collapsed upper lateral cartilage by fixation to the nasal bone periosteum. Clocking sutures may be placed between the septum and upper lateral cartilages to unfurl the twisted dorsal septum. Septocolumellar sutures secure a scored or weakened caudal septum to a rigid columellar strut.[12] With each of these approaches, the sutures reorient the cartilaginous portion of the framework in the desired direction. Camouflaging onlay grafts will help to mask minor, residual asymmetries.

LOWER THIRD OF THE CROOKED NOSE

Although tip refinement can be performed through an endonasal approach, the external approach affords the best opportunity for success in addressing a severely deviated or twisted nasal tip. Prior to refining the tip, a displaced caudal septum should be secured in the midline so as to provide a stable foundation, and any resection should be performed conservatively. The nasal tip is straightened and sculpted with grafting or suture-based techniques, and tip support mechanisms are reconstituted. The 5-0 polydioxanone (PDS) suture affords sufficient durability to maintain position and is subsequently resorbed, thereby avoiding a persistent nidus for chronic inflammation. Grafts are placed in precise pockets or fixated with sutures.

NASAL STABILIZATION

Rhinoplasty is an inherently destabilizing procedure, and the nose is fragile in the immediate postoperative period. Although a structural approach emphasizes preservation or reconstitution of nasal support structures, internal and external stabilization is often helpful. Septal splints, secured with a nylon stitch, flank the septum, help to stabilize the midline, and prevent formation of synechiae during the first postoperative week. If there is concern that a nasal side wall is unstable, an intranasal stent is secured in position with sutures that pass up through the skin of the lateral nose and are tied to a soft dressing. Taping of the nasal dorsum and placement of a nasal cast obliterates dead space, stabilizes the nose, and prevents inadvertent injury during the initial phase of healing. Because dissection is performed in avascular planes, bleeding should be minimal and internal nasal packing is not needed.

SUMMARY

Surgical correction of the crooked nose is deceptively complex. A detailed understanding of its pathogenesis facilitates proper diagnosis and treatment. Systematic identification of the structures responsible for the deviation is a prerequisite for correction. Usually a combination of structural reorientation and camouflaging techniques is required. In our experience, the presence of nasal obstruction, marked septal deformity, and tip asymmetry all favor an external approach to correcting the crooked nose. Preservation and reconstitution of nasal support mechanisms remain paramount.

REFERENCES

1. Byrd HS, Salomon J, Flood J. Correction of the crooked nose. *Plast Reconstr Surg.* 1998;102:2148–2157
2. Rhee SC, Kim YK, Cha JH, et al. Septal fracture in simple nasal bone fracture. *Plast Reconstr Surg.* 2004;113:45–52.
3. Hsiao YC, Kao CH, Wang HW, Moe KS. A surgical algorithm using open rhinoplasty for correction of traumatic twisted nose. *Aesthet Plast Surg.* 2007;31:250–258.
4. Metzenbaum M. Replacement of the lower end of the dislocated septal cartilage versus submucous resection of the dislocated end of the septal cartilages. *Arch Otolaryngol.* 1929;9:282.
5. Seltzer AP. The nasal septum: Plastic repair of the deviated septum, associated with a deflected tip. *Arch Otolaryngol.* 1944;40:433.
6. Kim DW, Toriumi DM. Management of posttraumatic nasal deformities: The crooked nose and the saddle nose. *Fac Plast Surg Clin North Am.* 2004;12:111–132.
7. Hall JA, Peters MD, Hilger PA. Modification of the Skoog dorsal reduction for preservation of the middle nasal vault. *Arch Fac Plast Surg.* 2004;6:105–110.
8. Hilger JA. The internal lateral osteotomy in rhinoplasty. *Arch Otolaryngol.* 1968;88:211–212.
9. Byrne PJ, Walsh WE, Hilger PA. The use of "inside-out" lateral osteotomies to improve outcome in rhinoplasty. *Arch Fac Plast Surg.* 2003;5:251–255.
10. Sheen JH. Spreader graft: A method of reconstructing the roof of the middle nasal vault following rhinoplasty. *Plast Reconstr Surg.* 1984;73:230–239.
11. Toriumi DM, Ries WR. Innovative surgical management of the crooked nose. *Fac Plast Surg Clin North Am.* 1993;1:63–78.
12. Pontius AT, Leach JL Jr. New techniques for management of the crooked nose. *Arch Fac Plast Surg.* 2004;6:263–266.

CHAPTER TWENTY-THREE

Saddle Nose Deformity

Kevin Brenner • Jay Calvert

A saddle nose deformity derives its name from the appearance of the nose on lateral view as the dorsal curve resembles the depression in a horse's saddle. The gross deficiency that exists in the dorsum of the nose, no matter the etiology, creates an obvious and progressive scooped-out deformity. When viewed frontally, an illusory excessive width exists across the bridge. The first paper written on the treatment of saddle nose deformity was John Orlando Roe's original article in 1887, "The deformity termed 'Pug-Nose' and its correction by a simple operation."[1] The first attempt at correction of saddle nose deformity occurred when Robert F. Weir implanted the breastbone of a duck into the shrunken nose of a syphilitic patient in 1892.[2] In 1896, Israel was the first to use a human bone graft to the nose.[3] Many authors have published articles detailing the etiology, classification, and treatment of this deformity.[1-28] Most recently, Daniel and Brenner published a classification of saddle nose deformity with a focus on septal saddling. In this article, the authors describe their approach to the treatment of these deformities as they address each component separately.

DEFINITION

The term "saddle nose deformity" is a pathologic entity resulting from loss of dorsal height, caused by a substantial decrease in the cartilaginous vault and/or bony vault. It may include any of a variety of features: (1) middle vault and dorsal depression, (2) loss of tip support and definition, (3) columellar retrusion, (4) shortened vertical length, (4) tip overrotation, and (5) retrusion of the nasal spine and caudal septum. Regardless of the etiology, the central underlying defect is lost integrity of the bony and cartilaginous dorsum resulting in a short nose with compromised support.

Saddle nose deformity can occur following a variety of nasal pathologic conditions. The majority of saddle nose deformities are acquired (secondary to trauma, septal hematoma, septorhinoplasty to correct traumatic injuries, cocaine abuse, infection, and cosmetic septorhinoplasty), but congenital causes do exist (i.e., Binder syndrome). Although it is difficult to assess the true prevalence of nasal saddling in any given population, certain groups of patients seem to be particularly prone. Facial trauma victims, cocaine abusers, and patients who have undergone previous septorhinoplasty, particularly following traumatic injury, seem to be at highest risk.

CLASSIFICATION

No matter which classification system is followed, nasal saddling exists along a spectrum. Tardy has described a three "M" category classification system: minimal, moderate, and major. *Minimal* saddling demonstrates modest tip–supratip differential with a supratip depression greater than the ideal 1 to 2 mm. The bony nasal hump is mildly accentuated, the nose is wide, and minimal columellar retraction exists. *Moderate* saddling shows depression secondary to lost dorsal height in the quadrangular cartilage. Columellar retraction results in an acute nasolabial angle. *Major* saddling is a more severe deformity often secondary to massive blunt frontal trauma, resulting in a twisted nose with severe septal deviation. Vartanian categorized saddling into four types, based on the degree of existing anatomic deficit. *Type 1* describes minor supratip or dorsal nasal depression with preservation of lower third projection. *Type 2* has moderate to severe dorsal depression with a prominent lower third. *Type 3* has moderate to severe dorsal depression and lower third deficits resulting in loss of tip support. *Type 4* refers to a pan-nasal defect with severe middle nasal dorsal deficiency, in combination with deficits of the upper and lower thirds.

Daniel recently expanded on these earlier classification systems, attempting to integrate the external appearance of the nose, the degree of compromise of septal support, and selection of surgical treatment into what is referred to as *septal saddle nose*. Septal support is determined by pressing the nasal tip inward—if the tip remains supported, then septal support is adequate; if the tip compresses against the premaxilla, then the support is inadequate. This classification system thus consists of a subset within the broader *saddle nose* classification systems and is defined by the combination of a dorsal depression and inadequate septal support:

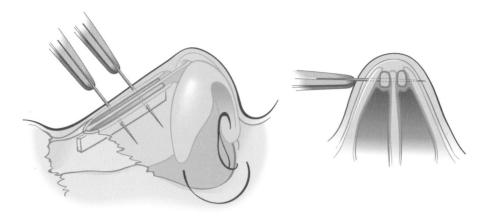

Figure 23-1 Standard placement of bilateral spreader grafts.

Type 0 (Pseudosaddle)

These patients present with depression of the cartilaginous vault following a prior rhinoplasty and is invariably due to over-resection of the cartilaginous vault, a relative depression of the cartilaginous dorsum due to a prominence of the bony vault, or a combination of the two. The etiology is not due to lost septal support but rather to aggressive dorsal changes. Septal support is excellent and there is a negative septal support test.

Type I (Minor—Cosmetic Concealment)

These cases have excessive supratip depression and columellar retraction but normal septal support. Cosmetic concealment is possible provided the septal compromise is static and not progressive.

Type II (Moderate—Cartilage Vault Restoration)

The dominant factor is compromise of septal support, which leads directly to cartilaginous vault collapse, columellar retraction, and loss of tip support.

Type III (Major—Composite Reconstruction)

In major cases, there is a total absence of septal support for the cartilaginous vault, columellar, nasal tip, and external valves. Flattening of the nose is obvious in all views.

Type IV (Severe—Structural Reconstruction)

These cases represent the end stage of septal collapse. They are compounded by bony vault disruption and severe contracture of the nasal lining often associated with major septal perforations. Septal collapse has occurred resulting in cartilage vault depression and columellar shortening. The nasal tip has lost its projection and the nostrils are broad. There is no support to the vestibular and nostril valves with dramatic compromise of the external airway. The nasal loblule is often rotated upward. The nose is short in absolute terms and further emphasized by an acute nasolabial angle. Depression of the bony vault is a major factor that may limit support for the reconstruction.

TYPE V (Catastrophic—Nasal Reconstruction)

The majority of these cases have progressed from reconstructive aesthetic rhinoplasty to aesthetic reconstruction of the nose and its adjacent tissues. Many will require forehead flaps for either lining or skin coverage. Equally significant, the bony deformity extends farther into the facial skeleton, warranting some type of degloving approach and extensive bone grafting and/or plating. These cases are best referred to surgeons who have a high degree of special expertise.

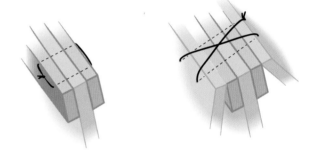

Figure 23-2 Securing spreader grafts. *Left,* Three-layer mattress suture technique. *Right,* Five-layer "figure-of-eight" technique that includes the upper lateral cartilage for security and narrowing.

TREATMENT

The surgical correction of saddle nose deformity should be approached and planned in the same intricate manner as any major nasal reconstruction case. Burget and Mennick have worked extensively to develop an algorithmic approach to rebuilding complex nasal defects.[18] Preoperative deficiencies in bony and cartilaginous support, internal nasal lining, and external coverage must all be determined. Less severe deformities, where supporting structures remain strong, can be simply treated with dorsal onlay grafts. When upper lateral cartilage weakness exists, middle vault integrity must be reestablished. Spreader grafts help restore the internal nasal valve (Figures 23-1 and 23-2); severe upper lateral cartilage collapse may require replacement Batten grafts. Obviously every patient will be unique in all of these categories, dictating a slightly different plan for each operation. The basic components to consider follow:

1. *Reestablishing support:* When the quadrangular cartilage is no longer able to support the nasal roof, it must be either buttressed or, better yet, replaced. Autologous rib cartilage is the ideal material for this purpose since it is abundant in supply and extremely strong in form.

2. ***Addressing the airway:***   As the degree of saddling becomes more severe, there appears to be an increasing need for restoration of both the internal and external nasal valves. Spreader grafts must be used as part of the reconstruction, frequently in concert with the septal support and/or replacement grafts. When external valve collapse occurs or the upper lateral cartilages are no longer sufficient, batten grafts should be used to reestablish the requisite support. With severe scarring, as occurs in the multiply operated patient and the advanced cocaine nose, large batten grafts from the eighth costal cartilage frequently work the best. For patients with compromised nasal lining and alar retraction, skin–cartilage ear composite grafts work well to augment the lining and prevent recurrent retraction. In severe cases, the addition of alar rim grafts may be necessary.

3. ***The nasal tip:***   Support is essential. With the exception of septal replacement grafts, the columellar strut is the most important determinant of long-term tip support and projection (Figure 23-3). In saddle noses, the scarring is severe and ear cartilage clearly lacks the requisite strength to resist the inevitable contractile forces of the skin envelope. A large post of costal cartilage works extremely well as a columellar strut. For the best aesthetic reconstruction, it is wise to place this graft as a stand-alone graft instead of incorporating it or attaching it to the septal replacement graft. Once the support is reestablished, then the tip structure can be defined by either suturing the existing alar cartilages or replacing them with tip grafts.

4. ***The dorsum:***   The dorsum must be considered as a separate component. We have found that reestablishing the dorsal line is difficult with carved cartilage grafts. The authors almost exclusively use deep temporal fascia grafts alone or in combination with diced cartilage as minor dorsal camouflage grafts or major augmentation grafts.

DISCUSSION

There appears to be a progression in difficulty with these cases as follows: (1) postseptoplasty, (2) posttraumatic, (3) secondary rhinoplasty, (4) secondary saddle deformity, and (5) the cocaine nose. The patient who saddles following a septoplasty has essentially normal tissue throughout the nose except for the compromised septum. Once the septum is restored, the tip and bony vault can be modified as desired using standard techniques. The question is whether to perform cosmetic concealment, structural restoration, or both.

Posttraumatic noses can be divided into primary and secondary cases. The nose that sustains severe septal trauma with saddling often requires a total septoplasty with restoration of the L-shape strut. In contrast, the posttraumatic nose that has had surgery with subsequent saddling may now include a septal perforation, significant resections, and additional scarring. The secondary rhinoplasty nose can have saddling due to overresection, loss of septal support, or both. Simple tip compression will help in defining the need for structural support versus aesthetic correction. The most difficult cases are patients with failed prior attempts at correcting their saddle deformity and cocaine noses. In addition to the challenges of support and aesthetics, one must contend with lining contracture, which often requires extensive composite grafts. The classical method of mobilizing the lining sleeve is often limited as it does not add to the destroyed tissue— hence, the need to add composite grafts of conchal cartilage and skin, which can resist the contractile forces.

As the deformities become more complex, the need for restoration of structure and support becomes critical for the shape of the nose and opening of the airway. The greater the problem, the less septal cartilage is usually available and the less adequate conchal cartilage becomes. Costal cartilage is virtually the only material with sufficient strength and volume to achieve the reconstructive goals. Cadaver cartilage is not an acceptable alternative unless the patient is medically unfit to withstand rib

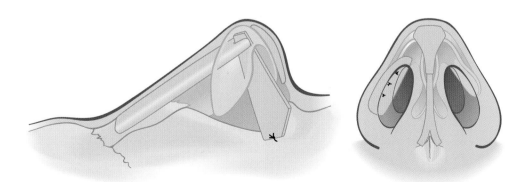

Figure 23-3 Total nasal reconstruction can require a dorsal replacement graft integrated with a septal replacement strut graft. Additional shield tip graft is shown. Some patients require an additional columellar strut independent of the septal strut.

cartilage harvest or has been shown to have extensive ossification of their costal cartilage rendering it useless. In our opinion, these complex cases deserve the best possible results, and patients will ultimately be better off if the surgeon elects to not compromise their choice of graft material in an effort to save the patient a short costal scar. In our experience, cadaver cartilage absorbs over time.

The goal in composite reconstruction is to restore the cartilaginous support to the nose. The problem is that large costal cartilage grafts carved to restore the dorsum are time consuming, frequently warp, and can provide a less-than-ideal dorsal appearance unless executed perfectly. Further, reconstruction of the columellar–tip complex if performed en bloc has a minimal margin of error (Figure 23-4). Composite reconstruction was designed to overcome many of these problems by splitting the operation into two separate components: a rigid deep foundation layer and a more superficial aesthetic layer. The *deep foundation layer* replicates the structural support provided by the septum/cartilaginous vault. The *superficial aesthetic layer* allows maximum flexibility in achieving the desired tip and dorsal contour. Fascia-wrapped diced cartilage grafts have become extremely useful for this purpose. The addition of a distinctly independent columellar strut allows one to push down the columellar labial angle, achieve additional nasal length, and project the nasal tip above the dorsal line.

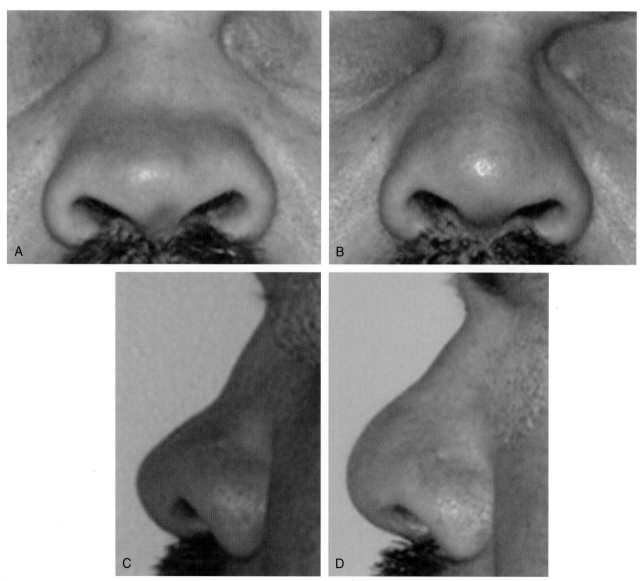

Figure 23-4 Pre- and postoperative photos of a patient with saddle nose repair.

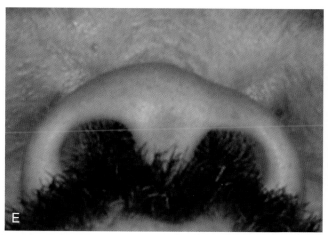
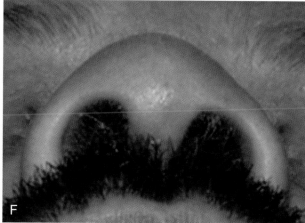

Figure 23-4, cont'd.

SUMMARY

Saddle nose deformity is perhaps one of the most challenging problem in all of rhinoplasty surgery. It requires correction of both form and function while providing the least amount of tissue to work with. The authors have found that composite reconstruction, using autogenous tissues, can provide excellent results for these very difficult problems.

Ultimately, autogenous rib reconstruction becomes the only option and it serves as both structural framework and aesthetic contour. One important question is, What is the reconstructive surgeon's obligation—to provide rigid support to the nose or simple cosmetic camouflage? It is our belief that the surgeon should re-create a strong supportive nose using the patient's own tissues that will last a lifetime.

REFERENCES

1. Daniel RK, Brenner KA. Saddle nose deformity: A new classification and treatment. *Fac Plast Surg Clin North Am.* 2006;14(4):301–312.
2. Shipchandler TZ, Chung BJ, Alam DS. Saddle nose deformity reconstruction with a split calvarial bone L-shaped strut. *Arch Fac Plast Surg.* 2008;10(5):305–311.
3. Mutaf M. The anatomic replication technique (ART): A new approach in saddle nose correction. *Ann Plast Surg.* 2008; 61(2):169–177.
4. Taylor SM, Rigby MH. The Taylor saddle effacement: A new technique for correction of saddle nose deformity. *J Otolaryngol Head Neck Surg.* 2008;37(1):105–111.
5. Acarturk TO, Kivanc O. Correction of saddle nose deformity in ectodermal dysplasia. *J Craniofac Surg.* 2007;18(5): 1179–1182.
6. Emsen IM. New and detailed classification of saddle nose deformities: Step-by-step surgical approach using the current techniques for each group. *Aesthet Plast Surg.* 2008;32(2): 274–285. Epub 2007 Sep 21.
7. Bilen BT, Kilinç H. Reconstruction of saddle nose deformity with three-dimensional costal cartilage graft. *J Craniofac Surg.* 2007;18(3):511–515.
8. Daniel RK. Rhinoplasty: Septal saddle nose deformity and composite reconstruction. *Plast Reconstr Surg.* 2007;119(3): 1029–1043.
9. Akikusa JD, Schneider R. Saddle nose deformity in a patient with Crohn's disease. *J Laryngol Otol.* 2006;120(3):253; author reply 253–254.
10. Converse J. Saddle noses, noses with a depressed dorsum, and flat noses. In: Converse J, ed. *Reconstructive plastic surgery.* Philadelphia: WB Saunders; 1977:1135.
11. Weir R. On restoring sunken noses. *N Y Med J* Oct 1892; 499.
12. Vartanian AJ, Thomas JR. www.emdicine.com/ent/topic121.htm
13. Tardy ME. *Rhinoplasty: The art and science.* Philadelphia: Saunders; 1997.
14. Gerow FJ, Stal S, Spira M. The totem pole rib graft reconstruction of the nose. *Ann Plast Surg.* 1983;11(4): 273–281.
15. Yabe T, Muraoka M. Treatment of saddle type nasal fracture using Kirschner wire fixation of nasal septum. *Ann Plast Surg.* 2004;53(1):89–92.
16. Drumheller GW. The push down operation and septal surgery. In: Daniel RK, ed. Aesthetic plastic surgery: Rhinoplasty. Boston: Little, Brown; 1973.
17. Tardy ME, Schwartz MS, Parras G. Saddle nose deformity: Autogenous graft repair. *Fac Plast Surg.* 1989;6:121.
18. Burget G. Aesthetic restoration of the nose. *Clin Plast Surg.* 1985;12:463.
19. Sessions DG, Stallings JO. Correction of saddle nose deformity. *Laryngoscope.* 1972;82(11):2000–2007.
20. Daniel RK, Calvert JC. Diced cartilage in rhinoplasty surgery. *Plast Reconstr Surg.* 2004;113:2156.
21. Daniel RK. Aesthetic plastic surgery: Rhinoplasty. Boston: Little, Brown; 1993.
22. Daniel RK. *Rhinoplasty: An atlas of surgical techniques.* New York: Springer, 2002.
23. Gunter JP, Rhorich RJ, Adams WP. *Dallas rhinoplasty.* St Louis: Quality Medical Publishing; 2002.
24. Sheen JH, Sheen AP. *Aesthetic rhinoplasty.* St Louis: Mosby; 1987.

25. Daniel RK. Rhinoplasty and rib grafts. Evolving a flexible operative technique. *Plast Reconstr Surg.* 1994;94:597.

26. Kim DW, Toriumi DM. Management of posttraumatic nasal deformities: The crooked nose and saddle nose. *Fac Plast Surg Clin North Am.* 2004;12:111–132.

27. Kelly MH, Bulstrode NW, Waterhouse N. Versatility of deiced cartilage-fascia grafts in dorsal nasal augmentation. *Plast Reconstr Surg.* In press.

28. Toriumi DM, Ries WR. Innovative surgical management of the crooked nose. *Fac Plast Clin.* 1993;1:63.

CHAPTER TWENTY-FOUR

The Large Nose

Minas Constantinides • Frank P. Fechner

Reduction rhinoplasty has been the main objective for the majority of cosmetic rhinoplasties performed in Caucasians over many decades. Rhinoplasty experts today have a much better understanding of the intricate relationships between anatomic changes and rhinoplasty outcomes than previous generations of nasal surgeons. Although Aufricht's observation that rhinoplasty is "an easy operation to do, but it is hard to get good results" still holds true, the end results of cosmetic nasal operations have become more predictable. Modern aesthetic goals for a normal looking nose have made today's "reduction rhinoplasty" a different operation than it was just 25 years ago. The goals of patients who are interested in cosmetic rhinoplasty reflect these modern insights. Today, patients specifically ask not to have pinched, scooped-out, or upturned noses, common consequences of older rhinoplasty techniques. Our informed patients are looking for better looking and better functioning noses devoid of signs of prior surgery. The request for a smaller nose is as commonplace today as it was in the past. The majority of primary rhinoplasty patients are concerned that their noses are too big. Only the nuanced discussion during the consultation will reveal that "too big" of today is not the "too big" of the past; it may simply mean poor tip definition or a nasal hump. Even African Americans or Asians who will benefit from augmentation rhinoplasty may describe their noses as large, for lack of a better descriptor. If used judiciously and honestly, preoperative photoanalysis and computer photoimaging can add value to the educational preparation for the patient and clarity for the surgeon.

DEFINITION

"A nose that is too big for the patient's face" is our definition of the large nose. We consider a nose large if the tip is overprojected *and* the dorsum is too high. Given these characteristics, the large nose is almost exclusively encountered in Caucasian patients. Commonly, other related issues need attention for a balanced outcome, including rotation and refinement of the tip, width of the nasal vault, and configuration of the alar base. Although a variety of bony and soft tissue facial dimensions have been established to describe facial size and proportions, most experienced rhinoplasty surgeons rarely use exact measurements to analyze a nose before rhinoplasty. It is rather their aesthetic sense and experience that most surgeons use to prepare for the operation. This "eye" of the rhinoplasty surgeon for what looks good reflects his or her knowledge of ideals in facial angles and dimensions, personal judgment, and aesthetic goals. A woman, for instance, with a prominent nose and receding chin may benefit from both reduction rhinoplasty and chin enhancement. It depends on her other facial characteristics, ethnicity, body habitus and height, as well as the surgeon's own aesthetic sense and biases. A surgeon's bias is rarely discussed as affecting their rhinoplasty result, but it is clear that a surgeon practicing in southern California often has a very different goal for their female rhinoplasty patient than if he or she had been practicing in New York. A surgeon's judgment is colored by the demands of what patients have requested over years of practice mixed with their own definition of beauty.

AESTHETICS AND ANALYSIS

Requests for correction of the large nose are commonly encountered in patients of southern European and Middle Eastern decent. Assessment of the large nose hinges on overall facial proportions, and the patient's stature, race, and gender. Men have more robust nasal features than women. The rotation of the male tip (90 to 95 degrees) should be less than the female (95 and 110 degrees). A tall and athletic man benefits from a nose that is on the large end of the spectrum of male aesthetics. A nose that is too small for a tall man will appear more unnatural and worse than a larger nose. For a petite woman, on the other hand, a rather small and delicate nose with tip rotation at the upper end of normal may appear just right.

Although experienced rhinoplasty surgeons rely on their judgment when considering overall nasal proportions, they also incorporate established norms in their nasal analysis.

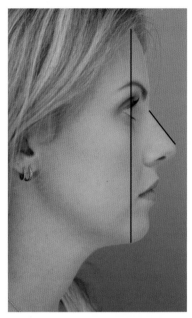

Figure 24-1 Nasal length, as measured from the nasion to the tip-defining point, should approximate the height of one-third of the face.

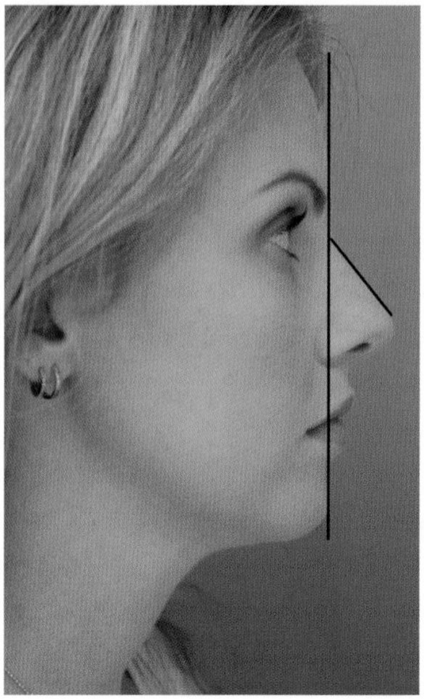

Figure 24-2 The aesthetic facial angle (as described by Joseph) is formed by the intersection of a vertical line dropped from the glabella with a line from the nasion to tip-defining point. Tip projection is optimal with an angle of 30 degrees.

NASAL PROFILE LENGTH

As measured from the nasion to the tip-defining point, nasal length should approximate one-third of the height of the face from hairline to menton (Figure 24-1).[1]

RADIX POSITION AND NASOFRONTAL ANGLE

The radix, or root, of the nose is a synonym for the nasion, the gentle depression where the nose meets the forehead. The angle that is formed by the forehead and nose is the nasofrontal angle. It is usually between 115 and 130 degrees. Too shallow an angle creates a "Greek" nose, with the forehead sloping directly into the nasal dorsum. Another useful angle is the nasofacial angle. This angle is formed between the dorsal line and a vertical line traversing the nasion. Called the aesthetic profile angle by Jacques Joseph (who actually had a device to measure it directly) and renamed the nasofacial angle today, this angle ideally measures from 30 to 35 degrees (Figure 24-2).[2]

More relevant is the relative height of the radix. The ideal level lies at the upper eyelash line in women and slightly higher in men. The height of the radix directly affects nasal length: the higher the radix, the longer the nose. Today (and throughout time) a long, elegant profile is the aesthetic ideal. Adjusting the height of the radix is an important step in achieving this ideal (Figure 24-3).

NASAL PROFILE PROJECTION

Projection of the tip is the actual measured distance from the alar–facial plane to the tip. A change in nasal projection requires either an increase or decrease in the distance the nasal tip extends from the vertical facial plane. The Goode method and the 3:4:5 triangle are the two most common ways of measuring projection.

THE GOODE METHOD

As described by Goode, nasal projection as measured from the alar–facial crease should be 60% of nasal length. A vertical axis is drawn from nasion to alar groove intersecting a horizontal line from the alar groove to the tip. A ratio can be expressed as ala-tip–nasion-tip equaling 0.55 to 0.60. This ratio correlates well with an aesthetically balanced nasal projection (Figure 24-4).[1]

THE 3:4:5 TRIANGLE

Crumley and Lanser demonstrated a relationship between nasal length and desired tip projection as forming a 3:4:5 right triangle. The vertical line is dropped from the nasion and the hypotenuse is a line drawn from the nasion to the tip. The ratio of the horizontal line (from vertical facial plane to tip) to the nasal dorsal line (hypotenuse) should be 3:5 or 0.60 (Figure 24-5).[3] This is in accordance with the measurements proposed by Goode.

NASAL TIP ROTATION

Simons describes rotation of the nasal tip as an arc with the radius maintained.[4] As the tip is rotated, there is some illusion of increased projection, although none exists

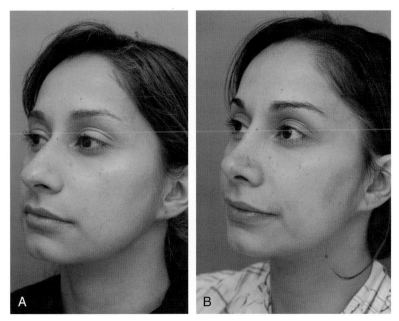

Figure 24-3 A, Preoperative left oblique view illustrating a low radix, making the bridge appear short. Since the apparent nasal start point is at the hump and the tip is dependent, the nose appears bottom-heavy. **B,** The 19-month postoperative left oblique view illustrating higher radix, with a longer, more elegant profile. The nose is no longer bottom-heavy, so attention is directed to the eyes. Radix augmentation was achieved with diced cartilage wrapped with temporalis fascia.

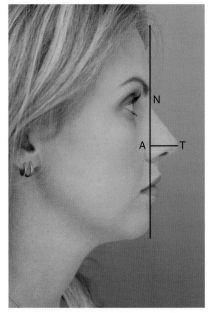

Figure 24-4 Goode's method. Vertical axis is from nasion to the alar groove. The horizontal line is from ala to the tip. Nasal projection should be 60% of nasal length. This is expressed as a ratio with ala-tip–nasion-tip equaling 0.55 to 0.60.

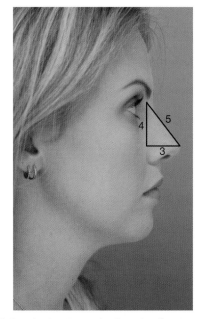

Figure 24-5 In the 3:4:5 triangle, the ratio of projection to length is represented by the ratio 3:5. In accordance with Goode's method, nasal projection is 60% of nasal length.

(Figure 24-6). Tip rotation is defined as the tip angle from the vertical alar crease through the tip. In women this angle is approximately 105 degrees, and in men, it is 100 degrees. The degree of rotation may be affected by the intrinsic properties of the nasal tip (lower lateral cartilages) or external properties (caudal septum).

NASOLABIAL ANGLE AND COLUMELLA

The nasolabial angle is the angle formed between the columella and upper lip. Ideally, the nasolabial angle is 90 to 95 degrees in men and 95 to 110 degrees in women (Figure 24-7).[5] It is affected by two major

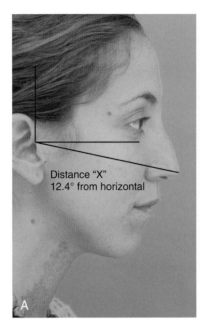
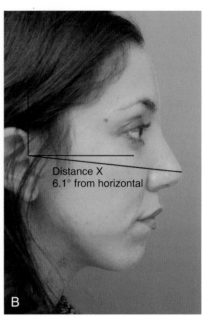

Distance "X"
12.4° from horizontal

Distance X
6.1° from horizontal

A

B

Figure 24-6 As described by Simons, as the nasal tip rotates through an arc, there is an apparent increase in nasal projection, although none exists. **A,** "X" is the distance from the tragus to the nasal tip. The angle from the horizontal is 12.4 degrees. **B,** The distance from tragus to tip remains the same while the angle from the horizontal significantly decreases to 6.1 degrees. The illusion is one of increased projection while all that has occurred is increased rotation.

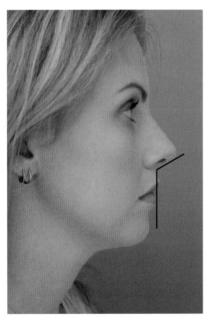

Figure 24-7 The nasolabial angle is formed between the columella and upper lip. Ideally, the nasolabial angle is 90 to 95 degrees in men and 95 to 105 degrees in women.

parameters—the caudal septum as it meets the nasal spine and the relative position of the columella. A prominent caudal septum and/or nasal spine will push the upper philtrum of the lip out, effacing the nasolabial angle and making it more obtuse (Figure 24-8). A deficient caudal septum at its posterior angle (as seen in platyrhine noses,

for example) creates a more retracted, acute nasolabial angle (Figure 24-9).

Columellar position may be classified as retracted, neutral, or hanging. Ideally, 2 to 4 mm of columellar show on lateral view is normal. A retracted columella occurs with upwardly displaced medial crura. This may occur from either a deficiency of the mid-portion of the caudal septum alone or in conjunction with a cephalically rotated tip. A hanging columella occurs either from an overdeveloped caudal septum pushing the medial crura inferiorly (as in a tension nose), or from weak medial crural support (typical of a full transfixion incision without subsequent re-support of the medial crural complex) (Figure 24-10).

OVERALL FACIAL APPEARANCE AND THE NOSE

Changes in the size of the nose immediately affect the appearance of other parts of the face, namely the lips and chin. On the contrary, alterations to the lips, chin, and even neck may influence apparent nasal size. It is relatively common to see a patient with a convex facial profile where the nose receives overwhelming attention. The large nose may appear more pronounced by limited forehead projection, microgenia, and submental fullness. By enhancing chin projection and neck definition, the overall prominence of the nose is seemingly decreased. Through these ancillary procedures, less dramatic nasal reduction may be required for a balanced facial profile (Figure

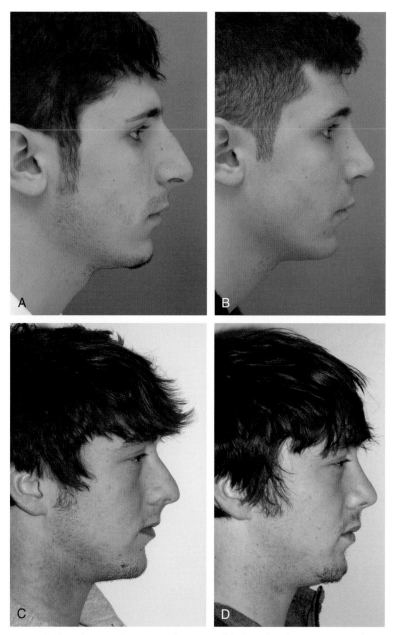

Figure 24-8 A, C, Preoperative right lateral views illustrating obtuse nasolabial angles due to excessively prominent posterior septal angle. **B, D,** Postoperative right lateral views illustrating more acute nasolabial angles, creating more attractive lines between nose and upper lip.

24-11). Similarly, in this situation, reduction rhinoplasty alone can help improve the facial balance and will make the weak chin less apparent. Because we prefer to strive for normal facial balance, we would recommend chin enhancement in conjunction with reduction rhinoplasty. Commonly, patients may not be aware of their microgenia but rather focus exclusively on the nose. Computer photoimaging can be extremely helpful in demonstrating the advantage of a balanced facial profile. At the very least, it uncovers the patient's own aesthetic preferences and ensures that both surgeon and patient share the same aesthetic and surgical goals.

PHYSICAL EXAMINATION

The preoperative examination will prevent many unsatisfactory results and establish a precise surgical plan. The nose is considered within the overall facial anatomy. Does the patient have rather bold facial features such as high cheeks, strong jaw, and full lips, or rather a delicate appearance? How do chin projection and the neck definition fit into the overall facial profile with the nose? How does the nose complement or detract from other features? In particular, does it distract from the beauty of the eyes?

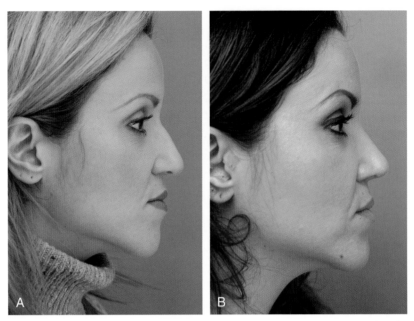

Figure 24-9 A, Preoperative left lateral view illustrating acute, deep nasolabial angle from congenitally underdeveloped posterior septal angle and nasal spine. **B,** One-year postoperative view illustrating improvement of appearance from both tip rotation and filling of nasolabial angle with cartilage grafts.

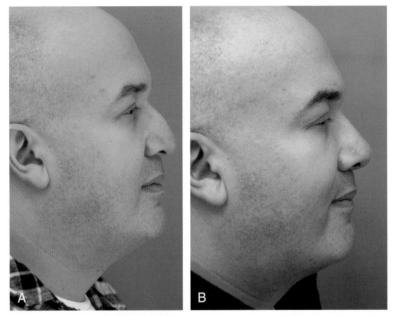

Figure 24-10 A, Preoperative right lateral view illustrating a hanging columella from weak medial crural strength. **B,** One-year postoperative view with improved columellar strength and length after tongue-in-groove and tip-grafting techniques.

The quality of the skin requires accurate assessment when considering reducing a large nose. If the skin is relatively thin and elastic, it may more readily follow structural changes made to the underlying bone and cartilage. But when the skin is thick and stiff, it may not contract readily around a smaller nasal skeleton, leading to poor tip definition. In thick-skinned patients, an overzealous reduction is ill advised.

Next, the nose is analyzed in the frontal view where straightness and width are assessed. This examination is best subdivided in thirds starting from the top. The top third is mostly represented by the bony nasal vault. Is the width appropriate or too wide? Both dorsal width and ventral width are considered. Dorsal width is the plateau of the nasal bones; ventral width corresponds to the nasofacial grooves. An upper third that is too narrow overall

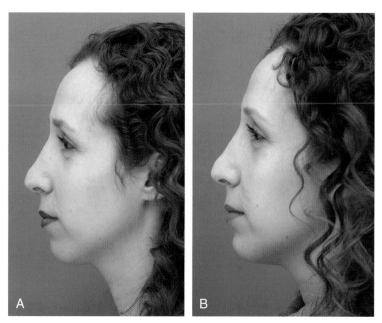

Figure 24-11 A, Retruded chin with a prominent nose exaggerates overall facial imbalance. **B,** Chin implantation alone will partially restore facial balance, even without rhinoplasty.

is extremely rare in primary rhinoplasty but may be seen in secondary cases. More commonplace is an upper third in which one nasal bone has been depressed by injury while the other has been elevated, creating a deviation to one side.

The middle third is largely determined by the relationship of the upper lateral cartilages to caudal ends of the nasal bones and the cartilaginous septum. Is it too wide, normal, or collapsed? What is the side wall's internal resilience? A collapsed or weak middle third may lead to internal valve collapse after reduction rhinoplasty if precautions are not taken.

The lobular lower third has to be assessed for tip configuration, symmetry, length, projection, and width. The need for alar base reductions can often be predicted during the initial examination.

Last, the profile view is studied. Starting from the top, the nasion, or radix, is evaluated. If too deep, it can be augmented. If too shallow, it can be carved out. A deep nasion commonly presents with a nasal hump. After filling of the nasion, less of a dorsal reduction may be needed for a straight profile of the upper two thirds.

COMPUTER PHOTOIMAGING

As with any cosmetic procedure, it is important to understand goals, desires, and expectations of the rhinoplasty patient. The patient needs to understand what he or she can expect from the cosmetic nasal operation. The patient's satisfaction after the procedure will in part be determined by the surgeon's success in laying out these goals beforehand. Photoimaging plays an adjunctive role in showing the patient a predictive image of his or her nose after a successful rhinoplasty. It is advisable for the surgeon to demonstrate a conservative result rather than an overly perfect one. Most patients understand that a computer-generated image is not real life, but they still may expect such a result. Computer imaging has proved useful to determine the extent of nasal reduction. Commonly, a patient bothered by his large nose will desire a nose that objectively may be too small for his face, and beyond what realistic surgery can achieve.

We image the nose in two views: the lateral and the worst oblique. Invariably, one oblique view will look better than the other; we choose the worst-looking one in order to show greatest possible improvement. This often corresponds to the side that the patient sees as his worst side when taking photographs. Many patients request frontal imaging, but this is often the most difficult view to image accurately with the least distortion. If helpful, base-view imaging can also be accurate and demonstrate improvements in tip symmetry, base and lobular width, and tip definition.

Imaging can also help solve certain planning dilemmas. If the radix is low, does the patient like the appearance of the dorsal line with the radix low or high? How much dorsal reduction looks good to the patient? Is a straight dorsal line desired, or does the patient prefer a supratip break? Does the middle third need to be substantially widened or just subtly supported? How much tip rotation looks best? Once the desired images are obtained, we typically either print them for the patient to take home, or burn them onto a CD as jpeg files. In patients who are dissatisfied with their surgical outcome, we have never found that it is because of the preoperative imaging.

Photoimaging is an excellent communication and planning tool that is invaluable during rhinoplasty planning for surgeon and patient alike.

ANESTHESIA

There are multiple anesthesia options available for a reduction rhinoplasty operation. Most commonly, the rhinoplasty surgeon has his or her personal preferences based on training and personal experience. Today, many surgeons prefer nasal surgery under general inhalation anesthesia. Advantages include total analgesia, hypnosis, and protection of the patient's airway. Side effects like intraoperative vasodilation and postoperative nausea and vomiting can jeopardize the outcome of a rhinoplasty. In addition, many patients perceive general anesthesia as risky and invasive.

We prefer conscious sedation via the intravenous route. Sometimes, local anesthesia with preoperative premedication can provide an attractive alternative to deeper modes of anesthesia. Independent of anesthesia mode, the decongestion and anesthesia of the nose are achieved with endonasal placement of 4% cocaine-soaked packs followed by injection of 1% to 2% lidocaine with 1 : 100,000 epinephrine as regional and local blocks. Appropriate management of the intraoperative blood pressure by an experienced anesthesiologist will further minimize bleeding. Placement of small tampons into the posterior nasal passages and choanae will provide appropriate minimization of posterior oozing into the pharynx. The tampon strings are kept attached and brought out of the nostril to prevent the tampon's inadvertent aspiration.

SURGICAL TECHNIQUE

The sequence that rhinoplasty surgery is performed varies from surgeon to surgeon. Some surgeons start creating the new dorsal line of the nose starting from the top down, with the nasal tip being addressed last. Alternatively, if the open rhinoplasty approach is used, tip projection can be set first and the upper third of the nose addressed at the end. In endonasal rhinoplasty, this bottom-up sequence is often not feasible given the difficulty of exposure after dome binding and tip definition have been completed. To facilitate a systematic discussion, we will address surgical technique questions by the three segments of the nose: upper, middle, and lower thirds.

UPPER THIRD OF THE NOSE

The upper nasal anatomy is determined by the bony nasal vault, which includes the maxillary frontal processes and the confluence of the nasal bones with the bony nasal septum. The large nose usually presents with a bony nasal

hump and wide nasal bones. Sometimes, the bony pyramid is shifted and requires straightening. The nasion may benefit from alterations.

Radix: Classically, the ideal position of the radix is at the level of the supratarsal crease when assessed in the side view. Although this guideline is helpful, minor deviations from the norm are common. Most commonly, the radix has acceptable position and depth before rhinoplasty and will not require alteration.

If the nasion is lacking depth, deepening can be achieved en bloc with the hump reduction (see later). To control the superior extent of the neoradix, a transcutaneous horizontal osteotomy with a 2-mm osteotome is helpful. Additional radix deepening can be achieved with radix rasps. The skin and soft tissue envelope of the radix is thicker than that of the remaining nose. Contracture of these soft tissues around a lowered radix is variable and it will not always lead to a one-to-one radix reduction.

For the deep radix, augmentation is indicated. Planning this maneuver before surgery is important because filling the deep radix is routinely performed after hump reduction. If hump removal is performed to the level of the radix, augmentation will not be possible or will lead to undesirable results. The preferred grafting material for nasion augmentation is autologous cartilage obtained from the nasal septum. In the rare case when no nasal septal cartilage is available (such as after a previous septoplasty), cartilage obtained from the cartilaginous nasal hump, cephalic trim, or ear concha can be used. The graft can be layered and sutured together to fill the deep nasal–frontal angle. The graft edges should be beveled or crushed to prevent the visibility of the radix graft. If concerns exist about postoperative graft shift or movement, a temporary transcutaneous suture is used. An even more novel radix graft may be created from temporalis fascia wrapped around diced cartilage. This graft shows great local stability, is moldable during early healing, and does not lead to a visible edge as in some solid radix augmentation grafts (see Figure 24-3).[6] The outcome of radix augmentation is more predictable than the reduction maneuver.

Bony hump: Reduction of a nasal hump is an integral part of rhinoplasty for the large nose. Virtually all nasal humps have a bony and a cartilaginous portion. Being part of the middle third of the nose, the cartilaginous hump is reduced sharply (see later) followed by bony reduction achieved with an osteotome, rasp, or the combination of both. Because most humps encountered in large noses require reduction by 2 mm or more, we favor the use of a flat osteotome (i.e., Rubin osteotome) first, followed by further incremental reductions with nasal rasps. The goal of hump removal is a straight nasal profile avoiding a stigmatizing overreduction. Performing hump reduction requires that the surgeon is able to follow the osteotome's path beneath the skin; even in the open approach, visualization of the bone cuts is limited. Once the osteotomy is completed and the reduction has been assessed, further bone reduction and smoothening are performed with nasal rasps. We prefer coarse and fine pull-action rasps used sequentially. Bone debris is aspirated and a smooth contour is ensured.

Nasal osteotomies: Usually performed at the completion of the rhinoplasty procedure, nasal osteotomies will narrow the upper nose. Because the nasal pyramid will appear wide after hump reduction, osteotomies play a vital role in reduction rhinoplasty by closing the "open roof" and producing an elegant nasal shape. Our most common osteotomy technique includes the high–to–low–to–high lateral bone cut followed by a possible medial osteotomy through an endonasal incision. Subperiosteal tunnels are developed to minimize postoperative bruising by periosteal rents and vessel injury. A curved, guarded 3-mm osteotome is used to create a continuous lateral osteotomy. Alternatively, a 2-mm straight unguarded osteotome may be used to create perforating osteotomies through an intranasal technique. Digital pressure applied to the nasal bones leads to the desired infracture of the bony segment. For a bone that does not produce the desired narrowing, we reconfirm that a complete lateral osteotomy was performed or outfracture the bony plate followed by a repeated infracture. Rarely, a 2-mm percutaneous osteotomy may be required to complete the osteotomy. Important in performing lateral nasal osteotomies is to stay rather posterior within the nasal process of the maxilla and not come too anterior lest the osteotomy be visible.[7]

MIDDLE THIRD OF THE NOSE

Aside from reduction of the cartilaginous hump, the middle third of the nose commonly requires limited work in management of the large nose. It rather follows somewhat passively changes produced by managing the upper and lower thirds.

Hump reduction: The cartilaginous dorsal hump is produced by the dorsal septal cartilage and its confluence with the upper lateral cartilages. Most of the hump is produced by the quadrangular cartilage; therefore, dorsal reduction of the septum after its separation from the upper lateral cartilages in the open rhinoplasty approach will produce effective hump removal. The integrity of the confluence is reestablished with 4-0 PDS sutures. Using the endonasal technique, separation of the upper lateral cartilages is not routinely performed. The horizontal aspect of the upper lateral cartilages is usually removed en bloc together with the dorsal septum. Entering the nasal cavity during hump reduction should be avoided.

Spreader grafts: Spreader grafts are routinely fashioned from autologous septal cartilage and placed between dorsal septum and upper lateral cartilages. They can serve four main goals: supporting weak upper lateral cartilages to maintain dorsal width, widening of the dorsal middle third width, opening of the internal nasal valve, and camouflaging or straightening of a curved dorsal septum. Spreader grafts can be layered for additional width and should be flush with the height of the septum after being secured in place with 4-0 PDS sutures. They are easier placed using the open approach. Endonasally, spreader grafts can also be placed into tight-fitting pockets between dorsal septal mucoperichondrium and septal cartilage without suturing (Figure 24-12).

LOWER THIRD OF THE NOSE

The nasal tip of the large nose commonly is overprojected and bulbous. In addition to deprojection and tip definition, goals of nasal tip improvements also commonly involve adjustments to tip rotation. Balanced relationships of columella to alar margins should be ensured but rarely require additional maneuvers in the large nose. Finally, appropriate alar width is ensured.

PROJECTION

Large noses are usually overprojected. Whenever the nasal tip is altered, special consideration has to be paid to tip support. Although various major and minor tip support structures have been identified, their individual importance varies from patient to patient.

Patients with a tension tip deformity have an overprojected nose secondary to an overdeveloped quadrangular cartilage, both dorsally and caudally. In a tension nose, the anterior septal angle represents the highest point of the nasal tip. Indeed, the height of the septum is the main tip-support mechanism in this case. When it is reduced as part of the hump treatment to a level below the domes, it alone will lead to effective deprojection. In addition, separating the medial crura from and shortening the caudal septum will further weaken tip support. Indeed, excessive loss of projection is a danger in these noses.[8] Often, the tension nose presents with a prominent posterior septal angle and/or nasal spine. Resection of this can improve definition of the lip–columella transition.

When the lower lateral cartilages are strong and prominent, tip deprojection and appropriate adjustment of rotation will need to be managed by alterations to this cartilage pair. Deprojection can be achieved by reducing the length and strength of the lower lateral cartilage. According to Anderson's tripod concept,[9] shortening the medial crura (i.e., resection or weakening of the footplates) will deproject the tip and decrease rotation. More commonly, we use the versatile lobule division followed by suture overlay of the lower lateral cartilages. The extent of overlay will determine deprojection and tip rotation. The location of lobule division (lateral, intermediate, or medial crus) will further influence rotation (Figures 24-13 and 24-14).[10]

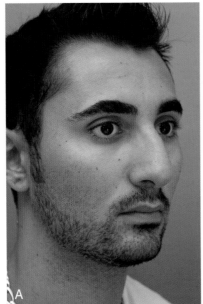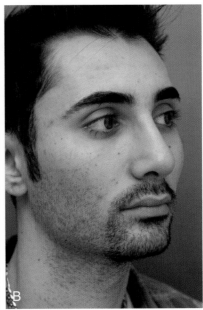

Figure 24-12 A, Right oblique preoperative view illustrating large nose with large bony and cartilaginous hump in a tension nose. **B,** One year postoperative view. Bony and cartilaginous hump reduction and lateral osteotomies were accompanied by spreader grafts to stabilize the upper lateral cartilages.

ROTATION

Conservative cephalic trims of the lateral crura usually represent the first step in tip modification. At least 7 mm of cartilage width should be maintained at the widest point. This maneuver by itself will lead to moderate tip definition and minimal tip rotation. Tip rotation can be further changed by strategic adjustment of the caudal septum: if a triangle of cartilage with its base at the dorsal septum is excised, the tip will rotate up; if the triangle base is posterior, caudal rotation will be the consequence due to weakening of the medial crural footplate attachments. Most commonly in the large nose, we prefer to alter rotation and projection simultaneously by lobule division techniques. After dividing the lateral crus and shortening the cartilage strip through overlap and suturing, rotation and deprojection will result. If the medial crus is divided, caudal rotation and deprojection will be controlled by the extent of crural overlay. Division of the intermediate crus leads to only small rotational changes and primarily decreases projection. A similar impact can be achieved by simultaneously dividing and shortening both the medial and lateral crura. The advantages of the lobule division technique include complete control of projection and definition while recreating a double-layer strong continuous cartilaginous strip. The domes are usually not divided to minimize risks for bossae and tip asymmetries.

TIP DEFINITION

Many large noses will present with a wide, bulbous, or boxy tip, making tip sculpting techniques imperative. After conservative cephalic trims have been performed and tip projection and rotation have been set, double-dome binding sutures are commonly used. These horizontal mattress sutures of 4-0 or 5-0 Prolene set the domes to the most desirable position. In thin-skinned patients, care is taken to ensure that the lateral crus lateral to the suture is not indented to guard against surface shadows, telltale signs of rhinoplasty (see Figure 24-15). Tip grafts are rarely necessary in the large nose. Final definition of the tip will in part be determined by the skin thickness.

ALAR BASE REDUCTION

Although the need for alar base reduction is usually determined preoperatively, this step is always performed at the end of the procedure. Because alar base reductions are virtually impossible to reverse, a conservative approach is best. If in doubt, it can also be performed as an office procedure once the first stages of healing are completed. Alar base reduction is useful in narrowing the alar width and/or decreasing nostril flare, which may increase with tip deprojection.

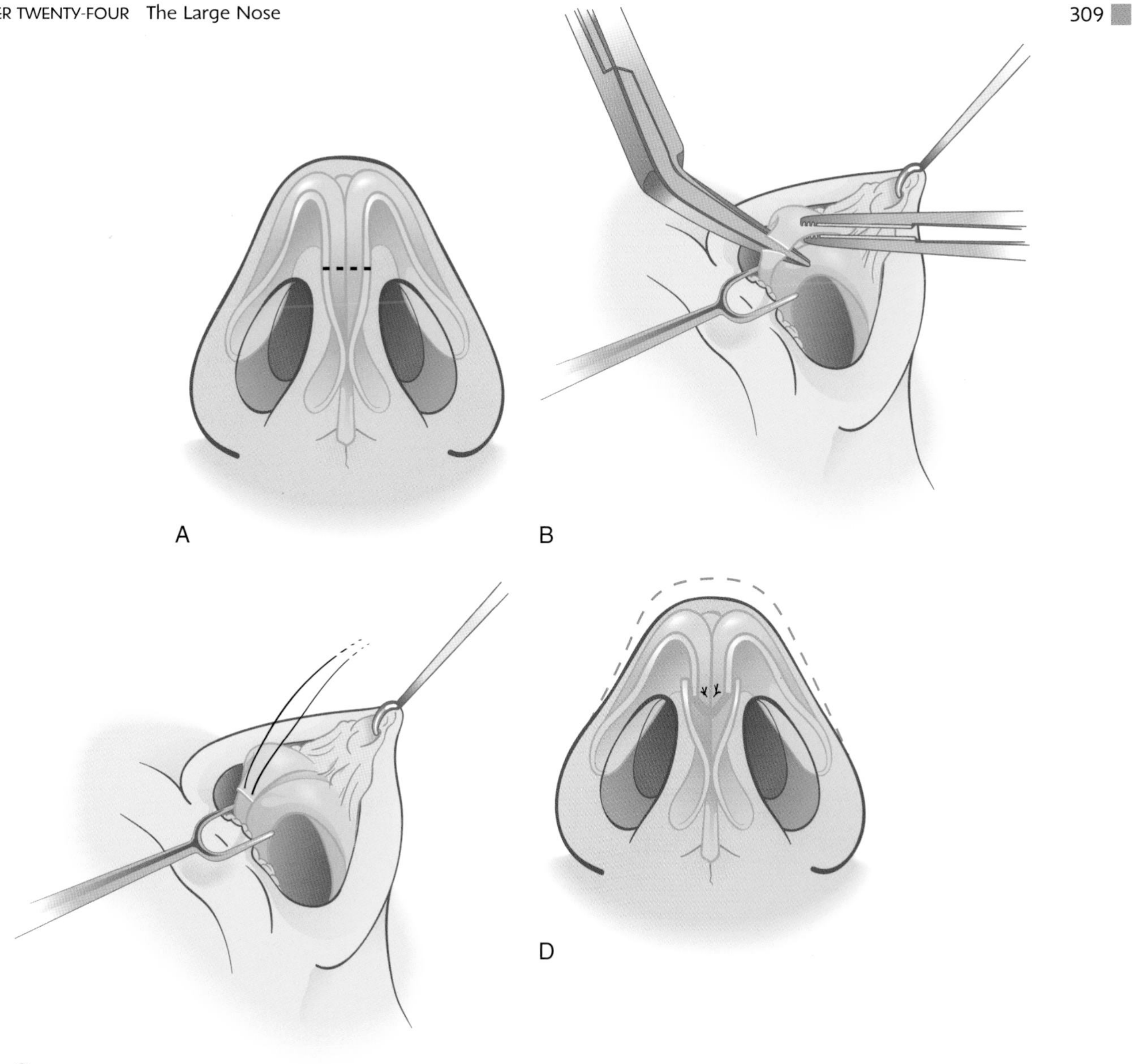

Figure 24-13 A, Schematic base view of the overprojected nose. **B,** The tip scissors have cut through the alar cartilage, dividing it at the angle, or the junction of the medial and intermediate crura. **C,** A horizontal mattress suture has been placed after the intermediate crus has been overlapped over the medial crus. Typically, 6-0 nylon is used. **D,** Base view shows the achieved deprojection.

The alar base is best reduced by creating a medial advancement rotation flap of the ala. A portion of the nostril sill can be excised, and then an incision carried laterally just above the alar–facial groove. The ala can then be rotated into the defect left on the sill. If flare is present, an additional excision of the caudal cut edge of the ala can be performed prior to closure.[11]

COMPLICATIONS SPECIFIC TO THE LARGE NOSE

Although general complications in rhinoplasty will be discussed extensively in other chapters of this book, there are specific complications of reducing the large nose that warrant discussing here.

UPPER THIRD COMPLICATIONS

Complications of the upper third are complications involving osteotomies. The most common is the open roof deformity, occurring most frequently after large hump reductions with a Ruben osteotome. When a high nasal dorsum is reduced, a gap is created between the nasal bones. If lateral osteotomies are insufficient to close the gap, a visible and palpable ridge will result where the overlying soft tissue is unsupported. If such a gap is noticed in the operating room, repeating the lateral osteotomy

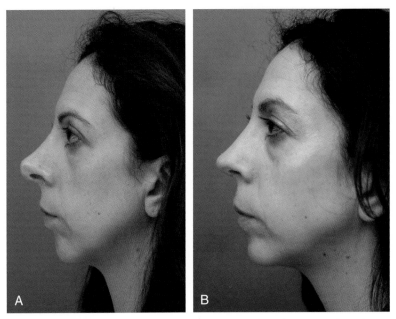

Figure 24-14 A, Preoperative left lateral view illustrating an overprojected, over-rotated tip after primary rhinoplasty, creating a nose that is too short. **B,** The 20-month postoperative view after vertical lobule division, creating a less-projected, less-rotated tip and a longer, balanced profile.

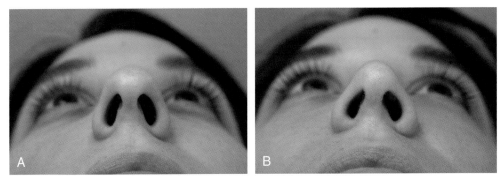

Figure 24-15 A, Preoperative base view with wide domal angle and convex lateral crura in thin-skinned patient. **B,** One-year postoperative base view after dome-binding and interdomal sutures. The domal angle is reduced but the crura lateral to the domes are flat, not concave, creating a strong, natural-appearing tip.

lower and performing complete medial osteotomies will often close the gap. If not, then the gap may be filled with either crushed cartilage or cephalic trim cartilage.

Such large gaps in the bones may also be accompanied by inadvertent resection of the mucosa beneath the bones, creating a fistula between the skin flap and the nasal cavity. Packing this area off with crushed cartilage or soft tissue will allow the underlying mucosal edges to seal themselves off from the nasal superstructure.

If the nasal bones are overly narrowed because of nasal bone collapse after osteotomies, then a pinched and abnormal upper vault will result. One effective way to stabilize the collapsing bone is to place a long spreader graft beneath it. If this is not feasible, then packing the bone up temporarily may suffice. One effective material is oxidized cellulose gauze (Surgicel, Ethicon, Somerville, NJ) moistened with antibiotic ointment.

Overly lowering the dorsum with a Ruben osteotome occasionally occurs to even the experienced surgeon. Indeed, one technique is to resect the bony dorsum, rasp the deep surface, and then replace the dorsal segment. Such a technique is more technically challenging than sequential dorsal lowering with rasps but is a valuable option in the event of overaggressive en bloc resection of the dorsum (Figure 24-16).

Overaggressive deepening of the radix with osteotomies can also yield surprises. Tardy described a technique by which an osteotomy is first made into the frontal bone in the midline to the radix, and then the dorsal osteotomy is carried up to meet.[12] With this procedure, care must be

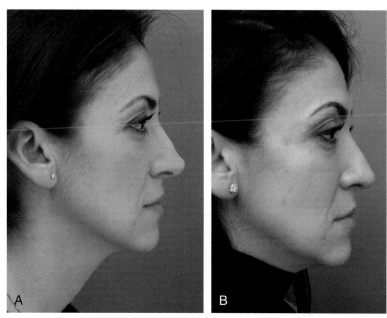

Figure 24-16 A, Preoperative right profile view illustrating high bony profile with supratip saddle due to trauma. **B,** Postoperative view. During the dorsal reduction with a Ruben osteotome, too much lowering was achieved. On the table, the excised dorsum was rasped on its undersurface and then replaced. The result illustrates an acceptable dorsal contour. Note that tip deprojection without rotation was achieved by vertical lobule division with overlap at the angle, the junction of the intermediate with the medial crus.

taken not to carry the osteotomy too acutely into a well-pneumatized frontal bone lest the frontal sinus be encountered.

MIDDLE THIRD COMPLICATIONS

Upper lateral cartilage destabilization leading to contour deformity, the most severe being the inverted-V deformity, is commonly seen with large nose rhinoplasty. Strong stabilization of the upper lateral cartilages with spreader grafts is almost always required after large dorsal reductions. Both this deformity, and nasal bone deformities discussed earlier, are amenable to correction with injectable fillers to mask the shadowing created by the instability.

LOWER THIRD COMPLICATIONS

In tension noses, inadequately stabilizing the medial crura will result in delayed postoperative tip ptosis with a resultant pollybeak. Overreducing tip projection in thick-skinned patients will result in loss of tip definition and a worse aesthetic outcome. Both of these problems are avoided when the medial crura are well stabilized and supported. Commonly, a columellar strut graft is used for this. However, in many tips even this is not adequate, and the more secure tongue-in-groove technique yields stronger support for a more predictable tip position.[13]

CONCLUSIONS

Although operating on the large nose is simply performing more reduction than a typical reduction rhinoplasty, there are unique challenges presented by this type of rhinoplasty. Communicating and making clear what surgery can and cannot do is aided by computer photoimaging. Surgical techniques that ensure stability and predictability are more likely to result in achieving the expected result. In the end, by creating a more balanced nose, the focus of the observer will revert to the eyes and improve how the whole face looks. Ultimately, this goal is what leads to the highest degree of patient satisfaction.

REFERENCES

1. Powell N, Humphreys B. *Proportions of the aesthetic face.* New York: Thieme-Stratton; 1984.
2. Joseph J. *Rhinoplasty and facial plastic surgery with a supplement on mammaplasty; English translation by Stanley Milstein.* Phoenix: Columella Press; 1987.
3. Crumley RL, Lanser M. Quantitative analysis of nasal tip projection. *Laryngoscope.* 1988;98(2):202–208.
4. Simons RL. Nasal tip projection, ptosis and supratip thickening. *J Ear Nose Throat.* 1982;61(8):452–455.
5. Pearlman SJ. Surgical treatment of the nasolabial angle in balanced rhinoplasty. *Fac Plast Surg.* 2006;22(1):28–35.

6. Daniel RK, Calvert JC. Diced cartilage in rhinoplasty surgery. *Plast Reconstr Surg.* 2004;113:2156.

7. Kortbus MJ, Ham J, Fechner F, Constantinides M. Quantitative analysis of lateral osteotomies in rhinoplasty. *Arch Fac Plast Surg.* 2006;8:369–373.

8. Constantinides M, Levine J. Managing the tension nose. *Fac Plast Surg Clin North Am.* 2000;8(4):479–486.

9. Anderson JR. A reasoned approach to nasal base surgery. *Arch Otolaryngol Head Neck Surg.* 1984;110:349–358.

10. Constantinides M, Liu E, Miller PJ, Adamson PA. Vertical lobule division in open rhinoplasty: Maintaining an intact strip. *Arch Fac Plast Surg.* 2001;3:258–263.

11. Bennet GH, Lessow A, Song P, Constantinides M. The long-term effects of alar base reduction. *Arch Fac Plast Surg.* 2005;7(2):94–97.

12. Tardy ME. *Rhinoplasty: The art and the science.* Philadelphia: WB Saunders; 1997:313–318.

13. Kridel RW, Scott BA, Foda HM. The tongue-in-groove technique in septorhinoplasty: A 10 year experience. *Arch Fac Plast Surg.* 1999;1(4):246–256.

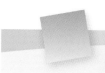

CHAPTER TWENTY-FIVE

The Underprojected Nose and Ptotic Tip

Vito C. Quatela • James M. Pearson

Surgery of the lower third of the nose represents one of the most challenging aspects of rhinoplasty. The nasal tip is a three-dimensional structure described in terms of projection, rotation, length, and shape. Each of these components must be considered to achieve an aesthetically pleasing result, which depends upon symmetry and proportion in relation to the rest of the nose and surrounding facial features.

The nasal tip is a dynamic structure, hinged by the upper lateral cartilages and by the recurvature of the lower lateral cartilages. Major and minor tip support mechanisms play a central role in tip stability and positioning. The nasal surgeon should be keenly aware of tip anatomy and also have a solid understanding of tip dynamics and factors that contribute to tip rotation and projection. He or she should appreciate the range of techniques available to affect tip position and possess the foresight to judge which techniques would be most advantageously applied to each case.

ANATOMY

The nasal tip is comprised of the paired lower lateral cartilages, or alar cartilages, which may be each divided into three crura: medial, middle, and lateral. Regarding terminology, the terms *medial segment of the lower lateral cartilage* and *medial crus* are synonymous. Likewise, the *lateral crus* is also called the *lateral segment of the lower lateral cartilage*. These terms are used interchangeably throughout the literature and in this chapter. The domal junction denotes the border between the lateral and middle crura, while the columellar junction separates the middle and medial crura. The dome itself is formed by the domal segment of the middle crus, which is situated adjacent and anterior to the lobular segment of the middle crus[1] (Figures 25-1 and 25-2).

A key component of nasal tip anatomy lies in the scrolled attachment of the cephalic margins of the lower lateral cartilages to the caudal margin of the upper lateral cartilages. This region is often affected during rhinoplasty, which results in weakening of this major source of tip support.

TIP UNDERPROJECTION AND UNDERROTATION/PTOSIS

Nasal tip projection is defined as the horizontal distance from the alar crease of the facial plane to the nasal tip on lateral view, or the posterior-to-anterior distance that the nasal tip extends in front of the facial plane as seen on basal view.[2] The analysis of tip projection may be undertaken using several different techniques.

One of the most commonly used measurements is the Goode method, which defines ideal tip projection as a ratio of the distance from the nasion to the tip-defining points. Using the Goode method, this ideal ratio of tip projection to nasal length is 0.55 to 0.6:1[3] (Figure 25-3, A). With Simons method, tip projection (defined as the distance between subnasale to the tip-defining point) should equal the height of the upper lip (subnasale to the vermillion border) (Figure 25-3, B). Crumley and Lanser described a right triangle with dimensions corresponding to nasal proportions; ideally projection:height:length is equal to 3:4:5. In other words, ideal tip projection is 75% of the nasal height, measured using a vertical line from the nasion to the nasal base (Figure 25-3, C). Powell and Humphries defined the ideal relationship between tip projection and nasal height as a 2.8:1 ratio (Figure 25-3, D). Byrd and Hobar proposed that ideal projection is two thirds of the ideal nasal length, which is itself ideally two thirds of the midfacial height.[3]

Nasal tip rotation is defined as movement of the nasal tip along an arc with constant distance from the facial plane[4] (Figure 25-4). A ptotic nasal tip may be otherwise described as underrotated. Thus, the terms *ptotic* and *underrotated* as applied to the nasal tip are used interchangeably.

Points of reference used when measuring tip rotation include the upper lip and the Frankfort horizontal plane. When the upper lip is referenced, the nasolabial angle is

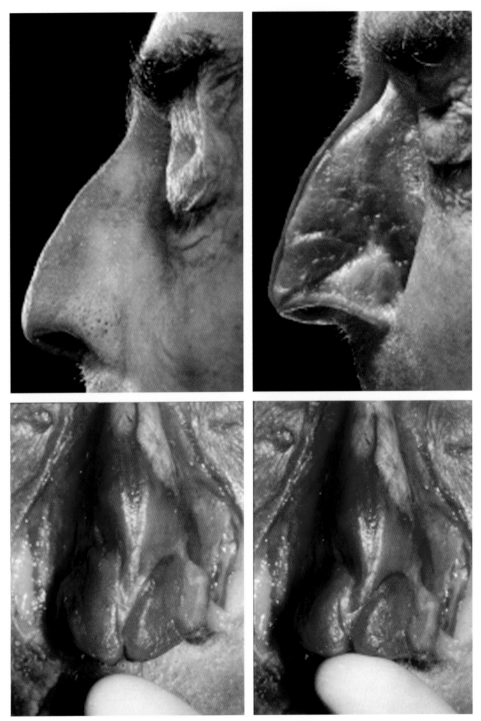

Figure 25-1 Anatomy of the nose. The nasal tip is a dynamic structure, hinged by the upper lateral cartilages and by the recurvature of the lower lateral cartilages. (Johnson Jr CM, Toriumi DM. Open Structure Rhinoplasty. Philadelphia: WB Saunders; 1990.)

the angle between the line of the nasal columella and the line of the upper lip.[5] The authors' preferred method is based upon the Frankfort horizontal plane and the long axis of the nostril (Figure 25-5). The long axis of the nostril is ideally oriented parallel to the columella (Figure 25-6), but often discrepancy exists between the two. When addressed surgically, the long axis of the nostril is first rotated to an angle favorable to the Frankfort

horizontal plane, and then the columella is brought into balance with the ala.[6] The ideal angle varies with gender; for women an angle between 10 and 30 degrees is favored, whereas for men an angle between 0 and 15 degrees is considered ideal.

The amount of rotation and projection demonstrated by a nose should be interpreted in relation to the overall nasal appearance. Individual nasal characteristics,

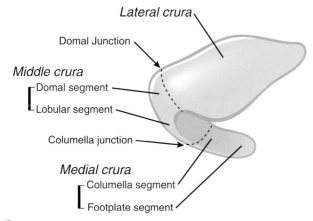

Figure 25-2 Anatomy of the lower lateral cartilage.

Lateral crura
Domal Junction
Middle crura
Domal segment
Lobular segment
Columella junction
Medial crura
Columella segment
Footplate segment

including rotation, projection, length, and height, do not exist in a vacuum and should not be evaluated in isolation. Their relevance derives from their contribution to the overall aesthetic balance and proportion of the nose and face. Similarly, illusion plays an important role in nasal appearance. For example, a ptotic nasal tip will appear to be elongated due to the loss of a distinct supratip break. Similarly, excessive dorsal height or a dorsal hump may cause an otherwise well-projected nose to appear to be underprojected as well as elongated. Other facial features contribute to nasal illusions as well; a retrodisplaced pogonion or an anteriorly sloping forehead lends to the illusion of an overprojected nose. These concepts were introduced and are discussed more completely in Chapter 3 of this text.

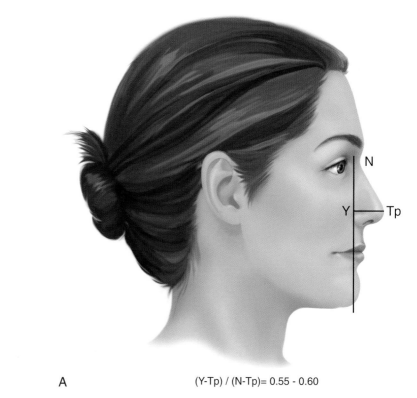

A

(Y-Tp) / (N-Tp)= 0.55 - 0.60

Figure 25-3 A, The Goode method defines ideal nasal tip projection as a ratio of 0.55 to 0.6 of the distance from the nasion to the tip-defining points. **B,** With Simons method, tip projection (Sn-Tp) should equal the height of the upper lip (Sn-Vs). **C,** Crumley and Lanser described a right triangle with dimensions corresponding to nasal proportions; ideally projection : height : length is equal to 3 : 4 : 5. **D,** Powell and Humphries defined the ideal relationship between tip projection and nasal height as a 2.8 : 1 ratio.

B   (Sn-Tp) = (Sn-Vs) = 1:1

C   (Y-Tp):(Y-N):(N-Tp)= 3:4:5

D   (N-X) / (X-Tp) = 2.8

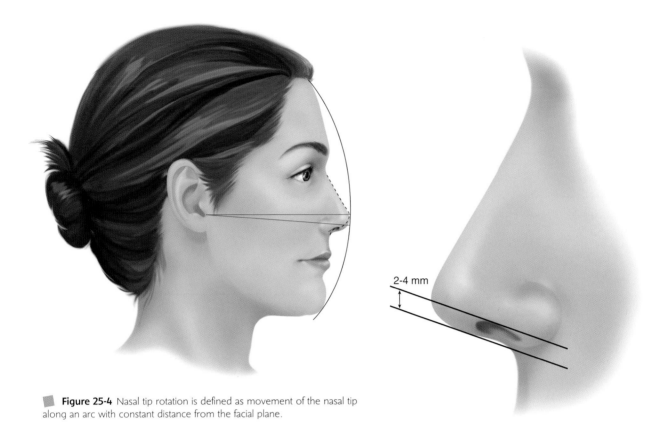

Figure 25-4 Nasal tip rotation is defined as movement of the nasal tip along an arc with constant distance from the facial plane.

Figure 25-6 The long axis of the nostril is ideally oriented parallel to the columella.

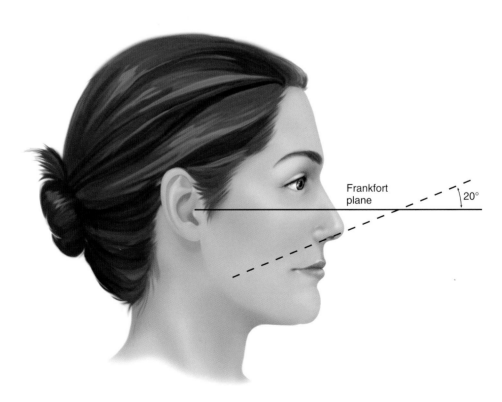

Figure 25-5 The degree of tip rotation is measured with reference to the Frankfort plane and the long axis of the nostril.

TIP SUPPORT

The structure and position of the nasal tip depend not just on the sum of its constituent parts but also on the support conferred by the upper lateral cartilages, nasal septum, and skin–soft tissue envelope (SSTE). Additionally, the combined effects of age, underlying medical conditions, trauma, and surgical interventions factor prominently in the ultimate appearance of the nasal tip.

To achieve the desired changes to the structure of the nasal tip, the surgeon must understand the factors contributing to tip support and dynamics. Nasal tip support derives from the inherent strength of the lower lateral cartilages, the nasal septum, and the various ligaments and fibrous connections between the alar cartilages and adjacent structures. By convention, support mechanisms are divided into major and minor groups. The three major tip support mechanisms include the size, shape, and resilience of the medial and lateral crura of the lower lateral cartilages, the attachment of the medial crural footplate to the caudal septum, and the scrolled attachment of the cephalic margins of the lower lateral cartilages to the caudal margin of the upper lateral cartilages. The minor tip supports generally include the dorsal septum, interdomal ligaments, membranous septum, anterior nasal spine, attachment of the lower lateral cartilages to the SSTE, the thickness of the SSTE, and the lateral crural attachment to the pyriform aperture (Table 25-1).

The interdomal ligament acts to support the nasal tip as a fibrous connection between both domes and the anterior septal angle. The contribution of this ligament is somewhat controversial in that some authors consider the interdomal ligament to be a fourth major tip support mechanism, whereas others consider it to be a minor one.

The tripod model proposed by Jack Anderson provides a mechanical model with which to understand the relationship between projection and rotation. Importantly, it can be used to predict the effects that alar cartilage–modifying maneuvers are likely to have on both tip projection and rotation.

The tripod concept postulates that nasal tip projection and rotation may be understood by considering the nasal tip as a tripod composed of the conjoined medial crura of the lower lateral cartilage as one leg and the two lateral crura as each remaining leg (Figure 25-7, A). By changing the length of one component of the tripod, a corresponding change in nasal tip projection and rotation can be anticipated. For example, shortening the two lateral crura would be expected to increase tip rotation along with slight deprojection (Figure 25-7, B). Likewise, lengthening the conjoined medial crura alone would increase both projection and rotation (Figure 25-7, C).

CAUSES OF TIP PTOSIS AND UNDERPROJECTION

Any condition that weakens the tip support mechanisms just delineated may lead to tip ptosis and underprojection. The range of possible etiologies includes congenital weakness of the nasal cartilages or other tip support mechanisms, infection, trauma, and iatrogenic damage.

For each patient, the etiology of ptosis and underprojection should be investigated to elucidate the contributing factors. To ensure success, the surgical plan must address the specific issues pertinent to each case.

Iatrogenic causes of tip ptosis and underprojection are common. Patients with a history of prior septorhinoplasty are at risk for developing tip sequelae due to surgical disruption of tip support mechanisms. Additionally, the effects of scar contracture of the disrupted SSTE further contributes over time to postoperative tip ptosis and deprojection.

Practically every maneuver associated with the endonasal approach compromises tip support mechanisms, including the intercartilaginous incision and the alar cephalic trim. A cadaveric study using objective measurements found that the intercartilaginous incisions and cartilage delivery techniques inherent to the endonasal approach caused a 35% loss of tip support.[7] Alar cartilage–splitting techniques and aggressive cartilage resection further compromise nasal structure and support mechanisms.

There is controversy as to the relative destructuring effects of the endonasal approach versus the nasal decortication undertaken with the open approach. The authors' opinion is that although the open approach to rhinoplasty is referred to as simply another approach, in reality it is another operation entirely. The open approach necessitates rebuilding injured tip support that is compromised as part of the decortication.

In the operated nose, ptosis and underprojection are typically not apparent in the early postoperative period. However, with passing time, the effects of scar contracture and gravity often create conditions that cannot be withstood by the diminished structure of the operated nose.

Table 25-1   Nasal Tip Support Mechanisms

Major Group	Minor Group
• Strength and shape of lateral crura	• Cartilaginous septal dorsum
• Strength, shape, length of medial crura	• Lateral crura-pyriform aperture
• Upper lateral union to lower lateral	• Skin thickness and its attachment to cartilage
• Medial crural-septal fibrous union	• Nasal spine
• Interdomal ligamentous sling	

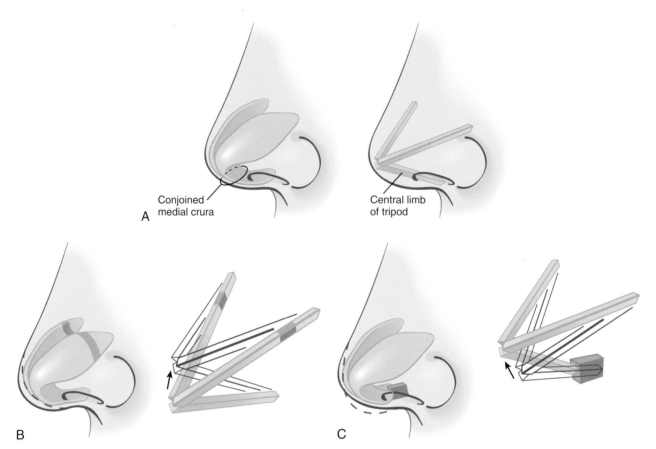

Figure 25-7 A, Tripod theory. The upper tripod legs are formed by the lateral crural complex and the lower tripod leg is formed by the conjoined medial crura. **B,** Here, shortening of the upper legs leads to movement of the tip of the tripod upward and slightly posteriorly, effectively increasing nasal tip rotation without a significant effect on tip projection. **C,** Lengthening the lower tripod leg increases both tip rotation and projection.

Likewise, the effects of skin envelope contracture are only seen over time and through hindsight the need for more structure is elucidated.

METHODS OF REPAIR

The authors prefer the open approach to the nose if any tip work is required, as is the case in the great majority of our nasal cases. Methods of repair may be divided into alar cartilage–modifying techniques and adjunctive maneuvers.[8]

Alar cartilage–modifying techniques to address tip underrotation and underprojection include placement of a columellar strut, tip grafting, lateral crural steal, lateral crural overlay, and the tongue-in-groove techniques. Adjunctive maneuvers include establishing proper dorsal height, addressing alar–columellar discrepancy, premaxillary grafting, alar cephalic trim, resection of an overdeveloped scroll region, and debulking the SSTE. Each of these options will be described next.

The surgical techniques described in this chapter may be used either independently or in combination depending on the findings and contributing factors present in each case, as well as on the degree of rotation or projection intended.

GRAFTING MATERIALS

Throughout the course of a rhinoplasty, often cartilaginous grafting material is needed to provide the structural support required to affect desired changes. The preferred grafting materials are septal cartilage followed by auricular cartilage, then costal cartilage. In the unoperated nose, sufficient septal cartilage is usually available to enable its use in most cases. In revision cases, the surgeon should investigate the status of the septal cartilage, while retaining a backup plan should insufficient septal cartilage be found at the time of surgery. A paucity of remaining septal cartilage requires that the surgeon find another source. As a matter of course, revision cases should be counseled about and consented for auricular and costal cartilage harvest in the event the need arises for alternative sources of cartilaginous grafting material.

When septal cartilage is found to be inadequate, auricular cartilage should be sought. A cartilage incision is made along the inner rim of the antihelical fold, while preserving a strip of intact cartilage between the cymba concha superiorly and the concha cavum inferiorly, which the authors prefer to harvest separately. Preservation of this auricular cartilage strut enables the healing auricle to resist contraction and deformation during healing, thus preserving the anteroposterior dimension of the conchal bowl.

The concha cavum is the preferred auricular substrate for tip grafting if septal cartilage is unavailable, while the cymba concha is the favored source of alar grafting material. When used for a columellar strut, the concha cavum or concha cymba is reinforced by folding it upon itself, with concave surfaces facing each other, and sutured together using multiple 5-0 nylon sutures in a horizontal mattress fashion.

COLUMELLAR STRUT

The columellar strut graft, along with septocolumellar fixation, provides the foundation upon which to build and refine the nose. This maneuver is the first tip-modifying step performed as part of the authors' preferred open technique. The structural integrity of the tripod segment formed by the conjoined medial crura is often compromised in noses undergoing rhinoplasty. That compromise may be due to congenitally weak crura or secondary to traumatic or iatrogenic damage to tip support mechanisms. Regardless of the etiology, the effects of diminished integrity of this inferior tripod segment cause the nose to collapse toward the face, effectively deprojecting and counterrotating the nasal tip.

A sturdy fragment of cartilage is desirable for columellar strut grafting. A favorable piece of septal cartilage can usually be harvested from along the floor of the nose where the cartilaginous septum joins the maxillary crest (Figure 25-8). After harvesting it, the graft is further trimmed to the appropriate size and shape using a No. 15 blade and a cutting block. A graft measuring 20 mm in length and 3 to 5 mm in width is typically adequate.

In the authors' preferred rhinoplasty sequence, septoplasty and harvest of septal cartilage are performed first, followed by opening the nose and dorsal reduction if indicated. Next, placement of spreader grafts is undertaken before the tip is addressed. Once the columellar strut graft is prepared, a pocket is dissected between the limbs of the medial crura in the direction of the nasal spine, while carefully preserving a layer of soft tissue overlying the nasal spine (Figure 25-9). The columellar strut is then implanted into this pocket, to a depth that preserves a soft tissue cushion between the deep aspect of the strut and the nasal spine. The columellar strut is then sutured to the medial crura using multiple 4-0 plain gut sutures in horizontal mattress fashion (Figure 25-10). Symmetric fixation of the medial crura to the strut graft is necessary to maintain symmetry between the left and right alar domes.

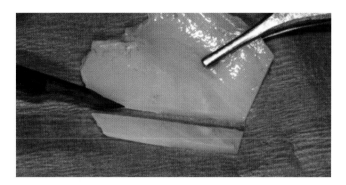

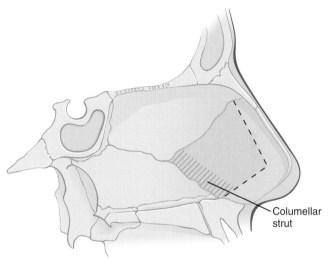

Figure 25-8 Columellar strut: a sturdy strut is harvested from along the inferior border of nasal septal cartilage.

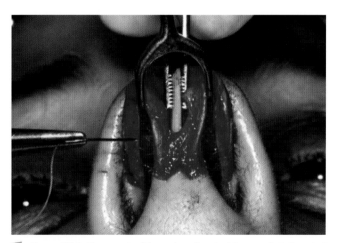

Figure 25-9 Placement of the columellar strut in a pocket dissected between the medial crura.

The columellar strut adds substantially to the stability of the nasal base. In a study that used objective measurements of nasal support in patients undergoing rhinoplasty, placement of a columellar strut alone increased nasal tip support 40% over baseline in the vector of the columella.[7]

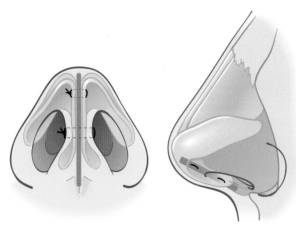

Figure 25-10 The columellar strut is inserted into a pocket dissected between the medial crura, to a depth that preserves a soft tissue cushion between the deep aspect of the strut and the nasal spine. The columellar strut is sutured to the medial crura using multiple 4-0 plain gut sutures in horizontal mattress fashion. (Adapted from Johnson et al.[6])

Once the columellar strut is secured, the surgeon can then closely evaluate the contribution of the lateral crura to tip rotation. Considering again the tripod model, disproportionately long lateral crura will tend to have a counterrotating effect on the nasal tip. At this juncture, the surgeon may wish to consider using one of two cartilage-modifying techniques described for this purpose: the *lateral crural steal* or the *lateral crural overlay*. Both maneuvers increase tip rotation. The choice as to which technique to employ depends on the existing tip projection, and the surgeon's decision based on this to modify tip projection. Both of these techniques are described in greater detail later.

NASAL TIP GRAFT

Tip grafting is a powerful tool that can provide additional structural support as well as projection to the nasal tip. The tip graft was developed to provide a stable and durable tip support that appeared natural over time.[9] The graft is fashioned from autogenous cartilage, preferably septal cartilage, and is secured at the caudal margin of the medial crura. It should extend from the proximal end of the conjoined medial crura to just beyond the domes. The tip graft can provide a small increase in tip projection as well as a refined tip contour that accentuates favorable nasal light reflexes.

The shape of the graft is roughly hexagonal, with the projecting end wider than the proximal end (Figure 25-11). It is carved intentionally longer than required and fixated to the caudal border of the medial crura using 6-0 nylon sutures. Once in place, its shape and size are refined using a No. 15 blade to shave the cartilage to the exact specifications indicated. Circumferential beveling should be performed to minimize visible edges. The projecting

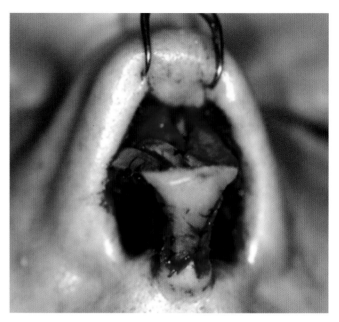

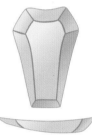

Figure 25-11 The shape of the tip graft is roughly hexagonal, with the projecting end wider than the proximal end. It is fixated to the caudal border of the medial crura using 6-0 nylon sutures.

end should be thinned adequately to allow it to take on a gentle anterosuperior curvature. Prior to making final adjustments, the SSTE can be redraped over the domal–tip graft complex and temporarily sutured at the columella to allow the surgeon to visualize the tip graft's effect on nasal tip contour and projection as well as to check for visible irregularities. If the SSTE is thin, the surgeon may choose to apply a crushed cartilage onlay graft to camouflage any visible edges. The tip graft is performed last in the sequence of tip-modification maneuvers.

LATERAL CRURAL STEAL TECHNIQUE

If increased tip rotation and projection are desired, the *lateral crural steal* technique may be employed. This maneuver entails placing an interdomal mattress suture in such a way as to advance the lateral crura onto the medial crura[10,12] (Figure 25-12). Two technical points warrant description. First, the vestibular skin must be dissected from the undersurface of the domal portion of the alar cartilages bilaterally. Otherwise, the mattress suture will traverse the mucosa and remain exposed within

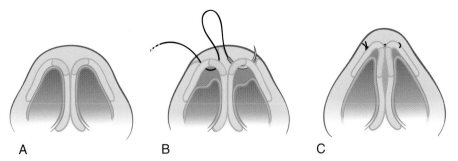

Figure 25-12 Schematic diagram of the lateral crural steal technique. The lateral crura are advanced medially onto the medial crura.

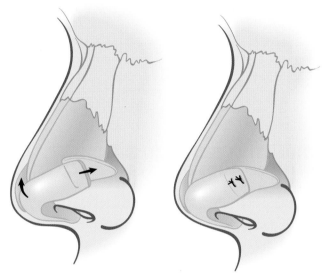

Figure 25-13 Schematic diagram of the lateral crural overlay technique. The middle section of the lateral crus is divided, and the margins are overlapped. (Adapted from Konior.[13])

the nasal airway. Such exposure increases the risk of postoperative infection, ulceration, or otherwise delayed healing. Second, the columellar strut may extend beyond the level of the native domes. If that is the case, the mattress suture should traverse the strut as well, at the intended height of the new tip. If the columellar strut still extends beyond the augmented domes, it is trimmed at that time to be 1 mm below the intended level of tip projection as established by the tip graft.

LATERAL CRURAL OVERLAY TECHNIQUE

If increased tip rotation along with decreased projection or maintenance of projection is desirable, the *lateral crural overlay* technique may be used (Figure 25-13). This maneuver involves dividing the lateral crura at its midsection and overlapping the proximal ends over the distal ends, then suturing the overlapped ends together using horizontal mattress sutures.[10] The degree of overlap is modified to impart the desired amount of tip deprojection and rotation. With regard to the tripod theory, lateral

crural overlap effectively shortens the upper tripod limbs, resulting in decreasing projection along with increasing rotation. If less deprojection or maintenance of projection is desired, less lateral crural overlap is used. As previously described for the lateral crural steal, the vestibular skin must be dissected from the undersurface of the domal and mid-body segments of the alar cartilages bilaterally as described earlier.

TONGUE-IN-GROOVE TECHNIQUE

The *tongue-in-groove* technique is another method of increasing tip rotation and controlling tip projection. The technique consists of advancing the medial crura cephaloposteriorly onto the caudal septum into a surgically created pocket between the crura.[2] The amount of tip rotation may be adjusted based upon the degree of superior advancement of the medial crura onto the septum. Similarly, tip projection may be decreased by positioning the medial crura posteriorly onto the septum.

This technique should only be used in patients who have a redundancy of the caudal septum that would otherwise require trimming.[11] Ideal patients for application of this technique include those with either a short upper lip or with columellar show, as this maneuver improves both conditions. When the *tongue-in-groove* technique is used, columellar strut placement is typically not required because the caudal septum takes the place of the columellar strut in stabilizing the medial crura and the base of the nose.

Performance of the tongue-in-groove maneuver begins with a transfixion incision made at the caudal border of the cartilaginous nasal septum. Caudal to that incision, a pocket is dissected between the medial crura of the lower lateral cartilages. Next, the medial crura are advanced cephalically and posteriorly onto the exposed caudal nasal septum. The amount of advancement in each direction is dictated by the intended degree of rotation and/or deprojection. Once the desired position of the lower lateral crura is achieved, fixation is accomplished using horizontal mattress sutures through the ipsilateral medial crura–caudal septum–contralateral medial crural complex (Figure 25-14).

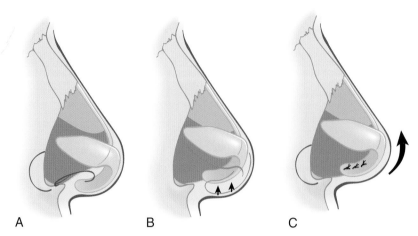

Figure 25-14 Schematic diagram of the tongue-in-groove technique. The medial crura are advanced cephalically and posteriorly onto the exposed nasal septum. The complex is suture fixated in the desired orientation.

Following suture fixation, excess caudal septum may still project beyond the medial crura–septum complex. Once the surgeon is satisfied with the new tip position, any excess caudal septum may be conservatively trimmed. Following this maneuver, redundant membranous septum may be present intranasally. This excess soft tissue should be grasped with forceps and gently retracted caudally, then trimmed and sutured such that the caudal portion of the membranous septum approximates with the transfixion incision. Not excising the redundant soft tissue in this region may predispose the patient to nasal airway obstruction due to membranous septum bunching postoperatively.

In addition to its usefulness for increasing tip rotation and controlling tip projection, the tongue-in-groove method may also be applied to improve columellar show and to aid in the correction of caudal septal deviation.[2] Advocates of this technique note the predictability of the final tip position in comparison to other cartilage-modifying techniques, which may be subject to changes with contracture during healing. Depending on the degree of rotation desired, additional maneuvers may be required to supplement the tongue-in-groove. In a series of 203 rhinoplasty patients who underwent the tongue-in-groove technique, 14 patients also required the employment of the lateral crural overlay to further increase rotation or to deproject the tip.[2]

With the tongue-in-groove technique, the effect on nasal tip projection and rotation is not necessarily predicted by the tripod model because the tripod concept describes only the changes brought about by lengthening or shortening the tripod limbs. With the tongue-in-groove, it is not the length but rather the position of lower tripod limb that is modified with respect to the septum and the upper limbs.

ADJUNCTIVE TECHNIQUES AND OTHER CONSIDERATIONS

ESTABLISHING PROPER DORSAL HEIGHT

The establishment of proper dorsal height should be accomplished prior to undertaking attempts at tip modification, as improper dorsal height fosters an illusion of tip malposition. For example, an overly high dorsum appears as a dorsal convexity on lateral view. This convexity creates the illusion of underprojection in an otherwise well-projected tip. The dorsum should follow a smooth, straight contour from the radix to the supratip break. Once dorsal height is established, the surgeon will more readily appreciate which adjustments, if any, may be indicated to the nasal tip position to achieve the desired result.

ALAR–COLUMELLAR DISCREPANCY

Excessive caudal projection of the septal quadrangular cartilage may contribute to alar–columellar discrepancy or "columellar show" resulting in apparent underrotation of the nasal tip (Figure 25-15). Similarly, excessive caudal projection of the medial crural cartilages may contribute to the same problem. When present, resection of the caudal septum or caudal margin of the medial crura may be indicated. The offending cartilage should be trimmed as needed to reduce columellar show to within the favorable 2- to 4-mm range and to reestablish harmony between the long axis of the nostril and the columella. Alternatively, the tongue-in-groove technique, described previously, may be applied to address alar–columellar discrepancy. This subject will be covered at length in a separate chapter.

PREMAXILLARY GRAFTING

Inadequate tip projection may arise from a lack of adequate support at the base of the lower tripod limb, where the medial crural footplates lie adjacent to the premaxilla. In that situation, the lower limb of the tripod is weakened and apparently foreshortened. A useful technique to address this finding is the premaxillary graft. A graft of septal or auricular cartilage is placed in a surgical pocket created at the base of the columella, beneath the feet of medial crura and overlying the central premaxilla.[9] This maneuver moves the lower limb of the nasal tripod anteriorly, effectively raising the height of the base of that tripod limb and contributing to tip projection (see Figure 25-7 C). Additionally, a premaxillary plumping graft can also be used to open (i.e., make more obtuse) an overly acute nasolabial angle. Bruised autologous cartilage can be placed just inferiorly to the soft tissue of the nasolabial angle, where it can add to the illusion of tip rotation.

ALAR CEPHALIC TRIM

Excessively wide lateral crura may contribute to tip ptosis. A simple alar cephalic trim of cartilage creates an area of dead space that, with scar contracture, rotates the tip upward to a more favorable position. The surgeon should be careful to preserve at least 8 mm of lateral crural width to ensure structural integrity of the lower lateral cartilage. Overresection of the lateral crura may result in weakened cartilages, which are predisposed to buckling with scar contracture, leading to bossae formation.

OVERDEVELOPED SCROLL REGION

The scroll is the region of overlapping attachment of the caudal border of the upper lateral cartilage to the cephalic border of the lower lateral cartilage. Overdevelopment of the scroll region can also contribute to tip ptosis. If indicated, conservative resection of the scroll can effectively shorten the length of the lateral crura (lateral tripod limbs) and consequently aid in rotating a ptotic tip (Figure 25-16).

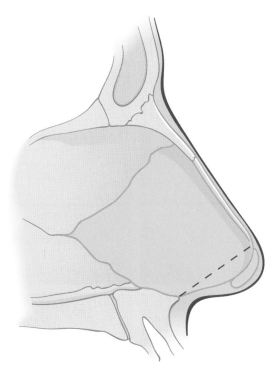

Figure 25-15 Excessive caudal projection of the septal quadrangular cartilage may contribute to "columellar show" resulting in apparent underrotation of the nasal tip. Resection of the caudal septum may be indicated to increase tip rotation.

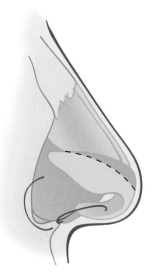
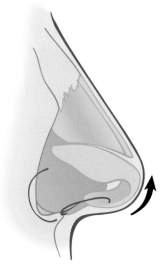

Figure 25-16 Conservative resection of an overdeveloped scroll can effectively shorten the length of the lateral crura (lateral tripod limbs) and consequently aid in derotating a ptotic tip.

SKIN–SOFT TISSUE ENVELOPE

In every rhinoplasty, the thickness of the nasal SSTE must be considered. In some cases, the SSTE may have a major influence on the appearance of the nasal tip. In other cases, it may have only a minor contribution. A thick SSTE provides additional mass, which may contribute to forces favoring tip counterrotation. Additionally, the inherent inelasticity of a thickened SSTE may prevent the overlying envelope from conforming to the underlying structure, thereby blunting and taking away from the definition of the nasal tip, despite an ideally defined underlying structure. Conservatively thinning the undersurface of the SSTE should be undertaken when indicated to minimize these effects. During healing, periodic treatments with subcutaneous long-acting steroid

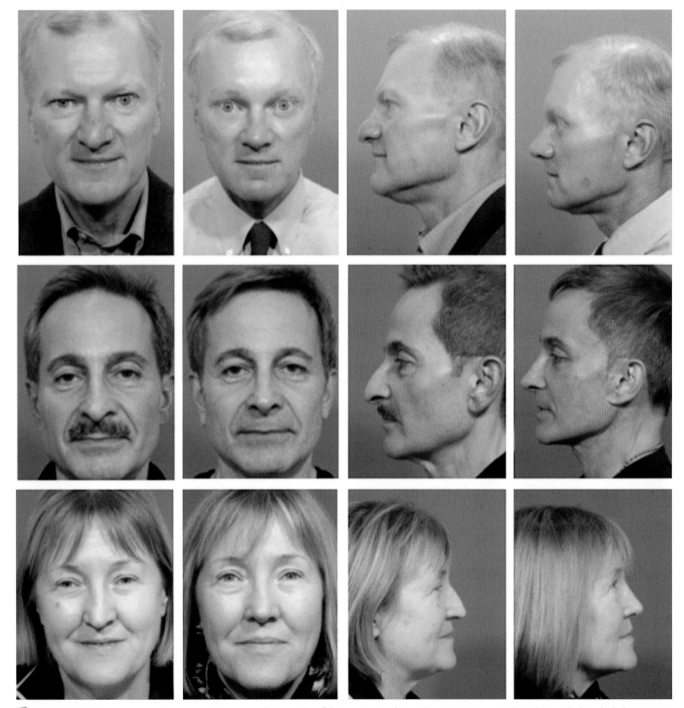

Figure 25-17 Preoperative and 1-year postoperative photographs of three patients who underwent open septorhinoplasty, which included correction of tip underprojection and underrotation in each case.

(triamcinolone acetonide 10 mg/mL) can aid in reducing edema and scar contracture of the tip.[6]

Once the tip work is completed, osteotomies are performed as needed. If septal work or cartilage harvest was performed, a 4-0 plain gut suture on a Keith needle is used to approximate the septal mucoperichondrial flaps. Splints made from Silastic sheeting are applied to each side of the nasal septum and sutured in place using a 2-0 silk suture anteriorly. The columellar skin incision is closed using 6-0 nylon sutures. The marginal incision is closed using 5-0 plain gut sutures. Polysporin-coated Telfa rolled onto itself is used to lightly pack the nasal cavity.

POSTOPERATIVE CARE

The patient is discharged home with a prescription for broad-spectrum antibiotics for a few days. The nasal packing is removed the following morning, and the patient is instructed to begin using saline nasal spray several times daily. The columellar sutures are removed on postoperative day 3 or 4, and the incision site is dressed with paper tape. If used, the Silastic splints are removed on postoperative day 7. If subtle irregularities or excessive edema are present, nasal exercises are started at this time. The patient is instructed to avoid exertion and aerobic exercise until the end of the third postoperative week. By the end of the fourth week, if excessive or asymmetric edema or scar tissue formation is present, subcutaneous injections of long-acting steroid (triamcinolone acetonide) are initiated typically in the supratip or side wall regions as indicated.

SUMMARY

The need to modify the underprojected and underrotated nasal tip arises regularly in patients seeking rhinoplasty. In fact, the majority of all cases involve some degree of such modification (Figure 25-17). Tip underrotation was observed in 72% of patients in a report of 500 consecutive rhinoplasty cases.[8] Of those, 85% required application of a cartilage-modifying technique to rotate the tip. The remaining 15% were surgically treated with adjunctive maneuvers alone, including cephalic trim of the lateral crura, excision of the overdeveloped scroll region, or lowering the height of the anterior septal angle.

The nasal surgeon has at his or her disposal several proven methods for addressing tip projection and rotation. A method of repair should be chosen based on the desires and needs of the patient and the anatomy of the nose in question. A case may call for increasing projection alone, increasing rotation alone, or increasing both projection and rotation. Different presentations may require differ-

ent procedures, as described. Further modifications can be made using adjunctive techniques as indicated.

Successful surgery of the nasal tip demands a thorough knowledge of anatomy, tip support mechanism, dynamics, and techniques. Factors contributing to tip rotation and projection are unique to each nose. A surgical plan should be tailored to the particular needs presented by each patient.

The techniques described herein are not intended to be an exhaustive review of the surgical options available to address the array of nasal tip characteristics that may be encountered. Instead, this chapter provides an overview of versatile and proven techniques that may be applied to the majority of cases and that have been found to effect predictable and lasting results.

The challenge presented to the nasal surgeon by tip rhinoplasty is to integrate a keen appreciation for nasal aesthetics with an intimate knowledge of tip anatomy and dynamics, the diagnostic insight to elucidate the etiology of tip malposition, and the surgical skill to apply a variety of techniques as needed to achieve a desired result.

REFERENCES

1. Daniel RK. The nasal tip: anatomy and aesthetics. *Plast Reconstr Surg*. 1992;89(2):216–224.
2. Kridel RWH, Scott BA, Foda HMT. The tongue-in-groove technique in septorhinoplasty. *Arch Fac Plast Surg*. 1999;1: 246–256.
3. Toriumi DM. Rhinoplasty. In: Park SS, et al., eds. *Facial plastic surgery: The essential guide*. New York: Thieme; 2005; 223–253.
4. Simons RL. Nasal tip projection, ptosis, and suptratip thickening. *J Ears Nose Throat*. 1982;61(8):452–455.
5. Orten SS, Hilger PA. Facial analysis of the rhinoplasty patient. In: Papel ID, et al., eds. Facial plastic and reconstructive surgery. New York: Thieme; 2002;361–368.
6. Johnson Jr CM, Toriumi DM. *Open structure rhinoplasty*. Philadelphia: WB Saunders; 1990.
7. Beaty MM, Dyer WK, Shawl MWW. The quantification of surgical changes in nasal tip support. *Arch Fac Plast Surg*. 2002;4:82–91.
8. Foda HM. Management of the droopy tip: A comparison of three alar cartilage-modifying techniques. *Plast Reconstr Surg*. 2003;112(5):1408–1417; discussion 1418–1421.
9. Pastorek N, Ham J. The underprojecting nasal tip: An endonasal approach. *Fac Plast Surg Clin North Am*. 2004; 12(1):93–106.
10. Foda HMT, Kridel RWH. Lateral crural steal and lateral crural overlay. *Arch Otolaryngol Head Neck Surg*. 1999;125: 1365–1370.
11. Toriumi DM. New concepts in nasal tip contouring. *Arch Fac Plast Surg*. 2006;8:156–185.
12. Kridel RWH, Konior RJ, Shumrick KA, Wright WK. Advances in nasal tip surgery: The lateral crural steal. *Arch Otolaryngol Head Neck Surg*. 1989;115:1206–1212.
13. Konior RJ. The droopy nasal tip. *Fac Plast Surg Clin North Am*. 2006;(14):291–299.

CHAPTER TWENTY-SIX

Thin Skin Rhinoplasty: Aesthetic Considerations and Surgical Approach

Michael J. Brenner • Peter A. Hilger

Thin nasal skin readily reveals imperfections of the underlying osseocartilaginous framework and has profound implications for the surgical planning and execution of rhinoplasty. Thin skin may be a normal variant or the result of prior surgery, trauma, or disease. The relative inattention to this subject in the literature is striking, particularly when one considers the small tolerance for error that exists when working with thin skin. One possible explanation is the misconception that relatively few techniques are available to improve surgical results in this difficult group. Another explanation for this conspicuous omission is the prevailing notion that the character of thin skin is largely immutable.[1] This chapter addresses these concerns and introduces a variety of techniques that we have found beneficial in patients with thin nasal skin.

In this discussion, "thin skin" and "thin nasal skin" more properly refer to a thin nasal skin–soft tissue envelope (SSTE). When anatomic reference to the skin of the nose *in isolation* is intended, we refer specifically to the epidermis, dermis, or cutaneous layer. We have chosen this potentially confusing terminology because most clinicians tacitly include the four layers of tissue between the skin and osseocartilaginous framework when they speak of patients with thin skin. Furthermore, this approach allows us to consider in our discussion of thin skin both patients with naturally fine skin as well as patients who have undergone prior rhinoplasty and have thin SSTEs with a parchment-like character. Several of the technical considerations in these two groups are similar. The aging nose, discussed in a separate chapter, also exhibits thinning of the SSTE and is briefly addressed in this discussion.

ANATOMY OF THE SKIN-SOFT TISSUE ENVELOPE

The anatomy of the SSTE and its relation to the nasal framework is of great interest to the rhinoplasty surgeon working with thin nasal skin. The thickness of the SSTE

varies, being thickest over the radix and supratip area and thinnest at the rhinion. There are four layers of tissue that reside between the skin and osseocartilaginous framework: the superficial fatty panniculus, the fibromuscular layer, the deep fatty layer, and the perichondrium or periosteum.[2] The fibromuscular layer contains the nasal superficial musculoaponeurotic system (SMAS), which is in continuity with facial SMAS, platysma, and galea. This layer provides structure and is flush to the underlying vascular supply of the SSTE. In the patient with thin nasal skin, extra care is taken to preserve the vascular supply of the SSTE by elevating a flap immediately superficial to the perichondrium.

The facial muscles exert dynamic forces on the nose that are often pronounced in patients with thin skin. The nasal muscles are innervated by the zygomatic branch of the facial nerve and have been divided into four groups: elevator, depressor, compressor, and minor dilator muscles. The elevator muscles, including the procerus, levator labii superioris alaeque nasi, and anomalous nasi, shorten the nose and dilate the nostrils. The depressor muscles, including the depressor septi and alar portion of the nasalis, lengthen the nose and dilate the nostrils. The compressor muscles, including the transverse portion of the nasalis and compressor narium minor, lengthen the nose and contract the nostrils. Last, the minor dilator muscle is the dilator naris anterior. These muscles have functional and aesthetic relevance to thin skin rhinoplasty, with their role in surgical treatment sometimes described as "dynamic rhinoplasty." Understanding these muscle actions allows for improved control of dorsum–tip–labial relationships.

TYPES OF THIN SKIN

NATURALLY THIN SKIN

In patients who have not undergone prior nasal surgery, the thickness of the supratip soft tissue is dictated by the density of sebaceous glands in the epithelium and the suppleness of the subcutaneous tissues. Patients with "thick skin," discussed in detail in Chapter 27 in the text, usually have sebaceous skin with dense underlying soft tissues that obscure nasal framework and resist surgical refinement. Patients with naturally fine skin have the opposite problem—skin that reveals too much—and subtle imperfections will "shine through" the delicate veil of the thin nasal covering. In such cases, absence of the usual buffer of skin and soft tissue will often draw attention to the contours of the underlying cartilaginous and bony nasal anatomy in an unflattering manner. Thin skin may occur irrespective of age, gender, or ethnicity; however, the prototypical thin-skinned patient in the senior author's practice is a young woman in her 30s, often of Nordic descent, with fair skin, blonde or red hair, and blue eyes (Fitzpatrick Type I or II).

PARCHMENT THIN SKIN

Thin skin is also seen in association with prior rhinoplasty.[3] The prototypical patient in this setting is a female with medium to medium-thin facial skin who relates a history of progressive changes to the character of the skin subsequent to one or more prior rhinoplasties. Examination of the skin and its underlying soft tissue elements demonstrates atrophic changes in association with scarring. Actinic changes or talangiectasias are usually present, often over the rhinion, and there is poor elasticity to the nasal covering. This skin is sometimes described as "parchment thin skin," a reflection of its fragile quality and its thin, almost translucent appearance.

In the previously operated nose, thin skin may be adherent to the underlying framework. As a result, the underlying cartilaginous and skeletal irregularities stand out in relief. Parchment preparation, which historically involved the stretching, scraping, and drying of skin under tension to create a stiff, translucent material, has much in common with the pathogenesis of iatrogenic thin skin in postrhinoplasty patients. Thinness of the SSTE—often unrecognized at time of original surgery—predisposes to development of this complication, but parchment thin skin usually indicates transection or injury of the nasal SMAS during dissection. This transgression permanently compromises skin quality and increases risk of alar retraction due to exaggerated scarification. Steroid injection compounds the problem.

AGING AND DISEASE-RELATED THIN SKIN

Last, normal aging and several disease entities cause thinning of the skin. These causes have an underlying physiology that differs from both innately thin nasal skin and from acquired parchment thin skin. Aging is associated with reduction of the skin's strength, thickness, and elasticity. Actinic changes and solar damage also alter the characteristics of the skin and contribute to thinning and premature aging of the skin. Corticosteroid excess, as may occur with diseases of the adrenal cortex, pituitary neoplasms, and exogenous corticosteroid use are additional factors associated with thinning, weakening, and delayed healing of the skin. Ehlers-Danlos syndrome and osteogenesis imperfecta, which are associated with defective collagen synthesis, result in abnormally thin skin with decreased tensile strength, as part of their clinical behavior. While the techniques presented herein for thin skin are highly versatile, the dynamics of healing in aging and disease are beyond the scope of this chapter.

PHILOSOPHICAL CONSIDERATIONS RELATED TO THIN SKIN

SMALL MARGIN OF ERROR

Identification of thin skin during the preoperative assessment is crucial in planning rhinoplasty so that the patient can be counseled appropriately and the surgical plan adapted to the special needs of thin skin. The potential margin for error is narrower in patients with thin nasal skin. While thin skin confers an excellent opportunity for achieving refinement of the nasal tip, subtle irregularities will be more difficult to conceal. Some patients have very strong or prominent cartilages whose entire cartilage outline is discernible.

THE SHRINK WRAP EFFECT

The "shrink wrap" effect that occurs after rhinoplasty is more profound in patients with thin skin. In contrast to thick skin, which limits the degree of resection that can be performed, thin skin allows for a greater degree of overall reduction and creation of a smaller nasal contour. On the other hand, such patients are at greater risk for disfigurement by the contractile forces of healing. During the postoperative course, patient with tight skin will notice that the nasal covering becomes even more constricted. The surgical plan must acknowledge that the toll of the "shrink wrap" effect may progress well beyond the first couple of postoperative years.

IMPLICATIONS OF THIN SKIN ARE DIFFERENT FOR EACH THIRD OF THE NOSE

The healing process in patients with thin skin exerts characteristic effects on each portion of the nose. Over the bony pyramid, thin skin predisposes to palpable and sometimes visible osteotomy sites. Small spicules of bone, minor bony irregularities, or asymmetric bone regrowth are poorly concealed. The late narrowing of the nasal midvault seen with typical reductive rhinoplasty is accentuated in these patients. In addition, imprecise correction of the open roof deformity and other irregular contours become progressively more conspicuous as the skin seats down tightly over the framework. Thin skin in this area resists attempts by the surgeon to camouflage significant structural abnormalities with onlay grafts. The thin skin over the rhinion is most prone to alterations in color, texture, and tone. Prior to surgery, many patients have actinic changes; these patients need to be counseled regarding the risk for development of telangiectasias. The skin may become shiny as it becomes taut. The lower third of the nose is particularly prone to deforming forces of the healing SSTE.

TECHNICAL CONSIDERATIONS

OVERVIEW

The presence of thin skin has implications for all major aspects of rhinoplasty. Thin skin necessitates extra care in the elevation and protection of the SSTE; it requires specific strategies for structural correction and camouflage of the osseocartilaginous framework, and it calls for special measures for prevention and treatment of bossae and other contour irregularities. Skin color changes can be minimized or treated, and this will be discussed later in this chapter. Crushed cartilage may be combined with a variety of other soft tissue grafting materials. Certain adjunctive techniques are beneficial for fine tuning after thin skin rhinoplasty, although injection of either fillers or steroids is best performed conservatively or avoided altogether. Each of these technical points is covered in the discussion that follows.

ELEVATION AND PROTECTION OF THE SSTE

In patients with thin nasal skin, it is important to elevate the SSTE in as thick a flap as possible. The plane of dissection is immediately superficial to the perichondrium over the upper and lower lateral cartilages and subperiosteal over the bony dorsum. If no bony dorsal surgery is required, elevation over the dorsum is avoided because such unnecessary dissection may provoke the unwanted shrink-wrap effect. Thick skin is comparatively forgiving of imprecise dissection, whereas failure to respect the vascular supply of the SSTE in the patient with thin skin results in excessive postoperative edema and a parchment-like character to the skin. Furthermore, transsection of the SMAS disrupts the anatomic barrier between the skin and structural framework, allowing adhesions to form between the framework and dermis. This impropriety can permanently compromise skin quality and also increases the risk of retraction and dimpling due to exaggerated scarification.

In cases of parchment thin skin, where the quality of the SSTE is compromised, we routinely place an implant that increases the thickness of the soft tissue between the skin envelope and the framework. When performing a secondary rhinoplasty, we will often harvest not only the conchal cartilage but also postauricular fibroconnective tissue, which is obtained from the conchal mastoid sulcus and over the mastoid process as shown in Figure 26-1. This tissue is flattened in a tympanoplasty press, creating a pliable sheet of soft connective tissue that can be placed over the nasal framework. This graft can be heavily compressed, but it is kept hydrated to improve viability. In our hands, this technique not only thickens the SSTE but may actually improve the *quality* of the scarified SSTE, making it more supple and natural appearing. Temporalis fascia is also useful for this purpose. Perichondrium provides a nice soft tissue cushion and is readily available if one is harvesting a rib graft. Acellular dermal matrix is an alternative,[4] but it does thin progressively over time, and in many cases virtually disappears.

STRATEGIES FOR CAMOUFLAGE, AUGMENTATION, AND STRUCTURAL CORRECTION

Most of the soft tissue grafts used as a buffering between the nasal covering and the framework serve the dual function of camouflage and protection of the SSTE. Temporalis fascia is effective for smoothing contour irregularities. When used alone, it does not add significant bulk. Due to its thick, fibrous consistency, the temporalis fascia provides excellent tissue cover. Fibroconnective tissue, perichondrium, and crushed cartilage are also useful for this purpose. Temporalis fascia and fibroconnective tissue may both be harvested with minimal concern for the donor site and, unlike crushed cartilage, are usually available in ample supply even in the case of revision surgery.

When performing surgery on the upper third of the nose in patients with thin skin, several technical pearls should be kept in mind. First, it is important to use a very fine rasp to smooth out any subtle irregularities. Although rather coarse rasps are used frequently in rhinoplasty, thin skin is unforgiving and requires a painstaking approach. It is especially important to vigorously irrigate out any debris that remains after dorsal reduction or osteotomies. Retained small particles of bone or cartilage can act as a nidus for inflammatory response and lead to unsightly postoperative irregularities that show through the skin.[5]

In a primary rhinoplasty, by far, our preferred graft material is crushed septal cartilage. A thin sheet of septal cartilage is reserved for a dorsal onlay graft that will extend from the radix to the supratip. The edge of the cartilage is beveled and placed in a cartilage crusher that has smooth surfaces and that will not macerate the graft. The cartilage is carefully crushed to create a pliable yet intact graft that is slightly larger than the original sheet of cartilage. At this point, the dorsum should already have been lowered approximately 0.5 mm below the

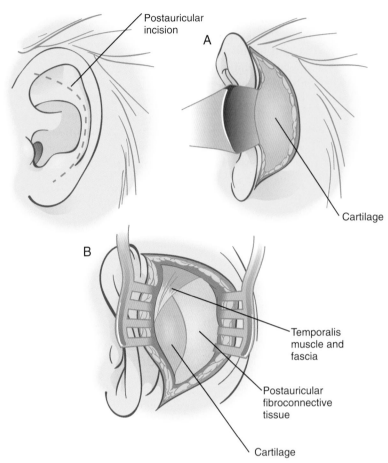

Postauricular
incision

A

Cartilage

B

Temporalis
muscle and
fascia

Postauricular
fibroconnective
tissue

Cartilage

Figure 26-1 Harvest of temporalis fascia and fibroconnective tissue. The postauricular approach used for harvest of conchal cartilage is easily adapted for harvest of either postauricular fibroconnective tissue or deep temporalis fascia.

desired profile to allow for the height added by the graft. The graft is then placed over the dorsum using bayonet forceps and may be secured in place, if desired. As with the patient shown in Figure 26-2, this technique is almost routinely used in a prophylactic fashion, and the objective is to provide a smooth structural interface with the SSTE.

When a smooth sheet of cartilage is not available for minor augmentation, one may consider wrapping diced auricular cartilage in fascia[6] or in Surgicel, as described in the "Turkish Delight" procedure.[7] When used in closed rhinoplasty, these rolled grafts have a tendency to drift from their intended position. Therefore, minimizing dissection plays an important role in providing a more precise pocket. With an external approach, such movement is of lesser concern since direct fixation with suture is possible. We avoid the use of Gore-Tex in revision rhinoplasty, particularly when the nasal vault has been reconstructed with spreader grafts or other techniques that require separation of the upper lateral cartilages from the septum. We have noted persisting erythema of the nasal skin when using Gore-Tex in these cases as a cushioning agent.

For major anatomic deformities, definitive structural grafting is indicated. Whereas crushed cartilage may conceal a multitude of imperfections in patients with thicker skin, thin skin rhinoplasty mandates precise structural alignment and contouring to avoid visible or palpable deformity. The previously discussed camouflage techniques should be applied over a carefully contoured framework. Grafts and implants are beveled and positioned precisely. Peripheral crushing of cartilage grafts may further assist with their camouflage. Sometimes, two different grafts confer similar functional benefits, but one is superior from an aesthetic standpoint. For example, strong alar batten grafts are excellent for resisting the weight of thick, heavy skin that would otherwise collapse the nasal valve, but such an approach yields an unacceptable aesthetic result with thin skin. Placement of lateral crural strut grafts, in contrast, is more appropriate for patients with thin skin, as in the patient shown in Figure 26-3. Lateral crural strut grafts will improve the nasal airway without untoward effects on the external appearance of the nose, since they are concealed underneath the alar cartilages.

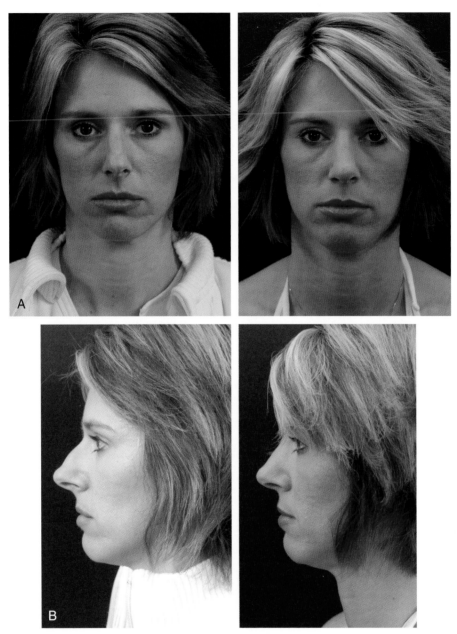

Figure 26-2 Use of crushed cartilage as a prophylactic measure in the patient with thin skin. This patient wished correction of a broad, overprojecting nose with dorsal convexity. Dorsal hump reduction was followed by laterally fading medial osteotomies and internal lateral osteotomies to close the open roof. A tongue-in-groove relationship was established between the medial crura. A crushed cartilage radix graft was followed by onlay of dorsal crushed cartilage to ensure smooth contour.

PREVENTION AND TREATMENT OF BOSSAE IN PATIENTS WITH THIN SKIN

Bossae are the most common postrhinoplasty deformity of the lower third of the nose and are one of the more common indications for revision rhinoplasty.[8–11] Patients with thin skin have a substantially increased risk for formation of bossae and other related deformities of the nasal tip. Bossae, illustrated in Figure 26-4, are knoblike protuberances of the alar cartilages that typically develop from months to years after rhinoplasty.[11] The classic triad of risk factors for bossae includes thin nasal skin, interlobular bifidity, and strong alar cartilages.[9,11] The presence of thin skin not only contributes to the pathogenesis of bossa formation (due to the "shrink wrap" effect) but also increases the likelihood that revision surgery will be necessary for their correction, since bossae range in severity and thicker skin may conceal subtler deformities.

Some authors have suggested that early and late bossae arise through distinct mechanisms.[11] According to

Michael J. Brenner • Peter A. Hilger

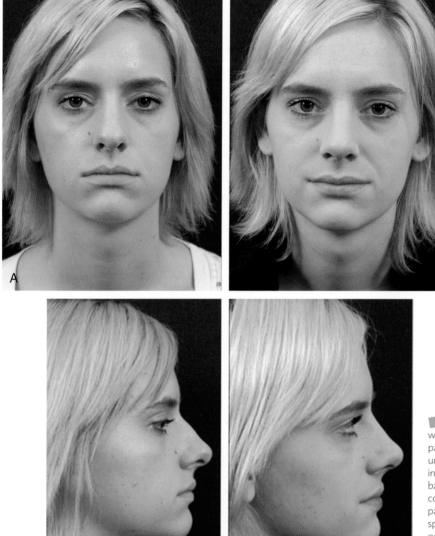

A

B

Figure 26-3 Lateral crural strut grafts in a patient with prominent nasal cartilages and thin skin. In this patient, lateral crural strut grafts were placed along the undersurface of the alar cartilages. These grafts are inconspicuous and preferable to more visible alar batten grafts. The lateral crural struts smoothed alar contour, corrected recurvature, and improved nasal patency. After hump reduction, the use of asymmetric spreader grafts, larger on right than left, closed the open roof and achieved aesthetic widening of the mid-vault with correction of deviation of the cartilaginous vault. A radix graft assisted in achieving a smooth dorsal contour, and crushed cartilage was used as softening agent over the infratip lobule and nasal dorsum.

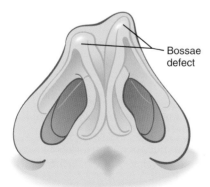

Bossae
defect

Figure 26-4 Bossa formation. A bossa is a knob-like prominence affecting the nasal tip that may develop after rhinoplasty. They may be unilateral or bilateral and often involve weakening of the lower lateral cartilages such that forces of scar contracture buckle the lateral crus resulting in distortion of the dome and alar rim.

this theory, early bossae result from inadequately corrected or iatrogenic asymmetries that become evident early in the postoperative course, as postsurgical edema resolves. In this situation, thin skin acts almost like a veneer that fails to buffer and may even accentuate asymmetries. Late bossae are the product of progressive scar contracture and fibrosis acting upon an attenuated cartilaginous scaffold. Here, the thin nasal covering, with its exaggerated contractile characteristics, not only heralds the development of the deformity but actively mediates the knuckling and contortion of the alar cartilages. Late bossae are often associated with alar retraction and other deformities, such as collapse of the alar rim.

Fortunately, if thin skin is identified at the outset, several useful approaches are available for prevention and treatment. Technical oversights that may predispose to late bossae formation are failure to reconstitute the domal unit with suture in a symmetric fashion; weakening of the cephalic margins of the lower lateral cartilages by crushing, scoring or overresection; and creation of sharp or irregular edges with resection. Conservative resection is advised, as the desired contour alteration can often be achieved with nondestructive techniques, such as suture sculpting. Beveling of cartilage is preferable to more traumatic methods. Use of a columellar strut or other structural grafting affords stability to the tip that may decrease the risk of bossa formation. In addition, placing crushed cartilage grafts or other softening agents, such as

perichondrium, over the nasal tip may decrease the risk of this complication.[9] Any weak areas that may buckle under the influence of contractural forces should be reinforced to decrease the likelihood of complication. Vertical dome division is to be avoided in patients with thin skin.

The surgical approach to correction of bossae in patients with thin skin emphasizes the same concepts that assist in prevention: reconstitution of the dome, strengthening of alar cartilages, and correction and camouflage of irregularities (Figure 26-5). As Daniel has emphasized, of cardinal importance is the question, "Is this a minor bump, or is it a major tip deformity?[8]" Bossae represent

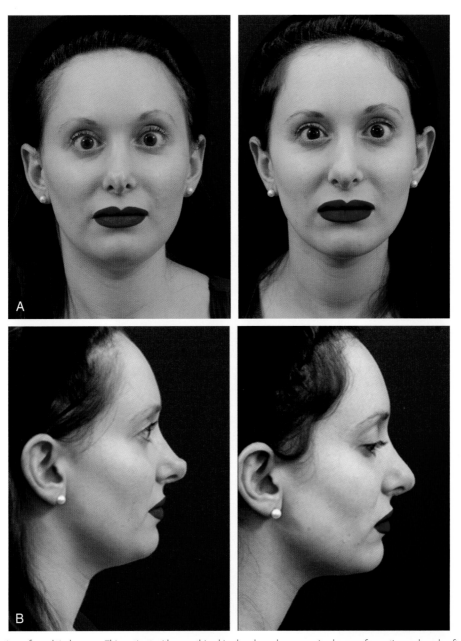

Figure 26-5 Correction of nasal tip bossae. This patient with very thin skin developed progressive bossae formation a decade after previous rhinoplasty. Bossae were exposed through an external approach. The tip was retrodisplaced through conservative shave of the medial crural footplates and a total transfixion incision. The use of postauricular fibroconnective tissue as softening agent was instrumental in restoring a smooth, natural contour to the nasal tip.

a range of deformities, and the extent of deformity may not be entirely evident before surgery. While some deformities may be improved with conservative trimming through an endonasal approach, others may be addressed with cartilage overlapping techniques. Severe deformities often necessitate structural grafting for tip reconstruction that may best be performed through an external approach. An often overlooked technical pearl is generous undermining of the vestibular skin. Failure to do so will leave the cartilage in its distorted mold, thereby causing the framework to fall back into a buckled configuration. In addition, with more severe deformities, the contraction of the bossa also causes collapse of the remaining lateral crus with resultant accentuation of the bossa and medialization of the alar rim.

REFINEMENTS AND ADJUNCTIVE TECHNIQUES

Certain adjunctive techniques may be of benefit after rhinoplasty in patients with thin skin. If the patient develops a very small cartilaginous area that is palpable through the skin, and the irregularity is caused by small cartilage excess, we would consider using a 16-gauge needle that we pass through the skin and then morsalize the small irregularity in situ. For the patients who develop erythema of their skin following rhinoplasty, we recommend pulse dye laser therapy. Careful avoidance of sun exposure and use of sun block will decrease the incidence and severity of this complication (Figure 26-6). It may also be advisable for patients to avoid use of isotretinoin, as its effects on collagen production and degradation influence the

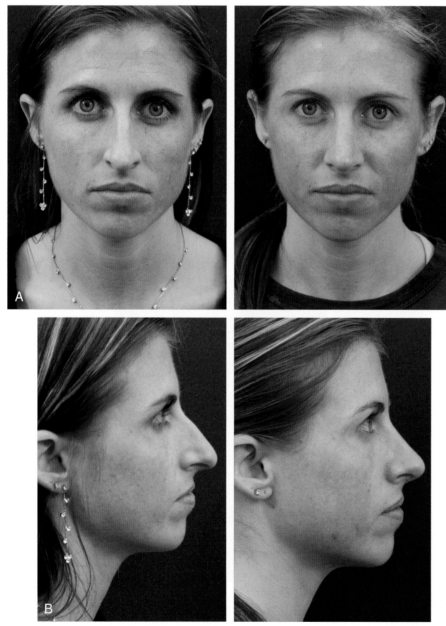

Figure 26-6 Maintenance of skin quality in a patient with fair, thin skin. Excessive freckling and change to skin color and texture were avoided by raising a thick skin flap, using crushed cartilage, and sunscreen use postoperatively. Correction of a ptotic, overprojected tip and dorsal convexity was achieved with a combination of conservative resection, structural grafting, and use of radix graft and crushed cartilage.

character of nasal skin and may increase the risk of late deformities.[12] Nasal exercises, involving manual massage to smooth areas of irregularity, may help settle areas of induration and liberate overly adherent skin from the underlying structural framework.

Some "minimally invasive" procedures, frequently thought to be innocuous, should be performed with the utmost caution in patients with thin skin. Most grafts will thin to some extent with passage of time, and we are inclined to observe small prominences initially. We are extremely cautious with injectable steroids or any other method to decrease soft tissue volume, even if there is initially a subtle contour irregularity from the cushioning technique. Use of fillers is generally ill-advised in patients with thin skin, particularly in the setting of revision rhinoplasty. Many patients will exhibit a bluish discoloration of the overlying skin prior to extrusion of the agent. Patients may pursue such treatments, wishing to avoid surgery, but the transient nature of the improvement and the often disappointing aesthetic result make these treatments generally unattractive options.

CONCLUSION

An understanding of thin nasal skin and its significance in nasal surgery is of great importance to the rhinoplasty surgeon. The predilection of thin skin to contract and to give rise to secondary deformities is an integral aspect of this subject. Identification of the thin skin preoperatively is crucial for surgical planning and prevention of disfigurement.

REFERENCES

1. Sheen J. Special problems: Thick skin, thin skin. In: *Aesthetic rhinoplasty*. St Louis:1987;1032–1043.
2. Letourneau A, Daniel RK. The superficial musculoaponeurotic system of the nose. *Plast Reconstr Surg.* 1988;82:48–57.
3. Baker TM, Courtiss EH. Temporalis fascia grafts in open secondary rhinoplasty. *Plast Reconstr Surg.* 1994;93:802–810.
4. Gryskiewicz JM. Waste not, want not: The use of AlloDerm in secondary rhinoplasty. *Plast Reconstr Surg.* 2005;116:1999–2004.
5. Parkes ML, Kanodia R, Machida BK, et al. Revision rhinoplasty. An analysis of aesthetic deformities. *Arch Otolaryngol Head Neck Surg.* 1992;118:695–701.
6. Kelly MH, Bulstrode NW, Waterhouse N, et al. Versatility of diced cartilage-fascia grafts in dorsal nasal augmentation. *Plast Reconstr Surg.* 2007;120:1654–1659.
7. Erol OO. The Turkish Delight: A pliable graft for rhinoplasty. *Plast Reconstr Surg.* 2000;105:2229–2241.
8. Daniel R. Nasal bossae. *Arch Fac Plast Surg.* 2003;5:424–426.
9. Gillman GS, Simons RL, Lee DJ, et al. Nasal tip bossae in rhinoplasty. Etiology, predisposing factors, and management techniques. *Arch Fac Plast Surg.* 1999;1:83–89.
10. Goodwin WJ, Schmidt JF. Iatrogenic nasal tip bossae. Etiology, prevention, and treatment. *Arch Otolaryngol Head Neck Surg.* 1987;113:737–739.
11. Kridel RW, Yoon PJ, Koch RJ, et al. Prevention and correction of nasal tip bossae in rhinoplasty. *Arch Fac Plast Surg.* 2003;5:416–422.
12. Allen BC, Rhee JS. Complications associated with isotretinoin use after rhinoplasty. *Aesthet Plast Surg.* 2005;29:102–106.

CHAPTER TWENTY-SEVEN

The Thick-Skinned Rhinoplasty Patient

Richard E. Davis

When it comes to the subject of rhinoplasty, many authors trivialize or overlook the role of nasal skin in cosmetic nasal surgery. Instead, interest is directed at the nasal skeleton and the various methods of modifying the underlying skeletal framework. Although skeletal modification is fundamental to a successful rhinoplasty, the nasal skin and its associated soft tissue components, often called the skin–soft tissue envelope (SSTE), also play a critical role in the surgical outcome. Indeed, for a small subset of rhinoplasty patients, soft tissues may prove the limiting factor in creating a more beautiful nose. At the very least, it is the nasal SSTE that transforms the unfamiliar shape of the raw nasal skeleton into the refined and elegant outer contour of an attractive human nose. Moreover, this transformation is far from simplistic. Owing to site-specific variations in skin thickness within the nose, the skin's contribution to nasal topography is nonlinear and indirect, making cosmetic nasal surgery a *translational* activity—exponentially more challenging than directly sculpting an object's surface contour. Furthermore, because the SSTE is susceptible to the capricious effects of contracture, fibrosis, and edema, unforeseen skin changes can alter the intended nasal contour and compromise the otherwise well-executed operation. In rare but extreme cases, soft tissue healing aberrations may become so severe as to negate the skeletal modifications entirely, resulting in even greater cosmetic deformity. Hence, to ignore the importance of the SSTE in cosmetic nasal surgery is to disregard a critical component of the surgical outcome.

VARIATIONS IN SKIN TYPE

While skin of any type can potentially spoil the rhinoplasty outcome, it is generally skin types on the extreme limits of thickness that are the most challenging for the cosmetic nasal surgeon. In patients with extremely *thin* nasal skin, the atretic covering offers scant camouflage or concealment, and the surgeon must render a flawless underlying skeletal contour to prevent visible imperfections in the surface topography. Moreover, both

telangiectasias and dyschromias are easily provoked with surgical dissection of thin nasal skin. On the other hand, delicate skin is generally much less prone to edema or excessive fibrosis, and skin incisions tend to heal favorably in thin-skinned individuals. In fact, the thin-skinned rhinoplasty patient will often experience a shorter-than-average length of recovery with far less soft tissue distortion.

In contrast to the thin-skinned nose, extremely *thick* nasal skin conceals all but the most conspicuous imperfections of the underlying nasal skeleton. However, the advantages of ultra-thick skin end there. In fact, excessive skin thickness is often regarded as one of the most formidable, and sometimes insurmountable, obstacles in cosmetic rhinoplasty. The reasons for this sinister distinction are numerous, and the hazards of thick nasal skin have prompted many surgeons to avoid treating this challenging patient population altogether. However, as ethnic diversity continues to increase throughout the United States, thick-skinned patients have become an increasingly prevalent segment of the rhinoplasty consumer demographic. Moreover, the growing popularity of cosmetic nasal surgery in places like South America and Asia, where thick nasal skin is common, ensures that thick-skinned patients will become more prevalent worldwide. Without question, the thick-skinned rhinoplasty patient will be seen with greater frequency in the future, and demands for effective ethnically appropriate outcomes will increase accordingly.[1]

ANATOMY OF NASAL SKIN

Histologic analysis of *nasal* skin reveals most of the same components and structures found elsewhere in the integument. However, several important differences are worth noting. Without question, the most profound difference is a discrete fibromuscular tissue layer that separates the nasal skin from the underlying skeletal framework. Comprised largely of skeletal muscle, this fibromuscular layer is functionally and anatomically analogous to the superficial musculoaponeurotic system (SMAS) seen elsewhere in the face.[2] Dubbed the "nasal SMAS," this fibromuscular layer also varies in thickness according to the individual skin type. In the thin-skinned nose, pores are small and both the dermis and the nasal SMAS are thin and delicate. In contrast, large pores and modest dermal thickening are often observed in thick-skinned noses. However, robust hypertrophic thickening of the nasal SMAS layer is considered to be the underlying cause of the thick-skinned nose.[3] In fact, hypertrophy of the nasal SMAS can more than double the thickness of normal nasal skin. Fortunately, the nasal SMAS is also a discrete tissue layer that can be excised with relative ease—a key feature in surgical management of the ultra thick-skinned nose.

Although dermal thickening and muscle hypertrophy are frequently observed in the thick-skinned nose, these characteristics are seldom distributed evenly (Figure 27-1). For example, hypertrophy of the nasal SMAS is typically most prominent in the nasal tip and immediate surroundings. In contrast, very little muscle hypertrophy is observed at the rhinion or columella, even in patients with ultra-thick skin. In the same way, fat is also more abundant in the thick-skinned nose. However, fat makes little contribution to overall flap thickness *except* in the nasal root and supratip regions. In conclusion, all noses have site-specific variations in flap thickness, but thick-skinned noses tend to have more fat, a thicker dermis, and markedly thickened fibromuscular tissues with comparatively few areas of thin, pliable soft tissue covering.

PHYSICAL LIMITATIONS OF THE THICK-SKINNED NOSE

As a consequence of its physical bulk and added weight, thick nasal skin poses a formidable challenge for the rhinoplasty surgeon. Perhaps the foremost challenge is the loss of surface definition created by *masking* of the underlying skeletal framework. Because thick nasal skin more effectively obscures topographic features of the underlying nasal skeleton, the delicate surface undulations which characterize a well-defined and attractive nose are lost. Moreover, a weak and underprojected nasal framework only serves to exacerbate the loss of surface highlights.

In addition to skeletal masking, ultra-thick nasal skin also burdens the cartilage framework with added *weight* relative to a thin nasal covering. Surgical modifications that undermine structural support are ill-advised, especially in thick-skinned noses, since progressive skeletal collapse and nasal deformity often ensue. Instead, cosmetic modifications must be accompanied by structural reinforcement to ensure both an attractive outer contour *and* a skeletal framework that can permanently support

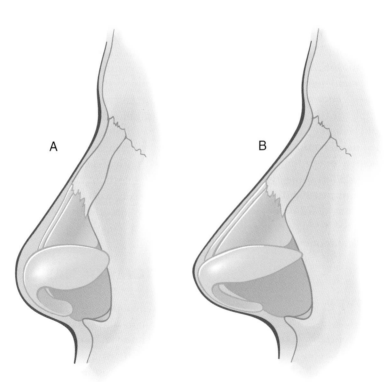

Figure 27-1 Schematic comparison of nasal skin thickness in the thick-skinned platyrrhine nose (**A**) and in the mesorrhine nose with intermediate skin thickness (**B**). In both types of nasal morphology, skin is thickest at the nasion and supratip. However, in the platyrrhine nose (**A**), the cartilage framework is typically weak and underprojected, with broad, soft alar cartilages that are covered by a comparatively thick skin–soft tissue envelope. In contrast, the mesorrhine nose (**B**) is characterized by a strong, well-projected skeletal framework and a more delicate skin–soft tissue envelope, giving rise to a more attractive outer contour.

the added burden of bulky nasal skin. Indeed, without a sturdy and structurally secure cartilage framework, a stable and more refined nasal contour is virtually impossible. Although rigid skeletal support does not by itself ensure a more beautiful nose, a strong nose with ample structural support is the first and foremost requirement for cosmetic enhancement in the thick-skinned patient.

In addition to safeguarding against structural col- ... l rigid skeletal framework ... nasal skin to further refine ... the nasal tip skin over a ... letal framework improves ... g, and thus thinning, the ... increases in nasal length ... lly improve surface high- ... not only a sturdy skeletal ... distensible skin envelope. ... *elasticity*, forceful attempts ... e may produce unsightly ... essive skin tension. In the ... al thickening, the resulting ... n stretching and prohibits ... In extreme cases, severely ... ent desired increases in tip ... wever, not all thick-skinned ... ity. In some thick-skinned ... ghly distensible despite its ... nning can be achieved with ... nsion. Therefore, skin elas- ... te with skin thickness, and ... nent of skin distensibility is ... nned patients, particularly ... ey determinant of surgical ... sal skin may become leath- ... previous nasal surgery, the ... is also vitally important in ... ent.

... elope is an important tool in ... inned nose, it is not without ... tension may restrict cutane- ... rculatory compromise or even ... l skin is stretched too tightly. ... reased by preexisting factors ... flow, such as tobacco use, ... caine-induced vascular com- ... that may compromise per- ... of electrocautery, reckless or ... and overly tight compression ... of the situation, nutrient blood flow ... ed by ensuring sustained capillary refill, particularly upon application of a tight compression dressing. Visible signs of vascular insufficiency, such as blanching, loss of capillary refill, or severe venous congestion, should prompt immediate intervention directed at the restoration of nutrient blood flow. Topical vasodilators, such as nitroglycerin paste or topically applied

nifedipine, may be useful in treating postoperative vasospasm,[4] but surgical intervention may be needed to reduce skin tension and restore perfusion when conservative measures prove ineffective.

Whereas the cosmetic merits of a rigid skeletal framework and a taut, tightly adherent skin envelope are irrefutable, optimization of surface definition will sometimes require a nose that is aesthetically too large for the face. Although this dilemma has no easy answers, an artfully proportioned and well-defined, if slightly oversized, nose is generally preferable to a smaller, yet amorphous one. In every case, a careful preoperative assessment of skin elasticity, coupled with a frank discussion regarding the limitations of thick skin, is imperative to establish appropriate cosmetic expectations.

Ironically, even though good skeletal support is paramount in the thick-skinned nose, most individuals with overly thick nasal skin also possess soft and exceedingly weak nasal cartilage. This is best exemplified in the *platyrrhine* nasal morphology known for its broad flat nasal contour. In addition to its hallmark shape, the platyrrhine nose is also characterized by thick inelastic nasal skin, soft underprojected tip cartilages, and a small underdeveloped nasal septum (see Figure 27-1). In fact, the distinctive architecture of the platyrrhine nose is widely regarded as one of the most difficult technical challenges in cosmetic nasal surgery. Paradoxically, the unfavorable combination of thick skin and weak cartilage is compounded by the need to substantially increase nasal tip projection in most platyrrhine noses. While the platyrrhine nose is arguably among the most challenging of all anatomic configurations, it is also among the most common nasal morphologies worldwide.

ADVERSE HEALING CHARACTERISTICS OF THICK NASAL SKIN

Although the physical properties of bulky inelastic skin often complicate its surgical manipulation, it is the adverse healing characteristics of thick skin that most profoundly distinguish it from other skin types. Although *all* surgically manipulated nasal skin exhibits a characteristic cycle of inflammation, repair, and recovery; thick nasal skin is far more prone to excessive inflammation, prolonged tissue distortion, and abnormal recovery. Unlike thin nasal skin which exhibits only modest edema and minimal fibrosis, in virtually all thick-skinned individuals, robust edema gives rise to unwanted cosmetic distortion and prolonged recovery. In the thin-skinned individual, rapid restoration of the lymphatic and capillary circulation leads to prompt reduction of lymphedema and softening of the firm and swollen nasal soft tissues. Often this process is complete in as little as 3 to 6 months. This in turn gives rise to a thin, delicate, and more tightly adherent skin envelope, producing a more attractive and better defined nasal contour. In contrast, for the thick-skinned individual, capillary and lymphatic channels are slow to recanalize and recovery is protracted, sometimes requiring as long as 18 to 24 months for complete recuperation. Soft-tissue edema temporarily obscures surface highlights and skeletal modifications often appear overly conservative or even imperceptible. In severe cases, swelling may never fully resolve as prolonged lymphedema may trigger subcutaneous fibrosis and permanent increases in skin thickness. Exogenous influences, such as sunburn, acne, allergic rhinitis, tobacco use, vigorous exercise, or prolonged dependent posture, may also exacerbate swelling and increase the risk of unwanted fibrosis, particularly in previously operated noses or noses undergoing extensive surgical dissection. For these challenging patients, subcutaneous fibrosis may occasionally prove difficult to control and may actually result in a larger and less attractive nose, particularly when the nasal skeleton has been aggressively reduced in size and/or when preventative measures have been neglected. Hence, the need to curtail runaway inflammation is paramount in the thick-skinned patient.

In addition to unwanted fibrotic thickening of the skin envelope, thick-skinned patients, like all rhinoplasty patients, are also susceptible to contracture of the nasal soft tissues. In extreme cases, contracture and adhesions triggered by subcutaneous fibrosis can severely distort the underlying nasal framework giving rise to progressive misalignment and unsightly nasal deformity. Patients with naturally weak or surgically compromised skeletal tissues are particularly prone to this undesirable wound-healing phenomenon, again underscoring the importance of secure skeletal support in the thick-skinned nose. Although the cosmetic ideal may dictate a reduction in nasal size, soft tissue complications such as fibrosis or contracture are far more common following aggressive size reductions. Thus, in the oversized thick-skinned nose, it is often prudent to sacrifice diminutive size in exchange for improved overall shape and enhanced definition.

PERIOPERATIVE MANAGEMENT

While surgical swelling is undesirable in all patients, it is often far more detrimental in the thick-skinned rhinoplasty patient. To minimize the threat of unfavorable wound healing, all reasonable efforts should be taken to prevent and/or contain surgical swelling and inflammation. Without question, this is best accomplished through a multifaceted approach. First, favorable anatomic dissection planes are exploited using delicate surgical dissection combined with meticulous soft tissue technique. This limits disruption of the lymphatic and capillary networks while minimizing the release of harmful inflammatory mediators. Suture materials prone to a robust

inflammatory response, such as catgut or Vicryl are avoided whenever possible, and tissue trauma is minimized with judicious use of electrocautery and tissue retraction. Prior to surgery, nasal soft tissues are also vasoconstricted with topical decongestants and infiltrated with adrenaline to minimize the extravasation of blood and fluid. Ancillary supportive measures, such as controlled hypotension, corticosteroids, icepacks, upright positioning, compressive bandaging, and emesis prevention, further help to prevent unwanted fluid extravasation.

Despite prudent measures to contain surgical inflammation, in a small number of thick-skinned patients, a vigorous and sustained inflammatory response may still develop. In the worst case scenario, the outcome is severe cosmetic distortion, often accompanied by nasal airway obstruction. While there is no conclusive means of identifying susceptible patients, the incidence is much higher in patients with darker skin tones, thick sebaceous skin, and a history of hypertrophic scars or keloid formation. Postoperative steroid treatment may negate the inflammatory response, but early intervention is essential, since it is often difficult or even impossible to reexpand the thickened and scarred soft tissue envelope.

SKELETAL AUGMENTATION

In addition to the mandatory adjunctive measures for controlling surgical inflammation discussed above, perhaps the single most important element in the thick-skinned rhinoplasty is secure structural support. Without question, achieving good surface definition is far more likely when thick skin has been stretched to its full capacity over a stable and shapely nasal framework. While this goal requires both a healthy cutaneous blood supply and rigid skeletal tissues, the cutaneous blood supply is largely predetermined, and only skeletal rigidity can be improved to any significant extent. However, a skeletal framework of sufficient rigidity is not easily achieved in the patient with naturally weak nasal cartilage. Not only must the framework bear the additional weight of thick skin, it must also provide sufficient strength to stretch the inelastic tissues and to resist the formidable deformational forces of postoperative swelling and contracture. Ironically, the thick-skinned nose, particularly the platyrrhine morphology, is often structurally deficient to begin with, and thick-skinned noses often lack cartilage of sufficient quantity or quality to create a secure skeletal framework. Consequently, autologous rib cartilage and/or conchal cartilage grafts are frequently needed to augment skeletal support and enhance nasal contour in the thick-skinned individual.

While the specifics of skeletal augmentation and structural fortification are beyond the scope of this chapter, a host of established and effective grafting techniques are now available to ensure a structurally secure and rigid nasal framework. Although skeletal reconstruction is sometimes a formidable task, particularly in the previously operated nose, modern structural rhinoplasty techniques have proved invaluable in the thick-skinned patient. In fact, owing to the reliability of these techniques, it is most often the lack of skin distensibility, rather than structural instability, that is the limiting factor in cosmetic enhancement of the thick-skinned nose.

Despite structural fortification of the thick-skinned nose with autologous cartilage, a satisfactory cosmetic outcome is not a foregone conclusion. In every nose, the tug-of-war between skeletal rigidity and soft tissue compliance is governed by a host of independent variables. The collective impact of soft tissue influences, such as elasticity, fibrosis, contracture, vascularity, immune function, and inflammation, serve to create either a hostile or favorable environment for the transplanted cartilage. Cartilage characteristics, such as size, shape, ischemic tolerance, susceptibility to warping, and fixation technique, also combine to influence the end result. Which forces will ultimately prevail is impossible to predict with absolute certainty, and favorable prognostic indicators are not a guarantee of success. However, when the complexion is smooth and healthy, when the skeletal tissues are abundant and firm, and when the soft tissue inflammatory reaction is modest, sound surgical principles are usually rewarded with a noticeably more attractive nasal contour.

Just as enlarging the skeletal framework will theoretically enhance nasal contour, so too, shrinking the skeletal framework may have the opposite effect. Perhaps the most difficult patient in rhinoplasty is the thick-skinned individual with a massively oversized nose. Although reduction rhinoplasty is needed to enhance facial aesthetics, the loss of skeletal volume creates copious dead space, often giving rise to edema, fibrosis, and additional thickening of the already thick skin. Instead of a tightly adherent skin envelope with enhanced contour and improved definition, the thick-skinned nose may appear amorphous, unstructured, and decidedly less attractive, despite its smaller size. Moreover, the capacity of nasal skin to shrink also declines with age, and is particularly poor in the older adult with inelastic skin. Because a *less* attractive nose is a very real possibility in this circumstance, it is often best to forego elective cosmetic rhinoplasty in this small subset of thick-skinned patients.

NASAL SKIN "DEFATTING"

While a sturdy and well-proportioned nasal framework remains the cornerstone of effective rhinoplasty, surgical thinning of the SSTE is a potentially safe and effective means of achieving additional definition and contour refinement in the ultra thick-skinned nose. Although nasal "defatting" has been advocated for decades, this term has been used to denote a group of dissimilar surgical techniques that are often risky and potentially harmful. Techniques that seek to promote skin flap shrinkage, such as dermal cross-hatching or CO_2 laser treatment of the flap undersurface, are ill advised since dermal thickening and decreased elasticity often result. Injuries to the subdermal plexus may also result from these techniques, potentially leading to vascular insufficiency and skin necrosis, particularly when combined with aggressive skeletal augmentation and/or comorbidities such as tobacco use. In contrast, careful excision of the fibromuscular tissue layer can provide a safe and effective surgical adjunct to cosmetic rhinoplasty in select thick-skinned individuals. In addition to restoring the skin envelope to a more favorable thickness, nasal SMAS excision may also improve skin distensibility to further improve surface highlights.

SMAS DEBULKING TECHNIQUE

Using the exposure afforded by the external rhinoplasty approach, the fibromuscular SMAS layer is accessed for surgical debulking. Following standard skin incisions, the nasal framework is degloved in the subperichondrial plane using mostly blunt (cotton swab) dissection to minimize disruption of the capillary and lymphatic networks. Once elevated, the full depth of the SSTE can be evaluated, and the contribution of the fibromuscular tissue layer can be assessed (Figure 27-2, A). In patients with ultra-thick nasal skin (usually 5-mm total thickness or more), the fibromuscular SMAS layer can be safely excised in areas where improved surface definition is desired—usually the tip, supratip, and infratip lobule. In order to maintain a uniform flap thickness and avoid injury to the subdermal plexus, the fibromuscular SMAS layer is excised en bloc using a combination of blunt and sharp dissection[5] (Figure 27-2, B–D). With careful and direct dissection of the SMAS layer, the subdermal plexus is left largely undisturbed, and the nutrient blood supply to the nasal skin is protected, a vitally important step if aggressive skin stretching is also planned. Special care is exercised near the alar groove where the predominant blood supply enters the subdermal plexus[6] (Figure 27-3). In addition to creating a uniform flap thickness, en bloc excision yields a slab of malleable graft material that can be used for augmentation of the radix or other deficient sites. While this procedure can sometimes be performed in revision rhinoplasty patients, previous surgical disruption of the soft tissues may make navigation far more challenging. Possible complications, such as inadvertent skin perforation or ischemic skin necrosis, are rare, but occur with

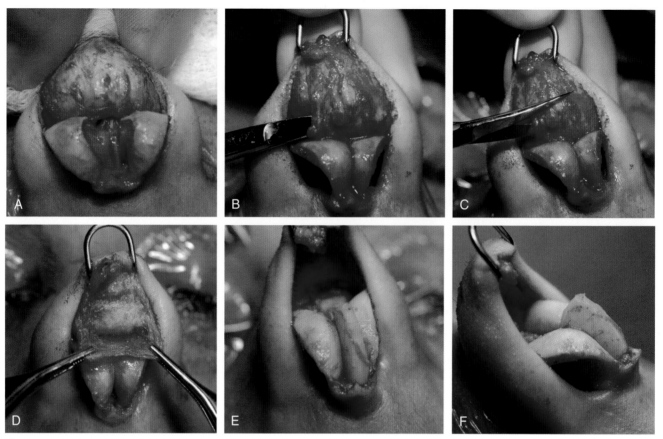

Figure 27-2 A–D, Intraoperative views showing en bloc excision of fibromuscular (nasal SMAS) tissue layer with preservation of underlying subdermal fat. **E, F,** Skeletal augmentation with septocolumellar extension graft.

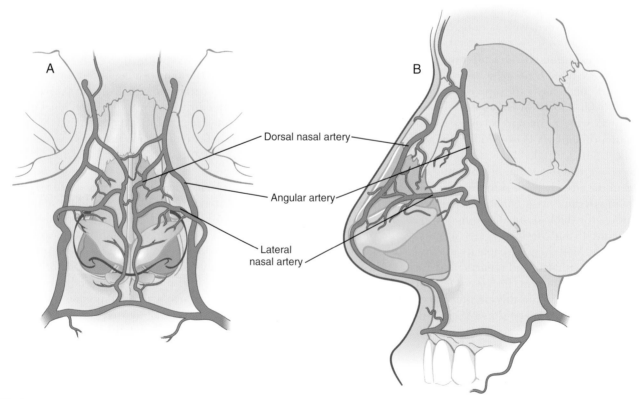

Dorsal nasal artery

Angular artery

Lateral nasal artery

Figure 27-3 Schematic illustration of predominant arterial blood supply to the nasal tip skin from the front (**A**) and lateral (**B**) perspectives. The nasal tip skin is perfused by a rich interconnecting vascular arcade derived from both the internal and external carotid systems. The proximal nose is supplied by terminal branches of the internal carotid artery: the angular artery (*AA*) and the dorsal nasal artery (*DN*). However, the nasal tip is supplied predominantly by the external carotid system via the lateral nasal artery (*LN*). As a terminal branch of the facial artery, the lateral nasal artery courses 2 to 3 mm above the alar groove and should be preserved during dissection to avoid compromise of nutrient blood flow.

greater frequency in the severely fibrotic revision rhinoplasty patient, especially those with preexisting comorbidities such as nicotine use.

COMPRESSION DRESSING

Immediately following surgical intervention the focus shifts to postoperative supportive care. For the thick-skinned rhinoplasty patient, supportive care can "make or break" the surgical outcome. Intraoperatively, supportive care begins with a firm yet gentle, cinch-type compression dressing. Binding the nose securely with hypoallergenic tape and a nasal splint limits nasal edema, minimizes dead space, and tamponades small vessel bleeding. Although an overly tight bandage potentially risks soft tissue ischemia, a gentle compression dressing restricts postoperative swelling and is an important tool in postoperative edema management. Capillary refill is monitored closely in the first 12 to 24 hours after dressing placement to ensure that nutrient blood flow remains intact, and ancillary supportive measures such as ice, elevation, rest, antiemetics, and blood pressure control are instituted to minimize swelling. While 6 to 7 days of gentle compression are generally most effective, the dressing is sometimes removed sooner in cases of vascular insufficiency or contact dermatitis.

POSTOPERATIVE STEROID TREATMENT

In general, all thick-skinned individuals should be considered at risk for dead-space fibrosis and cutaneous thickening regardless of nasal size. In addition to a well-designed compression dressing and aggressive perioperative edema management, long-term avoidance of sunburn, excessive salt intake, prolonged recumbent posture, and strenuous activity will help to facilitate shrinkage of the swollen skin envelope. In the event that supportive measures are unsuccessful, adjunctive treatment measures may also prove beneficial. Such treatments include massage, stenting, compressive taping, topical steroid administration, and steroid injection. Of these, by far the most effective, yet also the most risky, is injection with triamcinolone acetonide suspension. This long-acting synthetic glucocorticoid acts to reduce edema and prevent fibrosis when injected into the subcutaneous nasal tissues. Commonly known by the brand name Kenalog (Bristol-Myers Squibb, Princeton, NJ), this powerful anti-inflammatory drug may also predispose to local tissue atrophy, such as dermal thinning, fat necrosis, or cartilage graft resorption. Triamcinolone may also predispose to localized infection or telangiectasias, and side effects are more common when used at full strength or frequent intervals. Fortunately, adverse reactions are usually avoided with a low starting concentration of 5 to 10 mg/ml, restricting the total dose to less than 5 mg, and gradually titrating to the desired effect. Treatment is best postponed in the first 2 to 3 months following surgery to prevent cartilage atrophy unless severe fibrosis or bony callus is evident. Prior to injection, triamcinolone acetonide is diluted in lidocaine containing epinephrine to minimize tissue spread and reduce injection site discomfort. Initial treatment results are usually evident within 3 to 4 weeks, but repeated monthly injections are often necessary before sustained clinical improvement is achieved. Although triamcinolone injection is a useful adjunct in the actively healing nose, it has little benefit in the fully healed nose—emphasizing the importance of timely intervention.

SUMMARY

The thick-skinned nose has long proved a difficult challenge for the cosmetic nasal surgeon. The challenge is even greater when thick skin is accompanied by a weak, underprojected cartilage framework. Although cosmetic expectations must be tempered, surgery in the thick-skinned patient often results in substantial cosmetic improvement when sound surgical principles are observed. The combination of a reinforced and well-proportioned nasal framework, coupled with a carefully thinned and taught nasal skin envelope, is often rewarded with surprisingly good cosmetic results in the favorable patient (Figure 27-4).

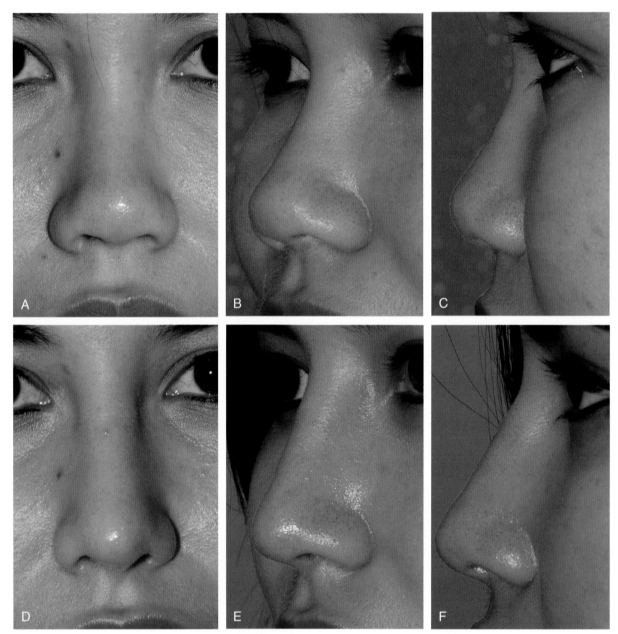

Figure 27-4 A–C, Preoperative views of thick-skinned platyrrhine nose prior to cosmetic rhinoplasty. **D–F,** Postoperative views after rib graft skeletal augmentation and nasal SMAS excision.

REFERENCES

1. Davis RE. Rhinoplasty and concepts of facial beauty. *Fac Plast Surg.* 2006;22(3):198–203.
2. Letourneau A, Daniel RK. The superficial musculoaponeurotic system of the nose. *Plast Reconstr Surg.* 1988;82:48–57.
3. Garramone Jr RR, Sullivan PK, Devaney K. Bulbous nasal tip: an anatomical and histological evaluation. *Ann Plast Surg.* 1995;34:288–291.
4. Davis RE, Wachholz J, Jassir D, et al. Comparison of topical anti-ischemic agents in the salvage of failing random-pattern skin flaps in rat. *Arch Fac Plast Surg.* 1999;1(1):27–32.
5. Davis RE, Wayne I. Rhinoplasty and the nasal SMAS augmentation graft: advantages and indications. *Arch Fac Plast Surg.* 2004;6:124–132.
6. Rohrich RJ, Gunter JP, Friedman RM. Nasal tip blood supply: an anatomic study validating the safety of the transcollumellar incision in rhinoplasty. *Plast Reconstr Surg.* 1995;95:795–799.

CHAPTER TWENTY-EIGHT

Short Nose

Michael M. Kim • *Tom D. Wang*

*"The very short nose is an atrociously eye-catching deformity, which attracts
ridicule and revulsion ... a plastic surgeon's nightmare."*
—D. Ralph Millard, Jr. M.D.[1]

Lengthening the short nose is one of the most difficult challenges in rhinoplasty. Etiologies for the development of a short nose include congenital, traumatic, iatrogenic (previous surgery), infectious, and granulomatous factors. Regardless of the cause, short nose correction requires the surgeon to precisely identify anatomical abnormalities and deficiencies and to perform an array of technically precise and difficult operative techniques.

THE SHORT NOSE DEFINED

There is no strict definition of what makes a nose "short," but multiple surrogate measurements exist. These proportions and measurements enable the surgeon to ascertain an "ideal" nasal length and shape that are harmonious with the rest of the face. The face in its vertical dimension may be divided into thirds, with the nose—measured from the glabella to the subnasale—comprising the middle third of the face. In a similar fashion, ideal nasal length measured from the radix to the subnasale should approximate 47% of the distance measured from the radix to the menton.[2]

Ideal nasal length can also be extrapolated through the use of various formulas devised to determine ideal nasal tip projection. Goode determined that the ideal ratio between nasal tip projection and length ranged from 0.55 to 0.6 : 1. The pitfall of using this ratio to extrapolate ideal nasal length is that one must assume ideal tip projection, a condition that is not universally met. In fact, many short noses feature poorly supported, underprojected tips.

Tip rotation is another determining factor in producing a short or short-appearing nose. Rotation is determined by the nasolabial angle or the angle between a line drawn from the subnasale along the columella and a line drawn from the subnasale down to the upper lip vermillion. Nasolabial angles are gender-specific in that an ideal male nasolabial angle ranges from 90 to 105 degrees, while the ideal female angle ranges from 95 to 115 degrees. Nasolabial angles greater than these ideal ranges are considered overrotated and can produce a "snub-nose" or "pig snout" appearance.

Additional factors that contribute to a short-appearing nose are a dorsal concavity, a long upper lip, an overprojected tip, and a low and deep nasion or nasal starting point.[3] In Caucasian patients, the nasal starting point should be at the level of the superior palpebral fissure, while in other ethnic populations, such as Asians, a lower starting point at a mid-pupillary level may be more appropriate.

A thorough understanding of ideal nasal proportions enables the surgeon to identify patient-specific anatomic deficiencies. As such, various operative maneuvers and techniques have been devised to lengthen a short nose into a more ideal shape.

A SHORT HISTORY OF SHORT NOSE CORRECTION TECHNIQUES

Jackson and Reid[4] and Millard[1] used full-thickness external incisions in the supratip area referred to as a "guillotine chop." The tip was then released inferiorly, creating a defect of the skin–soft tissue envelope (SSTE). This cutaneous defect was then replaced with tissue provided by a paramedian forehead flap. The placement of cartilage grafts was staged and done only when extra support was deemed necessary.

Dingman and Walter[5] emphasized the augmentation of inner lining through the use of composite grafts. Bilateral, curved conchal cartilage composite grafts were placed within bilateral intercartilaginous incisions. The septal portions of the flaps were sewn together such that the two grafts were "gull wing"–like in appearance. The juxtaposition of the septal portion of the grafts essentially created a four-layer composite graft. If the SSTE was deficient, cutaneous releasing incisions in conjunction with forehead flap reconstruction were used.

Kamer's technique also featured the use of composite grafts in short nose correction.[6] He described the inferior release of the bilateral mucoperichondrial flaps through the use of staggered septal incisions. The mucoperichondrial void created within the inferiormost incision was filled with a composite cartilage graft, while the superiormost void was left to heal by secondary intention. As with Dingman's technique, the grafts were not fixated to the underlying cartilaginous substructure.

In 1987, Giammanco described the use of a pedicled chondromucosal flap in short nose correction.[7] This flap emanated from the dorsal septal cartilage and was rotated to reside along the caudal edge of the septal cartilage. This maneuver, in conjunction with bilateral composite grafts placed between the upper and lower lateral cartilages, served to lengthen the nose by creating additional septal extension.

Gruber's preferred technique featured the release of the lower lateral cartilages from the upper lateral cartilages.[8] Depending on the amount of release and correction necessary, intervening auricular composite grafts (with the skin side replacing a vestibular defect) may be used as an interposition graft. Subsequent placement of a batten graft secured to the caudal septal cartilage served to brace the tip into its new, lower position.

Through an endonasal delivery approach, Gunter and Rohrich[9] performed a similar tip release maneuver between the upper and lower cartilages. In addition, they resected a small wedge-shaped portion of the posterior septal angle. Therefore, the nose gained absolute length via the tip release maneuver while apparent length was afforded by the posterior septal angle excision. Both maneuvers serve to counter rotate—and consequently lengthen—the nose. Additional apparent lengthening through modest deprojection is afforded by the transfixion portion of the incision. They described this technique as a "less aggressive" approach to lengthening that would obviate the need for flaps, grafts, and implants, while acknowledging that that this operation was mostly suitable for minor to moderately short noses.

MODERN LENGTHENING TECHNIQUES

Many different nasal lengthening techniques have been described. As is the case with many surgical challenges, the fact that many operative techniques exist illustrates that there is not one single ideal technique. However, despite their differences, most modern and successful short nose operations often exhibit the following: (1) extensive undermining of the SSTE, (2) release, mobilization, or replacement of the inner lining, and, most importantly, (3) the construction of a stable cartilaginous or bony framework that can resist the relentless forces of contraction exhibited by the healing nose.[3]

Recent descriptions of nasal lengthening techniques build upon the work of the aforementioned pioneers. Currently, many of these surgical descriptions emphasize open structure techniques and increasingly stable reconstructions of the cartilage framework designed to resist the contractile forces associated with healing.

Increased nasal length can be achieved by anchoring grafts to the existing septal cartilage. An example is the caudal septal extension graft. These extension grafts can be fashioned into a wedge shape such that the wider end is placed anteriorly. This placement serves to counter rotate the nasal tip and add absolute length to the nose.[10] Due to this graft's unilateral nature, it is preferably sutured to the nondeviated side to achieve balance (Figure 28-1).

Alternatively, extended spreader grafts—which extend past the anterior septal angle—may be used for increased length in conjunction with an extended columellar strut. Fixation of these two structures can create a longer and more stable cartilaginous L-strut. The dorsal portion of the strut, which is composed of the paired extended spreader grafts, is suture-fixated to the existing dorsal septum and the paired upper lateral cartilages. The caudal portion of the L-strut is then either placed to reside within a columellar pocket or anchored to the nasal spine. Once the L-strut is in place, then the medial crura of the lower lateral cartilages are sutured to the columellar strut in a tongue-and-groove manner. Placement of the lower lateral cartilages can be tailored to reside in a less rotated position.

Multiple versions of this L-strut have been described with relatively minor differences.[11,12] However, one special case deserves mention. In cases where saddle deformity is concomitantly present, a canoe-shaped cartilage graft crafted from autologous costal cartilage can be used for both dorsal augmentation and lengthening. Fixation of this graft can be achieved by cutting a notch in the caudal end of the graft and interdigitating a columellar strut graft. The result is an L-strut with the benefit of having the additional dorsal bulk required to augment the saddle-nose deformity.[13]

Despite the interest in open structure techniques, many simple, less aggressive maneuvers are available to lengthen the short nose. Because nasal length is measured from the tip-defining points to the nasal starting point, it would follow that placing the nasal starting point in a more cephalic position and the tip-defining points in a more caudal position would provide additional length. The former can be achieved by placing radix grafts in patients who have a low and deep radix. This is done while keeping in mind that the ideal nasal starting point in Caucasians is approximately at the level of the superior palpebral fissure, while certain ethnic populations, such as Asians, feature ideal nasal starting points at the mid-pupillary level.

At the tip of the nose, grafts can be placed to move the tip-defining points to a more inferior position while simultaneously providing apparent counter rotation. On occasion, stacking multiple layers of tip grafts may be necessary to achieve the desired amount of correction. Additional derotation can be achieved by a conservative wedge-shaped resection of the membranous septum with the wider portion of wedge resection positioned anteriorly. The clear benefit of these less aggressive techniques is that

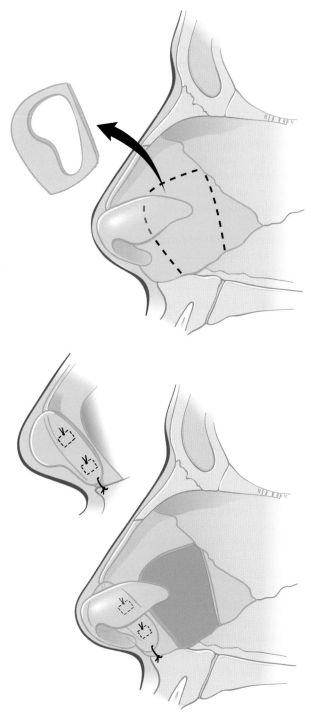

Figure 28-1 A caudal septal extension graft harvested from septal cartilage. The wedge shape allows for counter rotation and consequent lengthening of the nasal tip.

tip support structures are maintained and thus do not need replacement or reconstitution.

GRAFTING MATERIALS

With the techniques described here, abundant grafting material is often required. Autologous sources of cartilage include auricular, septal, and costal cartilage. Advantages

of using auricular cartilage include minimal donor site morbidity, minimal resorption, the possibility of simultaneous harvest, and the possibility of composite grafting. However, auricular cartilage often lacks the rigidity to provide meaningful strength and support for structural purposes, but can be useful in fashioning tip grafts. Septal cartilage may have adequate strength and stability, but it is often absent or insufficient secondary to harvest from a prior operation. If present, septal cartilage can be used to fashion tip grafts, columellar struts, and/or spreader grafts. Autologous costal cartilage has the advantage of potentially providing abundant amounts of rigid grafting material. Some potential disadvantages include donor site pain, scarring, and the possibility of pneumothorax and graft warping. However, with technical refinements, many of the potential complications related to rib cartilage harvest have been minimized. The use of homologous, irradiated cadaveric costal cartilage in lengthening is less ideal in light of its relatively higher resorption rates.[14]

Alloplastic materials such as expanded polytetrafluoroethylene (Gore-Tex; Implantech Associates, Ventura, CA) and porous polyethylene (Medpor; Porex Surgical, Newnan, GA) can also be used in the short nose. Layered Gore-Tex sheets or blocks can augment dorsal and radix deficiencies, while the structural rigidity of Medpor allows for its use as a stable columellar strut or caudal septal extension grafts. Although alloplastic materials are easy to work with and obviate the need for a separate donor site, their increased rates of infection and extrusion relative to autologous materials have limited their popularity within the United States.

PREOPERATIVE CONSIDERATIONS

The importance of the preoperative history and physical cannot be overemphasized. Notably, the patient's past medical and surgical history may impact the surgeon's ability to achieve optimal results. Previous rhinoplasty or nasal procedures can make surgical correction extremely challenging as many of the problems associated with the postrhinoplasty short nose stem from the overzealous resection of cartilage and support structures. For instance, the removal or overresection of lateral crura can cause overrotation of the nasal tip as predicted by the "tripod" concept described by Anderson.[15] Similarly, overresection of a prominent nasal dorsum may cause iatrogenic saddling, another feature contributing to a short nose. These factors, in addition to changes to the SSTE after nasal surgery, can make revision short nose surgery technically demanding.

A thorough examination of the nose facilitates the identification of patient-specific anatomic deficiencies. Assessment of the degree of tip support should be performed as these elements may require replacement or strengthening during the upcoming surgery. An intranasal examination should ascertain the presence or absence of internal lining as a paucity of septal mucosa (e.g., septal perforation) and vestibular skin may require replacement or at least wide elevation and release. Last, the mobility and quality of the SSTE deserve close evaluation. Toriumi et al.[13] caution others with regard to the presence of a significantly immobile and scarred envelope as this may limit the amount of nasal lengthening possible. In those patients, they advocate a preoperative program of vigorous massage to aid in stretching and loosening the SSTE.[13]

Standard, seven-view preoperative studio-quality photographs should be taken to compare the patient's nasal shape to previously mentioned ideals. Some practitioners perform computer imaging to predict or estimate nasal changes following surgical correction. Discussion of these images with the patient may be helpful to explain the surgery and set expectations so long as conservative computer modifications are made. If one is to use computer-altered imaging, it is important to show realistic modifications because changes are infinitely easier to perform at the computer table than in the operating room.

The patient's anatomy will guide the surgeon with regard to what techniques or combination of techniques will be required. However, an algorithm devised by Naficy and Baker attempts to simplify this process.[3] The crucial decision-point in their short nose algorithm concerns the status of tip rotation. If the nasal tip is overrotated, maneuvers such as the "flying buttress graft" or L-strut, interposition grafts between the upper and lower lateral cartilages, wedge-shaped caudal septal extension grafts, and layered tip grafts may be appropriate. On the other hand, if the tip is underrotated or has normal rotation, techniques such as radix grafting, full-length tip grafts, and rectangular caudal septal extension grafts may be used when appropriate. Regardless of the system used by the surgeon, treatment must be individualized based on correcting each patient's specific deficiencies.

OUR TECHNIQUE IN DETAIL

After general anesthesia is induced, the patient is intubated and turned toward the surgeons. Two cotton pledgets soaked in 4% cocaine are placed within each side of the nose. A 1:1 local anesthesia mixture consisting of 1% lidocaine with 1:100,000 of epinephrine and 0.5% bupivacaine with 1:100,000 of epinephrine is infiltrated under the SSTE, nasal base, and bilateral septal mucoperichondrial flaps. The patient is then prepped and draped in a sterile fashion. Bilateral marginal incisions and an inverted-V transcolumellar incision are made with a No. 15 scalpel. The columellar skin is carefully elevated by scissor dissection without damaging the intimately associated medial crura of the lower lateral cartilages. Often the paired columellar arteries must be cauterized for optimal hemostasis. Elevation of the SSTE from the remaining portions of the lower lateral cartilages is done via

a three-point retraction technique. At this point of the procedure, the surgeon may encounter previously placed grafts, especially in the case of revision surgery. These grafts should be removed and may be potentially reused if appropriate.

Continued elevation of the SSTE in a subnasal superficial musculoaponeurotic system plane (SMAS) is carried up to the rhinion. At that juncture, elevation of the envelope in a subperiosteal plane is achieved with a Joseph elevator. Excessive lateral and cephalic extension should be avoided. On occasion, only a small precise pocket should be elevated to accommodate radix or dorsal only grafts, minimizing the possibility of postoperative migration.

In cases where minimal lengthening is needed, this amount of dissection may be sufficient as the placement of radix grafts, dorsal only grafts, and tip grafts may be done with little difficulty and without disrupting potentially intact tip support elements. Septal cartilage can be harvested through a Killian incision or hemitransfixion incision. At least 1 cm of septal cartilage along the dorsal and caudal portions of the cartilage is retained to preserve an important support structure.

Auricular cartilage can be harvested from the conchal bowl through an anterior or posterior approach based on surgeon's preference. Our preference is to harvest through an anterior approach due to the ease of harvest and the virtually inconspicuous nature of the antihelical scar. Additional local anesthesia mixture is infiltrated under the anterior and posterior skin attached to the conchal bowl. This hydrodissection is avoided in cases where a composite graft is required. An anterior skin incision along the antihelical fold is made and extended superiorly and inferiorly to reside within the periphery of the concha. The skin is then elevated off of the conchal cartilage. Tip grafts are preferably shaped like an isosceles triangle and therefore the anterior portion, or base of the triangle, should be thickest as it is transplanted in an anterior position to help with derotation. Therefore, the base of the triangle is preferentially harvested closest to external auditory canal as this is the thickest portion of conchal cartilage. Other portions of the conchal cartilage may be harvested for grafting as well, but retention of a "shoulder" of cartilage medial to the antihelical fold will minimize the potential postoperative appearance of palpable and visible cut edges of cartilage. Closure is achieved with a running, locking 6-0 fast absorbing gut with subsequent placement of anterior and posterior Telfa bolsters secured in a through-and-through manner with 4-0 nylon suture.

In noses requiring more aggressive modification, both domes are grasped with Brown-Adson forceps and the intervening interdomal ligaments are separated. The anterior septal angle is identified and bilateral mucoperichondrial flaps are raised through an open septoplasty approach. Septal cartilage, if present, can be harvested for grafting material, and deviations of septal cartilage and bone can be addressed simultaneously. Great care should be taken during this portion of the procedure, especially in the case of revision surgery, as the risk of perforation between two directly apposed mucoperichondrial flaps is very high.

Often the paired upper lateral cartilages need to be separated from the midline septal cartilage so as to further identify the status of the septum and for additional inner lining release. This maneuver also facilitates the placement of extended spreader grafts, a prerequisite if a "flying buttress" L-strut is to be constructed. The placement of extended spreader grafts is particularly helpful in those noses with a pinched middle-third or an inverted-V deformity. The caudal portion of the L-strut can be fashioned by a columellar strut graft placed in a precise pocket along the columella and between the medial crura of the lower lateral cartilages. The columellar graft interdigitates between the paired, caudal portions of the extended columellar grafts and is fixed into position with 6-0 Prolene suture. Subsequently, the paired medial crura are fixed to the intervening columellar strut in a tongue-and-groove manner with 4-0 plain gut on a Keith needle. This relationship may be altered to provide additional counter rotation if required.

If the middle third is of adequate width, a caudal septal extension graft can be attached to the existing caudal septum with 6-0 Prolene mattress sutures. Because many short noses are overrotated, a wedge-shaped graft with the wide side anterior can confer counterrotation. Once again, the paired medial crura are fixed to the caudal septal extension graft in a tongue-and-groove manner. The use of caudal septal extension grafts is our preference when a large increase in nasal length is required as it is relatively simple to perform with potentially more predictable long-term results.

When concomitant saddling is present in addition to deficient nasal length, augmentation may be achieved through a variety of methods including costal cartilage grafting or the placement of alloplastic materials. If costal cartilage harvest is chosen, it can be performed with minimal associated complications or morbidity and has the added benefit of potentially serving as the dorsal portion of an L-strut if fixed to a columellar strut.

Once stability of the cartilaginous framework is ensured, nonstructural elements such as radix grafts and tip grafts can be placed. Layered tip grafts can be constructed to have more mass anteriorly and serve to counter rotate the nose and place the tip-defining points in a more caudal position.

While placing multiple grafts, the SSTE should be serially redraped over the modified cartilaginous scaffold, because the restricted mobility of a scarred SSTE may limit the amount of correction possible. The use of a single monocryl or Vicryl stitch in the center of the transcolumellar incision may be helpful in relieving tension from the redraped SSTE. Subsequent 6-0 fast-absorbing gut is used to close the remaining portions of the transcolumellar incision, while 5-0 chromic gut suture reapproximates the bilateral marginal incisions. The paired mucoperichondrial flaps are put in direct apposition with 4-0 Vicryl rapide in a running, quilting fashion.

At the conclusion of the procedure, skin adhesive followed by paper tape is placed on the dorsum so as to exert slight compression over the supratip area and provide modest cephalic support to the tip. A thermoplastic nasal splint is applied and tape is then placed over the splint. Bacitracin-coated Telfa packs are placed in the nose and are removed after 30 minutes while the patient is in the recovery room. Patients are typically seen on postoperative days 1 and 7.

ILLUSTRATIVE CASES

CASE 1

Patient 1 is a 32-year-old African American woman who had undergone four previous rhinoplasties. Her nose exhibited a widened dorsum, overrotated tip, and inadequate nasal length (Figure 28-2). Due to her previous rhinoplasty procedures, septal cartilage was unavailable for grafting.

The patient's nose was opened with bilateral marginal incisions and a transcolumellar incision. After elevation of the SSTE, the presence of bilateral spreader grafts was noted. Because she had excessive width in the middle third, the spreader grafts were removed. Subsequently, lateral osteotomies were performed to provide additional narrowing.

Auricular cartilage was harvested from the patient's left ear through an anterior approach. The donor site incision was closed and bolstered in front and back. Three layers of conchal cartilage were stacked and placed as a tip graft to affect a decreased nasolabial angle (Figure 28-3). The nose was closed in a standard fashion.

CASE 2

A 27-year-old man presented with a congenitally short, upturned nose. The tip was overrotated with excess nostril show and inadequate nasal length (Figure 28-4).

After the SSTE was elevated, bilateral dome division was performed via wedge resections with subsequent resuturing to affect additional caudal inclination of the lateral crura. The lower lateral cartilages were separated and septal cartilage was harvested through an open approach. A columellar strut graft was created from the septal cartilage and placed in a precise columellar pocket. The lower lateral cartilages were then sutured to the columellar strut in a tongue-and-groove fashion.

A "reverse" wedge of membranous septum was resected and the nasal spine was reduced. Both maneuvers combined to decrease the nasolabial angle. Last, auricular cartilage was harvested for a multilayered tip graft.

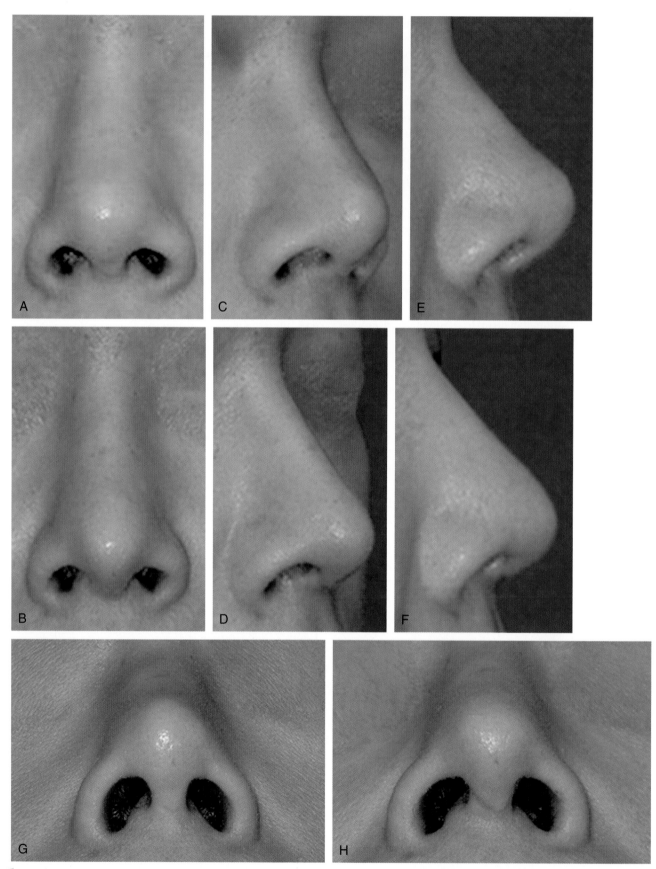

Figure 28-2 Preoperative (**A, C, E, G**) and 2-month postoperative (**B, D, F, H**) photographs of a 41-year-old woman after revision rhinoplasty which included removal of previously placed spreader grafts, bilateral lateral osteotomies, and placement of a layered conchal cartilage tip graft.

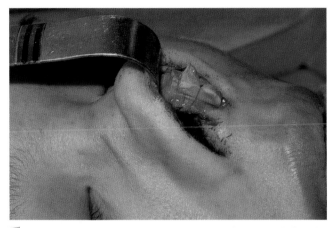

Figure 28-3 Placement of a three-layered tip graft comprised of autologous conchal cartilage.

Closure and dressing of the surgical site were done in the usual fashion.

CASE 3

A 32-year-old woman had undergone two previous reduction rhinoplasty procedures to "make the nose smaller." She presented with an excessively shortened nose and overrotated tip. She also had a deep and low nasion that started caudal to her superior palpebral fissure (Figure 28-5). The goal was to correct her severely retracted nose.

The nose was recessed and the SSTE was elevated. Exposure of the lower lateral cartilages revealed bossae of the right intermediate crus, and this was conservatively reduced. Autologous costal cartilage was simultaneously

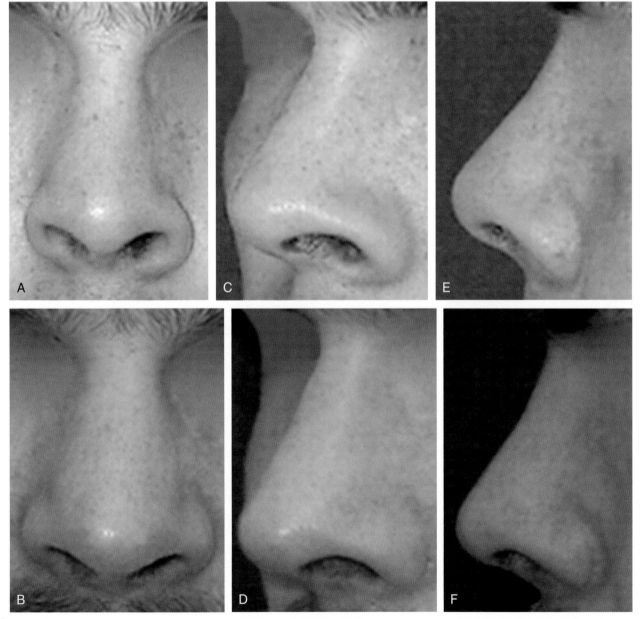

Figure 28-4 Preoperative (**A, C, E**) and 12-month postoperative (**B, D, F**) photographs of a 30-year-old man with a congenitally short, upturned nose after dome division, wedge resection of membranous septum, and placement of a columellar strut and a multilayered conchal cartilage tip graft.

harvested. An obliquely oriented incision over the left eighth rib was made with a No. 15 blade. Dissection of the musculature was achieved by spreading down to the level of the rib cartilage. The anterior portion of perichondrium and costal cartilage was incised medially and laterally. The posterior perichondrium was left intact while the cartilage was removed from the patient in a subperichondrial plane. Saline irrigation was poured into the wound, and a Valsalva maneuver was provided by the anesthesia team. After confirming the absence of an air leak, the wound was closed in layers.

The outer cortex of the costal cartilage was removed off from the central core. The remaining cartilage was allowed time to warp. Once the cartilage had stabilized to its natural curvature, a canoe-shaped dorsal graft and a columellar strut were fashioned and placed over the dorsum and into a columellar pocket, respectively. A wedge was resected from the caudal aspect of the dorsal graft to accommodate the anterior-most portion of the columellar graft. These were then sutured in place to create a stable L-strut. Then, the lower lateral cartilages were stabilized onto the columellar graft in a tongue-and-groove manner. Subsequently, a multilayered tip graft was placed and the nose was closed and dressed.

CASE 4

A 63-year-old Asian woman presented 45 years after augmentation rhinoplasty performed in Japan with a dorsal Silastic implant. She featured a severely retracted and overrotated nose and refused to consent for costal cartilage harvest (Figure 28-6). After an open approach and

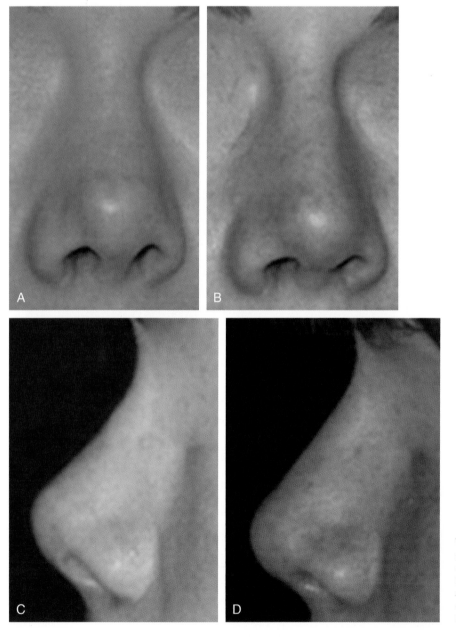

Figure 28-5 Preoperative (**A, C**) and 6-month postoperative (**B, D**) photographs of a 27-year-old woman after revision rhinoplasty, which included costal cartilage harvest for placement of a dorsal augmentation graft with interdigitating columellar strut and a layered cartilage tip graft. Bilateral malar implants were also placed.

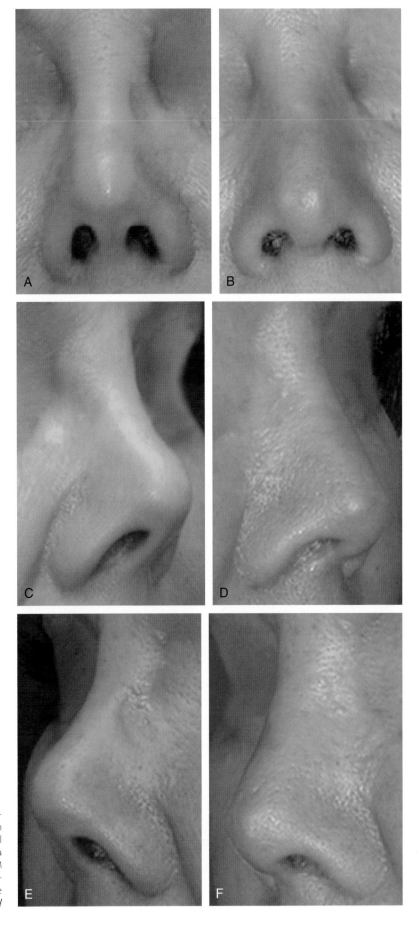

Figure 28-6 Preoperative (**A, C, E, G**) and 5-month postoperative (**B, D, F, H**) photographs of a 63-year-old woman following revision rhinoplasty, which included the removal of a previously placed Silastic implant and placement of a MedPor sheet for columellar grafting and a Gore-Tex SAM implant for dorsal reaugmentation. The patient also underwent concomitant revision blepharoplasty and revision face and neck lift. *Continued*

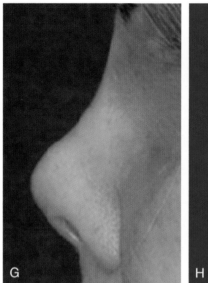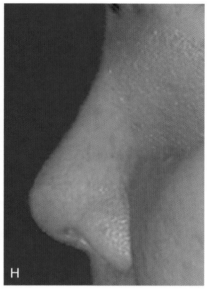

Figure 28-6, cont'd.

elevation of the SSTE, a displaced dorsal Silastic implant was removed. An open septoplasty was performed exposing the caudal end of the septal cartilage. A Medpor sheet was cut in a triangular shape and sutured to the septal cartilage as a caudal septal extension graft. Subsequent tongue-and-groove fixation of the lower lateral cartilages to the extension graft was performed. Last, a layered tip graft created from autologous auricular cartilage was placed and the dorsum was reaugmented with a carved Gore-Tex SAM dorsal implant. The nose was then closed and dressed in the usual fashion. The patient also underwent concomitant revision blepharoplasty and revision face and neck lift.

SUMMARY

Lengthening the short nose is one of the most challenging problems facing rhinoplastic surgeons, and many different nasal lengthening techniques have been described. As is the case with many surgical challenges, the presence of myriad operative techniques underscores the fact that there is not one single ideal technique. However, a working knowledge of using these operative maneuvers alone and in combination is necessary to produce optimal outcomes.

REFERENCES

1. Millard DR. Three very short noses and how they were lengthened. *Plast Reconstr Surg.* 1980;65:10–15.

2. Powell N, Humphreys B. *Considerations and components of the aesthetic face.* In: Smith JD, ed. Proportions of the Aesthetic Face. New York: Thieme-Stratton Inc; 1984:20–26.

3. Naficy S, Baker SR. Lengthening the short nose. *Arch Otolaryngol Head Neck Surg.* 1998;124:809–813.

4. Jackson IT, Reid CD. Nasal reconstruction and lengthening with local flaps. *Br J Plast Surg.* 1978;31:341–348.

5. Dingman RO, Walter C. Use of composite ear grafts in correction of the short nose. *Plast Reconstr Surg.* 1969;43: 117–123.

6. Kamer FM. Lengthening the short nose. *Ann Plast Surg.* 1980;4:281–285.

7. Giammanco PF. Lengthening the congenitally short nose. *Arch Otolaryngol Head Neck Surg.* 1987;113:1113–1116.

8. Gruber RP. Lengthening the short nose. *Plast Reconstr Surg.* 1993;91:1252–1258.

9. Gunter JP, Rohrich RJ. Lengthening the aesthetically short nose. *Plast Reconstr Surg.* 1989;83:793–800.

10. Toriumi DM. New concepts in nasal tip contouring. *Arch Facial Plast Surg.* 2006;8:156–185.

11. Dyer WK, Beaty MM, Prabhat A. Architectural deficiencies of the nose: treatment of the saddle nose and short nose deformities. *Otolaryngol Clin North Am.* 1999;32:89–112.

12. Guyuron B, Varghai A. Lengthening the nose with a tongue-and-groove technique. *Plast Reconstr Surg.* 2002;111: 1533–1539.

13. Toriumi DM, Patel AB, DeRosa J. Correcting the short nose in revision rhinoplasty. *Facial Plast Surg Clin North Am.* 2006; 14:343–355.

14. Burke AJ, Wang TD, Cook TA. Irradiated homograft rib cartilage in facial reconstruction. *Arch Facial Plast Surg.* 2004;6:334–341.

15. Anderson JR. A reasoned approach to nasal base surgery. *Arch Otolaryngol Head Neck Surg.* 1984;110:349–358.

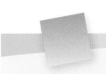

CHAPTER TWENTY-NINE

Asian Rhinoplasty

Samuel M. Lam

Cosmetic surgery for the Asian nose stands in marked contradistinction to that for the Western nose in that its objectives can be the opposite in many cases (i.e., augmentation rather than reductive rhinoplasty). However, an Occidental ideal for rhinoplasty has often been used for the Asian patient, leaving an individual with too high a nasal dorsum and too narrow a tip for his or her ethnicity. This monograph will introduce modified standards for the ethnic nose so that a surgeon who is unfamiliar with the Asian patient can create an aesthetically pleasing result that is ethnically sensitive but, even more important, that appears natural. A dimension that should not be ignored during the preoperative evaluation is the unusual cultural motivations that may drive an Asian patient's decision to undergo aesthetic rhinoplasty among other facial enhancement procedures. For example, a higher dorsum may signify wealth and fortune for an individual and a distinctly visible nostril show from a frontal view has been thought to indicate the potential for monetary loss. Although a Western surgeon may regard these ideas as unfounded, failure to explore this perception explicitly before surgery may lead to dissatisfaction postoperatively. Finally, a strategy will be developed for both primary and revision rhinoplasty for the Asian nose, taking into consideration the widespread popularity of solid silicone implants in Asia and the need to understand the role and results of this alloplast even if the surgeon does not desire to use this material (as I myself no longer do).

CULTURAL ISSUES

The first priority for surgeons should be to understand the patient before trying to understand the operation. What has emerged as a frequent comment from my colleagues is the failure to comprehend the enigmatic nature of the Asian patient and that miscommunication has led to surgical failure even when the surgical result may have been deemed a technical success. This lack of clear communication may only be partly blamed on the language barrier of some first-generation immigrants. There are two glaring failures that may in fact underscore the miscommunication: a lack of cultural sensitivity and a lack of

understanding ethnic identity. This section will cover the former aspect of the purported problem.

Some of the folkloric cultural beliefs that inform Asians—who either live abroad, who have recently immigrated to the West, and even for those who are several generations later born and reared in the West—should be explored herein. As alluded to in the introduction, some Asian patients may desire undergoing aesthetic rhinoplasty solely for nonaesthetic reasons. For instance, the larger nose has been regarded as a sign of wealth and fortune for the bearer of this feature, or by turns offers the individual who acquires this attribute even via surgery to attain that level of monetary gain. I clearly recall a Chinese chef who ascribed his job promotion to his higher nose bridge and was more elated with his enhanced fortune in life brought on, in his view, by his higher nasal dorsum, than with the aesthetic outcome of his rhinoplasty surgery. However, with regard to the height of the nasal dorsum, the surgeon should always respect the parameters that would preserve a natural result. This topic will be discussed in the following section. The second most common request or desire that may have cultural underpinnings is to have less visible nostril show from a frontal view. Accordingly, anything that would lead to greater nostril show (no matter how narrow the nostrils are to begin with) could lead to patient dissatisfaction. That is why a dome-binding suture that leads to nasal tip refinement may not be a wise surgical option in many Asian patients. Besides the unaesthetic feature of widely visible nostrils, the motivating factor for the Asian patient may be the folkloric belief that visible nostrils may engender monetary loss. I recall a Vietnamese patient of mine who was born and raised in the United States but who wanted to have a higher bridge and less visible nostrils because a fortuneteller had informed him of the importance of doing so to change his fortune in life. He also desired nasal enhancement for aesthetic reasons and with preoperative imaging appeared to have realistic goals. However, the surgeon who is contemplating proceeding with surgery in the patient who is profoundly motivated by cultural beliefs risks the uncontrollable outcome that a patient has not attained the desired station in life perhaps due to a surgeon's failure to accomplish sufficient structural change to the nose. These cultural elements should almost always be explored to determine the candidacy for undertaking rhinoplasty based on mutually aligned and attainable goals.

Other examples of folkloric beliefs related to the face may be illustrative and impart further insight for the Western surgeon who desires to work on the Asian patient. Freckles may be considered an endearing feature in the West, but any skin blemishes for the Asian patient may be remarked as unattractive and further thought to affect adversely one's good fortune. Like a large nose, large ears are also believed to designate the bearer as an individual who holds great wealth and wisdom. Consequently, reductive otoplasty is less commonly undertaken in the Far East. Dimples are thought to impart fertility and increase one's marriage prospect. Exploring these complex and multilayered motivations may help establish and align realistic objectives with the patient.

PRESERVING ETHNICITY IN THE ASIAN PATIENT

Many patients select me as a surgeon simply because of my own ethnicity. They believe that as a fellow Asian (I am Chinese), I will be more sensitive to their own cultural motivations and ethnic features. Perhaps this may be true. However, through this chapter, every surgeon attempting Asian rhinoplasty can attain this level of sensitivity. This section will focus primarily on what constitutes an ethnically sensitive rhinoplasty that preserves rather than effaces ethnicity. Following the trend of Asian eyelid enhancement over the past two decades, the creation of a supratarsal crease has moved away from the unnatural "Westernized" look that dominated in the 1980s where the crease was made very high and significant postseptal fat was removed. Today, the crease is much lower and the fullness is preserved. The same trend can be spotted in most ethnic surgeries with the current goal to be ethnic *preservation* rather than effacement. In the same way the Middle Eastern nose should not be overly reduced, the Asian nose should not be overly elevated in height.

What exactly are the standards for ethnically sensitive surgery then? For the nose, the dorsal height should not in most cases exceed the mid-pupil as the starting point for the radix. In many cases, the Occidental surgeon uses the Occidental standard of the supratarsal crease as the proposed radix height. This often can be too high for the Asian individual. Of course, facial features, like the depth of the nasofrontal angle, etc. will dictate aesthetic goals, which can be modified based on artistic judgment and communication with the prospective patient. The nasal tip can also be made too sharply defined and could appear unnatural for the Asian patient. Strategies of varying degrees of nasal tip definition from slightly rounder to slightly sharper will be elaborated upon later in this chapter. Finally, the alar base has often been considered

a very important area to narrow in order to achieve the optimal aesthetic results. In reality, I rarely perform an alar base reduction, as I find it unnecessary unless the alar base is extremely broad.

Using photographs of Asian models and reviewing a surgeon's "before and after" results can be helpful to any prospective Asian patient seeking to align aesthetic goals with a surgeon. There are two caveats that should be expressed: at times a patient can be more enamored with the overall composite of a model's face and not necessarily just the nose itself and the same pitfall may arise when reviewing a surgeon's results if the patient likes the face more than the nose. Assuming that an individual is wholly embracive of maintaining ethnicity can also be erroneous. Today's globalized marketplace has placed an emphasis on models of mixed racial heritage. Also, with increased interracial marriage rates, offspring can strike a more ethnically blended aesthetic. I have also observed anecdotally that Asians who are partnered with Caucasians may seek to blunt their ethnic features to appeal more to their significant other. However, many Caucasians are drawn to Asians who exhibit more ethnic features and may not want those attributes significantly softened. At times, an open conversation including the prospective patient's significant other may be a wise decision when electing aesthetic rhinoplasty or any facial enhancement procedure in the Asian patient.

When I perform Asian rhinoplasty (or almost any aesthetic endeavor for that matter), I rarely make great accommodations to a patient's wishes if those desires do not align well with my own aesthetic judgment. It is not out of fear of betraying my own sense of ethnicity but more out of reticence to make a result that would compromise my own aesthetic philosophy.

USE OF SILICONE FOR AUGMENTATION RHINOPLASTY

Augmentation rhinoplasty with a single solid silicone implant has remained the most popular choice throughout Asia. When I started my career in Asian rhinoplasty, I was heavily influenced by this technique that appeared to be so pervasively the choice in the Far East where I had spent 5 months of apprenticeship. However, after a couple of years of using solid silicone implants, even very soft and tapered versions, I found multiple problems with them which have encouraged me to abandon this technique entirely. Nevertheless, any surgeon contemplating undertaking Asian rhinoplasty must understand the nature of a silicone implant since he or she will encounter a patient for revision rhinoplasty who already has a silicone implant that must be addressed.

Many of my senior colleagues in Asia have had remarkable success with solid silicone so I am not here to cast a shadow on their accomplishments. I only want to express the limitations that I have personally encountered which have compelled me to abandon use of the material. I will take ownership for any technical errors that I may have committed that may have contributed to my failure. Here are the problems that I witnessed with solid silicone. Because the implant tends to undergo encapsulation under very thin nasal skin, the edges can become visible over time and make the implant more visible-imparting an almost "shrink-wrapped" appearance. The thickness of the implant even when shaved paper thin with the added encapsulation that occurs over time made most of my efforts appear too high for my aesthetic taste. I am much more conservative with dorsal augmentation, as discussed previously. The major problem I encountered was distal migration of the implant downward over the nasal tip after a year or two (or sometimes sooner) that could occur spontaneously for no apparent reason (i.e., no history of inciting trauma could be elicited in many cases). The weight of silicone as compared with expanded poly-tetrafluoroethylene (ePTFE), which will be discussed, can predispose to eventual descent of the implant. I was taught to scrape the periosteum of the nasal bone vigorously immediately before implant insertion to minimize this consequence. Despite diligent attention to this surgical maneuver, I still found many instances when the implant shifted downward over the nasal tip.

Because of my prior use of silicone implants, I have become more experienced with handling the complications that can arise, which the reader should be familiar with. Often, the first instinct with an overly augmented silicone implant (which I find most of them are) is to remove it and simultaneously replace it with a smaller dorsal implant. If the bridge is only slightly too high or of appropriate nasal height, a simultaneous revision rhinoplasty may be warranted (Figure 29-1). However, what I have found is that removal of the implant can often be all that is needed to restore a patient to a more pleasing nasal configuration without need for a revision rhinoplasty (Figure 29-2). Many individuals worry that implant removal alone will lead to a return to their former nose shape. This is rarely the case. The scar tissue and remaining encapsulation lead to a result that lies somewhere halfway between the original nose and the overaugmented nose with a silicone implant.

The major caveat that the patient should be aware of is the risk of pressure necrosis that a large silicone implant can impart to the nasal tip cartilages. Removal of an implant can expose the mangled nature of the nasal tip cartilages that may require surgical intervention to correct. This problem should be diligently explained to the patient who may not be aware of this potential outcome. Because I use liquid silicone microdroplets to correct minor nasal deformities, I can often camouflage the problem without having to proceed to surgery. However, major loss of nasal tip projection and or deformity would mandate a surgical remedy.

Why then go through an extra procedure of nasal implant if the likelihood for a revision rhinoplasty is high? First, it may not be if the surgeon has a more conservative perception of how an Asian nose should appear, especially within the context of a previously overaugmented nose. Second, more important, silicone implant removal should

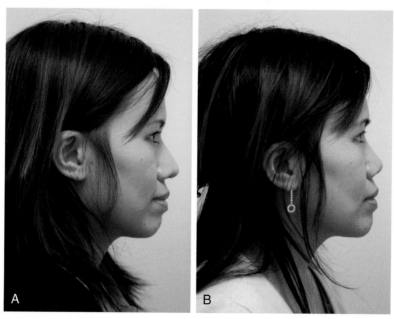

Figure 29-1 The patient had a previous solid silicone augmentation rhinoplasty that was removed and underwent a simultaneous revision rhinoplasty using a two-ply sheet of ePTFE intended for dorsal augmentation rhinoplasty and a double-layer onlay septal cartilage tip graft. (From Lam SM. Revision rhinoplasty for the Asian nose. Semin Plast Surg. Reprinted by permission.)

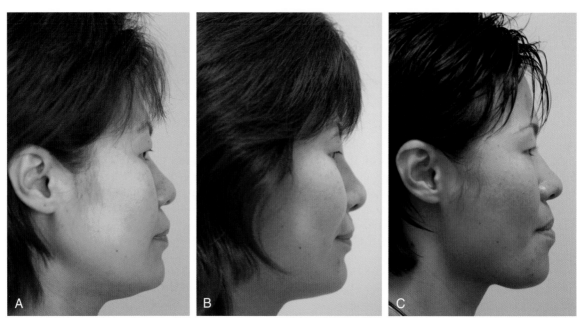

Figure 29-2 The patient is shown before augmentation rhinoplasty with a "one-piece" solid silicone implant (**A**), after rhinoplasty (**B**) with the nasal bridge profile aesthetically too high, and after removal of the implant (**C**) with a result that lies somewhere between the before and after results, at a height that is aesthetically conservative and attractive. (From Lam SM. Revision rhinoplasty for the Asian nose. Semin Plast Surg. Reprinted by permission.)

be a 5-minute office procedure under local anesthesia with no sedation. For the right-handed surgeon, the right marginal incision is more easily approached. After a topical anesthetic is applied within the nasal vestibule on the right side, 1% lidocaine with 1:100,000 epinephrine (typically 1 to 2 ml is sufficient) is infiltrated through the marginal incision into the nasal tip to blanch it and to achieve adequate anesthesia. Of course, a small 30-gauge needle is used and the anesthesia very slowly infiltrated so that the patient does not feel any discomfort. The surgeon need not anesthetize the entire nasal dorsum.

After 10 minutes are allowed to elapse for adequate vasoconstriction and anesthesia, a No. 15 Bard-Parker blade is used to incise the marginal incision just along the vestibular recess, about 1 cm in length. The incision does not need to be continued all the way across the inferior aspect of the lower lateral cartilage. Metzenbaum scissors are used blindly to "feel out" the implant (i.e., dissect above and below the implant to break the encapsulation). A curved hemostat is inserted through the marginal incision and is blindly (i.e., by palpation) used to take a firm grasp of the implant. One should not take a partial, tenuous grasp of the implant. It will otherwise tear and make removal close to impossible. With a firm grasp, the implant is slowly and deliberately tugged until the entire implant is removed in one piece. A very slow, deliberate and constant application of traction will release the entire implant from its recessed position. If the implant is not easily grasped, tiny double-hook retractors are used to gently lift the marginal incision upward, and with direct

visualization using a headlight, the surgeon can grasp the observed implant. The incision is then closed with interrupted 5-0 chromic sutures.

The only exception to an easy implant removal is the presence of calcifications along the dorsum. The skin surface of the nose should be palpated, and if irregularities are observed, the patient may need sedation; if the dorsum is not too high, then a simultaneous revision rhinoplasty may be a wiser option. I have personally taken out silicone implants laden with calcifications in the office, and it is never an enjoyable experience. With careful and tedious dissection, the implant can be removed in its entirety in 30 to 45 minutes rather than the otherwise to be expected 5 minutes.

One of the most devastating complications that can arise with previous silicone implant is a foreshortened nasal tip. The pressure that the silicone implant creates on the nasal-tip tissue can lead to one of three problems: distorted loss of the underlying cartilage (as mentioned), pressure changes to the overlying skin if not frank penetration, and a foreshortened nasal tip. Often the patient who undergoes repeated silicone implantation in the past with or without episodes of infection is more likely to experience this devastating outcome. With the foreshortened nose, revision rhinoplasty is mandated, which is not an easy task.

An open rhinoplasty technique is the preferred method of surgical approach with a transcolumellar incision made near the columellar–labial junction so as to permit recruiting white upper lip tissue as needed to extend the contracted columella. Extended spreader grafts are then necessary to relengthen and maintain the position of the contracted lower lateral cartilages in a more normalized position. The lower lateral cartilages can also be distorted and require reconstruction. Often, the septal cartilage remains intact since the surgeon who typically uses silicone implants does not rely on septal cartilage as grafting material. Use of conchal onlay grafts may likely be necessary as well. In the face of graft depletion, costal harvesting for this purpose may be required. At times, the infratip lobular skin can be contracted upward and bunch up in the supratip region to cause an excess of skin in that region. I have a recently published paper that I have co-written with an esteemed Korean colleague, which discusses a novel rotation flap aimed at correcting this deformity.

SURGICAL STRATEGY FOR ASIAN RHINOPLASTY

Although completely autogenous materials can be used for Asian rhinoplasty, I prefer a combination of alloplast for the dorsum and autograft for the nasal tip. ePTFE is the preferred material for dorsal augmentation and septal cartilage for tip grafting with or without use of conchal cartilage in rare conditions where additional grafting material is required. The interesting trend in the Far East recently has been away from "one-piece augmentation" with solid silicone in favor of "two-piece augmentation" with solid silicone only for the dorsum and autogenous cartilage for the nasal tip. I do not have any personal experience with the latter technique but moved from one-piece augmentation with solid silicone to my current strategy of using ePTFE for the dorsum and autogenous cartilage for the nasal tip.

Almost all my rhinoplasty procedures are performed via an external transcolumellar incision for ease of access and operative visualization. A standard inverted-V incision is preferred. This chapter will not reiterate the basic techniques of external rhinoplasty. Instead, this technique section will focus more on philosophical approach and the pertinent details of how this technique differs from Occidental rhinoplasty. The section on operative technique will encompass technical specifications on dorsal augmentation and methods for nasal tip improvement.

As mentioned, ePTFE is my preferred method for dorsal augmentation. ePTFE in the form of flat sheets, formerly marketed as SAM sheets by W.L. Gore (Flagstaff, AZ), is preferred over solid block implants of the same material. Now that W.L. Gore has stopped manufacturing Gore-Tex, two other manufacturers have stepped in to fill this void in the market, viz., Surgiform (Columbia, SC) and Implantech (Ventura, CA). ePTFE sheets of 1, 2, and 3 mm can be used to create the dorsal height that is desired. Stacking sheets of ePTFE can attain various modifications to the bridge height. The ePTFE sheet is cut into a rectangle to fit the nasal dorsum with a gently

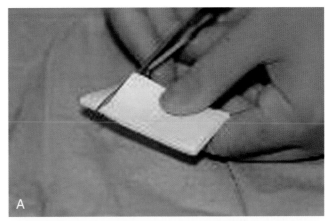

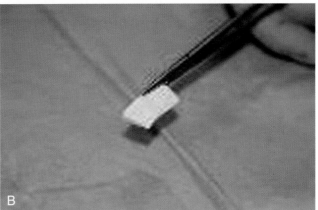

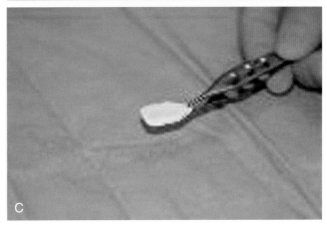

Figure 29-3 A, A 3-mm ePTFE sheet is cut into a rectangle to fit the nasal dorsum. **B,** The edges are crimped with a needle driver in order to create a smoother transition from the augmented implant to the unaugmented sides of the nose. **C,** The implant is shown crimped and cut to the requisite shape for insertion with a gently rounded superior aspect and a triangular point to be recessed between the medial crura inferiorly.

rounded contour in the superior aspect and an arrowed triangular shape inferiorly to fit between the medial crura (Figure 29-3). All edges of the implant are crimped along the outer 1-mm border using an empty needle driver before insertion. With a Converse-style retractor elevating the skin pocket, the implant can be inserted by using a variety of instruments based on the surgeon's preference.

A standard DeBakey forceps or Bayonet forceps will adequately do the job. It is important after implant placement that the implant edges be observed for any folding or crimping that can be seen by looking directly into the pocket and then by palpating the dorsal skin for any uneven edges with the skin flaps returned down to their resting position. As stated, the inferior aspect of the implant should rest between the medial crura as a triangular inset. No osteotomies are necessary for Asian rhinoplasty and would otherwise flatten the nasal profile or disrupt the position of the dorsal implant.

The dorsal implant insertion is completed before approaching the nasal tip. The principal method for nasal tip projection and definition in most cases relies on various onlay grafts rather than a cephalic lower-lateral cartilage trim and dome-binding suture. This lies in contradistinction to the technique typically used for the Occidental nose. With the very thin skin of the Caucasian nose, in most cases a cephalic trim and dome-binding suture can be very effective, whereas an onlay graft may become visible over time as the skin "shrink-wraps" down over the new architecture. The opposite is true in the Asian nose. Reducing the architecture of the nose through a cephalic trim under the thick nasal tip skin in the Asian patient can at times lead to scar production and a thicker nasal shape. With the wider stance of the nasal base, a dome-binding suture may cause untoward rotation of the nasal tip and lead to unintended nostril show, which can be both unaesthetic and also unlucky (as discussed). Instead, the nasal architecture must be built forward to push against the very thick nasal skin so as to create sufficient nasal tip projection and definition.

There are two major methods for nasal-tip definition depending on a few factors. For the individual who desires a softer and rounder shape, the nasal tip can be augmented by using oval-shaped septal onlay grafts immediately over the nasal tip (Figure 29-4). This method achieves a less angular look to the nasal tip, which can be desirable. Multiple, stacked onlay grafts can be used to achieve the desired degree of tip projection. As an alternative, for a slighter and sharper appearance to the nasal tip, a shield graft that has its distal aspect rest 1 to 2 mm anterior to the native lower-lateral cartilage domes can be used to create a more favorable nasal tip definition and projection (Figure 29-5). The shield graft can also be beneficial to correct columellar retraction that is often present in the Asian patient with a premaxillary retrusion. Of course, both techniques can be combined as needed to achieve the desired degree of projection and definition. Often, the supratip fat can be debulked from the undersurface of the supratip skin in order to decrease the round appearance of the nasal tip in the Asian patient. For added projection when cartilage grafting is depleted, the removed supratip fat can be used as the final augmentation material over the stacked onlay grafts (Figure 29-6).

An alternative method for nasal tip refinement uses Fernando Pedroza's conchal seagull graft that literally replaces the native lower lateral cartilages with conchal versions of them. This method for nasal tip enhancement can prove particularly useful when the entire framework to the lower lateral cartilages has been compromised by trauma or prior silicone implant (Figure 29-7). The technique employs the cymba concha of one ear (Figure 29-8) that is divided in turn lengthwise into two equal halves (Figure 29-9). These halves are trimmed so that one end resembles the narrower medial crus and the other end the broader lateral crus (Figure 29-10). A 5-0 Vicryl suture is used as a mattress to bend one end of each cartilage piece to resemble the natural curvature of the medial and lateral crus (Figures 29-11 and 29-12). The two pieces are sutured together (Figure 29-13) to create an entirely new lower lateral cartilage to be used in an onlay fashion over the partially attenuated native cartilages (Figure 29-14).

The alar base is the final topic of discussion. In my opinion too many alar base reductions are performed unnecessarily. It is very important to evaluate the width of the nasal lobule relative to the alae. With a very broad nasal lobule, reduction of the side alae can cause the relative size of the lobule to look even larger (i.e., worse). Care should be undertaken to ensure that the nasal lobule remains in good proportion to the alar width. There are two techniques for alar base reduction that can be performed depending on what is necessary. A nasal sill reduction can reduce a broad nostril that has a long nasal sill (Figure 29-15). A Sheen flap can be used to reduce the flare of the outer alar margin. At times, a nasal sill reduction performed in isolation can increase the lateral curvature of the nose that would in turn mandate the use of a Sheen flap. At times, simply lengthening the nasal tip and elevating the nasal dorsum are sufficient to create the impression of narrowing the nose without having to do so. As the nose tip is lengthened and the bridge raised, the alar width appears relatively smaller in size. By avoiding an alar-base reduction in many circumstances, the surgeon avoids two major pitfalls: overly narrowing the base can appear unnatural for the Asian individual and prolonged if not indefinite scarring that is more likely along the alar side wall from alar-base reduction.

CONCLUSIONS

Asian rhinoplasty requires an entirely different philosophical approach and surgical armamentarium than for an Occidental counterpart. Hopefully, this chapter has helped elucidate some of the fundamental aspects of cultural biases, ethnic sensitivity, and technical execution that are inherent features of any successful cosmetic rhinoplasty endeavor, whether for primary or revision surgery in the Asian individual.

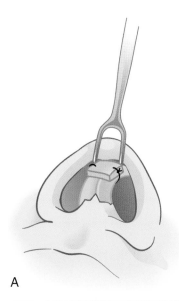

A

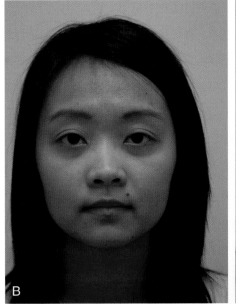

B

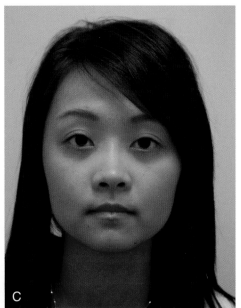

C

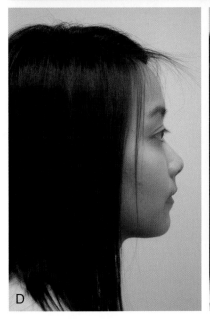

D

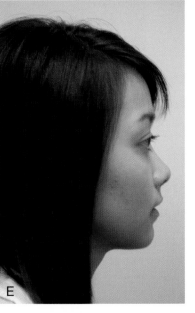

E

Figure 29-4 A, Onlay septal tip grafts are used to increase tip projection but to maintain a softer, rounded appearance to the nasal tip. **B–E,** This patient is shown before (**B, D**) and after (**C, E**) single-layer ePTFE onlay graft for the dorsum and a double-stacked onlay tip graft with septal cartilage. (From Lam SM. Revision rhinoplasty for the Asian nose. Semin Plast Surg. Reprinted by permission.)

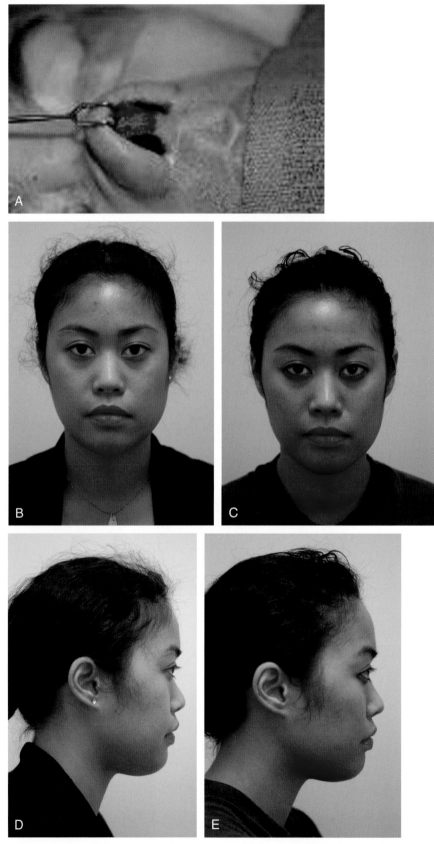

Figure 29-5 A, Shield grafts made of septal cartilage are used to attain a more defined nasal tip configuration than onlay grafts can. Also, shield grafts help to create a more favorable columellar show in the patient with a retruded premaxilla. **B–E,** This patient is shown before (**B, D**) and after (**C, E**) external rhinoplasty and full facial fat transfer. She had a shield graft and single-layered blocking graft placed to her tip and a two-ply 1-mm ePTFE sheet to the dorsum. She had fat transferred to her brow, anterior cheek, lateral cheek, and anterior chin to narrow the shape of her face and to provide more dimensionality to it. (From Lam SM. Asian rhinoplasty. Fac Plast Surg 2008;24[3]. Reprinted by permission.)

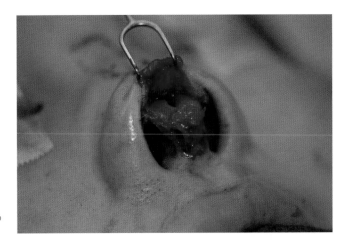

Figure 29-6 At times, the debulked supratip fat can be sutured on top of the cartilage onlay grafts for added nasal tip projection.

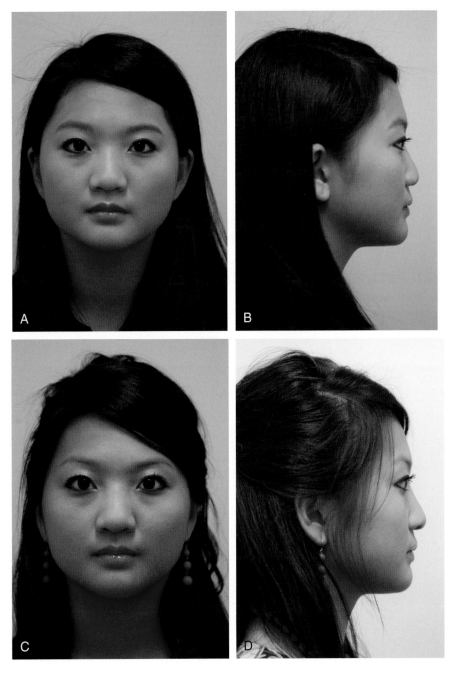

Figure 29-7 This 16-year-old Korean girl sustained traumatic injury to her nasal tip that caused loss of nasal tip projection through possibly a septal hematoma and consequent erosion of her inferior septum. She underwent a seagull reconstruction of her nasal tip (see Figure 29-8 and beyond) that rebuilt her deprojected lower lateral cartilages and also helped her to breathe much better.

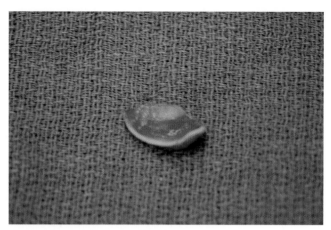

Figure 29-8 The cymba concha cartilage is shown removed as an intact single piece to be used to reconstruct the lower lateral cartilage by Pedroza's method that he calls the "seagull" graft. (From Lam SM. Asian rhinoplasty. Fac Plast Surg 2008;24[3]. Reprinted by permission.)

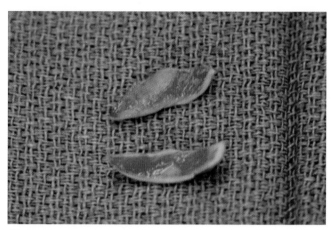

Figure 29-9 The conchal cartilage is then divided lengthwise into approximately equal halves. (From Lam SM. Asian rhinoplasty. Fac Plast Surg 2008;24[3]. Reprinted by permission.)

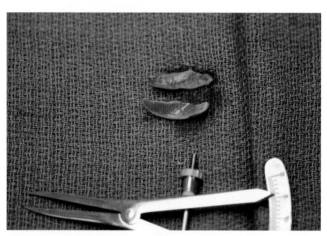

Figure 29-10 The two pieces are then trimmed so that they are of equal size and so that one narrower end resembles the medial crus. Calipers are used to ensure accurate measurements for symmetry. (From Lam SM. Asian rhinoplasty. Fac Plast Surg 2008;24[3]. Reprinted by permission.)

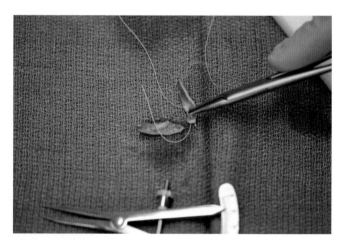

Figure 29-11 A 5-0 Vicryl suture is used as a mattress to bend the narrower end over to create the new dome. (From Lam SM. Asian rhinoplasty. Fac Plast Surg 2008;24[3]. Reprinted by permission.)

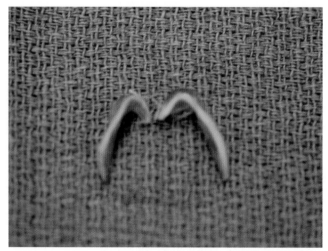

Figure 29-12 The two sutured pieces are shown adjacent to one another in the configuration that they will assume as the new lower lateral cartilage replacements. (From Lam SM. Asian rhinoplasty. Fac Plast Surg 2008;24[3]. Reprinted by permission.)

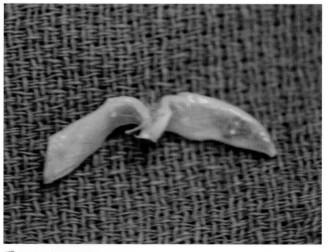

Figure 29-13 The medial crura are then sutured together to form the natural joined arc of the newly fashioned lower lateral cartilages. (From Lam SM. Asian rhinoplasty. Fac Plast Surg 2008;24[3]. Reprinted by permission.)

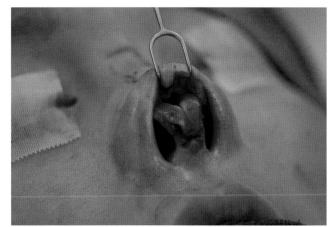

Figure 29-14 The graft is shown sutured as an onlay over the existing lower lateral cartilages. (From Lam SM. Asian rhinoplasty. Fac Plast Surg 2008;24[3]. Reprinted by permission.)

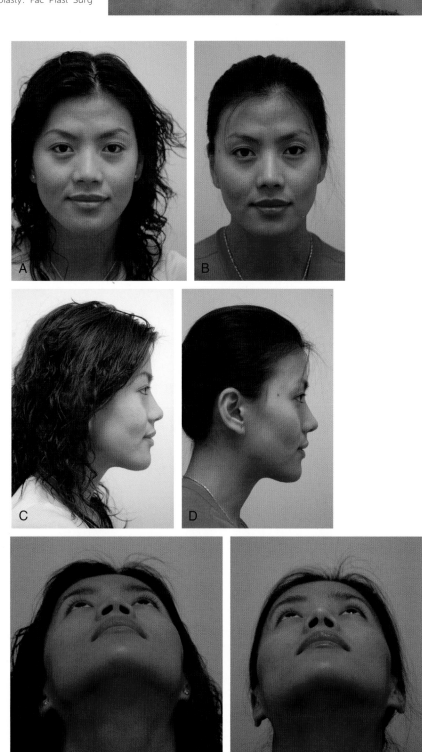

Figure 29-15 The patient is shown before (**A, C, E**) and after (**B, D, F**) external rhinoplasty that involved a single-ply 1-mm ePTFE sheet for the nasal dorsum, a one-layered septal cartilage onlay graft, and a septal columellar strut that was positioned lower than her natural medial crura to extend her columella inferiorly. She also had a nasal sill reduction. (From Lam SM. Asian rhinoplasty. Fac Plast Surg 2008;24[3]. Reprinted by permission.)

SUGGESTED READINGS

1. McCurdy Jr JA, Lam SM. *Cosmetic surgery of the Asian face.* 2nd ed. New York: Thieme Medical Publishers; 2005.

2. Lam SM. Aesthetic facial surgery for the Asian male. *Fac Plast Surg.* 2005;21:317–323.

3. Pedroza F, Anjos GC, Patrocinio LG, et al. Seagull wing graft: a technique for the replacement of lower lateral cartilages. *Arch Fac Plast Surg.* 2006:8:396–403.

4. Jung DH, Moon HJ, Choi SH, Lam SM. Secondary rhinoplasty of the Asian nose: correction of the contracted nose, *Ann Plast Surg.* 2004;28:1–7.

5. Lam SM, Kim YK. Augmentation rhinoplasty of the Asian nose with the 'bird' silicone implant. *Ann Plast Surg.* 2003;51: 24–56.

6. Shirakabe Y, Suzuki Y, Lam SM. A systematic approach to rhinoplasty in the Japanese nose: a thirty-year experience. *Aesthet Plast Surg.* 2003;27:397–402.

7. Jung DH, Choi SH, Moon HJ, Lam SM. A cadaveric analysis of the ideal costal-cartilage graft for Asian rhinoplasty. *Plast Reconstr Surg.* 2004;114:545–550.

8. Jung DH, Lin RY, Jang HJ, Claravall HJ, Lam SM. Correction of pollybeak and dimpling deformities of the nasal tip in the contracted, short nose by the use of a supratip transposition flap. *Arch Facial Plast Surg.* 2009;11(5):311-319.

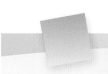
African American Rhinoplasty

Paul S. Nassif

Rhinoplasty in the African American population presents a unique set of challenges, including skin and soft tissue envelope thickness, alar base width, and inherent ethnic considerations. A delicate balance of patient satisfaction, achieving an aesthetically pleasing result, and maintaining a natural appearance are three goals to stay focused on during the surgical planning and execution phases of these procedures. Among these, meeting the patient's expectations can sometimes require redirecting and demonstrating alternatives to patients with unrealistic expectations who may at first desire an overly narrow Caucasian nose. Some patients may even choose to bring celebrity photographs to the consultation, requesting a particular result, despite the absence of a match with the subject's face, skin type, body habitus, or ethnic background. Occasionally, one of the surgeon's most important tasks is to demonstrate to patients that their requested result is unrealistic, nonfunctional, aesthetically incongruous, or out of harmony with the patient's facial or other features and is at times in fact outright unachievable given their skin characteristics. Morphing software may serve as a visual aid in this demonstration. Only after this task is accomplished should the surgeon proceed with a careful review of the history and physical examination. A comprehensive understanding of nasal anatomy, function, and surgical techniques is paramount. Having an extensive preoperative discussion encompassing patient expectations, surgical goals, and a detailed list of potential complications with the patient preoperatively can prevent miscommunication. This is best accomplished by reviewing the exam, previous operative summary, photographs, nasal analysis sheet, problem list, and surgical plan preoperatively before proceeding with the surgical treatment.

African American rhinoplasty can be one of the most difficult and challenging of the multitude of ethnic rhinoplasty procedures primarily because of the imbalance between the weak nature of the cartilaginous framework and thick skin–soft tissue envelope. One of the most common pitfalls in African American rhinoplasty occurs while attempting to accomplish a less bulbous nasal tip. The experienced rhinoplasty surgeon will be in tune with this inherent anatomic imbalance and avoid aggressive lower lateral cartilage over-resection. Aggressive lower lateral cartilage reduction usually results in:

- Loss of tip support
- Decreased tip projection
- Counterrotation (ptotis)
- Decreased tip definition (and, in fact, more pronounced bulbosity)
- Possible nasal tip contour irregularities
- Proclivity for long-term collapse after primary rhinoplasty

For all rhinoplasty procedures, especially ethnic rhinoplasty, aggressive cartilage removal is a procedure of the past. Concepts such as limited cartilage excision and adding nasal support with structural grafting and tip suturing techniques are being taught in both training programs and meetings. Proceeding in this fashion may lead to a decrease in the need for a future secondary rhinoplasty.

This chapter will discuss some of the nuances of the anatomy of the African American nose, followed by goals, preoperative nasal evaluation with surgical planning, surgical sequence and techniques, postoperative nasal care, risks and complications, pearls, as well as preoperative and postoperative photography techniques.

ANATOMY

A brief description of the African American nose is discussed and the descriptions described are present in the majority, but not all, of the typical African American noses (Figure 30-1). These include the following characteristics:

- The skin–soft tissue envelope is thick with abundant fibrofatty tissue.
- The radix is deep, low, and inferiorly set.
- The nasal bridge and dorsum feature short, wide, and flat nasal bones.
- The nasal tip is bulbous, thick-skinned, poorly projected, and counterrotated (ptotic) with abundant fibrous nasal superficial musculoaponeurotic system plane (SMAS) and broad domes; it has minimal tip definition and weak lower lateral cartilages.

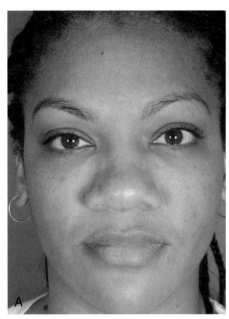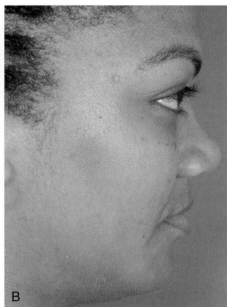

Figure 30-1 A, Frontal view of an African American female nose. **B,** Lateral view.

- The columella is short and retracted with minimal columellar show.
- The alae are wide, thick, and horizontal and the nostrils are flared.
- Nasolabial junction: retracted, acute nasolabial angle (<90 degrees), underdeveloped nasal spine.
- Maxilla: retruded and/or hypoplastic.

GOALS

The usual primary goals in African American rhinoplasty can include the following:

- Bridge: moderately thinner on frontal view.
- Dorsum: augmented height on lateral view.
- Tip: improve definition, increase projection, increase rotation.
- Base: vertical-oblique nostrils and nasal base approximating an equilateral triangle.
- Columella: Increased columellar "show" and length.
- Nasolabial junction: obtuse nasolabial angle (>90 degrees).
- Maxilla: less retruded.
- Skin–soft tissue envelope: moderate thickness that allows good tip definition.

PREOPERATIVE NASAL EVALUATION AND SURGICAL PLANNING

Excellent physician-patient communication is one of the most important features of the consultation process. While a detailed history is performed, listen very carefully to the patient's wishes and goals. Does he or she have realistic expectations? This is one of the most important details that the astute surgeon needs to focus on from the interview. What is the focus of the patient's dissatisfaction—a bulbous tip or a low dorsum? During the history, the surgeon should be able to identify if the patient is a good surgical candidate. Will your conservative rhinoplasty make the patient happy? Poor patient selection can lead to an unhappy patient and considerable amount of stress to both patient and surgeon.

Ascertain if the patient has nasal obstruction, although this symptom is uncommon. If nasal obstruction is present, is it static or dynamic? Is it present with normal or deep inspiration? What alleviates and worsens the nasal obstruction? What are the characteristics of the nasal obstruction? The physical examination follows.

For the physical examination, I use a nasal analysis worksheet (Figure 30-2) and perform a detailed visual and tactile evaluation of the nose. Visualize the bilateral paramedian vertical light reflexes along the dorsum and look for symmetry. I then use an ungloved finger to palpate the nose, examining the bony and cartilaginous skeleton, tip, and skin–soft tissue envelope characteristics in frontal, head-down, oblique, lateral, and base views.

In patients with nasal obstruction, whether for a primary or revision rhinoplasty, I observe them during normal and deep inspiration on frontal and basal views. Often, the diagnosis is easily identifiable as supra-alar, alar, and/or rim collapse (slitlike nostrils) during static or dynamic states. External valve collapse (lower lateral cartilage pathology) can be evaluated by supporting the area of nasal obstruction with the firm end of a cotton swab while occluding the contralateral nostril. Often, nasal obstruction in the supra-alar region may signify an overly

Patient Name:_____   Date: _____

- **Skin Quality:**   Thin   Medium   Thick   Sebaceous   Telangiectasias
- **Primary Description:**   Big   Twisted   Large Hump   Boxy   Pinched   Bulbous

FRONTAL VIEW

- **Dorsum:**   Twisted   Deviated   Straight   Convex: **R L**   Bony
                                             Bony-Cartilaginous   Cartilaginous
- **Width:**   Narrow   Wide   Normal   Wide-Narrow-Wide   Depressed   L   R
- **Tip:**   Normal   Deviated   Bulbous   Asymmetric   Amorphous
                                             Pinched   Parenthesis Deformity
- **Support:**   Normal   Weak
- **Medial Canthal–Alar Relationship:**   Wide   Normal   Narrow   Sill   Weir
- **Tip-Defining Points:**   Uni   Double   Narrow
- **Nasal Bones:**   Short   Normal   Long
- **Middle Vault/Upper Lateral Cartilages:** Narrow   Normal   Subluxed   Asymmetric

BASE VIEW

- Trapezoidal   Triangular
- **Tip:**   Deviated   Bulbous   Wide   Bifid   Asymmetrical
- **Base:**   Wide   Narrow   Normal   Dislocated Caudal Septum: No   Yes   R   L
- **Rim Aperture:**   Narrow   R   L   Normal
- **Columella:**   Columellar/ Lobule Ratio (2:1)   Normal   Abnormal
- **Medial Crural Footplates:**   Wide   Normal

LATERAL

- **Nasofrontal Angle:**   Shallow   Deep   Normal
- **Nasal Starting Point:**   High   Low   Normal
- **Nasal Length:**   Normal   Short   Long
- **Dorsal Hump:**   Y   N   Bony   Cartilaginous   Over-resected   Bone   Cartilage
- **Tip Projection:**   Normal   Decreased   Increased   Ratio (.55–.60)_____ (TDP-
                                             AFJ/Nasion-TDP)
- **Alar-Columellar Relationship:**   Normal   Abnormal   A-C Show _____mm
- **Naso-Labial Angle:**   Obtuse   Acute   Normal   _____ degrees
- **Infratip Lobule:**   Over-rotated   Counter-rotated   Normal
- **Supratip Break:**   Y   N
- **Nasal Ptosis:**   Y   N   With Smiling: Y   N
- **Infratip Break:**   Y   N
- **Chin:**   Normal   Microgenia   Macrogenia
- **Columella:**   Normal   Hanging   (Septum   Medial Crura   Soft Tissue)
                                             Retracted   (Base)
- **Ala:**   Normal   Hanging   Retracted   R   L
- **Pollybeak:**   Y   N   Cartilaginous   Soft Tissue

Figure 30-2 Nasal analysis worksheet. (From Nassif PS. Asian rhinoplasty. *Fac Plast Surg Clin North Am* 2010;18:153-171.)

INTRANASAL

- **Septum:**　　　　　　　　　　　**Deviated　Y　N　Spur　R　L**
  Caudal Deviation　Y　N　R　L
  _____% Obtsruction　R
  _____% Obstruction　L
  Edematous Mucosa　Y　N　Erythematous Mucosa　Y　N
  Perforation　Y　N　If yes, where _____
- **Turbinates:**　　　　　　　　　 **Hypertrophic　Y　N　R　L　Normal**
- **Internal Nasal Valve:**　　　　 **Narrow　Normal**
- **External Nasal Valve:**　　　　 **Collapsed　Intact**
- **More Prominent Ear:**　　　　 **R　L**

PROBLEM LIST/PLAN:

Alar Batten Grafts　L　R　Alar Rim Grafts　L　R　Lateral Crura Strut Grafts　L　R
Columellar Strut　Infratip Lobule Graft　Dome Graft　Shield Graft　Plumping Grafts
Composite Grafts　L　R　Medial Crural Overlay　Lateral Crural Overlay　Dome Sutures
Tongue-In-Groove　Spreader Grafts　L　R　Septal Extension Graft　Reposition LLC
Conchal Cartilage　L　R　Costal　Temporalis Fascia　L　R
Onlays:　Lateral Nasal Wall　L　R　Radix　Bony Vault　Middle Vault
Alar Base Reduction:　Sills　Weir　I　II1　Septoplasty　Turbinoplasty
Osteotomies　Double　R　L　Hump Reduction　Bone　Cartilage

Functional:　　　　　　　　　　　　　　　　　　　Cosmetic:

_____　　　　　　　　　　　　　　_____

Paul S. Nassif, MD, FACS　　　　　　　　　　　　　　　　Date

Figure 30-2, cont'd.

narrowed pyriform aperture secondary to low lateral osteotomies. Elevate the ptotic nasal tip and see if this helps alleviate the nasal obstruction. The Cottle maneuver can help assess internal valve collapse. Although this test is generally nonspecific, internal nasal valve pathology caused by supra-alar pinching or a narrowed angle between the upper lateral cartilage and septum can be diagnosed. On basal view, examine the medial crura feet and the recurvature of the lower lateral cartilage to identify if these impinge into the nasal airway.

Following a thorough external nasal evaluation, the endonasal examination ensues. At a minimum, perform anterior rhinoscopy. Evaluate the nasal septum for perforations, deviation, and septum characteristics, as the African American patient will usually have a short septum with insufficient cartilage for grafting. Other causes of nasal obstruction to identify are hypertrophic inferior turbinates, synechiae between the lateral nasal wall and septum, nasal masses, and middle turbinate abnormalities (concha bullosa, among others).

As the examination progresses, create a list of problems with solutions, followed by documentation on your nasal analysis sheet, such as (1) bulbous, poorly projected tip with a plan of open rhinoplasty, (2) low dorsum with a plan of augmentation with diced cartilage wrapped in deep temporalis fascia, and (3) wide ala with a plan of bilateral alar base reduction. If structural grafting is necessary, decide what material may be used. A thorough understanding of the types of autologous (septal, conchal, costal cartilage and deep temporalis fascia) or alloplastic grafting is needed as well as being facile with the harvesting techniques required for each one.

Computer imaging and morphing software may be an extremely useful method of communication if patients are made well aware that the final image will not represent their postoperative photograph. However, despite proper notification and consent, there have been reports of lawsuits filed by patients for outcomes that are different than what was generated by the surgeon. Computer imaging can give clues to the patient's expectations. Unrealistic expectations can be identified when a conservative image is generated by the surgeon and the patient desires a radical change. Therefore, computer imaging can be a powerful tool in evaluating patients for surgery. There have been numerous instances when I have decided not to perform rhinoplasty surgery secondary to the patients having unrealistic expectations only being identified by the computer morphing. An additional use for the computer image is to use it as a goal in surgery. Often in African American rhinoplasty, the patient has microgenia, and a chin implant would benefit the overall aesthetic appearance. Computer imaging will help the patient make a decision to have a chin implant. Prior to surgery, standardized rhinoplasty photographs are taken.

SURGICAL SEQUENCE AND TECHNIQUES

The sequence I find useful is to start with the septoplasty with septal harvesting and possible inferior turbinoplasty. This is followed by rhinoplasty incisions and skeletonization; I favor the external approach primarily—nasal tip surgery with harvesting/placement of autologous grafts, osteotomies as needed, dorsal augmentation with autologous and/or alloplastic grafts, and finally alar base reduction.

SEPTOPLASTY AND INFERIOR TURBINOPLASTY

Rarely will an African American nose have a deviated septum. If a deviated septum is present, a standard septoplasty is performed. If the septum is not deviated, septal cartilage harvesting is performed leaving approximately 10 mm of a caudal and dorsal strut. Commonly, a small amount of cartilage will be available to harvest and patients are always informed that the need may arise to harvest auricular or costal cartilage if dorsal grafting is to be performed. The details regarding the septal harvest and correction of the deviated septum are covered elsewhere. Commonly, hypertrophic turbinates will be present and the turbinoplasty of choice will be performed. Turbinectomy is disfavored as it carries the risk of empty nose syndrome and ozena.

EXTERNAL APPROACH RHINOPLASTY

INJECTION

In the majority of African American rhinoplasties, an external rhinoplasty is performed. The nose is infiltrated with local anesthetic (lidocaine 1% with epinephrine 1:100,000) to assist in hydrodissecting the cartilage framework from the skin–soft tissue envelope and to aid in hemostatic control. Subdermal dissection over the nasal tip is performed to leave the SMAS lying dorsal to the cartilage mucoperichondrium. Once the skin–soft tissue envelope has been elevated, I find repeating the

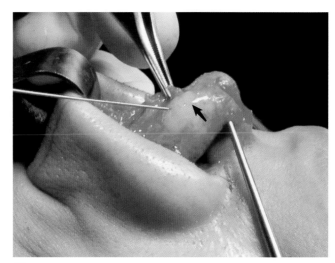

Figure 30-3 Local injection used to hydrodissect mucoperichondrium from the right lower lateral cartilage (*arrow*). (From Nassif PS. Asian rhinoplasty. *Fac Plast Surg Clin North Am* 2010;18:153-171.)

infiltration of local anesthetic helps me hydrodissect the perichondrium off the lower lateral cartilages (Figure 30-3). This technique will aid in dissecting the SMAS/perichondrium (Figure 30-4) from the nasal tip to use as an onlay or camouflage graft and assist in fine-tuning nasal tip definition. A subperiosteal dissection over the nasal dorsum is performed if dorsal augmentation is to be performed.

NASAL TIP SURGERY

Surgery of the nasal tip is among the most critical and challenging aspects of rhinoplasty in the African American patient. Trying to achieve definition, a narrower tip, increased projection (the more projection, the narrower the tip will appear), and rotation are frequent goals. Commonly, the infratip lobule is overrotated; this can be nicely addressed using a bruised infratip lobular graft. I primarily use a combined septal extension/columellar strut and a shield graft to provide maximum projection.

A conservative cephalic trim of the lateral crura of lower lateral cartilages can be carried out, making sure to leave at least 7 mm of cartilage in vivo (Figure 30-5). Next, I find undermining the vestibular tissue from the posterior surface of the alar cartilages (lateral and medial crura) (Figure 30-6) will release any constraints from the cartilage and possibly enable natural projection facilitating the lateral crural steal procedure.[1] This technique increases nasal tip projection and tip rotation. The lateral crura are advanced onto the medial crura, thereby projecting and rotating the nasal tip. The lateral crura are advanced adjacent to the domes medially (Figure 30-7). Finally, bilateral interdomal and transdomal sutures are placed using 5-0 absorbable suture material.

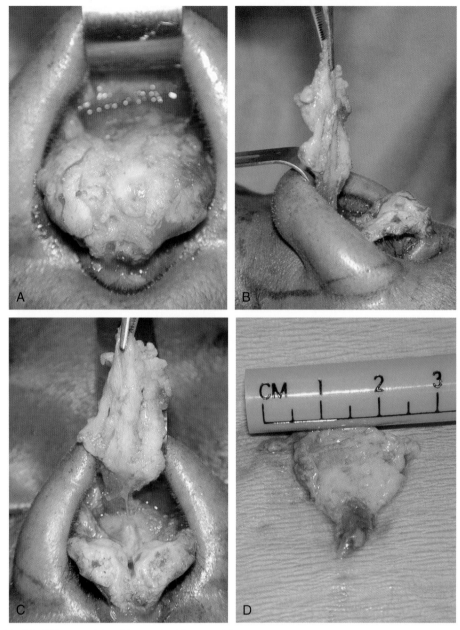

Figure 30-4 A–D, Nasal SMAS/mucoperichondrium excised from nasal tip.

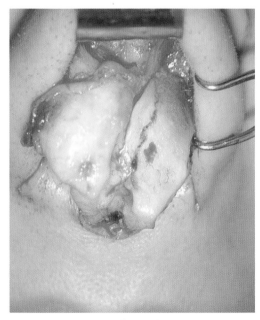

Figure 30-5 Cephalic trim performed, leaving a 7-mm caudal remnant of lower lateral cartilage. (From Nassif PS. Asian rhinoplasty. *Fac Plast Surg Clin North Am* 2010;18:153-171.)

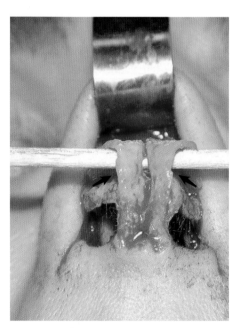

Figure 30-6 Released lower and medial lateral cartilages (*arrows*) from the adherent vestibular tissue to aid in increasing tip projection. (From Nassif PS. Asian rhinoplasty. *Fac Plast Surg Clin North Am* 2010;18:153-171.)

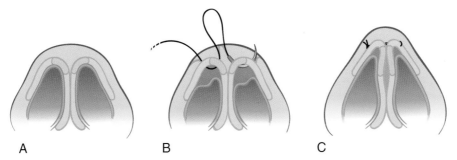

Figure 30-7 Lateral crural steal aids in increased nasal tip projection and rotation. The lateral crura are advanced onto the medial crura to project the nasal tip and to rotate the tip. The lateral crura are advanced adjacent to the dome medially. Finally, bilateral interdomal and a transdomal suture is placed with 5-0 absorbable suture of choice.

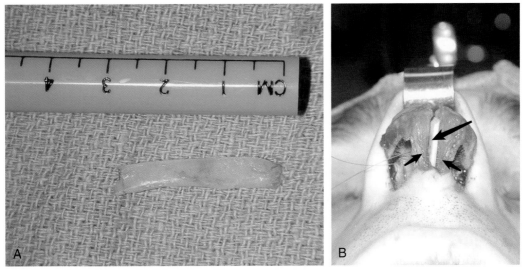

Figure 30-8 A, B, Columellar strut (*large arrow*) carved from septal cartilage placed in a pocket between the medial crura (*small arrows*). (From Nassif PS. Asian rhinoplasty. *Fac Plast Surg Clin North Am* 2010;18:153-171.)

Releasing the lower and medial lateral cartilages from the adherent vestibular tissue, as described earlier, with the placement of an extended or basic columellar strut may be all that is necessary to increase tip projection. Numerous grafts may modify tip projection such as a basic columellar strut (Figure 30-8), a shield tip graft (Figure 30-9), bruised onlay dome and/or infratip lobular grafts (Figure 30-10), or a combination of these grafts. In nearly 100% of the ethnic rhinoplasties I perform, a columellar strut is placed. This sets the foundation for tip projection as the nasal tip is rebuilt. I favor carving the columellar strut from septal cartilage, although auricular cartilage or rib cartilage can also be used. If the patient has undergone a septoplasty in the past, preoperative intranasal palpation of the septum may help determine if any significant cartilage remains available. In many instances, cartilage is present along the dorsal septum. In addition to the endonasal approach, dorsal septal cartilage may be harvested from the open approach by elevating the middle vault mucoperichondrium from the septum following

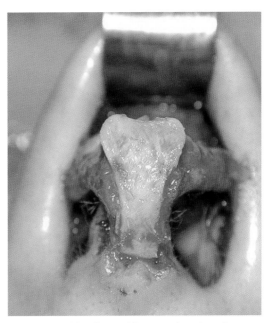

Figure 30-9 Shield graft carved from septal cartilage. (From Nassif PS. Asian rhinoplasty. *Fac Plast Surg Clin North Am* 2010;18:153-171.)

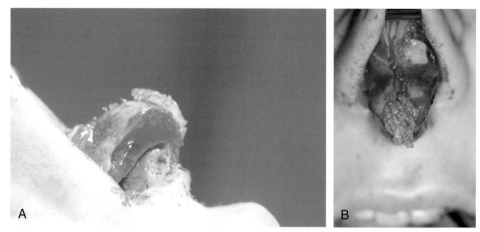

Figure 30-10 Lateral (**A**) and frontal (**B**) views of a bruised infratip lobular graft. (From Nassif PS. Asian rhinoplasty. *Fac Plast Surg Clin North Am* 2010;18:153-171.)

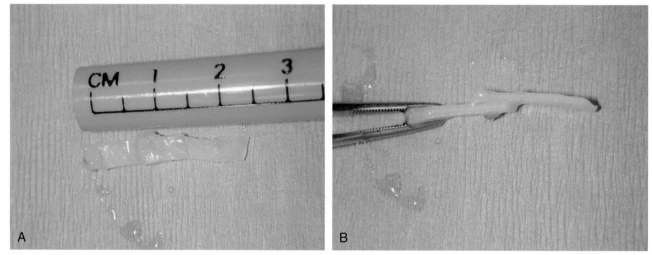

Figure 30-11 A, B, Two short segments of septal cartilage sutured to one another toward their distal ends, creating a columellar strut. (From Nassif PS. Asian rhinoplasty. *Fac Plast Surg Clin North Am* 2010;18:153-171.)

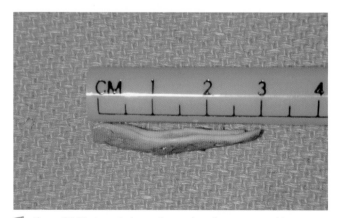

Figure 30-12 An auricular cartilage columellar strut created by suturing a double-layered segment with the concave sides facing one another. (From Nassif PS. Asian rhinoplasty. *Fac Plast Surg Clin North Am* 2010;18:153-171.)

release of the caudal end of the upper lateral cartilages. Dorsal septum may be harvested without loss of dorsal support as long as at least 1 cm of septum is preserved. If the septal cartilage harvested is short, two segments may be sutured to one another toward their distal ends (Figure 30-11). To augment the nasolabial region or subnasale, plumping grafts or a posterior septal extension graft may be used.

A columellar strut may be created with auricular cartilage by suturing a double-layered segment with the concave sides facing one another (Figure 30-12). In addition to adding tip projection, a shield graft or infratip lobular graft will add length to the infratip lobule and create the proper tip-defining points. Shield grafts made from auricular cartilage are usually less rigid than septal grafts but either will suffice. If the graft extends a moderate amount above the native tip, a

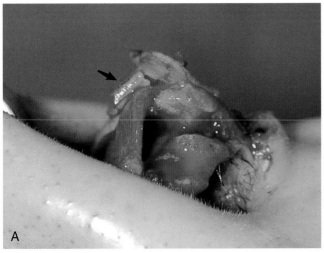

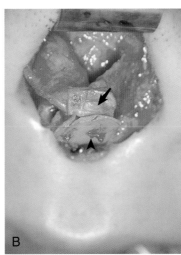

Figure 30-13 Lateral (**A**) and straight-on (**B**) views of a buttress graft (*arrow*) preventing bending of a shield graft (*arrowhead*). (From Nassif PS. Asian rhinoplasty. *Fac Plast Surg Clin North Am* 2010;18:153-171.)

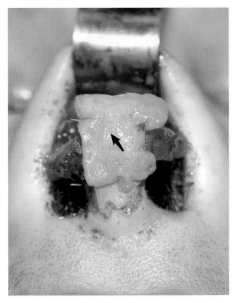

Figure 30-14 Mucoperichondrium (*arrow*) placed over a shield graft to prevent visibility of the graft through the skin. (From Nassif PS. Asian rhinoplasty. *Fac Plast Surg Clin North Am* 2010;18:153-171.)

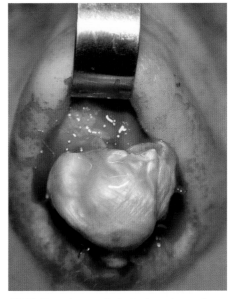

Figure 30-16 Deep temporalis fascia draped over the nasal tip and grafts. (From Nassif PS. Asian rhinoplasty. *Fac Plast Surg Clin North Am* 2010;18:153-171.)

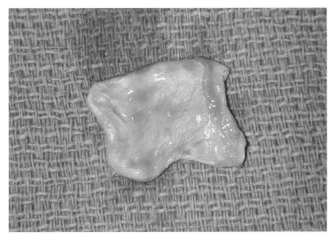

Figure 30-15 Deep temporalis fascia used for augmentation or to cover cartilage grafts. (From Nassif PS. Asian rhinoplasty. *Fac Plast Surg Clin North Am* 2010;18:153-171.)

buttress graft (Figure 30-13) is placed behind the shield graft to prevent "bending" of the graft. Additionally, rim grafts may be added to create a balanced alar–dome contour. Once all grafts are sutured into place, either SMAS/mucoperichondrium (Figure 30-14) or deep temporalis fascia (Figure 30-15) can be placed over the tip complex (Figure 30-16) to prevent skin contraction with eventual visibility of the grafts through the skin.

The tongue-in-groove technique may also be used.[2] In essence, the medial crura are advanced on the anterior caudal septum using 5-0 permanent suture. This can also increase tip projection and rotation as desired (Figure 30-17).

If additional cartilage is needed, autologous cartilage is the preferred choice. Auricular cartilage (Figure 30-18) harvesting from the concha cavum and cymba concha

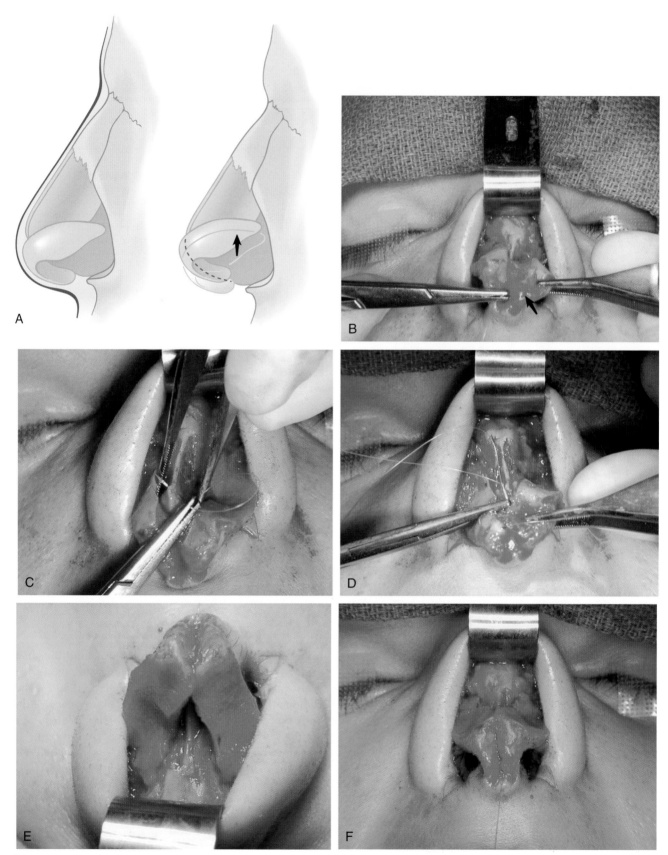

Figure 30-17 A, Diagram of the tongue-in-groove technique. **B,** The 5-0 PDS suture is being passed through the posterior caudal medial crural ligament (*arrow*) from the outside to the inside (toward the septum). The suture can also be passed through the posterior medial crura cartilage. **C,** The suture is passed through the anterior septal angle. **D,** The suture is finally passed in the opposite direction exiting the medial crural ligament (shown here) or the medial crura cartilage. Overhead (**E**) and frontal (**F**) views of the tip with increased tip projection. (From Nassif PS. Asian rhinoplasty. *Fac Plast Surg Clin North Am* 2010;18:153-171.)

may be approached from the anterior (Figure 30-19) surface; however, it is usually harvested from the posterior surface (Figure 30-20) (>90% of my cases). Costal cartilage (Figure 30-21) is my autologous cartilage of choice for dorsal reconstruction. Costal cartilage harvesting has been well described in many publications and will not be discussed here; however, it is worth mentioning for logistical purposes that while I harvest the temporalis fascia graft (which I use in the majority of cases), a second team of surgeons harvest the rib.

OSTEOTOMIES

Conservative management of the nasal bones should be considered since many African American patients have low nasal bones. Osteotomies in patients with low nasal

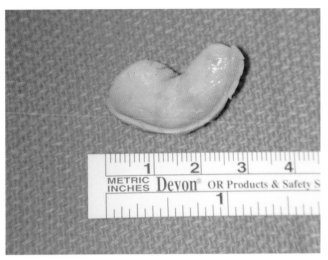

Figure 30-18 Convex auricular cartilage used for tip reconstruction. (From Nassif PS. Asian rhinoplasty. *Fac Plast Surg Clin North Am* 2010;18:153-171.)

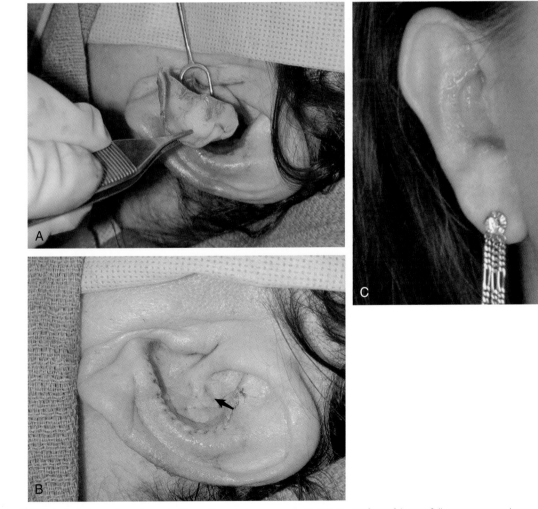

Figure 30-19 A, Auricular cartilage harvested from the anterior approach. **B,** Anterior surface of the ear following incision closure and coapting sutures placed through the concha cavum and cymba (*arrow*). **C,** Healing anterior auricular incision. (From Nassif PS. Asian rhinoplasty. *Fac Plast Surg Clin North Am* 2010;18:153-171.)

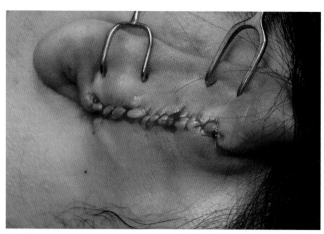

Figure 30-20 Postauricular closure following conchal cartilage harvesting. (From Nassif PS. Asian rhinoplasty. *Fac Plast Surg Clin North Am* 2010;18:153-171.)

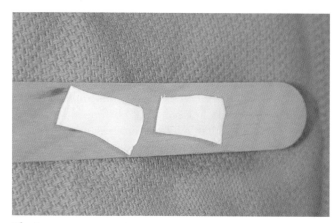

Figure 30-22 Layered 1- to 2-mm polytetrafluoroethylene sheeting. (From Nassif PS. Asian rhinoplasty. *Fac Plast Surg Clin North Am* 2010; 18:153-171.)

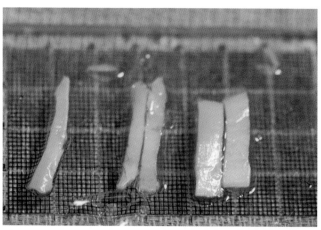

Figure 30-21 Costal (rib) cartilage carved into a columellar strut (*left*), rim grafts (*middle*), and alar batten grafts (*right*). (From Nassif PS. Asian rhinoplasty. *Fac Plast Surg Clin North Am* 2010;18:153-171.)

bones are typically difficult to perform and carry a higher than average risk of being asymmetric. If osteotomies are to be performed, infiltrating the nasal mucosa medial to the pyriform aperture with a solution containing local anesthetic and epinephrine will aid in hemostasis. I usually find that performing low-to-low osteotomies followed by fading medial osteotomies and ensuring bones are mobile and infractured will prevent green stick fractures or rocker deformities.

RADIX AND DORSAL AUGMENTATION

The pocket for the graft must be of adequate size or just larger than the graft. Autologous grafts, including septal, conchal, or costal cartilage, are preferred to alloplastic grafts such as layered 1- to 2-mm polytetrafluoroethylene (PTFE) sheeting (Figure 30-22). I prefer not to use silicone implants (Figure 30-23) because of the higher risk of infection and subsequent extrusion. For minimal radix

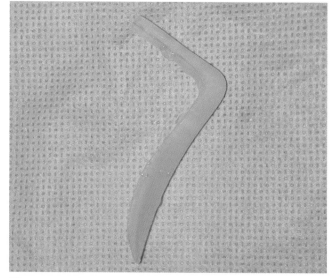

Figure 30-23 Typical silicone L-strut used for dorsal augmentation. (From Nassif PS. Asian rhinoplasty. *Fac Plast Surg Clin North Am* 2010; 18:153-171.)

and/or dorsal augmentation, my preference is to use nasal SMAS/mucoperichondrium or deep temporalis fascia (see Figure 30-15). For moderate radix and/or dorsal augmentation, bruised cartilage (septal, conchal, or costal) is placed posterior to the harvested scar tissue/mucoperichondrium or wrapped in deep temporalis fascia (Figure 30-24). Diced cartilage wrapped in fascia (DCF) (Figure 30-25) popularized by Calvert et al.[3] has become my preference for significant dorsal augmentation. The diced cartilage is placed in a 1-ml tuberculin syringe with the distal end of the syringe removed. Enlarging the distal end of the syringe will allow the diced cartilage to flow easily through the syringe. Deep temporalis fascia is wrapped around the syringe and secured with a running 5-0 chromic suture. To create a smooth dorsal augmentation, the DCF graft should extend to the cephalad supratip region. En bloc cartilage grafts placed over

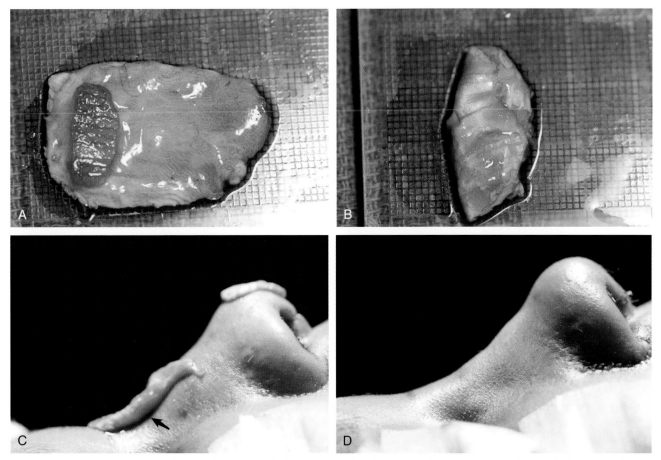

Figure 30-24 A, Bruised cartilage placed on deep temporalis fascia. **B,** Bruised cartilage wrapped in deep temporalis fascia. **C,** (Before) bruised cartilage wrapped in deep temporalis fascia used as a radix/cephalad dorsal graft (*arrow*) and fascia placed over the dome. **D,** After view. (From Nassif PS. Asian rhinoplasty. *Fac Plast Surg Clin North Am* 2010;18:153-171.)

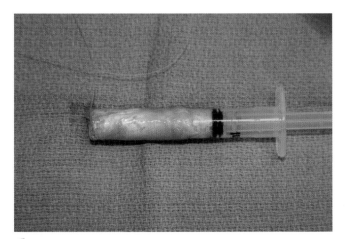

Figure 30-25 Diced cartilage wrapped in deep temporalis fascia (DCF). The diced cartilage is placed in a 1-ml tuberculin syringe with the distal end of the syringe removed. Enlarging the distal end of the syringe will allow the diced cartilage to flow easily through the syringe. Deep temporalis fascia is wrapped around the syringe and secured with a running 5-0 chromic suture. (From Nassif PS. Asian rhinoplasty. *Fac Plast Surg Clin North Am* 2010;18:153-171.)

the dorsum may warp, look unnatural, or reabsorb; therefore, I prefer not to use them in my practice.

ALAR BASE REDUCTION

In brief, alar base reduction in the African American patient can be subdivided into techniques that narrow the alae with or without modifying the vestibular component (nostril), the nasal sill/floor, or a combination of these. Rarely do I encounter the need to carry out an excision of the nasal sill region within this patient population. Furthermore, I find that this maneuver narrows the nostril and nasal floor with subsequent narrowing of the airway without reducing the alar lobule (Figure 30-26). With this technique, the only way to obtain some alar reduction is to make the standard sill incision at the junction of the ala and nostril. This is demonstrated in Figure 30-27 in an Asian patient. If the African American patient refuses to undergo a standard alar lobule reduction, the described technique may be used with limited results. In my experience and for the majority of my patient population, the

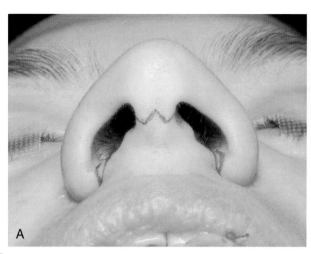 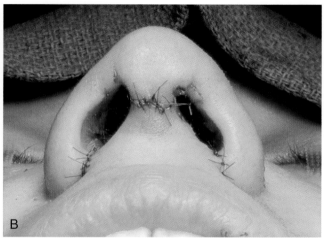

Figure 30-26 A, Preoperative base view of the standard nasal sill incision. **B,** Postoperative view of the nasal sill procedure revealing a narrowed nostril and nasal floor with subsequent narrowing of the airway without reducing the alar lobule. (From Nassif PS. Asian rhinoplasty. *Fac Plast Surg Clin North Am* 2010;18:153-171.)

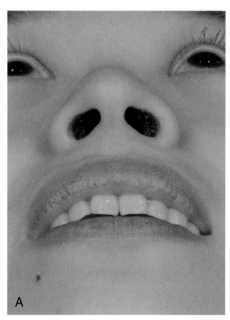 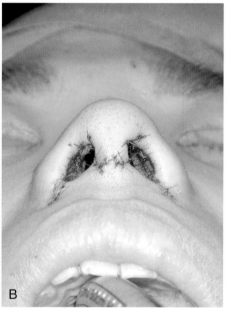

Figure 30-27 A, Preoperative base view of the lateral nasal sill/alar incision. **B,** Postoperative view of the lateral nasal sill/alar incision with a mild to moderate amount of alar lobule reduction. The nostril is also narrowed with subsequent narrowing of the airway. (From Nassif PS. Asian rhinoplasty. *Fac Plast Surg Clin North Am* 2010;18:153-171.)

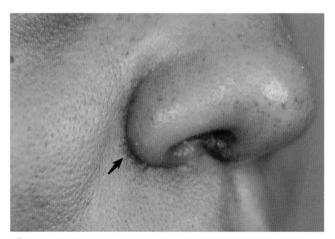

Figure 30-28 Minimally visible lateral alar base scar (*arrow*).

alar lobule needs to be reduced to achieve harmony and balance during the African American rhinoplasty.

Sheen[4] has described several ways to reduce the alar lobule and nostril, which, if performed properly, will create an aesthetically pleasing result with a minimally visible scar (Figure 30-28). To make this simple, vestibular (nostril) = decreased nostril size and cutaneous (alar lobule) = modified alar lobule and contour. Two frequently encountered types of alar base configuration in the African American nose (Figure 30-29) are described:

- Type I: Larger than ideal alar lobule with appropriately sized nostrils
- Type II: Larger than ideal alar lobule with larger than ideal nostrils

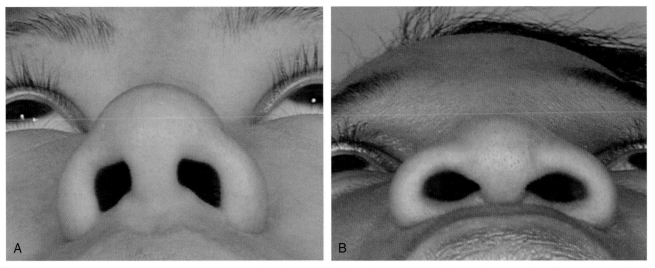

Figure 30-29 A, Base view of Type I: excessive alar lobule with normal sized nostrils. **B,** Base view of Type II: large nostrils and excessive alar lobules. (From Nassif PS. Asian rhinoplasty. *Fac Plast Surg Clin North Am* 2010;18:153-171.)

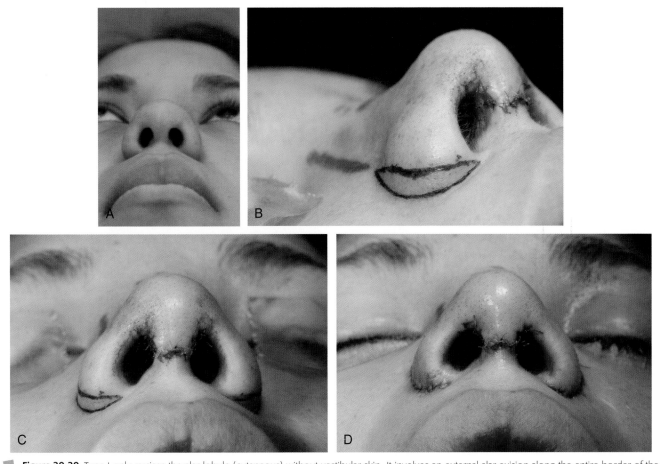

Figure 30-30 Type I only excises the alar lobule (cutaneous) without vestibular skin. It involves an external alar exision along the entire border of the alar lobule. (From Nassif PS. Asian rhinoplasty. *Fac Plast Surg Clin North Am* 2010;18:153-171.)

Addressing the Type I configuration involves cutaneous excision of the alar lobule (cutaneous) without vestibular skin by means of an alar base excision along the alar groove (Figure 30-30). In general, 3–4 mm of reduction will provide a significant degree of change; however, it is prudent to be conservative with this very powerful technique until significant experience has been accrued with it. For unique situations, I have removed as much as 5 mm of alar lobule, which is not common practice.

Addressing the Type II configuration involves excising primarily the alar lobule (cutaneous incision) with a limited amount of vestibular tissue (although significantly less than the cutaneous component). The same types of incision and amounts of resection are performed as during a Type I incision, with the exception that the incision extends into the vestibular lining of the nose, resecting a limited amount of vestibular tissue. The techniques described do not include routine nostril sill/floor excisions, which may be incorporated into either of the described alar base reduction techniques (Figure 30-31).

To obtain the most aesthetically pleasing scar, the following pearls should be considered. Traditional teaching instructs that the incision be approximately 1 mm on the nasal side of the alar–facial junction. After noticing on occasion a few visible scars at the cephalad alar lobule due to the placement of the incision despite meticulous closure techniques, I now make the incision in the alar–facial junction, which heals beautifully. The incision is beveled and a medial flap technique is used when vestibular tissue is resected. The medial flap technique (Figure 30-32) involves making the alar–facial incision initially while extending medially along the alar base and stopping short of the last 2 to 3 mm. A back cut that preserves a small triangular (medial) flap is made followed by the superior cut. A wedge of tissue is excised and the natural continuity of the lateral nasal sill is preserved. Figures 30-33 and 30-34 demonstrate a female and male patient's nasal base view following the medial flap technique.

Bipolar cautery can be used sparingly for hemostasis followed by subcutaneous closure using 5-0 Vicryl for the deep tissues and a running 6-0 Prolene for the skin closure. If any vestibular resection is performed, 5-0 chromic is used in a running or interrupted pattern. The sutures are typically removed in 7 days.

POSTOPERATIVE NASAL CARE

- Meticulous cleansing of incisions
- Basic saline nasal sprays
- Suction bulb to suction nose as needed
- Head elevation
- Cold compresses
- Postoperative nighttime taping for 6 to 10 weeks
- A mixture of 0.4 mL 5-fluorouracil and 0.04 mL of Kenalog 5 mg/mL is injected after 4 weeks as needed

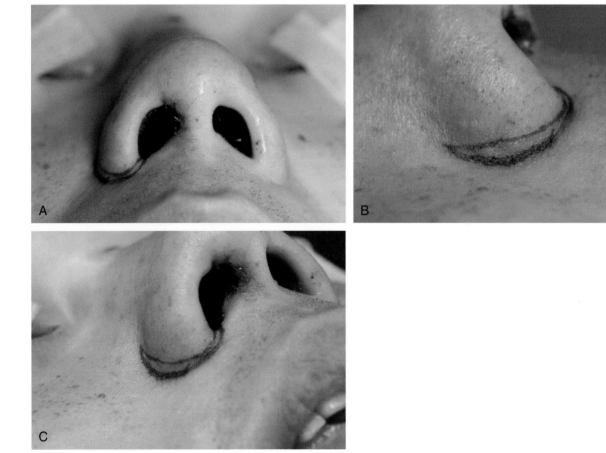

Figure 30-31 Base view of combined alar lobule and nostril sill/floor alar base reduction technique. (From Nassif PS. Asian rhinoplasty. *Fac Plast Surg Clin North Am* 2010;18:153-171.)

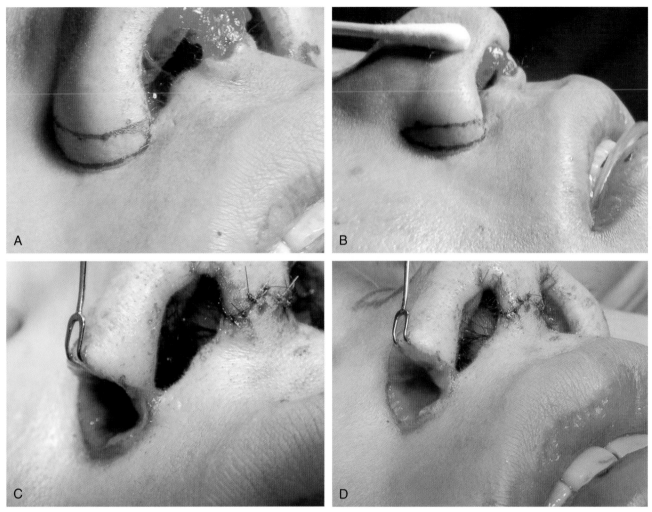

Figure 30-32 Surgical markings of the lateral base (**A**) and lateral view (**B**) of the medial flap technique. **C, D,** The medial flap is preserved following removal of the alar lobule. (From Nassif PS. Asian rhinoplasty. *Fac Plast Surg Clin North Am* 2010;18:153-171.)

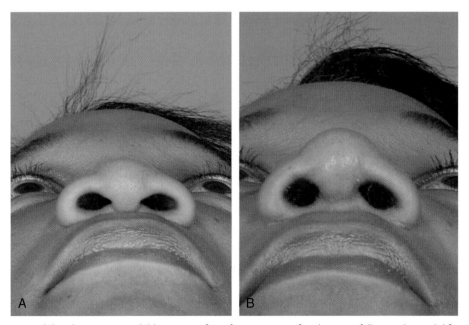

Figure 30-33 Preoperative (**A**) and postoperative (**B**) base view of an African American female's nose following the medial flap technique for alar base reduction. Note the natural continuity of the alar lobule is maintained.

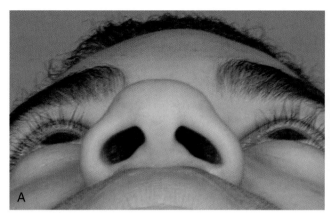 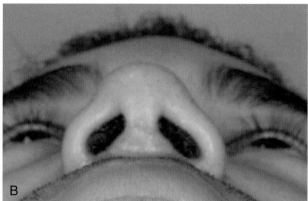

Figure 30-34 Preoperative (**A**) and postoperative (**B**) base views of an African American male's nose following the medial flap technique for alar base reduction. Note the natural continuity of the alar lobule is maintained.

RISKS AND COMPLICATIONS

- Overaggressive cartilage removal, causing loss of projection and ptosis
- Prolonged bruising or hyperpigmentation
- Infection
- Prominent alar scarring
- Excessive alar reduction
- Abnormal appearing ala
  - Flat ala with loss of natural base curves
- Nasal asymmetry, graft irregularity, displacement and extrusion
- Graft absorption
- Prolonged swelling

PEARLS

- Carefully evaluate the nasal anatomy, physiology, and the patient's expectations.

- Establish realistic goals for the patient and for yourself.
- Prepare a detailed preoperative evaluation and surgical plan.
- Maintain or improve nasal airway function.
- Perform revision procedures only when truly warranted.

REFERENCES

1. Kridel RWH, et al. Advances in nasal tip surgery: The lateral crural steal. *Arch Otolaryngol Head Neck Surg.* 1989;117:1206–1212.
2. Kridel RWH, et al. The tongue-in-groove technique in septorhinoplasty. *Arch Facial Plast Surg.* 1989;1:246–256.
3. Calvert JW, Brenner K, DaCosta-Iyer M, et al. Histological analysis of human diced cartilage grafts. *Plast Reconstr Surg.* 2006;118(1):230–236.
4. Sheen JH. Adjunctive techniques. In: *Aesthetic Rhinoplasty.* St. Louis (MO): The Mosby Company; 1987:255-258.

CHAPTER THIRTY-ONE

Middle Eastern Rhinoplasty

Babak Azizzadeh • Grigoriy Mashkevich

Aesthetic rhinoplasty in patients of Middle Eastern extraction poses a specific set of challenges for the rhinoplasty surgeon. As is true in other geoethnic groups, several unique anatomic features define the appearance of the "Middle Eastern nose" and require a tailored approach to achieve aesthetic refinement. Implicit in the surgical methodology for this group is the prevention of "Westernization rhinoplasty" and preservation of the native ethnic look (the word "ethnic" is used loosely throughout text and refers to all ethnicities of the Middle East). Middle Eastern rhinoplasty also highlights the fundamental surgical tenets of cartilage sparing and structural grafting. These are particularly applicable to this group of patients, who consistently demonstrate inherent cartilaginous weakness as well as thick overlying nasal skin. This chapter explores the common nasal characteristics shared by people of the Middle Eastern origin and reviews the essential elements of a rhinoplasty consultation. Various surgical techniques that have been found effective by authors in the aesthetic refinement of the Middle Eastern nose are discussed in detail.

BACKGROUND AND DEMOGRAPHICS

While the term "Middle East" refers to a geographic region, its precise borders have been poorly defined and blurred over the centuries by migration and intermixing of various populations. The phrase "Middle East" has its origins in the United Kingdom at the turn of the twentieth century and refers to regions of Western Asia and North Africa. Numerous modern nations presently comprise this subcontinent and are home to almost a billion people[1] (Table 31-1). Some historians argue that several large adjacent countries, such as Armenia, Afghanistan, Pakistan, and India, also belong in the Middle Eastern category. While this discussion is beyond the scope of the present chapter, it is not surprising that people inhabiting these neighboring countries certainly share many of the nasal characteristics reviewed in detail here.

The Middle East is also home to a wide range of ethnic and religious diversity. This may partially explain variations in the aesthetic desires for rhinoplasty between various geographic areas within Middle East. For instance, it has been suggested that people living outside of the Arabian Peninsula and Gulf regions (Saudi Arabia, Kuwait, Qatar, UAE, Oman, and Iran) desire more significant changes from rhinoplasty, such as greater dorsal reduction and tip projection.[2]

In the United States, the estimated size of the Middle Eastern diaspora varies according to the source, but nevertheless provides a sense of its demographic impact. According to a recent population census, more than 1.2 million people of strictly Middle Eastern origins reside in United States.[3] This number expands to "at least 3.5 million" as per the Arab American Institute.[4] While the residence of this ethnic group has been documented in all 50 states, an overwhelming 94% reside in large metropolitan areas (Los Angeles, Detroit, and New York are the top three cities).

VISUAL AND ANATOMIC CHARACTERISTICS OF THE "MIDDLE EASTERN" NOSE

Several unique features define the ethnic appearance of a Middle Eastern nose (Table 31-2, Figure 31-1). These can be readily appreciated in some of the well-known political figures from the Middle East (Figure 31-2).

One of the chief distinguishing characteristics of a Middle Eastern nose is its relatively thick overlying skin–soft tissue envelope (SSTE). Numerous pilosebaceous units dotting its surface produce an oily texture and further contribute to skin thickness. These anatomic properties of SSTE significantly influence the appearance of the lower third of the nose by effectively blunting the configuration of the underlying cartilaginous framework. Specific findings include an effacement of the supratip region and concealment of tip definition. This results in an overall amorphous appearance of the nasal tip. In the postoperative period, the above-mentioned features of SSTE promote scarring, which in turn predisposes to contracture forces and formation of a pollybeak deformity.

Table 31-1 Present Middle Eastern Nations and Their Respective Population Estimates

Country	Population	Country	Population
Algeria	32,930,091	Oman	3,102,229
Bahrain	698,585	Palestine	3,889,248
Egypt	78,887,007	Qatar	885,359
Iran	68,688,433	Saudi Arabia	27,019,731
Iraq	26,783,383	Sudan	41,236,378
Israel	7,260,000	Syria	18,881,361
Jordan	5,153,378	Tunisia	10,175,014
Kuwait	2,418,393	Turkey	70,413,958
Lebanon	3,874,050	UAE	2,602,713
Libya	5,900,754	Yemen	21,456,188
Morocco	33,241,259	**Total**	**465,263,512**

Source: mideastweb.org, cia.gov

Both of these can be controlled with specific surgical maneuvers and steroid injections respectively, as outlined in sections that follow.

High radix and a strong dorsum, with an associated dorsal hump, commonly frame the upper two thirds of a Middle Eastern nose. This visual feature is almost always accentuated by the underprojected and hanging nasal tip, thereby enhancing an illusion of increased dorsal height. As such, elevating tip position goes a long way in visually reducing the dorsum. Moreover, establishing an improved nasal harmony by elevating the tip avoids an overresection of the nasal dorsum.

Table 31-2 Common Visual Features Associated With a Middle Eastern Nose

Skin–soft tissue envelope	Thick skin with numerous pilosebaceous units, contributing to an amorphous appearance of the nasal tip and supratip fullness.
Upper third	Overprojecting bony dorsum and high radix; excessive and sometimes irregular dorsal width resulting in poor brow-tip dorsal aesthetic line.
Middle third	Widening of the osseous and cartilaginous vaults.
Nasal tip	Amorphous and hanging nasal tip, cephalic orientation of the lower lateral crura, weak medial crura, acute nasolabial angle.
Nostrils	Variable degree of alar flaring.

Weak structural integrity of the lower lateral cartilages represents an additional defining property of the nasal tip. Medial crura are typically thin and contribute minimal support to the tip. The lateral crura are commonly rotated in a cephalic orientation and variably contribute to tip fullness. Overactive depressor septi nasi muscle and alar flaring are also frequently seen, especially in people from the West African regions of the Middle East.

RHINOPLASTY CONSULTATION

The initial rhinoplasty consultation for a Middle Eastern patient allows the surgeon to form a fertile ground for understanding patient concerns, goals, and motivations for surgery. The concept of maintaining ethnic identity should be clearly communicated on both sides of the table. A surgeon should be wary of patients requesting a drastic change in their appearance, which may cause an unnatural result (or "Westernization") down the line and result in an unsatisfied patient.

It is generally a good idea to include a family member in the consultation process. His or her opinion may represent important feedback and help avert a potential misunderstanding. Digital photography and morphing can greatly assist in conveying the proposed changes and help communicate more effectively. These should be used as a point of reference, without implicit guarantees as to the result. Various points discussed in the previous and later sections should be kept in mind when altering patient images (Table 31-3). If requested, "before and after" photographs of previously operated patients can be used as well. This may also help in clarifying the differences

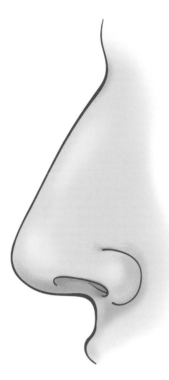
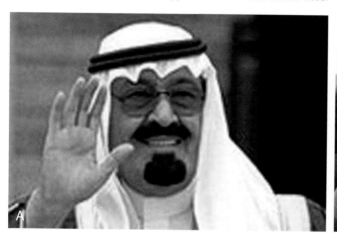

Figure 31-1 Unique features define the ethnic appearance of a Middle Eastern nose.

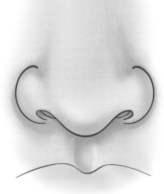
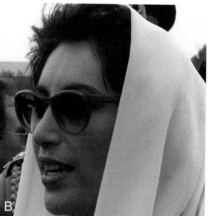

Figure 31-2 Nasal features in some of the well-known Middle Eastern political figures, exemplifying typical visual attributes of a Middle Eastern nose. **A,** Prince Abdullah of Saudi Arabia. (This image is from Wikimedia and is a work of an employee of the Executive Office of the President of the United States, taken or made during the course of the person's official duties. As a work of the U. S. federal government, the image is in the public domain. http://commons.wikimedia.org/wiki/File:Saudi_Crown_Prince_Abdullah_and_George_W._Bush.jpg). **B,** Benazir Bhutto. (This image is from Wikimedia and is courtesy of SRA Gerald B. Johnson, United States Department of Defense. This image is a work of a U. S. military or Department of Defense employee, taken or made during the course of an employee's official duties. As a work of the U. S. federal government, the image is in the public domain. http://commons.wikimedia.org/wiki/File:Benazir_bhutto_1988_cropped.jpg).

Table 31-3 Surgical Concepts and Techniques Commonly Used for Aesthetic Refinement of the Middle Eastern Nose

Skin–soft tissue envelope	Defatting into the subdermal plane, especially in the supratip region; postoperative observation and conservative Kenalog (triamcinolone acetonide) injections to prevent pollybeak formation.
Upper third	Maintenance of high radix during dorsal hump reduction; elevation of the tip to create a harmonious dorsum–tip relationship, rather than aggressive reduction of the dorsum.
Middle third	Medial and lateral osteotomies; placement of spreader grafts to avoid internal valve narrowing and an inverted-V deformity.
Nasal tip	Cartilage-sparing maneuvers with preferential use of suture techniques for the dome region; placement of strong supporting grafts (columellar strut or septal extension graft, shield or cap grafts); possible placement of lateral crural batten grafts and alar rim grafts.
Nostrils	Alar base modification as needed

in rhinoplasty goals for Caucasian and Middle Eastern noses.

MIDDLE EASTERN RHINOPLASTY

The basic tenets of Middle Eastern rhinoplasty include the avoidance of overresection and preservation of ethnic appearance.[5,6] Westernization, through application of standards suitable for a Caucasian nose, should be avoided in this patient group. Not adhering to this concept carries a risk of establishing a disharmonious and unnatural nasal–facial relationship. General concepts, discussed in detail later, include a very conservative lowering of the radix and dorsum, providing adequate tip projection, and rotating the nasal tip while maintaining a hint of an acute nasolabial angle (less than 95 degrees). These and other goals for the Middle Eastern rhinoplasty are summarized in Table 31-3.

The authors prefer an external rhinoplasty approach in this patient group, as it affords superior visualization of internal structures and allows precise modification of the tip and osseocartilaginous framework. An endonasal approach is used only when patients have natural tip aesthetics with good tip support requiring only dorsal modification. In the authors' experience, the columellar scar from an external approach heals exceptionally well in this patient group, making an open incision not an issue. This observation has been corroborated by Foda,[7] who performed a columellar scar analysis on 600 patients of Arabic extraction. In his series, only 1.5% of patients found the columellar scar to be unacceptable (cited reasons were scar widening, hyperpigmentation, and columellar rim notching).

The philosophy of open structure rhinoplasty underlies the surgical approach to the Middle Eastern nose. It is imperative to add sufficient structure to the cartilaginous framework, in light of the weak inherent cartilage strength and thick overlying SSTE. The latter structure becomes a significant risk factor in the postoperative period for soft tissue contracture, which can easily overwhelm any unaltered native cartilage.

Following an open rhinoplasty exposure, the upper two thirds of the nose are addressed with a conservative dorsal hump and radix modification (Figure 31-3). Maintenance of sufficient dorsal height, in harmony with a high radix, is critical in preserving an ethnic appearance in a Middle Eastern nose. These structures must be conserved to a greater extent than in a Caucasian nose. Gender differences in the height of the radix must also be carefully considered with male patients requiring a higher radix than their female counterparts. Overall, a low radix can accentuate the dorsal height. Correction of the radix-dorsum disproportion improves the overall dorsal balance and reduces its prominence. A crushed cartilage graft is an effective means of filling the radix bed and can be

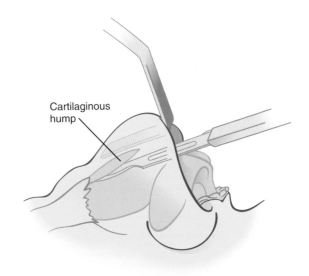

Cartilaginous hump

Figure 31-3 Dorsal hump reduction

guided into position with a 6-0 chromic suture on a Keith needle. A knot is then tied over the skin at the site of the transcutaneous suture placement, further securing the graft in the postoperative period. This suture can be removed in approximately 1 week.

In most cases where patients have dorsal hump reduction, the authors place spreader grafts to avoid internal valve narrowing and an inverted-V deformity.

As previously discussed, a dependent position of the nasal tip partially contributes to the appearance of excessive dorsal height. Judicious tip projection and rotation, in turn, create an illusion of a lowered dorsum. Tip modification is almost always necessary in a Middle Eastern rhinoplasty, allowing for a more conservative reduction of the nasal dorsum.

After dorsal hump modification and middle nasal vault reconstruction, the lower lateral cartilages are examined for inherent weakness. Nasal tip reconstruction begins by placing a columellar strut and securing it to both medial crura. Kridel's tongue-in-groove technique or septal extension graft can be used in place of strut as deemed appropriate for the nose.[8,9] When projecting the tip, it should be kept in mind that the supratip break should never be as prominent as in the ideal Caucasian nose. In male patients, it is especially desirable to only have a minimally visible break in the supratip region. Cartilage suturing techniques (intradomal sutures, lateral crural steal dome sutures, etc.) and additional grafting as necessary (shield or cap grafts) are used to improve tip projection and definition.[10–12] Judicious nasal skin de-fatting may be performed at this point, in the subdermal plane (Figure 31-4).

Minimal resection of the cephalic margin of the lower lateral cartilages should be performed. Lower lateral cartilages are typically weak structures and minimally contribute to tip fullness. The authors prefer to reinforce the

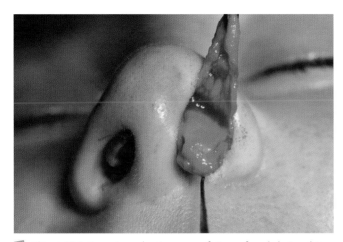

Figure 31-4 Excessive subcutaneous soft tissue found during rhinoplasty in patients of Middle Eastern extraction. Endonasal approach is shown with the delivery of lower lateral cartilages. Soft tissue overlying the cartilage is elevated to depict its thickness.

tip cartilages with lateral crural strut grafts and place rim grafts along the alar margin.[13,14] These maneuvers provide an additional layer of protection against postoperative collapse of the vestibule, as well as against alar rim notching and retraction. The key factor is to create a straight structurally sound lateral crura avoiding excessive convexity or concavity. Figure 31-5 highlights structural techniques commonly used in Middle Eastern rhinoplasty.

Tip rotation should be conservative and aim to create a nasolabial angle of approximately 95 degrees or less. This can be achieved in most instances with a combination of strut placement, dome suturing, and a conservative triangular caudal septal excision with the base at the anterior septal angle. Vertically oriented lateral crura may prevent cephalic rotation of the tip tripod, necessitating an additional lateral crural overlay[15] or caudal repositioning of the lateral crura. If either scenario is used, lateral crural strut grafts are used for reinforcement.

At the conclusion of the procedure, medial and lateral osteotomies are performed. Medial osteotomies

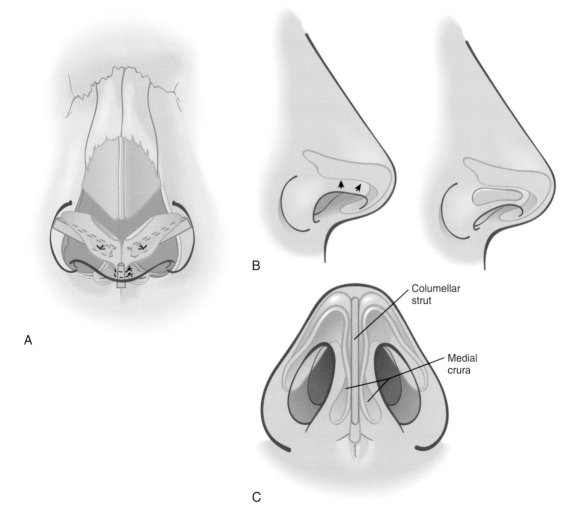

Columellar strut

Medial crura

A

B

C

Figure 31-5 Structural techniques commonly utilized in Middle Eastern rhinoplasty: **A,** lateral crural strut grafts; **B,** alar rim grafts; **C,** columellar strut grafts, and **D,** middle nasal vault reconstruction.

Continued

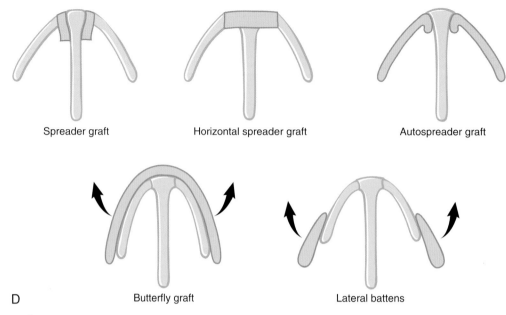

Spreader graft   Horizontal spreader graft   Autospreader graft

D   Butterfly graft   Lateral battens

Figure 31-5, cont'd.

are performed in a lateral fading fashion at the osseocartilaginous junction (Figure 31-6). If the patient has open roof deformity, medial osteotomy is avoided. Lateral osteotomies are performed in a high–low–high fashion.

If necessary, alar base modification is completed following osteotomies, keeping in mind that mild alar flaring is an important feature of the Middle Eastern nose (Figure 31-7). The type of alar base modification will depend on two key factors: alar flaring and interalar–intercanthal distance. If the patient has normal interalar–intercanthal relationship (usually should be 1:1), then "alar wedge resection" is performed. Alar wedge resection avoids sill incision. If the patient's interalar distance is significantly wider than intercanthal distance, then a sill incision will also be necessary. Sill incisions must be made medial to the nostril axis. Middle Eastern patients can tolerate to keep the alar base slightly wider than the intercanthal distance.[16]

COMPLICATIONS AND PITFALLS

Several undesirable outcomes may complicate the Middle Eastern rhinoplasty. These usually arise from a combination of factors, not the least of which is surgical execution.

In both men and women, overly aggressive resection of the dorsum and/or excessive lowering of the radix can take away an important ethnic characteristic of a Middle Eastern nose. Reestablishing adequate tip projection should avoid the need to significantly lower the dorsum.

Pollybeak deformity represents a real concern in this patient group due to excessive thickness and elevated glandular content of the SSTE. Avoiding overresection of

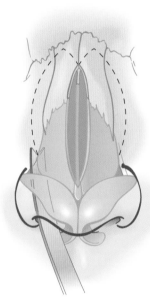

Figure 31-6 Medial and lateral osteotomies. Medial osteotomies typically fade laterally. Lateral osteotomies are performed in a high-low-high fashion.

the dorsum in combination with defatting of the supratip region in the subdermal plane and vigilant observation in the immediate postoperative period can help avoid this dreaded complication. Of particular assistance is triamcinolone acetonide (Kenalog-10; Bristol-Myers Squibb, Princeton, NJ).[17] Triamcinolone acetonide can be injected as soon as 1 week postoperatively. Injections can be repeated once every 4 weeks for several cycles until the desired effect is attained. The judicious use of smaller volumes and lighter concentrations of triamcinolone acetonide should reduce complications such as cutaneous

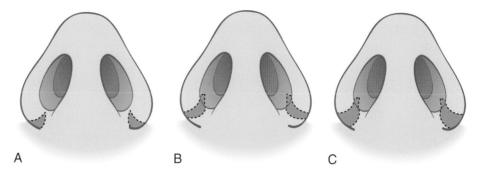

Figure 31-7 Alar base modification is completed following osteotomies, keeping in mind that mild alar flaring is an important feature of the Middle Eastern nose. **A,** Alar wedge resection; **B,** Alar sill resection; **C,** Alar wedge and sill resection.

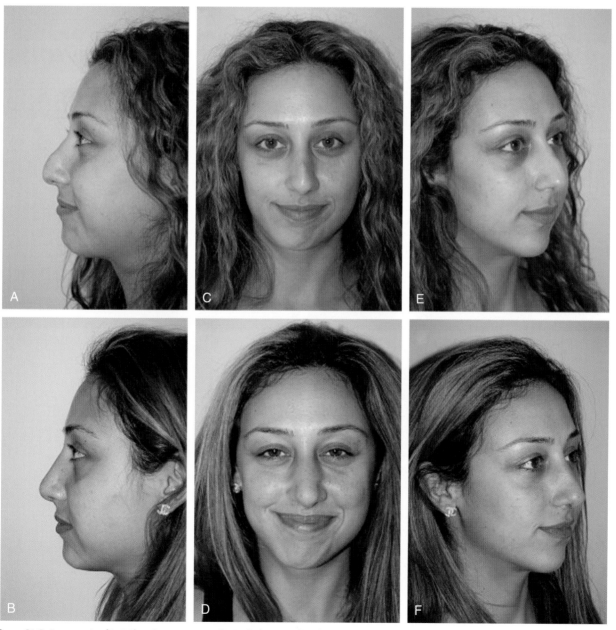

Figure 31-8 Preoperative **(A, C, E)** and postoperative **(B, D, F)** photographs of revision rhinoplasty in a Middle Eastern patient. (Azizzadeh B, Mashkevich G. Middle eastern rhinoplasty. In: *Fac Plast Surg* 2010;18[1].)

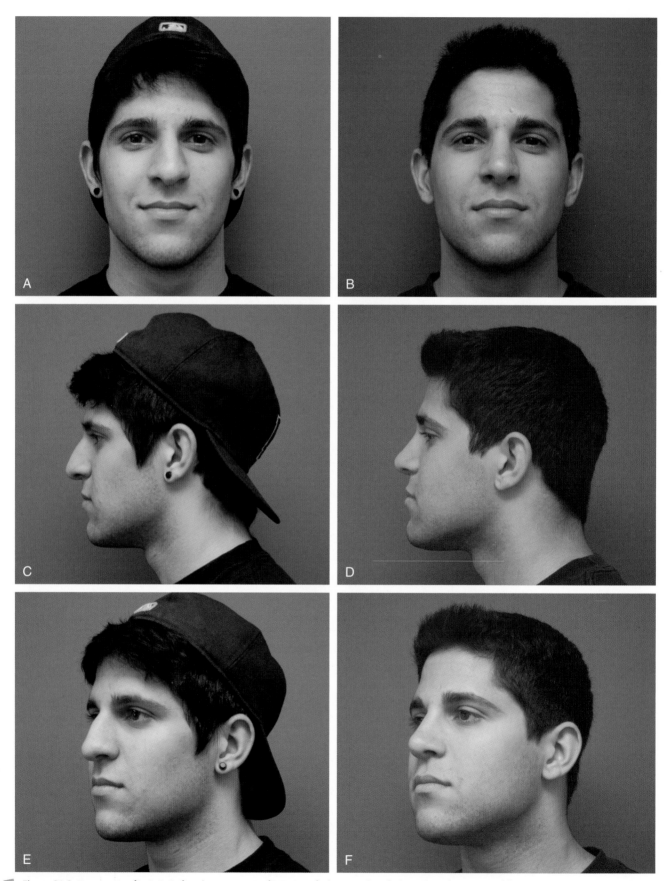

Figure 31-9 Preoperative **(A, C, E, G, I)** and postoperative **(B, D, F, H, J)** photographs of ethnic rhinoplasty in a Middle Eastern patient.

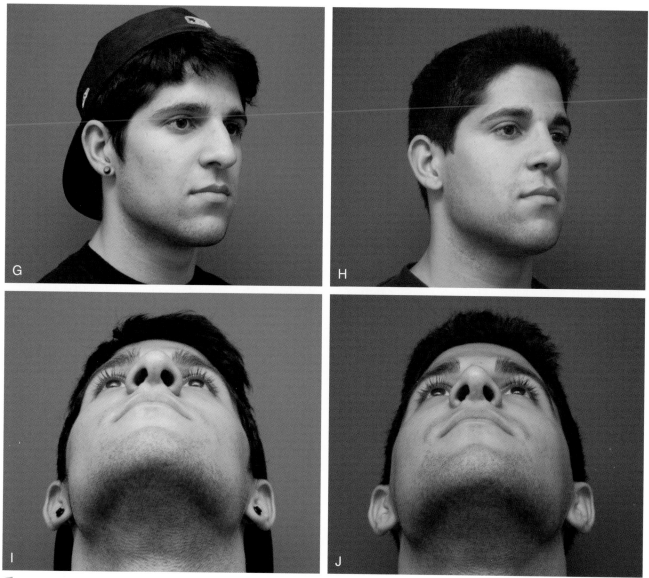

Figure 31-9, cont'd.

atrophy and pigmentary skin changes. We rarely use steroid injections but do reserve it for this purpose.

Tip descent may occur secondary to inadequate structural grafting of the columella and failure to preserve sufficient native cartilage. Placement of a strong columellar strut with concomitant medial crural binding sutures, septal–columellar tongue-in-groove technique, and/or placement of a septal caudal extension graft is essential to counteract forces of scarring and preserve tip projection postoperatively.

Aggressive rotation of the tip, resulting in an obtuse nasolabial angle, can create an unnatural appearance for this patient population. While tenets of Caucasian rhinoplasty dictate an ideal nasolabial angle of 95 to 110 degrees in women, the same angle in a Middle Eastern nose risks overrotation and an incongruous appearance.

A practical goal of less than 95 degrees of rotation should be followed to avoid this complication.

Figures 31-8 and 31-9 represent preoperative and postoperative photographs of Middle Eastern individuals who underwent successful ethnic rhinoplasty.

CONCLUSION

Aesthetic rhinoplasty in patients of the Middle Eastern extraction epitomizes primary goals of ethnic nasal surgery, which include avoidance of aggressive maneuvers, preservation and modification of native structures, and addition of supporting grafts capable of withstanding postoperative forces of contracture. These same guidelines, in the framework of a conservative and methodical surgical approach, underlie the basic tenets of Middle Eastern rhinoplasty. Preservation of native racial features through approaches described in this chapter should help achieve a natural aesthetic refinement in patients undergoing the "Middle Eastern" rhinoplasty.

REFERENCES

1. The World Factbook. United States Central Intelligence Agency. http://www.cia.gov. http://www.mideastweb.org

2. Bizrah MB. Rhinoplasty for Middle Eastern patients. *Fac Plast Surg Clin North Am.* 2002;10(4):381–396.

3. US Census Bureau. Census 2000. http://www.census.gov/prod/2003pubs/c2kbr-23.pdf

4. The Arab American Institute. Demographics. http://www.aaiusa.org/arab-americans/22/demographics

5. Rohrich RJ, Ghavami A. The Middle Eastern nose. In: Gunter JP, Rohrich RJ, Adams WP, eds. *Dallas rhinoplasty: nasal surgery by the masters.* St Louis: Quality Medical Publishing; 2007:1139–1165.

6. Romo T 3rd, Abraham MT. The ethnic nose. *Fac Plast Surg.* 2003;19(3):269–278.

7. Foda HM. External rhinoplasty for the Arabian nose: a columellar scar analysis. *Aesthet Plast Surg.* 2004;28(5):312–316.

8. Kridel RW, Scott BA, Foda HM. The tongue-in-groove technique in septorhinoplasty. A 10-year experience. *Arch Fac Plast Surg.* 1999;1(4):246–256.

9. Byrd HS, Andochick S, Copit S, et al. Septal extension grafts: a method of controlling tip projection shape. *Plast Reconstr Surg.* 1997;100(4):999–1010.

10. Baker SR. Suture contouring of the nasal tip. *Arch Fac Plast Surg.* 2000;2:34–42.

11. Rohrich RJ, Adams WP. The boxy nasal tip: classification and management based on alar cartilage suturing techniques. *Plast Reconstr Surg.* 2001;107(7):1849–1863.

12. Toriumi DM. New concepts in nasal tip contouring. *Arch Fac Plast Surg.* 2006;8(3):156–185.

13. Gunter JP, Friedman RM. Lateral crural strut graft: technique and clinical applications in rhinoplasty. *Plast Reconstr Surg.* 1997;99(4):943–952.

14. Rohrich RJ, Raniere J, Ha RY. The alar contour graft: correction and prevention of alar rim deformities in rhinoplasty. *Plast Reconstr Surg.* 2002;109(7):2495–2505.

15. Foda HMT, Kridel RWH. Lateral crural steal and lateral crural overlay. An objective evaluation. *Arch Otolaryngol Head Neck Surg.* 1999;125:1365–1370.

16. Kridel RW, Castellano RD. A simplified approach to alar base reduction: a review of 124 patients over 20 years. *Arch Fac Plast Surg.* 2005;7(2):81–93.

17. Hanasono MM, Kridel RW, Pastorek NJ, et al. Correction of the soft tissue pollybeak using triamcinolone injection. *Arch Fac Plast Surg.* 2002;4(1):26–30.

CHAPTER THIRTY-TWO

Mestizo Rhinoplasty

Roxana Cobo • William Numa

Most individuals have an interest in being perceived by others as attractive, regardless of their ethnic heritage, racial background, or country of origin. Over time, migratory movements have contributed to the ethnic and racial melting pot responsible for the diversity we have come to expect in major metropolitan areas. Industrialized countries in the world today constantly receive immigrants from developing countries seeking more freedom or better working opportunities than they experienced in their country of origin.[1] Latin America has not been the exception to this phenomenon. The United States, Canada, and, to a lesser degree, Europe have seen significant migratory movements arising from Latin American countries. Today one of the fastest growing and largest minority groups among these recipient countries are the "Hispanics" or "mestizos."[2]

Among the number of available aesthetic facial plastic surgical procedures, rhinoplasty is one of the most popular procedures. Elective aesthetic procedures have become more accessible to people of different parts of the world and from different socioeconomic backgrounds. Even though paradigms of beauty have shifted throughout the years, some publications still hold the "Caucasian" or "Western" features as ideals for aesthetic standards of beauty. In many textbooks and medical articles, the ideal nose is still defined as moderately thin, angular, tapered, and slightly projected.

Facial plastic surgeons today contend with the fact that the established standards, and proportions once conceived with the Caucasian ideals of beauty in mind, do not necessarily hold true across different ethnic backgrounds, including Hispanic patients. It behooves us to accurately redefine the ethnically correct standard of beauty so that patients can be delivered a surgical result that is in line and closer to their aesthetic ideal.[3]

MESTIZO RACE

"Hispanic" is a term derived from *Hispania*, a Greek word for the Iberian Peninsula (modern-day Spain, Portugal, Andorra, and Gibraltar) that is commonly used to describe Spanish-speaking people from Spain and Central and South America. Patients originating from territories once under the rule of the Spanish crown, especially countries from Latin America, are referred to as Hispanic patients. This population is also known as "Latinos" or "mestizos."[4] The U.S. Census Bureau does not consider Portuguese-speaking individuals as Hispanic.

The term "mestizo" is defined as a mixture of races. In Latin America, this meant the mixture of the local Indian tribes with the Caucasian European conquerors during the fifteenth and sixteenth centuries. The introduction of the African slave trade in the eighteenth century added a new ethnic and racial variation, and the term meant the mixture of three predominant races: Indian, Caucasian, and black.[5] Today, the mestizo race is characterized by distinct phenotypical features without a predominant racial pattern in Latin America. Racial features vary depending on the geographic zone. Mexican patients typically have a stronger Indian influence; some parts of Central America typically have a stronger African influence; Argentina is predominantly European; other countries such as Colombia have a heterogeneous mix of all of these.[6,7]

The Hispanic population in the United States is composed of mestizo patients who migrate mainly from Mexico, Central America, the Caribbean (including Cuba and the Dominican Republic), and South American countries. This mix of populations had initially established communities along the southwestern U.S. border, Florida, and New York City but have since transcended these territories, and they can be found throughout the nation and across international borders.[2]

MESTIZO FACIAL AND NASAL CHARACTERISTICS

Mestizo facial and nasal characteristics are different from the universally accepted ideal "Caucasian" proportions. Although phenotypical variations are as diverse as the origins of the racial backgrounds leading to them, the mestizo face tends to be broad with a relatively small underprojected, ptotic nose. The skin tends to be thicker and more sebaceous with a resulting skin–soft tissue envelope (SSTE) that is thicker and harder to redrape and for whom changes will be less noticeable. Malar eminences tend to be slightly more prominent and eyelids have a heavier look with more lid hooding. *Heavy skin* is a term that can commonly be used when describing these patients.

The noses of patients of Hispanic origin will tend to have an underlying cartilaginous architecture showing poor structural support. Nasal bones can be small, short, and slightly wide, with weak cartilaginous vaults. Tip support is poor due in part to a weak caudal septum, a small nasal spine, and soft alar cartilages. Externally, the Hispanic nose can exhibit a wide nasal bridge, a low nasion, a wide nasal base, a short columella, an acute nasolabial angle, and nostrils that tend to have a more flaring and horizontal shape[4] (Table 32-1, Figure 32-1).

PREOPERATIVE EVALUATION

CONSULTATION

It is important to be able to have the time and the ability to communicate with the patient in an adequate manner. The following points should be covered during the consultation:

1. Acknowledgment of the patient's ethnic background with explanation of key issues
2. Understanding of the patients' desires and expectations: a more balanced result preserving some of the patient's nasal ethnic features or a

more dramatic change resembling the "Caucasian" ideal
3. Complete history and physical exam (including disclosure of all previous nasal procedures as well as an internal and external nasal examination)
4. Discussion of a realistic surgical plan and discussion of potential complications and limitations

PHYSICAL EXAMINATION

FUNCTIONAL EVALUATION

A complete external and internal nasal examination must be performed to evaluate the function of the nose. The examination is usually performed through palpation, as well as with a nasal speculum, and can be complemented with nasal endoscopy.

Functionally, the following aspects should be noted:

1. Alar collapse
2. Compromise of internal or external nasal valve
3. Septal deviations/availability of septal cartilage for harvesting
4. Turbinate hypertrophy
5. Sinus disease

Aesthetic Evaluation

When evaluating a mestizo patient for aesthetic rhinoplasty, several criteria must be defined to delineate an adequate surgical plan (Table 32-2):

1. General facial characteristics
2. Skin type/thickness of soft tissue envelope
3. Nasal characteristics: upper third, middle third, lower third of nose
4. Underlying structural framework
5. Diagnosis of deformities and asymmetries

Once the consultation and physical exam have been completed, it is important to obtain a set of standard rhinoplasty photographs. This set includes frontal view, basal view, right and left lateral views, and right and left oblique views. Computer imaging is indispensable to demonstrate the existing challenges and to demonstrate a plan of how to overcome them with surgery. It is critical to have the patient understand the limitations of the procedure and be able to define a surgical plan within the context of realistic expectations and clear lines of communication.

Photography is useful for both the presurgical consultation and an intraoperative reference. Postsurgical results are also evaluated photographically, and photographs should be obtained ideally at 6 months and 12 months after surgery. This serves to help critically analyze aesthetic outcomes as well as surgical techniques.

Table 32-1 Mestizo Nasal Characteristics

	Mestizo Noses	Caucasian Noses
Type of skin	Oily, thick SSTE	Normal to thin SSTE
Upper third of nose	Wide nasal bridge	Normal nasal bridge
	Normal to low radix	Normal to high radix
	Short nasal bones	Normal to long nasal bones
Middle third of nose	Weak upper lateral cartilages	Normal upper lateral cartilages
Lower third of nose	Weak, unsupportive alar cartilages	Normal to thick alar cartilages
	Normal to acute nasolabial angle	Normal to obtuse nasolabial angle
	Poor tip recoil	Normal tip recoil
	Flaring, horizontally shaped nostrils	Oval-shaped nostrils

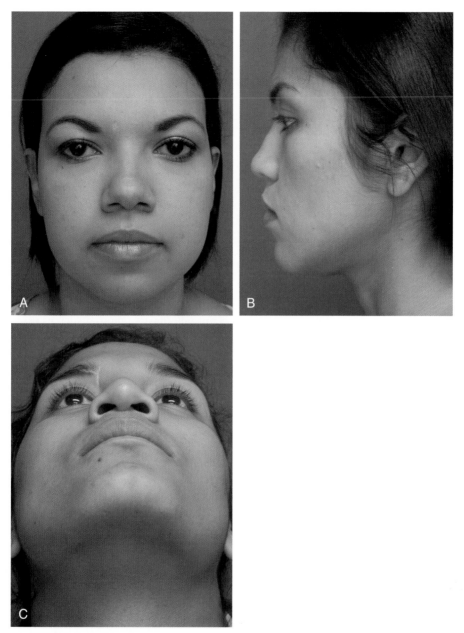

Figure 32-1 Mestizo nasal characteristics. **A,** Broad faces with an SSTE that tends to be thicker and slightly more oily; noses tend to be small with wide nasal bridge and short nasal bones; nasal tips typically look bulbous and undefined. **B,** On the lateral view, the radix tends to be low and is often associated with a small bony hump; the nasolabial angle tends to be acute. **C,** Base view: short columella with nostrils that tend to be more horizontally shaped and flaring.

All documentation from patients, including photography, must be kept as part of the medical record and serve as future reference for both medical and legal matters, should the latter arise.

APPROACHES TO THE MESTIZO NOSE

When evaluating mestizo patients, there are great anatomic variations depending on the predominant race of the patient. This makes it difficult to categorize these patients into a specific group. When defining what

possible approaches and surgical techniques could be used with these patients, it is easiest to do so by focusing on the different problems encountered. Pertaining to usual generalizations, these patients tend to have:

1. Thick skin
2. Short nasal bones
3. Bulbous undefined nasal tips
4. Weak alar cartilages
5. Weak bony and cartilaginous support structures of the nose

In general, mestizo patients seek noses that look smaller and more defined. This typically means a narrower dorsum, a more defined and projected nasal tip, and a narrower base. Our challenge as surgeons is to carry out surgical techniques that give defining structural support without making the nose look much bigger. The external rhinoplasty approach is used in most of these patients. Surgical techniques will be discussed focusing on the areas of the nose where the most important problems are encountered.

UPPER THIRD OF THE NOSE

Mestizo patients tend to prefer a smaller dorsum to a high profile nose with a prominent tip.[4] The dorsum in these

Table 32-2 Cosmetic Evaluation Sheet

- General facial characteristics: facial asymmetries, nose-chin balance
- Skin type: thin, thick/oily, dry
- Nasal dorsum: high, low/hump/deviation/depression
- Nasal bridge: wide or narrow
- Middle third of nose (upper lateral cartilages): wide/narrow/unilateral depression
- Nasal tip (alar cartilages): strong, flimsy/wide, narrow
- Nasolabial angle: acute/obtuse
- Nasal base: wide, normal, narrow
- Nostril orientation: vertical, horizontal, oval/flaring, nonflaring
- Tip support: weak, strong/tip recoil

patients are frequently low and wide and can have small convexities.

Surgically, the dorsum can be managed in several ways: To narrow a wide dorsum without an existing hump, medial and lateral osteotomies are performed routinely. In cases where there is a shallow radix with a small dorsal convexity, instead of lowering the hump to the level of the radix, a radix cartilage graft is used with excellent postsurgical results.[8] This helps give the appearance of a stronger dorsum without making the nose much larger[12] (Figure 32-2).

One of the problems with ethnic patients is that significant amounts of cartilage are usually needed for structural grafting of the nose and usually the septum does not have enough to address all the essential regions. When dorsal augmentation is needed and if there is enough cartilage, dorsal onlay grafts are used, preferably from septal cartilage. If an insufficient amount of cartilage is available and the required dorsal augmentation is significant, alloplastic material such as expanded polytetrafluoroethylene (ePTFE, Gore-Tex; Implantech Associates, Ventura, CA) or porous high-density polyethylene implants (Medpor; Porex Surgical, Newnan, GA), which have excellent long-term outcome with low complication rates, can be used as alternatives in patients who prefer not to undergo a costal cartilage graft harvest.[1,13]

MIDDLE THIRD OF THE NOSE

Mestizo noses very frequently have short nasal bones and weak upper lateral cartilages. This is a real problem for the surgeon if the cartilages are not strengthened properly.

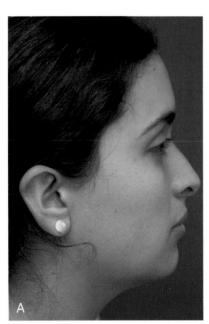
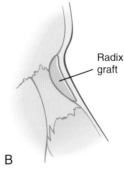
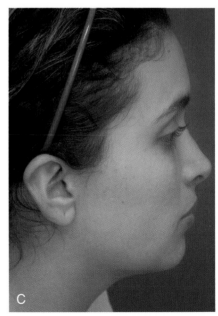

Radix graft

B

A

C

Figure 32-2 Approach to the upper third of the nose. **A,** Lateral presurgical view showing a low radix with a small osteocartilaginous hump and small nasal bones. **B,** Illustration of radix graft. **C,** Lateral postsurgical view after placement of radix graft harvested from septum and conservative hump removal.

Patients with small nasal bones, weak upper lateral cartilages, and dorsal septal deviations are at greater risk of resulting in inverted-V deformities, deviation of the middle vault, and collapse of the upper lateral cartilages with a resulting compromise of the internal nasal valve.[9] The use of bilateral spreader grafts as a preventive surgical technique strengthens the middle nasal vault, maintains a normal contour of the middle third of the nose, and avoids the formation of a postsurgical inverted-V deformity (Figure 32-3 and 32-4). In cases where dorsal hump removal is going to be performed, strengthening of the middle third of the nose becomes imperative to avoid late postsurgical deformities.

NASAL TIP PROCEDURES

The lower third of the nose can be divided into two categories: the base of the nose and the nasal tip lobule. When modifying the lower third of the nose in mestizo patients, several principles must be followed. A stable nasal base must be created to guarantee a strong foundation, to support the necessary tip modifications. The least disruptive surgical techniques must be used on the tip lobule to obtain predictable aesthetics; aggressive techniques should be reserved for more prominent deformities. The alar cartilages must be analyzed in the vertical and horizontal planes; surgical options should be based according to anatomic findings. Finally, the techniques performed should be planned, starting with simple procedures and evolving gradually toward more complex and aggressive ones (Table 32-3).

Following these principles will help prevent postsurgical loss of tip projection, asymmetries, tip deviations, or visible bossae formation. Although there are no standard tip procedures used in mestizo patients, some techniques

are used more often than others. The desired outcome is to increase rotation, projection, and definition of the nasal tip lobule.

PROCEDURES FOR THE NASAL BASE

Creating a stable nasal base is critical when dealing with mestizo noses. Most of our patients have weak structures lacking support in the nasal lobular complex. If left unsupported, loss of projection will likely occur postsurgically. The techniques used most frequently include columellar struts or the caudal septal extension grafts.[4,12]

The columellar strut has been used routinely in rhinoplasties carried out through the external approach to stabilize and add support to the medial crura and create an adequate medial crural–septal relationship. The strut is carved according to the patient's needs, placed in a pocket dissected between the medial crura, and fixed in place with 5-0 Vicryl sutures. Fixation should not be placed too anteriorly in the medial crura to preserve the natural double break of the columella. If a long strut that extends to the nasal spine is going to be used, this is secured inferiorly so that it does not move from the nasal spine. This strut gives additional support to the tripod, corrects any asymmetries or buckling of the medial crura, and helps maintain or increase tip rotation and projection.

The caudal extension graft has a special indication in mestizo rhinoplasty patients. This graft is extremely useful

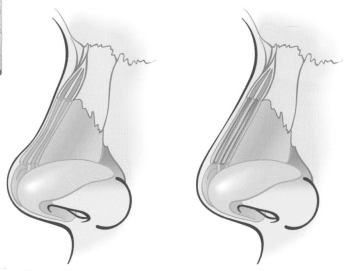

Figure 32-3 Illustration depicting placement of a bilateral spreader graft.

Table 32-3 Nasal Tip Surgical Procedures

Procedures aimed at addressing the nasal base
- Columellar strut
- Caudal extension graft
- Fixation of medial crura to caudal septal border

Procedures aimed at addressing the nasal tip lobule

Intact strip procedures
- Cephalic trim of the lateral crura
- Transdomal suture narrowing technique
- Double-dome unit technique
- Lateral crural steal

Incomplete strip procedures
- Lateral crural overlay technique
- Medial crural overlay technique
- Grafts
  - Shield graft
  - Shield graft + cap graft
  - Lateral crural strut grafts
  - Plumping premaxilla grafts
  - Alar rim grafts
  - Morselized cartilage over the tip
  - Alar batten grafts

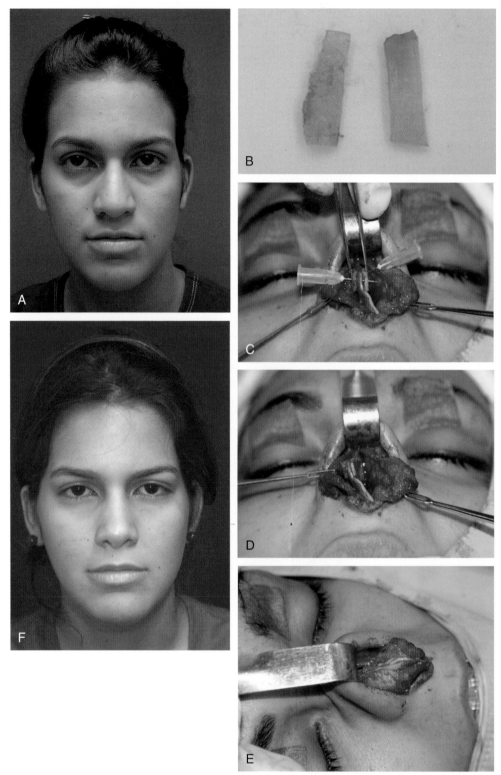

Figure 32-4 Approach to the middle third of the nose. Placement of bilateral spreader grafts. **A,** Frontal view of mestizo patient with short nasal bones, narrow middle third of nose with weak upper lateral cartilages. **B–E,** Surgical views of placement of bilateral spreader grafts. **F,** Postsurgical photograph after bilateral spreader graft placement and medial and lateral osteotomies.

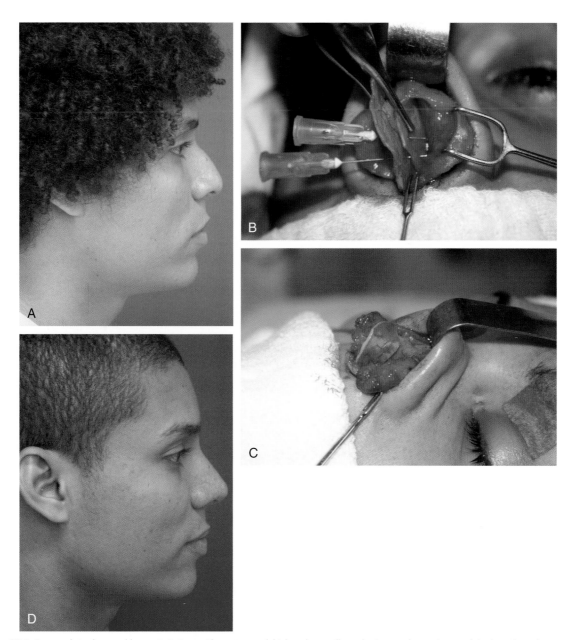

Figure 32-5 Approach to the nasal base. **A,** Patient with acute nasolabial angle, small nasal spine, and retrusive caudal edge of nasal septum; the nasal tip has caudal orientation as well as poor projection and rotation. **B–C,** Surgical views detailing placement of caudal extension graft. **D,** Postsurgical result after placement of caudal extension graft harvested from patient's cartilaginous septum; nasolabial angle is less acute and tip has gained rotation and projection. (From Cobo R. Hispanic/Mestizo rhinoplasty. *Fac Plast Surg Clin North Am* 2010;18:173-188.)

in patients with acute nasolabial angles, underprojected tips, poor tip support, short caudal septums, and/or inadequate alar/columellar relationship.[10,11] The graft ideally should be harvested from septal cartilage and should be a relatively straight piece of cartilage. It is placed overlapping the caudal edge of the patient's nasal septum and is fixed securely with 3-0 Vicryl sutures superiorly and inferiorly at the level of the nasal spine. The feet of the medial crura are then fixed to the caudal edge of this graft, and its height is set depending on how much tip rotation and projection the patient needs (Figure 32-5).

Once the tripod has been strengthened properly, the nasal tip lobule can be addressed in a proper fashion. Tip grafts should only be used with a stable nasal base. The SSTE of mestizo patients tends to be heavier, and if a stable base is not created, the underlying structures will tend to collapse with time.

CONTOURING THE NASAL TIP

Tip defining techniques in mestizo patients are challenging. Alar cartilages tend to be weak and relatively wide

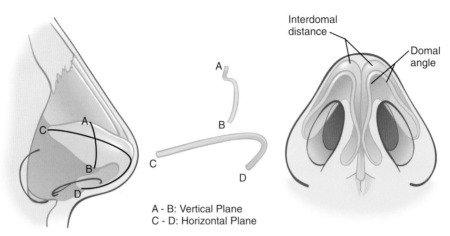

Figure 32-6 Vertical and horizontal components. Vertical plane is defined as the distance from *A* to *B*: width and curvature (concave, convex, flat) are primary considerations. The horizontal plane is defined as the distance from *C* to *D*. It is important to define the interdomal distance (distance from dome to dome) and characterize the domal angle (acute or obtuse).

without providing any meaningful structural support. Often, when these cartilages are sutured, they are so flimsy that postsurgical pinching can be seen at the level of the lobule. When managing the nasal tip, the alar cartilages must be analyzed from its horizontal and its vertical component. The vertical component is defined as the distance from its caudal to its cephalic margin. The horizontal component is defined as the distance of the alar cartilage from the foot of its medial crura to its lateral crus (Figure 32-6).

When evaluating the vertical component of the tip cartilages, one must define their width, curvature (flat, convex, concave), and strength (flimsly or strong). The horizontal component is used to determine the length of the alar cartilages, the characteristics of the domal angle (acute or obtuse), and the interdomal distance.

Surgical techniques can be divided into various categories:

- Remodeling of the alar cartilages: cephalic trim or cartilage suturing techniques that help refine, project, and rotate the nasal tip
- Division of the alar cartilages: division of the alar cartilages such as the lateral crural overlay method
- Grafts on nasal tip lobule: used to elongate, define, project, and give additional support to the alar cartilages

MANAGEMENT OF THE VERTICAL COMPONENT

A very common complaint of mestizo patients is that their tip is wide and bulbous and undefined. An "easy" way of dealing with this problem is to perform a cephalic trim of the alar cartilages and suture the domes to decrease the interdomal distance. If this is not done properly, it can create numerous problems postsurgical for these patients.

Cephalic trim of alar cartilages is only used when necessary to avoid postsurgical alar pinching and internal nasal valve collapse. If cephalic trimming is to be performed, this is usually performed at the level of the anterior lateral crura, taking care not to extend the excision laterally to avoid supralar pinching or collapse of the lateral nasal wall. When the scroll area is excised aggressively, this can also create pinching and compromise the internal nasal valve. Thus, cephalic trim is rarely performed in these patients, and the bulbosity of the tip is managed with suturing techniques that mainly affect the horizontal component of the alar cartilage.

MANAGEMENT OF THE HORIZONTAL COMPONENT

Suturing Techniques

Suturing techniques are the first steps in managing the bulbous undefined nasal tips. Of the different surgical options, the lateral crural steal is probably one of the most useful techniques.[4] Projection and rotation are obtained by lengthening the medial crura at the expense of the lateral crura. The vestibular skin is dissected to be able to mobilize the cartilage freely. The new domes are defined by placing independent 5-0 Prolene sutures lateral to the original existing domes. These "newly created domes" are then fixed in the midline with a continuous mattress 5-0 Prolene suture. This technique rotates the tip superiorly, increases projection, and creates a more triangular base. The use of a columellar strut with this type of suture creates a very stable, triangular nasal tip complex (Figure 32-7).

Other suturing techniques commonly used are the transdomal suture narrowing technique[14] and the double-dome unit technique.[15] The transdomal suture narrowing

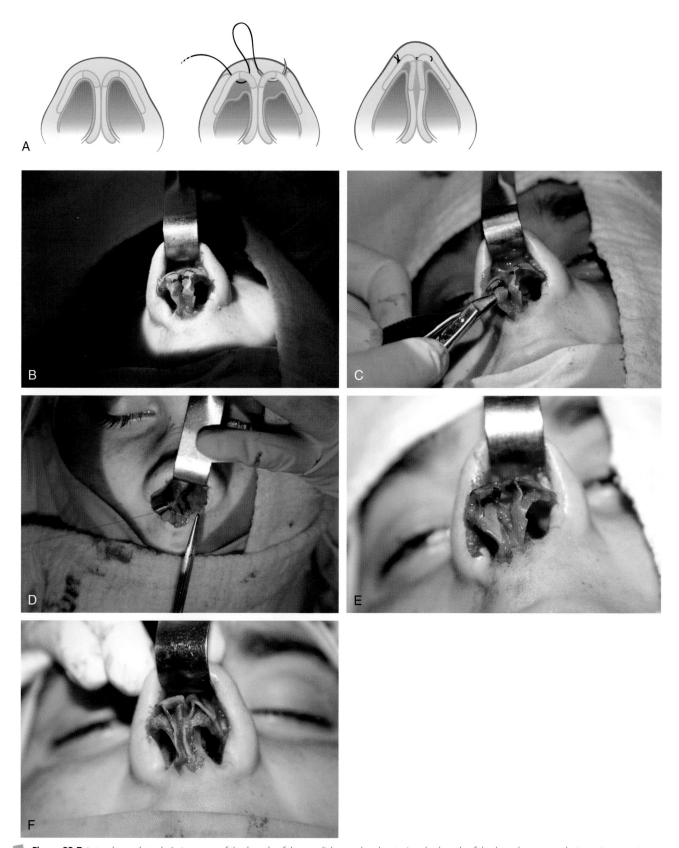

Figure 32-7 Lateral crural steal. **A,** Increase of the length of the medial crura by shortening the length of the lateral crura results in an increase in rotation and projection of the nasal tip. **B–D,** Surgical case where a columellar strut has been sutured in place and lateral crural steal has been performed. There has been an increase in tip rotation and projection at the expense of the lateral crura. (**B–F,** From Cobo R. Hispanic/Mestizo rhinoplasty. *Fac Plast Surg Clin North Am* 2010;18:173-188.)

technique is useful in nasal tips that are broad and trapezoidal in shape. It helps improve tip support and enhances tip projection. A 5-0 Prolene suture is passed through the domes and is tied in the midline. This suture creates a more triangular shape to the tip (Figure 32-8). The double-dome suture technique not only increases tip projection and support but also can be a more aggressive approach in lobular refinement. A 5-0 mattress suture is used to "define" each dome independently, creating a more acute interdomal angle. A third continuous suture is then passed through the "newly defined domes," securing them at the midline. Both of these techniques create a more triangular nasal lobule, increase tip projection, and result in a narrower nasal tip (Figure 32-9).

Division of the Alar Cartilages

Many mestizo patients have acute nasolabial angles and ptotic nasal tips with a long horizontal component of the alar cartilages. In many of these patients, suturing techniques are not sufficient to increase rotation; therefore, more aggressive techniques such as division of the lateral component of the alar cartilage are often required. The lateral crural overlay technique is an excellent option to increase rotation and to shorten an overlong nose without

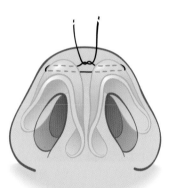

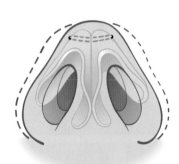

Figure 32-8 Transdomal suture narrowing technique. A continuous Prolene mattress suture is passed slightly lateral to the existing domes and knotted in the midline. This maneuver brings the domes together in the midline creating an adequate interdomal distance. This creates a more triangular tip and base. Tip projection is usually increased slightly or maintained.

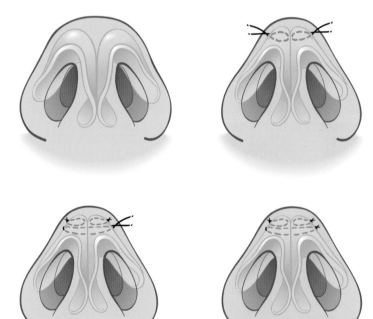

Figure 32-9 Double-dome unit technique. This technique is used with tips that are very bulbous and undefined and with a very thick SSTE. Each dome is defined and sutured independently. A third continuous horizontal mattress suture is passed slightly lateral to the newly defined domes and is sutured in the midline. This creates a triangular nasal base and increases projection and rotation slightly.

losing support.[16] Alar cartilages are divided lateral to the domes, and the cut segments are superimposed and sutured using 5-0 Prolene or nylon mattress sutures. This technique reconstructs the divided alar cartilage, thereby creating a new intact strip with increased support at the level of the overlapped lateral crura. The division should be carried out symmetrically to avoid postsurgical tip asymmetries. The domes are then defined with the suturing techniques mentioned earlier (Figure 32-10 and 32-11).

Grafts in the Nasal Tip

Tip grafts are used to improve definition and help increase support and projection to many of the bulbous, undefined, thick-skinned mestizo tips.[12] These grafts should not be used in excess and patients have to be chosen carefully because they tend to become visible over time if one is not careful to camouflage them adequately. Mestizo patients generally want noses that do not appear big or overbuilt but rather those that look narrower and more defined. Often, the only way to achieve this result is by using grafts to help build up the support structures that lie under a very thick SSTE.

The shield graft is very useful to help define and project a thick bulbous tip. It is ideally carved from septal cartilage, although ear cartilage can also be used with good results. Each shield graft is carved according to the patient's needs. Edges should be beveled and sutured with 6-0 Prolene to the caudal margins of the medial/intermediate crura–columellar strut complex. The leading edge of the graft should always be at or just slightly above the level of the existing domes regardless of the thickness of the SSTE. This leading edge is then covered with morselized cartilage or perichondrium to prevent visibility in the future (Figure 32-12).

Alar rim grafts are very helpful in patients with weak alar cartilages.[10] In mestizo patients, after dome-binding sutures and other suturing techniques are performed, it is not infrequent to see a small concavity form in the lateral crus of the alar cartilage that can later result in pinching of the nasal tip and notching of the alar margin. This is often due to the natural weakness of the lower lateral cartilages in these patients. Alar rim grafts are placed in a pocket at the caudal edge of the marginal incision. These grafts help contour the alar margin and give the tip lobule a more symmetrical appearance (Figure 32-13).

Frequently, after suturing techniques have been performed, morselized cartilage is placed over the nasal tip lobule. This cartilage helps hide any irregularities and gives the tip a softer, more rounded look. Morselized cartilage can also be used to fill in any gaps in the middle third of the nose.

Many other grafting options exist for the nasal tip (see Table 32-3). Grafts should be placed carefully and ideally sutured in place to avoid postsurgical shifting, which can create noticeable asymmetries.

ALAR BASE REDUCTION

Alar base reduction can be used to decrease alar flare, alar base width, or both. It is not a routine procedure in mestizo patients and should be performed only at the end of the operation if necessary. The medial incision is typically placed in a natural crease at the junction of the nasal sill and ala. The lateral incision should not extend into the alar facial groove as this could leave an unsightly scar especially in patients with thick oily skin. Incisions are closed using 6-0 Prolene or nylon sutures and sutures are removed after 8 days (Figure 32-14).

POSTSURGICAL FOLLOW-UP

Postsurgical follow-up is absolutely necessary in mestizo patients. Skin types vary but in general they tend to be thicker and more oily. Patients should be warned that edema of the nasal tip will be present for several months,

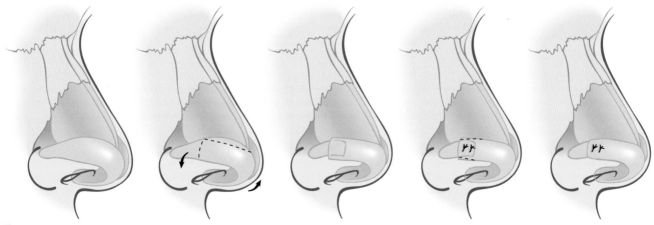

Figure 32-10 Illustration of lateral crural overlay technique.

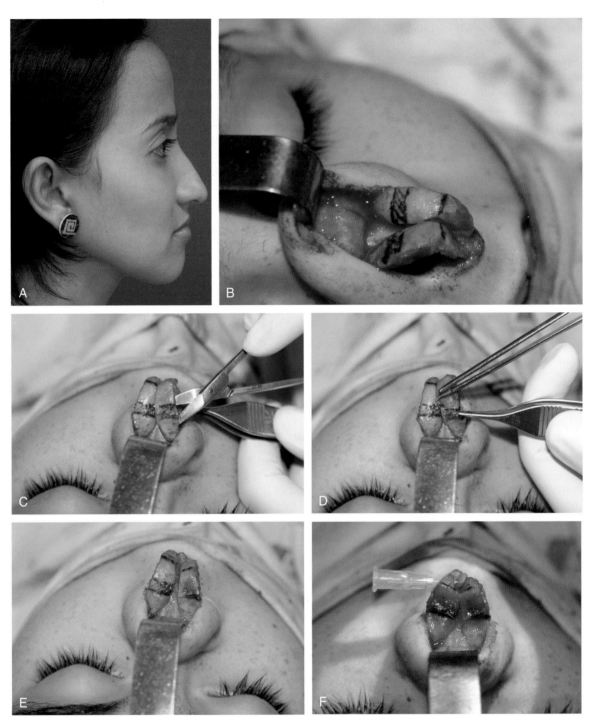

Figure 32-11 Patient photos of lateral crural overlay technique. **A–B,** This technique is useful in patients with a very long horizontal component of their alar cartilages that creates long ptotic noses with an acute nasolabial angle. **C,** Alar cartilage is dissected from the vestibular skin. If necessary a very conservative cephalic trim of the lateral crura is performed leaving at least 9 to 10 mm of cartilage in its vertical component. The cartilage is transected 10 mm lateral to the dome-defining point. **D,** Transected fragments are superimposed with the long medial segment placed on top of the short lateral segment. **E,** The segments are fixed with 5-0 Prolene sutures. The edges are beveled and regularized. **F,** A new intact strengthened strip has been created. This rotates the tip upward and shortens the long nose. (**B–F,** From Cobo R. Hispanic/Mestizo rhinoplasty. *Fac Plast Surg Clin North Am* 2010;18:173-188.)

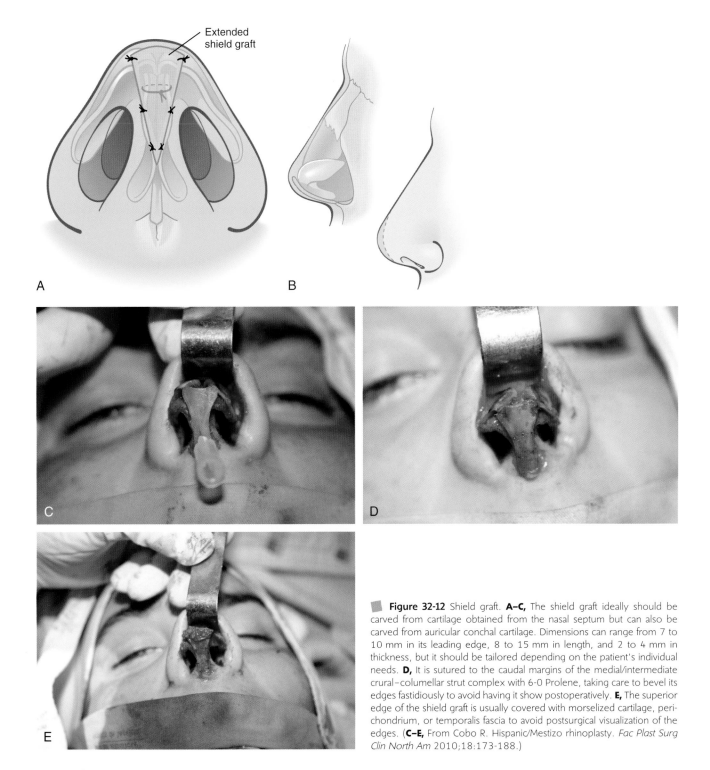

Figure 32-12 Shield graft. **A–C,** The shield graft ideally should be carved from cartilage obtained from the nasal septum but can also be carved from auricular conchal cartilage. Dimensions can range from 7 to 10 mm in its leading edge, 8 to 15 mm in length, and 2 to 4 mm in thickness, but it should be tailored depending on the patient's individual needs. **D,** It is sutured to the caudal margins of the medial/intermediate crural–columellar strut complex with 6-0 Prolene, taking care to bevel its edges fastidiously to avoid having it show postoperatively. **E,** The superior edge of the shield graft is usually covered with morselized cartilage, perichondrium, or temporalis fascia to avoid postsurgical visualization of the edges. (**C–E,** From Cobo R. Hispanic/Mestizo rhinoplasty. *Fac Plast Surg Clin North Am* 2010;18:173-188.)

and because of the skin pigmentation, dark periorbital circles can be accentuated and will be prominent for several months after the surgery. It is important for these patients to avoid sun exposure.

Persistent edema in the supratip region can be effectively treated with 1 mg to 2 mg of triamcinolone acetonide injections (Kenalog) subdermally. If necessary, these injections can be started as early as 2 weeks postsurgery and can be repeated every 6 weeks, taking care to tape

the nose following these injections. Care should be taken not to inject too frequently as this can produce permanent subcutaneous and cutaneous atrophy.

Following patients closely will help strengthen the doctor-patient relationship. It will help patients understand that time is their ally and that the postsurgical results will not be appreciated for at least 6 to 12 months. This is especially true in thick-skinned patients (Figures 32-15 and 32-16).

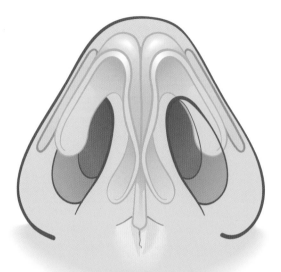

A

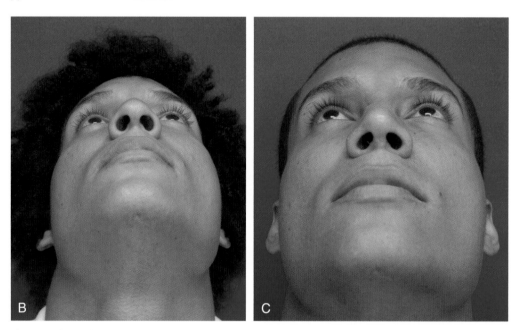

Figure 32-13 Alar rim grafts. **A,** Placement of alar rim grafts in a pocket that is made following the marginal incision. **B, C,** Preoperative and postoperative basal view of patient with placement of shield graft and alar rim grafts.

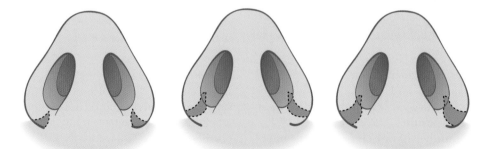

Figure 32-14 Alar base reduction. **A,** Reduction of alar flare: Reduction of the lateral portion of the alar base without resecting the nasal sill. **B,** Resection of the more medial segment of the alar base will decrease the width of nasal sill or base with less reduction in alar flaring. **C,** Combined resection will decrease alar flaring and the base width, giving the nostrils a more elongated look.

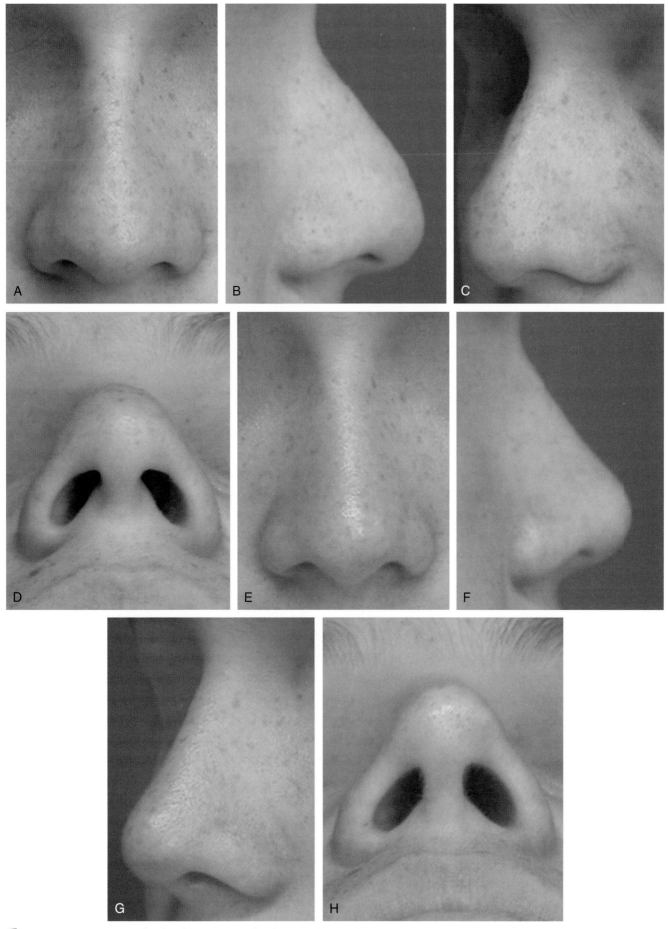

Figure 32-15 Preoperative **(A–D)** and postoperative **(E–H)** patient photographs.

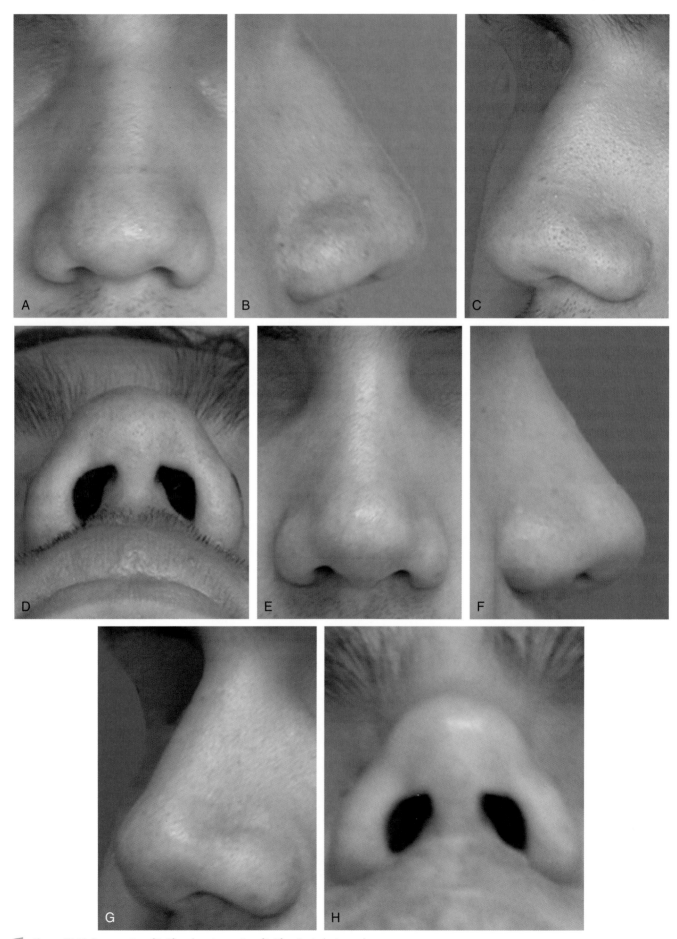

Figure 32-16 Preoperative **(A–D)** and postoperative **(E–H)** patient photographs.

CONCLUSIONS

Surgical techniques in mestizo patients are oriented to create definition and increase support, rotation, and projection without increasing size or volume dramatically. Support structures are reinforced, suture techniques and/or grafts are placed in a precise manner, and very little tissue is resected. The objective is to obtain a balanced nose that blends in with the patient's features. The results must withstand the natural healing process. If executed correctly, this will in most cases give patients a nose that is closer to their aesthetic ideal without changing their ethnic features dramatically.

REFERENCES

1. Romo III T, Abraham MT. The ethnic nose. *Fac Plast Surg.* 2003;19(3):269–277.
2. Leach J. Aesthetics and the Hispanic rhinoplasty. *Laryngoscope.* 2002;112.
3. Leong S, White P. A comparison of aesthetic proportions between the healthy Caucasian nose and the aesthetic ideal. *J Plast Reconstr Aesthet Surg.* 2006;59:248–252.
4. Cobo R. Mestizo rhinoplasty. *Fac Plast Surg.* 2003;119(3): 257–268.
5. Ortiz F, Olmedo A. Rhinoplasty on the mestizo nose. *Clin Plast Surg* 1977;4(1).
6. Ospina W. *América Mestiza—El país del Futuro.* Bogotá, Colombia: Villegas Editores; 2000:23–38.
7. Daniel RK. Hispanic rhinoplasty in the United States with emphasis on the Mexican American nose. *Plast Reconstr Surg.* 2003;112:244–256.
8. Becker D, Pastorek NJ. The radix graft in cosmetic rhinoplasty. *Arch Fac Plast Surg.* 2001;3:115–119.
9. Toriumi D. Management of the middle nasal vault in rhinoplasty. *Opin Tech Plast Reconstr Surg.* 1995;21:16–30.
10. Toriumi DM. New concepts in nasal tip contouring. *Arch Fac Plast Surg.* 2006;8:156–185.
11. Swartout B, Torimi DM. Rhinoplasty. *Curr Opin Otolaryngol Head Neck Surg.* 2007;15:219–227.
12. Cobo R. Facial Aesthetic surgery with emphasis on rhinoplasty in the Hispanic patient. *Curr Opin Otolaryngol Head Neck Surg.* 2008;16:369–375.
13. Godin MS, Waldman SR, Johnson CM. Nasal augmentation using Gore-Tex: A 10 year experience. *Arch Fac Plast Surg.* 1999;1:18–121.
14. Tardy ME, Cheng E. Transdomal suture refinement of the nasal tip. *Fac Plast Surg.* 1987;4:317–326.
15. McCollough EG, English JL. A new twist in nasal tip surgery: an alternative to the Goldman tip for the wide or bulbous lobule. *Arch Otolaryngol Head Neck Surg.* 1985;111: 524–529.
16. Konior RJ, Kridel R. Controlled nasal tip positioning via the open rhinoplasty approach. *Fac Plast Surg Clin of North Am.* 1993;1:53–62.

CHAPTER THIRTY-THREE

Rhinoplasty in the Aging Patient

Ryan M. Greene • Dean M. Toriumi

Aesthetic and reconstructive rhinoplasty is commonly acknowledged as the most demanding and difficult of the plastic surgical procedures. Although many technical advances have occurred throughout the past century, its fundamental philosophy remains constant. This philosophy involves significant planning and conservative surgical changes to achieve a natural-appearing result. Initially, the operation generally involved a tissue reduction procedure with excision of various nasal anatomic components. More recently, rhinoplasty has evolved into a procedure that involves tissue reorientation and augmentation, with careful attention to long-term surgical outcome.

PERSONAL PHILOSOPHY

Rhinoplasty is a complex operation that requires precise preoperative diagnosis to select the appropriate surgical technique. Owing to variations in nasal anatomy and aesthetic expectations, no single technique is appropriate for all patients. Each rhinoplasty patient presents the surgeon with a diversity of nasal anatomy, contours, and proportions that require a series of organized maneuvers tailored to the patient's anatomic and functional needs. The surgeon must also be skilled at manipulating and controlling the dynamics of postoperative healing to attain optimal long-term aesthetic results. A necessary prerequisite is the skill to visualize the ultimate long-term healed result while manipulating the nasal structures.

ANATOMY

Aging of the nasal structures and external contour of the nose is influenced by a variety of genetic and environmental factors. Additionally, the nasal shape changes over time as well. In children, the nasal dorsum is typically concave and assumes a more straight or convex shape in early adult life. This convexity is further enhanced in midlife by the development of a drooping, ptotic tip. In addition to these changes to the appearance of the nose,

nasal function tends to deteriorate over time as the nasal airway changes.

As patients age, the skin thins with loss of elasticity, subcutaneous fat deposits resorb, and the underlying soft tissues atrophy. With these changes, the underlying support structures of the nose, such as the lower lateral cartilages and nasal bones, become skeletonized or visible. In addition, skin hydration is diminished, and the skin becomes less pliable.[1] This affects the skin's ability to contract and redrape after the cartilaginous and bony structures of the nose are reduced.

The most significant changes over time occur in the upper and lower lateral cartilages. These cartilages are connected by a fibrous union at the cephalic margin of the lateral crura, the scroll region.[1] As the nose ages, the upper and lower lateral cartilages begin to separate and fragment.[2,3] This may result in collapse of the internal nasal valve and lateral wall. As one ages, the middle nasal vault will tend to collapse as the upper lateral cartilages move inferomedially. Loss of support of the medial crura and stretching of the fibrous attachments from the posterior septal angle and nasal spine to the medial crural footplates result in their posterior movement and retraction of the columella.[3] These changes also occur by loss of the fat pad below the medial crura and resorption of the premaxilla.[2] With loss of support of the medial crura and separation of the lateral crura from the upper lateral cartilages, the nasal tip may become ptotic, with an appearance of increased length and a more acute nasolabial angle.

With aging, the nasal bones may become brittle and are more readily fractured.[4] Care must be taken during osteotomies to avoid excessive narrowing of the bony vault or comminuted fractures of the nasal bones. Periosteal elevation is not recommended in the aging patient and, if used, should not extend to the point of the intended lateral osteotomies, to avoid loss of periosteal support.[4] Although undesirable in the younger patient, greenstick fractures can be effective in the older patient.[4] Finally, dorsal hump reduction must be executed with great precision to minimize irregularities of the bony nasal vault as the skin over the dorsum tends to be very thin.

PREOPERATIVE ASSESSMENT

Preoperative assessment of the rhinoplasty patient includes the assessment not only of the anatomic and functional components but also the emotional and psychological factors.[5] As with all facial aesthetic surgery, it is important for the physician to discuss motivation and aesthetic goals of rhinoplasty surgery with the patient. It is critical to elucidate what aesthetic changes the patient desires. Older patients have developed a self-image over many years and must be prepared for the planned surgical changes. Many older patients do not want to look dramatically different, and thus conservative changes are generally most appropriate. Patients who desire dramatic changes warrant careful evaluation prior to consideration as surgical candidates.

In this age group, a thorough preoperative medical examination is mandatory. Many of these patients have comorbid medical conditions. A careful medical history and physical examination are critical prior to performing this type of surgery. It is often a good idea to consult with the patient's primary care physician prior to scheduling surgery. Many of these patients take medications that can affect clotting; these medications should be stopped at least 2 weeks before surgery.

SURGICAL TECHNIQUE

PREOPERATIVE CONSIDERATIONS

The surgical approaches to the nose include nondelivery techniques (cartilage-splitting or retrograde approach), delivery of bilateral chondrocutaneous flaps, and the external rhinoplasty approach. Selection of the approach should be based on both operative objectives and surgical experience. When only conservative volume reduction of the lateral crura and dorsal hump reduction are planned, a nondelivery approach (cartilage-splitting or retrograde approach) will suffice. However, when more complex nasal tip work is required, delivery of bilateral chondrocutaneous flaps or the external rhinoplasty approach should be used. The external approach is preferred when complex tip grafting or middle nasal vault reconstruction is planned. Regardless, the surgeon should select the least invasive approach possible to avoid disruption of nasal support mechanisms and maximize the functional and aesthetic result.

External incisions can be used with greater frequency in older patients because the skin is less likely to scar unfavorably.[6] Nasal skin in the aging patient also has multiple rhytids that can aid in camouflage. Even though it is rarely necessary, direct excision of skin from the nasal dorsum or supratip can be performed to aid redraping of the skin or elevating the severely ptotic nasal tip.[7-9]

Because of the thin skin found in the aging nose, even the smallest irregularities or asymmetries can become noticeable. As a result, debulking of underlying subcutaneous fat and muscle tissue should not be performed. This subcutaneous tissue should be preserved to maximize camouflage of the cartilage and bone. Tip grafts should also be limited unless the patient has medium to thick skin.[10] If they are used, they should be carefully sculpted and camouflaged to avoid visible edges. With thin skin, a thin layer of perichondrium or superficial temporal fascia can be applied over the graft, with an understanding that it will create temporary edema of the grafted area that should resolve over 6 to 12 months.

When treating the aging nose, the nasal tip should be managed first to set tip projection and rotation before completing profile alignment. After setting appropriate tip projection, dorsal hump reduction may not be needed. Frequently, older patients will also benefit from augmentation of the radix to create a straight profile. This strategy of increasing tip projection and raising the radix allows the surgeon to preserve a high dorsal profile while also creating a favorable tip-supratip relationship (Figure 33-1). As mentioned earlier, only conservative changes should be made in the nasal contour because older patients tend to have a set self-image. The nose should also be in harmony with the patient's other facial features.

THE EXTERNAL APPROACH

The patient is first injected with 1% lidocaine with 1:100,000 epinephrine into the nasal tip, between and around the domes, down the columella, along the site of the marginal incision, and along the lateral wall of the nose. Additional injections high on the nasal septum and along the osteotomy sites are then placed. An inverted-V columellar incision is then marked, midway between the base of the nose and the top of the nostrils. A transcolumellar incision is executed with a No. 11 blade. Care must be taken to avoid damaging the caudal margin of the medial crura. Marginal incisions are then made along the caudal margin of the lateral crura, which are extended to meet the columellar incision.

After completing the incisions, angled Converse scissors are used to elevate the skin off the medial crura. Once the columellar flap is elevated off the medial crura, dissection is advanced laterally to expose the lateral crura. A thin layer of perichondrium is left on the surface of the lower lateral cartilages. The anterior septal angle is identified, with exposure of the middle nasal vault in the midline. Blunt dissection is continued to the rhinion, which may be followed by subperiosteal dissection of the skin off the nasal dorsum up to the nasion if profile alignment is necessary. If a radix graft is planned, then a narrow pocket should be dissected in the midline over the radix. This narrow pocket will prevent shifting of a radix graft if radix augmentation is necessary.

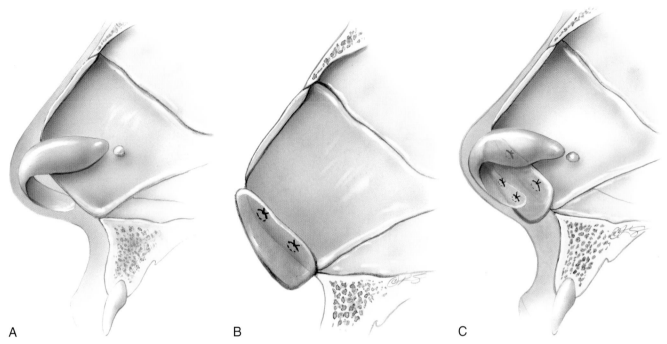

A   B   C

Figure 33-1 A, Profile of an aging patient. Note the underprojection of the nasal tip. **B,** Placement of a caudal extension graft with septal cartilage overlapping the existing nasal dorsum. **C,** Note the increased tip projection to create a straight dorsal profile.

SEPTAL SURGERY

When performing septal surgery in the older patient, dissection of the mucosal flaps should be limited because the mucoperichondrium is thinner and drier. A substantial L-shaped septal strut should be preserved to support the lower two thirds of the nose. We prefer to leave at least a 2-cm anterior septal strut and 1.5-cm caudal strut for support. Extra cartilage should be left at the osseocartilaginous junction to avoid loss of dorsal septal support. A Killian incision is preferred because of its excellent exposure without compromise of the support attachments between the feet of the medial crura and the caudal septum. A hemitransfixion incision can be used if exposure of both sides of the caudal nasal septum is required. The hemitransfixion or full transfixion incision can sometimes lead to a loss of support due to disruption of some of the attachments between the medial crura and caudal septum. When a decrease in tip projection is desired, a full transfixion incision can be used to disrupt these attachments.

When exposing the septal cartilage in the aging patient, it is generally preferable to raise a mucoperichondrial flap on only one side of the septum, to preserve the vascular supply of the contralateral side and minimize chances of hematoma formation. After completion of the septal surgery, a running 4-0 plain catgut mattress suture is used to approximate the mucoperichondrial flaps and prevent fluid collection and hematoma formation. By limiting septal surgery, nasal packing can be minimized

or avoided. The surgeon should be aware that the septal cartilage may be partially calcified, which leaves the surgeon with less cartilage for harvesting or grafting.

In some patients, it may be necessary to dissect between the medial crura to access the caudal septum. Patients with a deviated caudal septum may benefit from this approach to allow correction of the deformity. Other patients with poor tip support could benefit from stabilization of the nasal base through this approach.

PTOTIC NASAL TIP

As the nose ages, the nasal tip frequently droops, creating a ptotic nasal tip. This change in nasal contour gives an elongated appearance. Patients that have shorter medial crura are more likely to develop tip ptosis due to lack of support. Patients with long medial crura that wrap around the nasal spine and caudal septum are less likely to develop tip ptosis (Figure 33-2). Severe ptosis of the nasal tip can also result in nasal airway compromise by altering the pathway of inspiratory air currents.[3] Correction of the ptotic nasal tip generally involves increasing nasal tip rotation and projection. As demonstrated by the tripod concept described by Anderson,[11] ptosis of the nasal tip can usually be corrected by supporting the medial and intermediate crura or by shortening the lateral crura.

We typically use a graduated approach for correction of the ptotic nasal tip by initially considering placing a sutured-in-place columellar strut between the medial

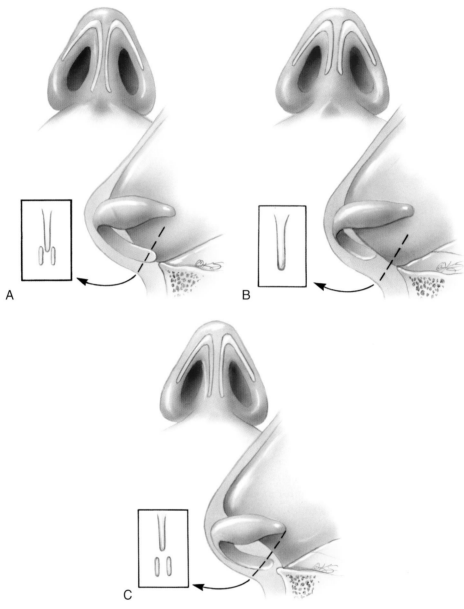

Figure 33-2 Relationship between medial crura and footplates to the caudal septum. **A,** Long strong medial crura extend to base of nose near posterior septal angle and wrap around caudal septum. **B,** This relationship provides excellent nasal tip support. Short medial crura do not extend to the nasal base and provide less tip support. **C,** Short caudal septum with separation of medial crura away from caudal septum results in loss of tip support.

crura. We have found this to be particularly effective if the dependent lobule is caused by buckling of the medial or intermediate crura. A sutured-in-place columellar strut both provides support and straightens buckled medial and intermediate crura. A straight rectangular piece of septal cartilage is placed in a precise pocket created between the medial and intermediate crura.[10] The columellar strut is fixed into position using a 5-0 plain catgut suture on a straight septal needle. The strut is easily applied using the external rhinoplasty approach, which allows maximal visualization, precise placement, and suture fixation of the graft. These struts can also be applied using a small endonasal incision placed just caudal to the caudal margin of

the medial crura. Once the incision is made, a precise pocket is made between the medial crura for graft placement and suture fixation.

In many patients, a columellar strut will not provide sufficient support to the nasal base. These patients will require more significant structural support. One option is to suture the medial crura to the caudal septum. This maneuver will shorten the nose and support the nasal base. This technique should be used only when the caudal septum is long and would otherwise require shortening. Another option is to use a caudal extension graft. Such a graft is typically overlapped and sutured to the existing caudal septum. Then the medial crura are sutured to the

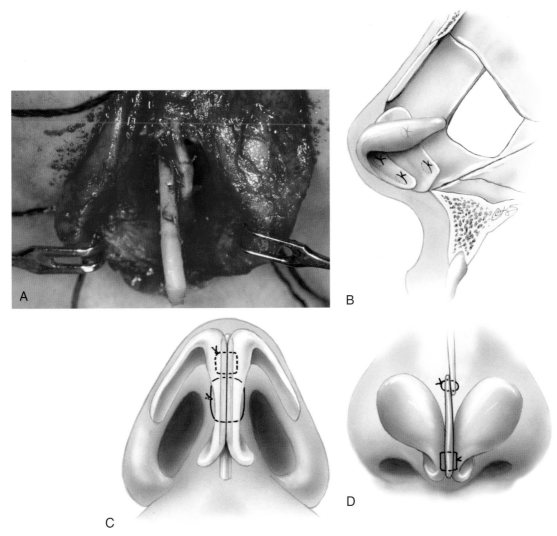

Figure 33-3 Caudal extension graft. **A,** The caudal extension graft is shown intraoperatively. **B,** The graft then is shown sutured into place. Note the harvesting site, maintaining the L-shaped support. **C,** The caudal view of the graft sutured into position. **D,** The superior view of the graft sutured into position. Note how the caudal extension graft typically overlaps the existing caudal septum. It is critical that the caudal margin of the extension graft is in the midline.

caudal margin of the caudal extension graft to stabilize the nasal base and reposition the nasal tip. The caudal extension graft must be in the midline and oriented to increase tip rotation. Fixation of the medial crura to the caudal septum or an extension graft provides increased tip support (Figure 33-3). Such fixation creates moderate rigidity of the nasal tip that can be discussed with the patient preoperatively.

If stabilizing the nasal base does not adequately correct the ptotic nasal tip, then additional surgical maneuvers must be used to increase tip rotation. The objective of these maneuvers is to rotate the nasal tip by recruiting lateral crura medially. Placement of a transdomal suture recruits lateral crura medially to increase tip projection and rotation.[12,13] Without violating the underlying vestibular skin, a 5-0 clear nylon suture is placed in a horizontal mattress fashion across both domes. To recruit the lateral crura medially, the lateral bite of the suture

extends lateral to the anatomic dome. This suture narrows the nasal tip by approximating the domes and creating a more acute domal angle, in addition to increasing tip projection and rotation. In some cases, the transdomal suture can further compromise the nasal airway if the lateral crura protrude into the airway. Such obstruction can be avoided by using an alar batten graft or lateral crural strut graft to lateralize the offending lateral segment of the lateral crus. If the transdomal suture does not correct the ptotic nasal tip, it may be necessary to perform a more aggressive maneuver that shortens the lateral crura.

The lateral crural overlay technique is a procedure that increases tip rotation by shortening the lateral crura. In this technique, the lateral crura are incised at the midpoint, and the medial segment is dissected from the underlying vestibular skin (Figure 33-4). The cut ends of cartilage are then overlapped (3 mm or 4 mm) and

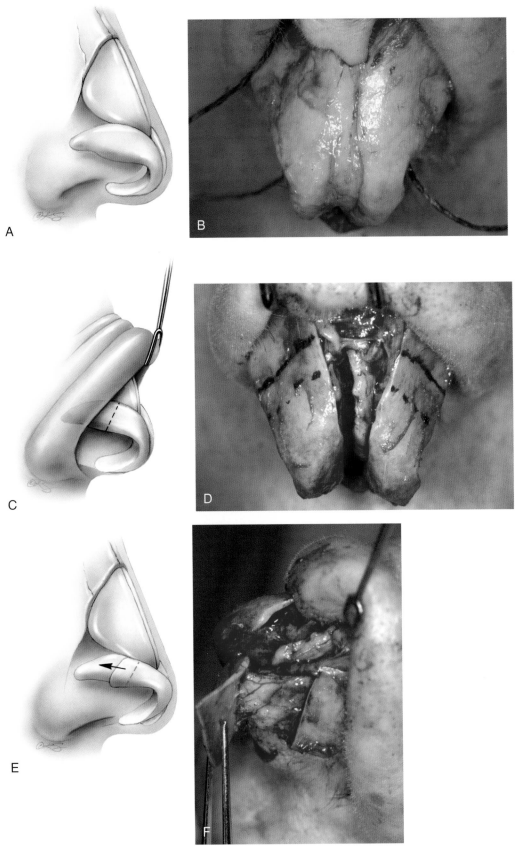

Figure 33-4 Lateral crural overlay technique. **A,** The overly long lower lateral cartilages. **B,** The overly long lateral crura are seen intraoperatively. **C, D,** The cartilages are marked for excision. **E,** Lateral crura overlap is depicted. **F,** An intraoperative photograph of cartilage dissected from underlying vestibular skin.

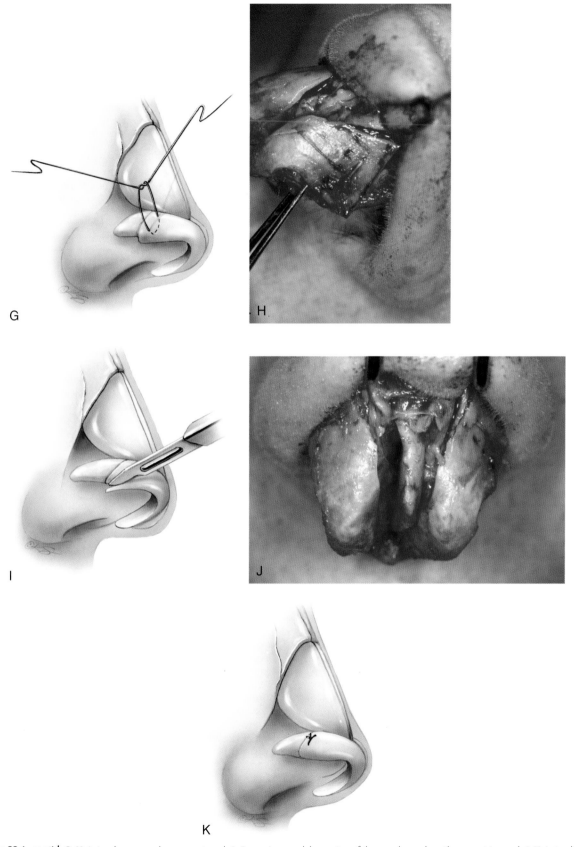

G

H

I

J

K

Figure 33-4, cont'd G, H, Lateral crura ends are resutured. **I,** Excessive caudal margins of the overlapped cartilage are trimmed. **J, K,** Lateral crura are realigned, symmetrical, and stable.

resutured with two 5-0 clear nylon mattress sutures to reconstitute the lateral crural segments into their shortened configuration. The degree of tip rotation is directly proportional to the degree of overlap (shortening) of the lateral crura. Symmetric alignment of the lateral crura must be achieved to avoid tip or alar margin asymmetry (Figure 33-5).

Another technique used in tip control involving the lower lateral cartilages is the lateral crural wedge technique (Figure 33-6). The wedge resection of the lower laterals is made to rotate the tip cephalad. In most cases, adequate correction of the ptotic nasal tip requires the use of more than one of the aforementioned techniques. An effective combination for correction of the ptotic tip is a lateral crural overlay with a caudal extension graft.

Once the ptosis of the nasal tip has been corrected, additional tip projection can be achieved by suturing a shield-shaped cartilage tip graft into position. A tip graft is sculpted from septal cartilage and sutured to the caudal margin of the medial and intermediate crura with 6-0 PDS (polydioxanone) suture (Ethicon, Somerville, NJ). The tip graft serves to provide additional tip projection, hide tip asymmetries, improve the shape of the lobule, and increase tip support.[14] The use of tip grafts should be limited in older patients, because maximal tip refinement is generally unnecessary. In addition, the leading edge of the tip graft will be more visible beneath the thinner skin of these patients and should be limited to patients with thicker skin. In thin-skinned patients, the leading edge of the tip graft should be camouflaged with crushed cartilage or soft tissue (perichondrium, fascia, etc.) (Figure 33-7).

Other nasal tip problems, such as an underprojected or bulbous tip, can be managed by other techniques commonly used in younger patients. However, care must be taken to preserve as much of the cartilaginous framework as possible. Emphasis should be placed on repositioning existing cartilage structures, rather than excising them. The weaker cartilages of the aging nose are also more prone to deformity (e.g., buckling, bossae) under the forces of scar contracture. When performing volume reduction of the lateral crura in the aging patient, resection should be primarily medial, leaving at least 8 to 10 mm of intact strip.

It is imperative that the surgeon anticipates the effects of scar contracture on the reduced cartilages. It is shortsighted to try to attain the ideal final result at the time of surgery, which neglects the additional refinement that occurs with resolution of edema and healing. Therefore, the surgeon can anticipate additional tip refinement that will result from postoperative forces of scar contracture. Finally, aesthetic changes should be conservative because older patients are more set in their self-image, as well as their perception of acceptable change in nasal contour.

NARROWED MIDDLE NASAL VAULT

In some older patients, an excessively narrow middle nasal vault can result when weak upper lateral cartilages collapse inferomedially. Severe collapse may also result in collapse of the internal nasal valve. These patients experience improvement in their nasal airway obstruction while performing the "Cottle maneuver" or with lateralization of the lateral nasal wall with an instrument. To correct this deformity, the surgeon can apply bilateral spreader grafts between the dorsal (anterior) margin of the nasal septum and the upper lateral cartilages.[14-16] These grafts are rectangular in shape and measure approximately 5 to 15 mm in length, 3 to 5 mm in width, and 1 to 2 mm in thickness. The majority of spreader grafts extend from a point just cephalic to the anterior septal angle to the osseocartilaginous junction. In most older patients with a functional deficit at the internal nasal valve or lateral wall, spreader grafts will be insufficient, and alar batten grafts should be used. These cartilage grafts are placed caudal to the existing lateral crura to support the lateral wall.

Spreader grafts can be applied via an endonasal approach into precise submucosal tunnels[16] or may be applied directly between the upper lateral cartilages and the nasal septum via the external rhinoplasty approach.[6,15] In the external rhinoplasty approach, the upper lateral cartilages are freed from the nasal septum after the middle nasal vault is exposed. The rectangular spreader grafts are then applied between the upper lateral cartilages and septum, and sutured into place with a 5-0 PDS mattress suture. With incorporation of the upper lateral cartilages in the suture, the middle nasal vault width is set and inferomedial collapse of the upper lateral cartilages is avoided. Patients with short nasal bones are at higher risk of collapse and will need thicker and longer spreader grafts. Careful attention must be given to the width of the middle nasal vault to avoid creating excessive width with the spreader grafts. If possible, the surgeon should try to avoid dividing the upper lateral cartilages from the septum, in order to preserve support in the older patient. Thus, if dorsal hump reduction is not needed, the spreader grafts may be placed into submucosal tunnels made via a small intranasal incision, with preservation of the attachment of the upper lateral cartilages to the septum.[6,16]

PROFILE ALIGNMENT AND NARROWING THE NOSE

Successful management of the bony nasal vault involves conservative dorsal hump reduction, preservation of a high dorsal profile, and avoidance of dorsal irregularities. Because the nasal bones in the aging patient can be thin and brittle, careful manipulation of the bony vault must be exercised in order to avoid comminuted fractures or excessive narrowing of the bony vault. Typically, conservative dorsal hump reduction is performed after tip

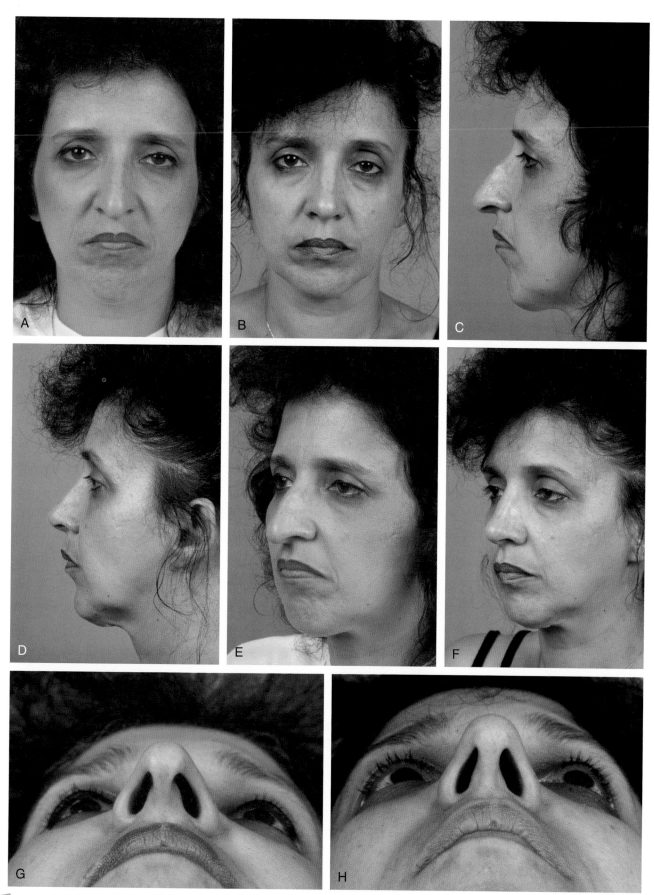

Figure 33-5 Patient with ptotic nasal tip. The lateral crural overlay technique was used to shorten the lateral crura and rotate the nasal tip. Preoperative (**A, C, E, G**) and postoperative (**B, D, F, H**) views.

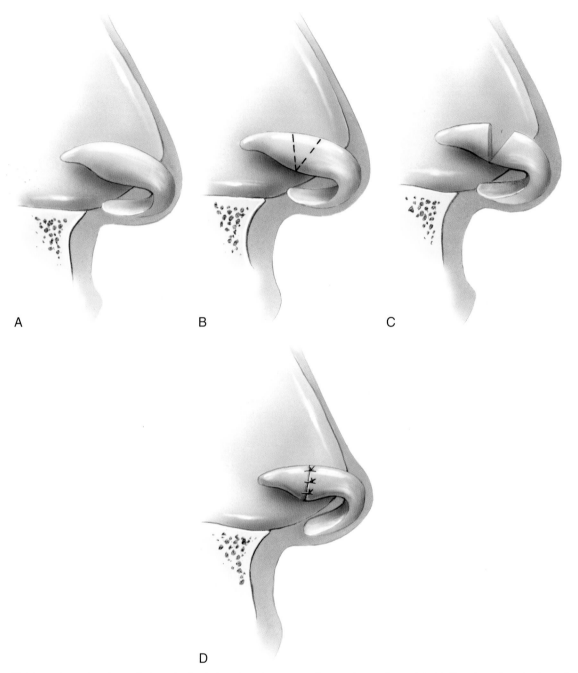

Figure 33-6 Lateral crural wedge technique. **A,** Overly long lateral crura contribute to the ptotic nasal tip. **B,** The planned wedge is outlined on the lateral crura. **C,** The lateral crura wedge is excised. **D,** Lateral crura are resutured, thus rotating the tip cephalad.

position is set. In patients with a deep nasofrontal angle, small crushed-cartilage radix grafts can be placed above a dorsal hump to create a straight profile (Figure 33-8). In many cases, dorsal hump reduction can be avoided if the profile can be corrected with the use of a radix graft in combination with an increase in tip projection and rotation. The surgeon should consider a radix graft in patients who demonstrate a deep nasofrontal angle with a low nasal starting point. The nasal starting point should be located at the level of the superior palpebral fold in female patients, with a slightly higher location in male patients.

For larger dorsal hump reductions, a Rubin osteotome can be used, while smaller dorsal humps can be managed with a fine rasp. With larger dorsal humps, wide undermining of the overlying skin–soft tissue envelope is necessary to accommodate for reduced skin elasticity and less rapid shrinkage and redraping. Because the thin skin of older patients shows even the smallest dorsal irregularity, special care must be taken to ensure a smooth dorsum.

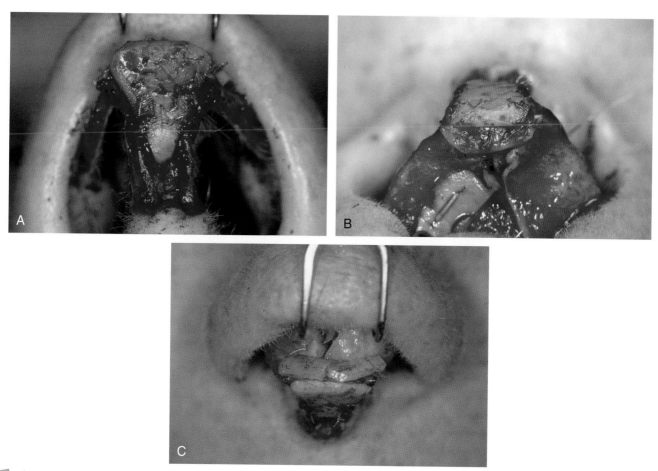

Figure 33-7 A, B, Tip graft camouflaged with a crushed cartilage graft behind the leading edge of the tip graft. **C,** Tip graft from the anterior view sutured in position.

Following profile alignment, lateral osteotomies can be performed using the smallest osteotome possible to minimize trauma and bleeding. Often, a 2- or 3-mm straight osteotome can be used to fracture the thin bone.[6,16] In most aging patients, medial osteotomies can be avoided as the bones are readily fractured.

EXTERNAL NASAL VALVE COLLAPSE

Older patients often present to the surgeon with complaints of nasal airway obstruction located primarily at the entrance to the nose (nostril margin). The nostrils may collapse on moderate to deep inspiration, with inadequate support of the lateral nasal wall and alae secondary to weak lower lateral cartilages. In some cases, the lateral crura are in a cephalic position and provide little support to the alar side walls.[15,17,18] This deficiency has been described as "external nasal valve collapse" and can be diagnosed by observing alar collapse on deep inspiration. These patients will characteristically experience improved nasal airflow if the alae are supported during nasal breathing.

Internal or external nasal valve collapse can be surgically corrected by applying bilateral alar batten grafts at the site of maximal lateral nasal wall collapse or near the nostril margin, respectively.[15,17,18] Alar batten grafts can be fashioned from curved cartilage of the nasal septum or of the cavum or cymba conchae of the ear. The concave surface of the batten graft is oriented medially to support the collapsing segment of the nostril (external valve collapse) or lateral nasal wall (internal valve collapse). To correct external valve collapse, the grafts are typically placed just caudal to the lateral crura and extend from the pyriform aperture to the lateral aspect of the lateral crura (Figure 33-9). For internal valve collapse, the grafts are placed at the point of maximal lateral nasal wall collapse, usually at the point of the supra-alar groove. As with spreader grafts, these grafts can be applied through either an endonasal incision or via the external rhinoplasty approach. Once the graft is in position, there should be an immediate improvement in support of the alar side walls as well as diminution of alar collapse during inspiration through the nose. We use splints in the nasal vestibule to support the alar battens and to help them heal in a lateral position.

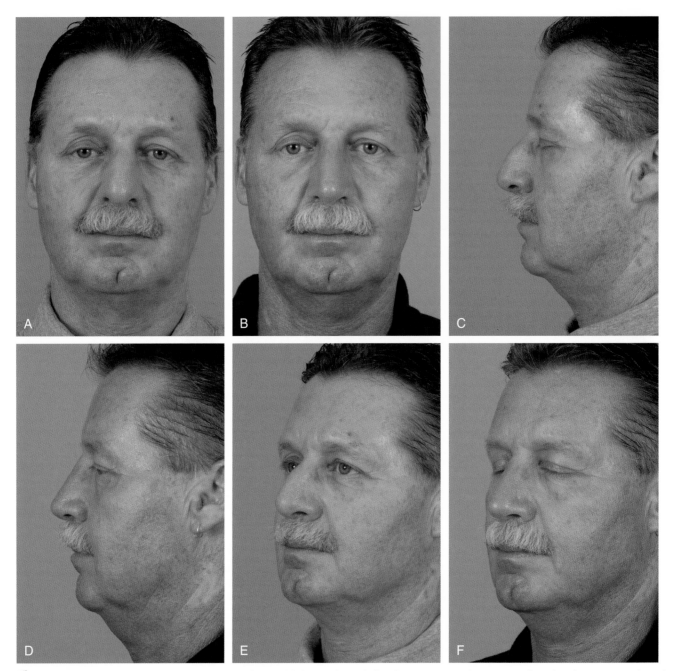

Figure 33-8 Patient with dorsal hump and deep radix. Double-layer radix graft placed into narrow pocket over nasofrontal angle to augment the radix and help create a straight dorsal profile. Preoperative (**A, C, E, G**) and postoperative (**B, D, F, H**) views.

ACUTE NASOLABIAL ANGLE OR RETRACTED COLUMELLA

Owing to posterior positioning of the feet of the medial crura, the older patient frequently has an acute nasolabial angle. Correction of this deformity adds support to the medial crural component of the tripod complex and improves the aesthetic appearance on lateral view. For minor augmentation, 1- to 2-mm pieces of cartilage can be placed into a small pocket between the feet of the

medial crura. This serves to support the lower lateral cartilages, preserve tip projection, and correct an acute nasolabial angle. With more significant deficiency of the medial crura, more aggressive maneuvers may be necessary. A sutured-in-place columellar strut may be sufficient. In most patients, however, a caudal extension graft will be necessary to support the nasal base and open the nasolabial angle.

The caudal extension graft is set in the midline and sutured between the medial crura. This maneuver moves

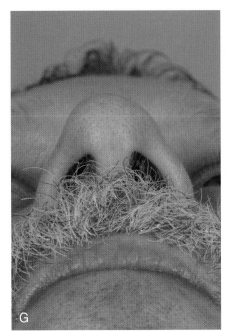
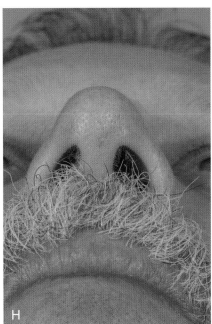

Figure 33-8, cont'd

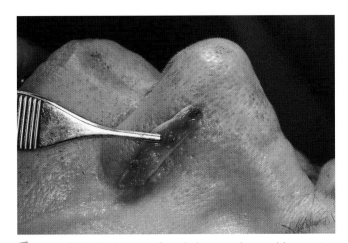

Figure 33-9 Alar batten graft applied into pocket caudal to existing lateral crura to support lateral wall.

the medial crura caudally and corrects the acute nasolabial angle or retracted columella.[19] A straight piece of septal cartilage is sutured to the stable caudal septum with 5-0 clear nylon mattress sutures (Figure 33-10). This allows extension of the graft into a pocket between the medial crura. The graft is then sutured between the medial crura with 5-0 clear nylon sutures. During this maneuver, care must be taken to set the proper tip projection, rotation, and columellar show. A more rigid nasal tip with less recoil results due to fixation of the medial crura to the caudal extension graft. If this grafting technique is planned, this rigidity and lack of recoil should be explained to the patient prior to the procedure. In addition, this graft may alter the length of the upper lip, which could change

the upper lip posture during smiling. This technique may be coupled with a tip graft to optimize the overall appearance of the lower third of the nose (Figure 33-11).

Many older patients present with a hanging columella deformity caused by loss of support or stretching of fibrous connections between the caudal septum and medial crura. Correction of this deformity may entail trimming of the caudal margin of the nasal septum or medial crura. This can also include excision of excess vestibular skin between the caudal septum and medial crura as well. If the caudal nasal septum is trimmed, there may be a loss of nasal tip support. A better option to correct the hanging columella is set-back of the medial crura on the overly long caudal septum. After dissecting between the medial crura, the medial crura can be sutured to the caudal septum with 5-0 clear nylon suture to set tip projection and alar–columellar relationship.

POSTOPERATIVE CARE

Careful postoperative care is critical to achieve an optimal result following rhinoplasty. In addition, patients should be monitored closely during the immediate postoperative period to ensure adequate oxygenation and hemostasis. To avoid life-threatening complications, the cardiac and pulmonary status of the patient should also be monitored. Finally, if nasal packing is used, it should be removed within 24 hours after surgery, with subsequent examination of the septal flaps to evaluate for a septal hematoma.

Columellar sutures should be removed on the seventh postoperative day. Postoperative edema that develops in

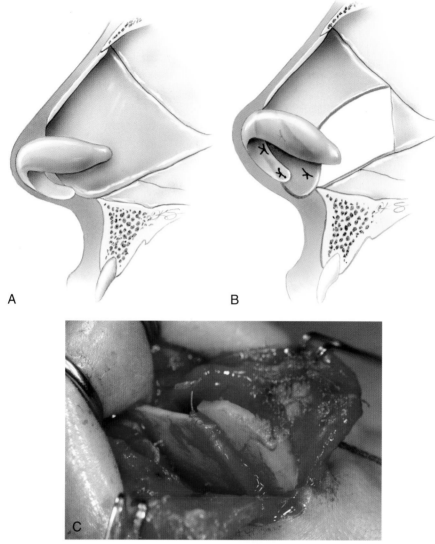

Figure 33-10 A, Short caudal septum. **B,** Caudal septal extension graft sutured in position. The graft is harvested with a standard septoplasty. **C,** Intra-operative photograph showing the graft sutured in place.

the supratip region can be treated with taping of the supratip. On rare occasions, subdermal injections (0.1 to 0.2 ml) of triamcinolone acetonide (Kenalog, 10 mg/ml; Westwood-Squibb, Buffalo, NY) can be placed into the supratip. Such injections should only be used in patients with thick skin. These injections may be administered 2 weeks after surgery, with no more than one injection per month. Dermal atrophy may result from either intradermal injections or frequent injections of higher concentrations of Kenalog.

COMPLICATIONS

Because rhinoplasty is considered to be an elective surgery, complications in the postoperative period can be particularly distressing. It has been estimated that complications occur in approximately 10% of cases.[20] This figure may actually be much higher if sequelae such as persistent swelling, ecchymoses, and skin discoloration are considered. Postoperative sequelae and complications of rhinoplasty generally fall into five major categories: infection, trauma, necrosis, functional problems, and iatrogenic difficulties.[5]

Rhinoplasty is considered by many to be the most difficult facial plastic operation, largely due to the intricate and highly variable anatomy. In addition, any surgical modification is likely to change over the lifetime of the patient, secondary to postoperative scar contracture and healing. For these reasons, primary rhinoplasty is often associated with a suboptimal outcome. It has been estimated that 8% to 15% of primary rhinoplasty patients eventually undergo revision surgery.[21] There are a number of nasal deformities that can result from primary

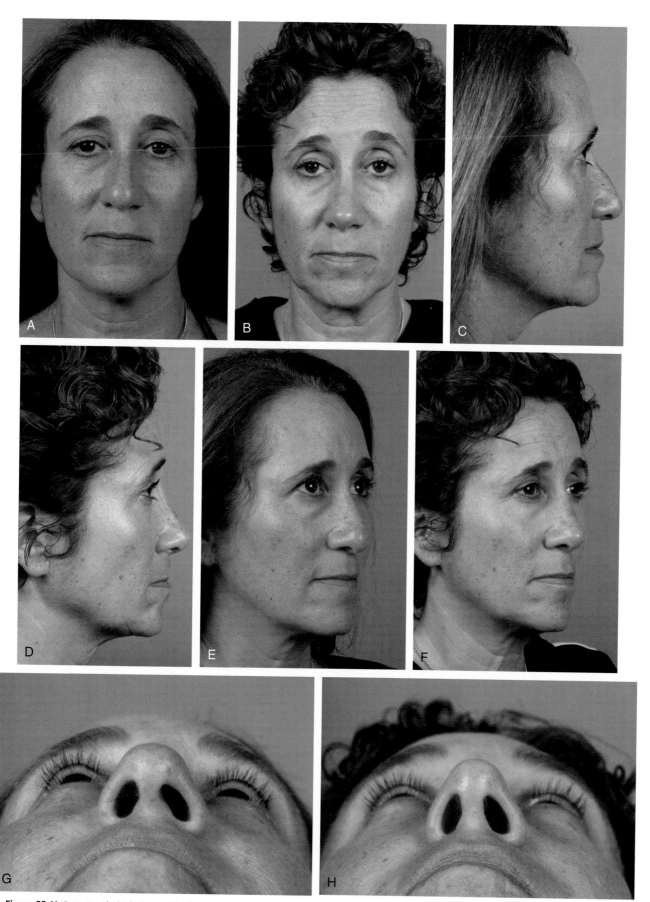

Figure 33-11 Patient with thick skin and bulbous nasal tip. In this patient, a tip graft was applied to increase tip projection. A caudal extension graft was used to support the nasal base. Preoperative (**A, C, E, G**) and postoperative (**B, D, F, H**) views.

rhinoplasty, including middle vault collapse, supra-alar pinching, and pollybeak deformity. Every surgeon should become familiar with these deformities.

FUTURE CONSIDERATIONS

The aging nose presents many unique challenges that must be considered to achieve a desirable result. In addition to addressing aesthetic changes, proper preoperative diagnosis is critical to identify all existing functional deficits. In this age group, aesthetic changes should be conservative, with extensive discussion prior to surgery. Because there is decreased structural support in the older patient, excision of supportive cartilaginous and bony structures should be minimized. Additional support should instead be provided with structural grafts to stabilize the nose and increase the likelihood of a favorable functional and aesthetic outcome.

REFERENCES

1. Janeke JB, Wright WK. Studies on the support of the nasal tip. *Arch Otolaryngol.* 1971;93:458–464.
2. Krmpotic-Nemanic J, Kostovic I, Rudan P, et al. Morphological and histological changes responsible for the droop of the nasal tip in advanced age. *Acta Otolaryngol.* 1971;71:278–281.
3. Patterson CN. The aging nose: Characteristics and correction. *Otolaryngol Clin North Am.* 1980;13:275–288.
4. Tardy ME. Rhinoplasty in midlife. *Otolaryngol Clin North Am.* 1980;13:289–303.
5. Holt GR, Garner ET, McLarey D. Postoperative sequelae and complications of rhinoplasty. *Otolaryngol Clin North Am.* 1987;20:853–876.
6. Toriumi DM. Surgical correction of the aging nose. *Facial Plast Surg.* 1996;12:205–214.
7. Larrabee WF. Rhinoplasty in the aging patient. In: Krause CJ, Pastorek N, Mangat DS, eds. *Aesthetic Facial Surgery.* Philadelphia: JB Lippincott; 1991:361–384.
8. Johnson CM, Anderson JR. Nose lift operation: An adjunct to aging face surgery. *Arch Otolaryngol.* 1978;104:1–6.
9. Kabaker SS. An adjunctive technique to rhinoplasty of the aging nose. *Head Neck Surg.* 1980;2:276–281.
10. Toriumi DM, Johnson CM. Open structure rhinoplasty: Featured technical points and long-term follow-up. *Facial Plast Surg Clin North Am.* 1993;1:1–22.
11. Anderson JR. Surgery of the nasal base. *Arch Otolaryngol.* 1984;110:349–358.
12. Tardy ME, Cheng E. Transdomal suture refinement of the nasal tip. *Facial Plast Surg.* 1987;4:317–326.
13. Toriumi DM, Tardy ME. Cartilage suturing techniques for correction of nasal tip deformities. *Op Tech Otolaryngol Head Neck Surg.* 1995;6:265–273.
14. Johnson CM, Toriumi DM. *Open Structure Rhinoplasty.* Philadelphia: WB Saunders; 1990.
15. Toriumi DM. Management of the middle nasal vault in rhinoplasty. *Opin Tech Plast Reconstr Surg.* 1995;2:16-30.
16. Sheen JH. Spreader graft: A method of reconstructing the roof of the middle nasal vault following rhinoplasty. *Plast Reconstr Surg.* 1984;73:230–237.
17. Tardy ME, Garner ET. Inspiratory nasal obstruction secondary to alar and nasal valve collapse. *Op Tech Otolaryngol Head Neck Surg.* 1990;1:215–217.
18. Constantian MB. The incompetent external nasal valve: Pathophysiology and treatment in primary and secondary rhinoplasty. *Plast Reconstr Surg.* 1994;93:919–931.
19. Toriumi DM. Caudal extension graft for correction of the retracted columella. *Opin Tech Otolaryngol Head Neck Surg.* 1995;6:311–318.
20. Weimert TA, Yoder MG. Antibiotics and nasal surgery. *Laryngoscope.* 1980;90:667–672.
21. Byrd HS, Hobar PC. Rhinoplasty: A practical guide for surgical planning. *Plast Reconstr Surg.* 1993;91:642–656.

CHAPTER THIRTY-FOUR

Cleft Lip Rhinoplasty

Jonathan M. Sykes

The cleft lip nasal deformity is a complex, three-dimensional problem that challenges any rhinoplasty surgeon. The extent of the nasal deformity is related to the severity of the original cleft malformation and ranges from mild to severe.[1]

The secondary cleft nasal deformity is related to several factors: (1) the original deformity, (2) any interim surgery performed on the nose, lip, and alveolus, and (3) growth pattern of the nose and midface. The decision to perform nasal surgery is determined by the amount of functional breathing issues and aesthetic concerns of the patient. This chapter describes the nasal deformities associated with congenital clefting and outlines the timing and techniques used to correct these deformities.

ANATOMY OF THE CLEFT NASAL DEFORMITY

The nasal deformities associated with congenital unilateral cleft lips have been well described and are consistent.[2,3] The extent of the typical nasal deformity is related to the degree of deficiency of alar base support on the cleft side. The typical characteristics of the unilateral cleft lip nose are described in Table 34-1.[4]

The hallmark of the unilateral cleft lip nasal deformity is a three-dimensional asymmetry of the nasal tip and alar base[4] (Figure 34-1). The columella and caudal nasal septum always deviate to the noncleft side, secondary to an asymmetric, unopposed pull of the orbicularis oris muscle. The cleft alar base is asymmetric and the cleft ala is displaced laterally, inferiorly, and posteriorly to its noncleft counterpart.[5] The nasal tip is also asymmetric, with the cleft side lower lateral cartilage (LLC) having a shorter medial crus and longer lateral crus than the LLC on the noncleft side (Figure 34-2). The weakened and malpositioned cleft side LLC produces a nostril that is wide and horizontally oriented.

The nasal septum in the unilateral cleft lip nose is deviated caudally to the noncleft side, and is bowed posteriorly to the cleft side[6] (Figure 34-3). In a study of 140 nasal septums in patients with unilateral lip clefting, Crockett and Bumstead[7] found that the bony septum was deviated into the cleft airway in 80% of these patients. Interestingly, most patients with clefting do not complain of nasal obstruction despite having significant deviation and abnormality of the nasal airway. In all likelihood, this tolerance of major abnormalities of the nasal septum can be attributed to the fact that cleft patients become accustomed to their nasal airway anatomy and associated impaired nasal breathing from a very young age.

The etiology of the asymmetry of the cleft alar base is a lack of skeletal support on the cleft side alar base.[5] Deformities of the bony skeleton near the pyriform aperture result in inadequate support of the alar base both medially (at the columella) and laterally (at the alar-facial groove). The lack of medial and lateral support causes introversion of the nasal ala and webbing of the nasal vestibule.[8] The contour of the lateral crus of the LLC is often concave, secondary to the lack of medial and lateral support.[9] Introversion of the cleft ala is defined as a posterior and inferior malposition of the cephalic border of the lateral crus of the LLC. The combination of the lack of skeletal support and the malposition of the cleft LLC causes weakness of the external nasal valve, often further compromising nasal airflow in the cleft patient.

The middle third of the nose in the unilateral cleft lip nasal deformity is also characterized by weakness of the upper lateral cartilages (ULCs) and malposition of these cartilages.[6] Again, this weakness results from inadequate skeletal support and is often manifest by concave ULC. This weakness typically affects the internal nasal valve on the cleft side.

BILATERAL CLEFT NASAL DEFORMITY

The bilateral cleft lip nasal deformity is also caused by a lack of skeletal support. The bilateral cleft lip nose is usually not grossly asymmetric. Of course, if a marked difference exists on the two sides of the lip, there can be gross asymmetry of the cleft nasal tip and alar base in the bilateral cleft lip patient.

The bilateral cleft lip nose is characterized by a lack of skin and cartilaginous support in the nasal tip.[10] The columella in bilateral deformities is typically short and there is inadequate projection of the nasal tip. The extent of columellar shortening is related to the size, shape, and position of the prolabium and to the severity of the cleft deformity (Figure 34-4). An abnormal junction between the columella and the central aspect of the upper lip is usually present. Characteristics of the bilateral cleft lip nasal deformity are listed in Table 34-2.

Table 34-1 Characteristics of Unilateral Cleft Lip Nasal Deformity

Nasal tip
Medial crus of lower lateral cartilage shorter on cleft side
Lateral crus of lower lateral cartilage longer on cleft side (total length of lower lateral cartilage is same)
Lateral crus of lower lateral cartilage may be caudally displaced and may produce hooding of alar rim
Alar dome on cleft side is flat and displaced laterally
Columella
Short on cleft side
Base directed to noncleft side (secondary to contraction of orbicularis oris muscle)
Nostril
Horizontal orientation on cleft side
Alar base
Displaced laterally, posteriorly, and inferiorly
Nasal floor
Usually absent
Nasal septum
Caudal deflection to the noncleft side and posterior deviation to the cleft side

The medial crura of the LLCs are short, and the lateral crura are both long in bilateral clefts (Figure 34-5). This results in underprojection of the nasal tip, and displacement of the alar bases in a posterior, lateral, and inferior location when compared to noncleft patients. If one side of the lip is more involved than the other side, the short columella is typically deviated toward the less involved side, pulling the tip toward that direction. The nostrils in bilateral cleft lip patients are more horizontal than those in noncleft patients. The nasal septum is usually midline, being deviated caudally to the less involved side if asymmetry exists. The middle nasal third exhibits poor cartilaginous support, compromising the internal nasal valve and affecting functional nasal breathing.

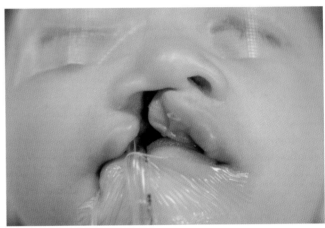

Figure 34-1 Intraoperative base view of a patient with a right complete cleft lip and cleft palate with significant cleft nasal deformity. This view shows the obvious alar base asymmetry and the caudal septum deviated to the noncleft side.

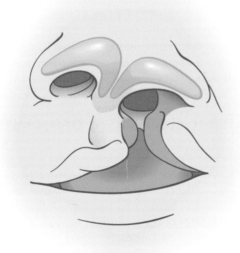

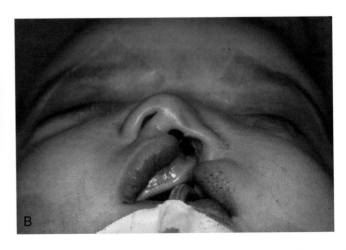

A   B

Figure 34-2 A, B, Schematic diagram and intraoperative photograph of a left complete cleft nasal deformity. On the cleft side, the medial crus is shorter and the lateral crus longer than the noncleft side counterpart.

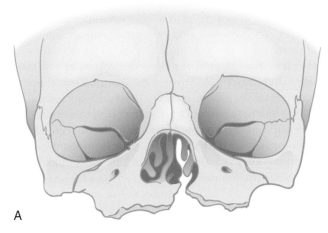
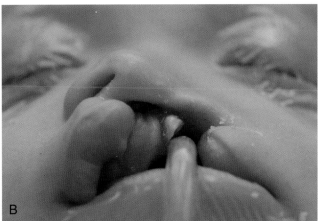

Figure 34-3 A, Schematic diagram of a left cleft nasal deformity showing the architecture of the caudal septum deviated to the noncleft side. **B,** Intra-operative photograph of this complete cleft lip and nasal deformity.

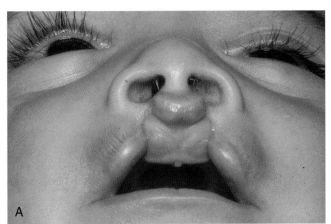
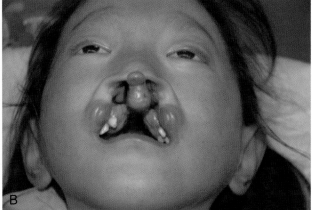

Figure 34-4 A, Basal view of a patient with incomplete bilateral cleft lip with good projection. **B,** Patient with severe bilateral complete lip and palate deformity showing obvious lack of columellar length and lack of normal tip projection.

TIMING OF CLEFT NASAL REPAIR

Cleft nasal reconstruction can be divided into primary and secondary repairs.[1] *Primary* rhinoplasty refers to nasal surgery performed at the time of the initial cleft lip repair. *Secondary* rhinoplasty refers to any cleft nasal surgery performed after the initial cleft lip repair. Secondary cleft rhinoplasty may be further subdivided into intermediate repairs, usually performed during childhood, and definitive repairs, occurring at the time of full nasal growth.

The decision to perform surgery on patients with cleft deformities is the product of many factors. These include the fact that the child with a nasal malformation is exposed to ridicule during childhood. This philosophy is counterpointed by the surgeon's knowledge that nasal and midfacial growth is not completed until the mid-to-late teen years. Early surgical intervention is thought to interfere with subsequent nasal growth. The philosophy that early nasal surgery affects subsequent nasal growth is supported by the experimental work of Sarnat and Wexler[11] and Bernstein,[12] who demonstrated nasal growth inhibition in animals after aggressive resection of the nasal septum and overlying mucoperichondrium.

Although traditional philosophy avoids aggressive early nasal surgery fearing nasal growth inhibition, there is a growing trend toward primary cleft nasal repair.[5,13] In many centers, rhinoplasty at the time of initial cleft repair is the accepted surgical treatment. This philosophy recognizes that maximizing nasal tip projection and nasal and alar base symmetry during lip repair allows the nose to grow in a symmetric fashion. For this reason, most contemporary cleft surgeons perform primary nasal repair on the tip and alar base.

PRESURGICAL MANAGEMENT OF THE CLEFT NASAL DEFORMITY

The traditional approach to management includes a single stage lip repair at 3 months of age, palatoplasty at approximately 1 year of age, alveolar bone grafting at 9 to 11 years, and definitive rhinoplasty after full facial growth has been reached. Nonsurgical repositioning of alveolar segments serves to lessen tension across the lip wound, improve nasal tip symmetry in wide unilateral clefts, and elongate the columella and expand the nasal soft tissues in bilateral clefts.[14] There have been many reports of presurgical devices designed to decrease the cleft gap and minimize the eventual lip and nasal deformity.[15,16] Presurgical nasoalveolar molding (PNAM) uses an intraoral alveolar molding device with nasal molding prongs[17] (Figure 34-6). Successful use of any presurgical orthopedic devices requires a team approach—a dedicated orthodontist, a flexible and patient surgeon, and an involved, responsive, cooperative, and compliant family

Table 34-2 Characteristics of Bilateral Cleft Lip Nasal Deformity

Nasal Tip
Medial crura of LLC short bilaterally
Lateral crura of LLC long bilaterally
Lateral crura displaced caudally
Alar domes poorly defined and widely separated, producing an amorphous tip
Columella
Short
Base is wide
Nostril
Horizontal orientation bilaterally
Alar base
Displaced laterally, posteriorly, and inferiorly
Nasal floor
Usually absent bilaterally
Nasal septum
In a complete bilateral cleft lip and palate, the septum is midline; however, if cleft on one side is incomplete, the septum deviates toward the less affected side.

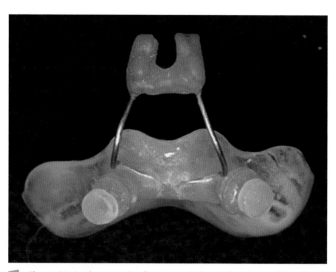

Figure 34-6 Photograph of a presurgical nasoalveolar molding device (PNAM).

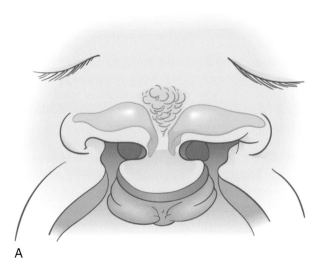

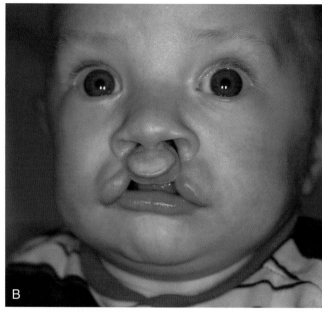

Figure 34-5 A, B, Schematic diagram and photograph of a patient with bilateral complete cleft lip deformity. The medial crus of each side of the nose is shorter and the lateral crus longer than in unaffected alar cartilage.

(Figure 34-7). If properly performed, PNAM can provide soft tissue expansion and mold the nasal infrastructure, thereby decreasing the nasal deformity.

PRIMARY CLEFT RHINOPLASTY

The goals of primary rhinoplasty are to maximize symmetry of the nasal tip and alar base. In that the base of the nose in the unilateral deformity involves gross asymmetries of both the skeleton and soft tissues, the soft tissue attachments of the alar base must be completely freed from the skeletal base (pyriform aperture).[5] This allows repositioning of the nasal and alar base in a more symmetric fashion.[13,18]

Dissection of the cleft alar base from the pyriform aperture involves an internal alotomy (Figure 34-8). Separation of the soft tissue attachments begins with an incision at the anterior portion of the inferior turbinate on the cleft side. After the cleft alar base is entirely separated from its skeletal attachments, the floor of the nose is approximated and the alar base is medialized, thereby creating improved three-dimensional symmetry.

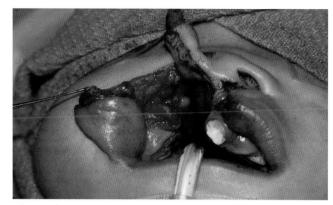

Figure 34-8 A, B, Schematic diagram and intraoperative photograph showing internal alotomy separating the cleft side nasal base from pyriform aperture.

The other component of primary rhinoplasty involves nasal tip plasty. The cutaneous attachments of the LLCs are separated. This is accomplished by creating medial and lateral tunnels using the incisions of the standard rotation–advancements lip repair[19] (Figures 34-9 and 34-10). Dissection on the undersurface of the LLC (between the cartilage and vestibular skin) is not performed. The medial and lateral tunnels are then connected.

After the lip is sutured closed and the alar base is repositioned, the LLC is molded into its new shape. This can be accomplished with interdomal sutures or with the application of nasal bolsters. The purpose of these maneuvers is to recreate the dome of the LLC into a more medial, projected position. Essentially, a "steal" from lateral crus to medial crus is performed to increase nasal tip projection and improve tip symmetry.[20] Complete release of the skin overlying the LLC prevents tethering and irregularities of the nasal tip. If a tip bolster is used, the suture is passed through a subcutaneous tunnel and tension is placed on the LLC, creating blanching of the nasal tip skin (Figure 34-11). Bolsters are typically removed at seven to ten days. Lastly, silastic nasal conformers are placed into the nostrils to help shape the LLC and reshape the nostril configuration (Figure 34-12). The conformers are left in place for 4 to 6 weeks, if tolerated by both the patient and family.

SECONDARY CLEFT NASAL RECONSTRUCTION

The cleft nasal deformity that is present during teenage years is a product of many factors including (1) the extent of the original nasal deformity, (2) the patient's growth, and (3) any intervening surgery and related scarring.

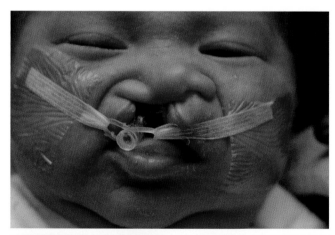

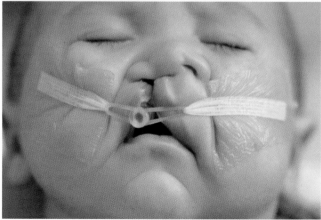

Figure 34-7 Patient with complete unilateral cleft lip and palate with the PNAM device in place.

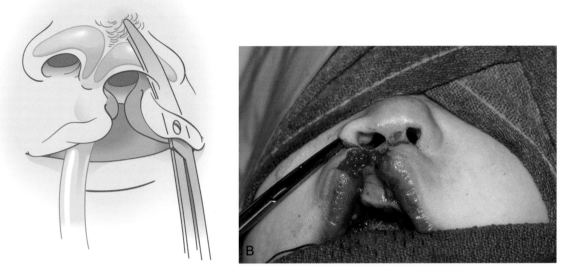

Figure 34-9 A, B, Schematic diagram and intraoperative photograph of the lateral nasal dissection separating the lateral crus of the lower lateral cartilage from the overlying skin.

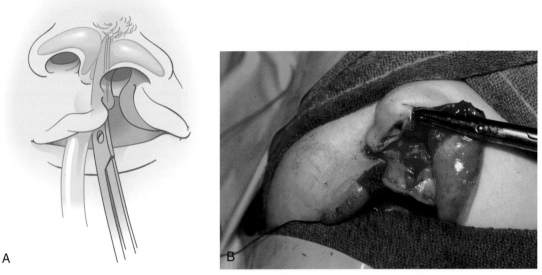

Figure 34-10 A, B, Schematic diagram and intraoperative photograph showing the medial dissection separating the medial crus of the lower lateral cartilage from the overlying skin.

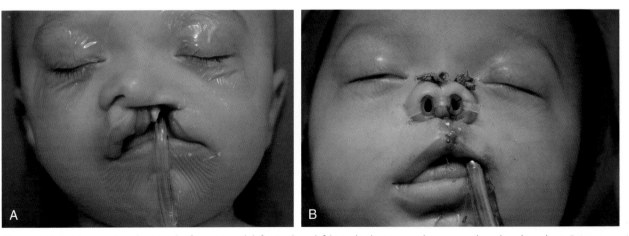

Figure 34-11 A, Intraoperative photograph of a patient with left complete cleft lip and palate prior to lip repair and nasal tip rhinoplasty. **B,** Intraoperative photograph after the completion of surgery with repair of the cleft lip and nasal tip rhinoplasty. Nasal conformers are in place as well as tip bolsters.

Therefore, the facial plastic surgeon must understand the anatomy of the standard nasal deformity associated with lip clefting, and be prepared for individual variations that can occur with intervening surgeries.

The timing of definitive cleft septorhinoplasty should account for several factors. These include midface and nasal growth, specific psychological patient desires, and any concomitant associated functional issues.[21] In general, nasal reconstruction in cleft patients is not performed prior to full nasal growth, which is approximately 16 years of age in females and 18 years of age in males. If significant dentofacial deformity exists, orthognathic surgery is usually performed prior to undertaking any nasal surgery.

INCISIONS

The approach used to perform cleft nasal reconstruction varies with the deformity. Although the endonasal

approach is used by some surgeons, the open or external approach provides additional exposure to diagnose deformities and perform various techniques to correct complex nasal deformities.

The incisions used to open the nose vary, but a combination of bilateral marginal incisions with an inverted-V mid-columellar incision is typically used.[22] However, if additional skin is needed in the columella, modification of the typical external columellar incision can be used. In the unilateral cleft nasal deformity, an asymmetric V-to-Y on the cleft side can be designed to increase columellar soft tissue (and length). If significant columellar deficiency is present in the bilateral cleft nose, a midline V-to-Y upper lip incision can be used, recruiting skin from the upper lip into the columella. An alternative incision choice is to use upper lip forked flaps[23] (Figure 34-13). These flaps have the advantage of narrowing the central segment while lengthening the columella. The sliding chondrocutaneous flap, first described by Vassarionov and modified by Wang, has been designed to advance both skin and cartilage into the columella and nasal tip while revising the cleft lip scar.[21]

SEPTAL RECONSTRUCTION

The cleft lip nose is usually associated with significant septal deformity. In the unilateral cleft nose, the pyriform aperture is very asymmetric and usually has a bony deficiency on the cleft side. This bony asymmetry, coupled with an unopposed pull of the orbicularis oris muscle results in a caudal nasal septum significantly deviated to the noncleft side. In the bilateral deformity, bony deficiency on both sides of the pyriform aperture causes a wide and poorly supported caudal nasal septum. This results in a wide and weakly supported caudal septal deformity.

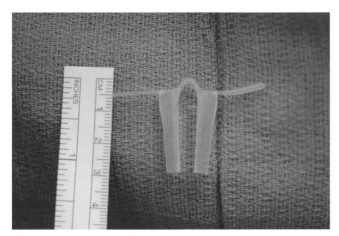

Figure 34-12 Close-up view of Silastic nasal conformers used at the conclusion of cleft repair.

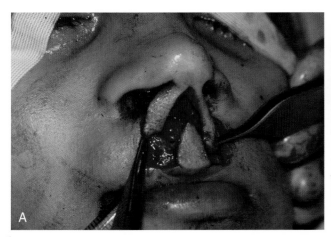
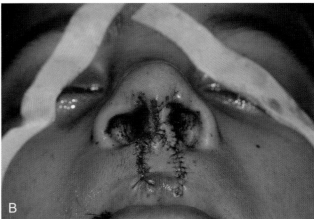

Figure 34-13 A, Bilateral forked flaps used to narrow philtral width in a bilateral cleft lip in lengthening the columella. **B,** Postoperative photograph of the same patient with fork flaps sutured into position lengthening the columella.

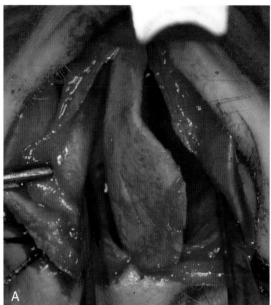 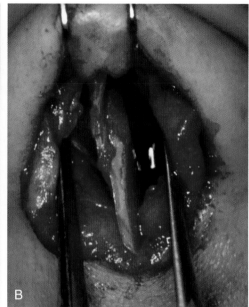

Figure 34-14 A, Deviated nasal septum in a patient with right cleft lip prior to reconstruction and repositioning. **B,** Intraoperative photograph of the patient after reconstruction of the nasal septum and suture repositioning to the nasal spine.

Nasal reconstruction begins with septal reconstruction and repositioning. If the caudal septum is dislocated, it must be freed from its bony and soft tissue attachments, and repositioned into the midline[6] (Figure 34-14). This often requires resection of a small amount of inferior cartilage from the maxilla and suture repositioning of the caudal septum. The caudal septum is usually sutured to the nasal spine with 4-0 monofilament long-acting absorbable suture. If the septum requires further stabilization or straightening, a caudal septal extension graft can be used. This provides support to the base of the nose, and can be a pillar upon which to suture and stabilize the nasal tip.

The posterior septal deformity should also be corrected to maximize the nasal airway and to obtain cartilage grafts. In the unilateral cleft nose, the posterior septum is usually deflected significantly to the cleft side. The septum is usually approached through an open septoplasty, by separating the LLCs. This allows correction of both the caudal and posterior deformities and gives access to obtain cartilage for graft material.

TREATMENT OF THE ASYMMETRIC ALAR BASE

The alar base on the cleft side is usually malpositioned. In the original congenital malformation, the position of the affected alar base is *posterior*, *lateral*, and *inferior* to the unaffected side. Once the lip is repaired, however, the alar base is repositioned. This new position may be symmetric with the noncleft side, but usually is in a new asymmetric position. The alar base width on the cleft side is often narrower than the noncleft side and malpositioned in either a superior or an inferior position versus the unaffected alar base.

An additional deformity that often presents with the secondary cleft defect is a lack of normal configuration of the affected nasal sill. During initial lip closure, the floor of the nose is reconstructed. A very small deformity (malposition) of the nasal sill (0.5 to 1 mm) at the time of lip closure usually creates a very noticeable deformity in the adult nose. At the time of definitive nasal reconstruction, the nasal sill and anterior floor should be closed in as symmetric a position to the noncleft side as possible. This often requires incision of the nasal sill and layered repair of the nasal floor. The cleft alar base is then repositioned in a symmetric fashion.

LOWER NASAL THIRD

After stabilizing the caudal nasal septum and providing three-dimensional alar base symmetry, the external rhinoplasty is performed. The lower third of the nose requires support and symmetry. Support and symmetry can be established by stabilizing the nasal tip complex to the nasal septum. This can be accomplished by (1) a tongue-in-groove technique, (2) extended spreader grafts, (3) a septal extension graft, or (4) a columellar strut to create three-dimensional symmetry.

After stabilizing the medial crura to the nasal septum, vertical division of the LLC can be performed lateral to the nasal dome. This allows an increase in nasal tip

projection. Reconstitution of the divided nasal tip cartilages is then performed with a 5-0 monofilament long-
acting absorbable suture. Camouflage of nasal tip
asymmetries is then accomplished with a shield-style
nasal tip graft.[24] The tip graft is sutured into position
with 6-0 monofilament permanent suture. In cleft nasal
deformities, tip grafts provide support, an increase in
nasal projection, and camouflage for tip asymmetries.

Vertical dome division both narrows the nasal tip and
provides elevation of the cleft side LLC. If there is residual
alar hooding of the cleft side LLC after completing division of the LLC, the LLC can be sutured superiorly to
elevate the cleft side alar rim. The LLC may be sutured
to the ipsilateral ULC for superior repositioning.

MIDDLE THIRD OF THE CLEFT NOSE

The middle third of the nose in cleft patients often is
weak, resulting in both aesthetic and functional issues.
Concavity of the cleft side ULC often results in internal
nasal valve dysfunction.[25] This weakness can be treated
with onlay grafts, spreader grafts, autogenous spreader
flaps, or flaring sutures (Figure 34-15). Unilateral, or
asymmetric spreader grafts, placed between the ULC and
the nasal septum, often improve nasal function and help
to straighten the deviated nose.

TREATMENT OF THE ALAR RIM (LATERAL CRUS OF THE LLC)

The cleft side LLC is poorly supported with lack of normal
skeletal support medially and laterally. This lack of
support usually causes malposition of the cleft alar rim.
The cleft side lateral crus of the LLC is concave and
results in an introverted alar contour.[26]

Various techniques exists to treat the LLC concavity.
These include suture techniques, underlay alar strut
grafts, onlay grafts, and autocartilage flaps.[27] Additionally, the lateral crus can be dissected from the underlying
vestibular skin, removed, flipped, and resutured in a
convex fashion (Figure 34-16). Alar strut grafts are placed
between the existing concave-outward LLC and the
underlying vestibular skin (Figure 34-17). This graft
strengthens the lateral crus of the LLC and flattens the
concave LLC.

Suture techniques such as horizontal mattress sutures
also strengthen and flatten the lateral crus of the LLC.
Last, the cephalic margin of the LLC can be made into
an advancement flap. This cartilage flap can be advanced
to support the remaining LLC. Each of these techniques

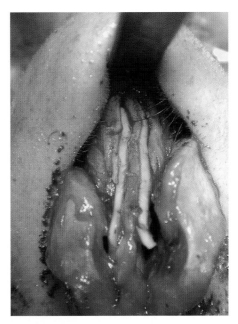

Figure 34-15 Intraoperative photograph of an open septorhinoplasty with middle third spreader grafts sutured into position.

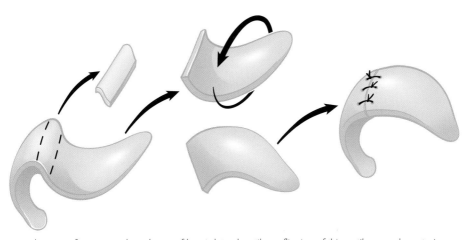

Figure 34-16 Schematic diagram of a concave lateral crus of lower lateral cartilage, flipping of this cartilage, and resuturing.

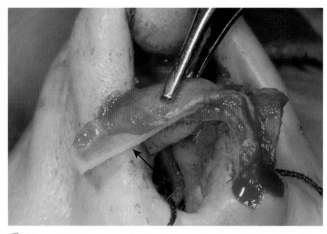

Figure 34-17 Intraoperative photograph of an open rhinoplasty with an alar strut graft sutured to the under surface of the lateral crus of the lower lateral cartilage.

supports the lateral crus of the LLC and strengthens the external nasal valve (Figures 34-18 and 34-19).

TREATMENT OF DENTOFACIAL DEFORMITIES

The incidence of dentofacial deformities in cleft patients is well known. The skeletal deformity includes maxillary hypoplasia. This affects maxillary growth in both antero-posterior and transverse dimensions.[28] Ross has shown that the development of maxillary hypoplasia is related to the type and timing of the palatoplasty procedure.[29] Maxillary hypoplasia results can result in class III malocclusion and significant midfacial skeletal deficiency (Figure 34-20).

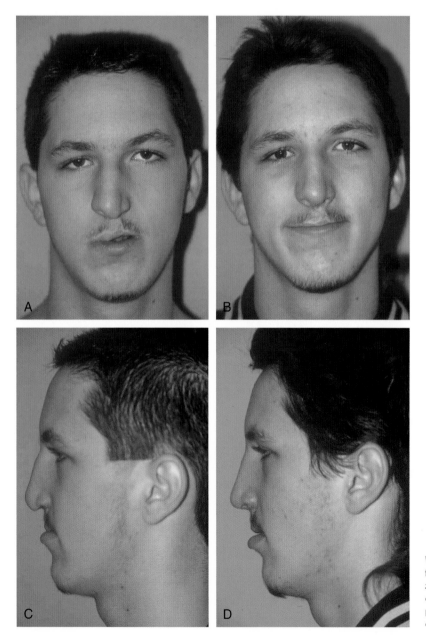

Figure 34-18 A, B, Preoperative and postoperative frontal photograph of a patient with complete left cleft lip and palate status post open septorhinoplasty. **C, D,** Preoperative and postoperative lateral photographs of the same patient who underwent open septorhinoplasty with lateral crural repositioning.

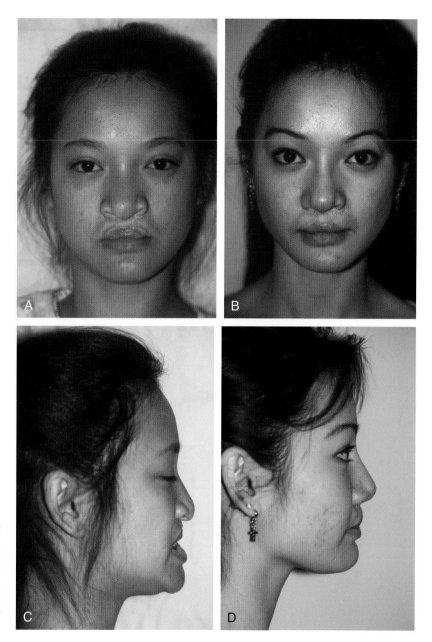

Figure 34-19 A, B, Preoperative and postoperative frontal photographs of a patient with bilateral cleft lip and palate after two procedures. The first procedure was a Le Fort I maxillary osteotomy with advancement and the second procedure, open septorhinoplasty with an autologous costal cartilage graft. **C, D,** Preoperative and postoperative photographs of the same patient before Le Fort I maxillary osteotomy and open septorhinoplasty after both of these procedures.

The dentofacial deformities associated with the treatment of cleft malformations result in poor support of the nasal base. To reconstruct the face of many cleft patients in an optimal fashion, both orthognathic surgery and rhinoplasty are required. If the dentofacial deformity is significant enough to necessitate orthognathic surgery, the skeletal surgery is usually completed prior to undertaking rhinoplasty.[30] Although some surgeons advocate simultaneous orthognathic surgery and rhinoplasty, staged surgery provides the most precise facial reconstruction and allows safe handling of the endotracheal tube. In severe Class III malocclusion with associated skeletal deformity, distraction osteogenesis, rather than traditional

Le Fort midface osteotomy of the maxilla, is performed (Figures 34-21 and 34-22).

SUMMARY

Reconstruction of cleft lip nose is extremely challenging. The congenital malformation involves all tissue layers, from the skeletal platform to the external nasal skin. Primary rhinoplasty is useful to maximize nasal symmetry and minimize psychological ridicule for the child. This also allows the nose to grow in a symmetric fashion. Definitive rhinoplasty is performed using an

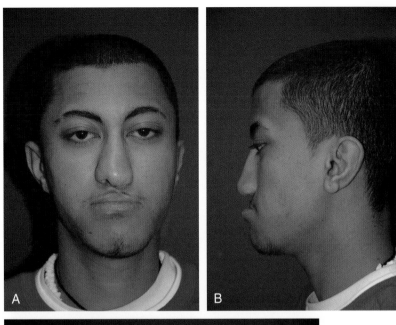

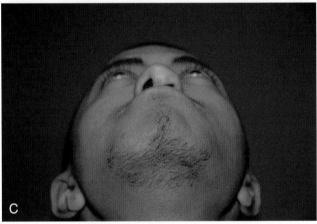

Figure 34-20 A–C, Frontal, left lateral, and basal view of a patient with left complete cleft lip and palate and significant nasal deformity. The patient has a significant skeletal disproportion with Class III malocclusion. On intraoral examination, the patient has 15 mm of underjet.

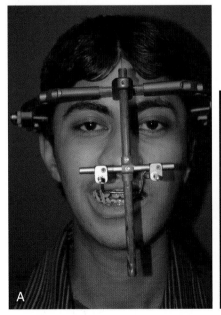

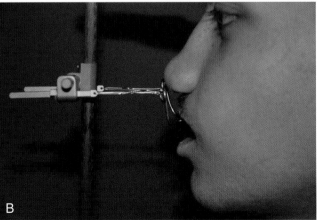

Figure 34-21 A, B, Frontal and close-up lateral photographs of the patient after a Le Fort I maxillary osteotomy and placement of a distraction osteogenesis device.

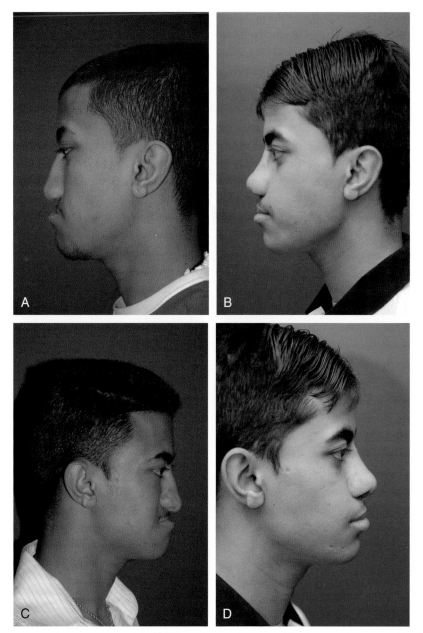

Figure 34-22 A–H, Preoperative and postoperative right and left lateral, right oblique, and basal views of the patient after distraction osteogenesis with and 16-mm maxillary advancement and open septorhinoplasty with autologous rib cartilage grafts.

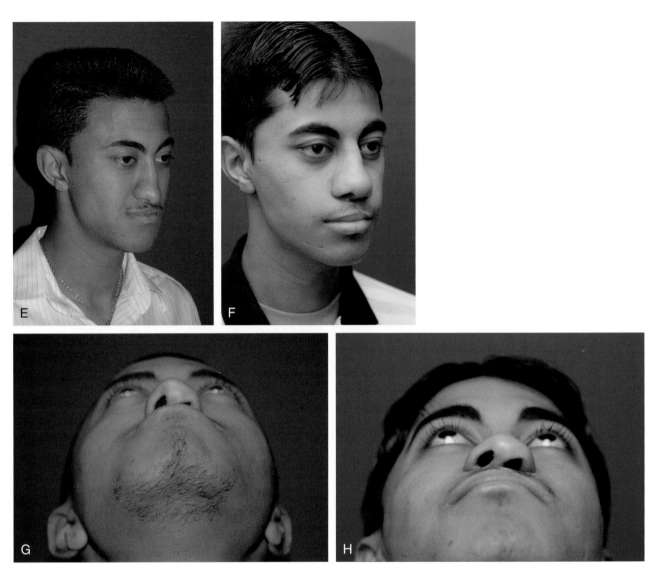

Figure 34-22, cont'd

external rhinoplasty approach with structural grafting. Structural grafting is used to maximize function, structure, support and symmetry.

REFERENCES

1. Sykes JM, Senders CW. Surgery of the cleft lip and nasal deformity. *Oper Tech Otolaryngol Head Neck Surg.* 1990;1:219–224.
2. Blair VP. Nasal deformities associated with congenital cleft of the lip. *JAMA.* 1925;84:185–187.
3. Huffman WC, Lierle DM. Studies on the pathologic anatomy of the unilateral hare-lip nose. *Plast Reconstr Surg.* 1949;4:225–234.
4. Sykes JM, Senders CW. Pathologic anatomy of cleft lip, palate and nasal deformity. In: Meyers AD, editor. *Biological basis of facial plastic surgery.* New York: Thieme; 1993.
5. Sykes JM, Senders CW. Surgical treatment of the unilateral cleft nasal deformity at the time of lip repair. *Fac Plast Surg Clin North Am.* 1995;3:69–77.
6. Jablon JH, Sykes JM. Nasal airway problems in the cleft lip population. *Fac Plast Surg Clin North AM.* 1999;7:391–403.
7. Crockett D, Bumstead R. Nasal airway, otologic and audiologic problems associated with cleft lip and palate. In: Bardack J, Morris HL, editors. *Multidisciplinary management of cleft lip and palate.* Philadelphia: WB Saunders; 1990.
8. Stenstrom SJ. The alar cartilage and the nasal deformity in unilateral cleft lip. *Plast Reconstr Surg.* 1966;38:223–231.
9. Avery JK. The unilateral deformity. In: Millard RD, editor. *Cleft craft: the evolution of its surgery.* Boston: Little, Brown; 1975.
10. Cronin TD. The bilateral cleft lip with bilateral cleft of the primary palate. In: Converse JM, editor. *Reconstructive plastic surgery.* Philadelphia, WB Saunders; 1964.
11. Sarnat BG, Wexler MR. Growth of the face and jaws after resection of the septal cartilage in the rabbit. *Am J Anat.* 1996;118:755–767.

12. Bernstein L. Early submucous resection of nasal septal cartilage: a pilot study in canine pups. *Arch Otolaryngol.* 1973;97:272–285.

13. McComb HK, Coghlan BA. Primary repair of the unilateral cleft lip nose: completion of a longitudinal study. *Cleft Palate Craniofac J.* 1996;33:23–31.

14. Grayson BH, Santiago PE, Beecht LE, Cutting CB. Presurgical nasoalveolar molding in infants with cleft lip and palate. *Cleft Palate Craniofac J.* 1999;36:486–498.

15. Liou EJW, Subramanian M, Chen PKT, Huang CS. The progressive changes of nasal symmetry and growth after nasoalveolar molding: a three-year follow-up study. *Plast Reconstr Surg.* 2004;114:858–864.

16. Maull D, Grayson B, Cutting C, et al. Long-term effects of nasoalveolar molding on three-dimensional nasal shape in unilateral clefts. *Cleft Palate Craniofac J.* 1999;36:391–397.

17. Grayson B, Cutting C. Presurgical nasoalveolar orthopedic molding in primary correction of the nose, lip, and alveolus of infants born with unilateral and bilateral clefts. *Cleft Palate Craniofac J.* 2001;35:193–198.

18. Mulliken JB, Martinez-Perez D. The principle of rotation advancement for the repair of unilateral complete cleft lip and nasal deformity: technical variations and analysis of results. *Plast Reconstr Surg.* 1999;104:1247–1249.

19. TerKonda RP, Sykes JM. Controversies and advances in unilateral cleft lip repair. *Curr Opin Otolaryngol Head Neck Surg.* 1997;5:223–227.

20. Ness JA, Sykes JM. Basics of Millard rotation-advancement technique for repair of the unilateral cleft lip deformity. *Fac Plast Surg.* 1993;9:167–176.

21. Wang TD. Secondary rhinoplasty in unilateral cleft nasal deformity. *Fac Plast Surg.* 2007;23:123–127.

22. Sykes JM, Senders CW, Wang TD, Cook TA. Use of the open approach for repair of secondary cleft lip-nasal deformities. *Fac Plast Surg.* 1993;1:111–126.

23. Millard DR Jr. Columella lengthening by a forked flap. *Plast Reconstr Surg.* 1958;22:545.

24. Toriumi DM, Johnson CM. Open structure rhinoplasty. *Fac Plast Surg Clin North Am.* 1993;1:1–22.

25. Park SS. Treatment of the internal nasal valve. *Fac Plast Surg.* 1999;7:333–345.

26. Park BY, Lew DH, Lee YH. A comparative study of the lateral crus of alar cartilage in unilateral cleft lip nasal deformity. *Plast Reconstr Surg.* 1998;101:905–919.

27. Chand MS, Toriumi DM. Treatment of the external nasal valve. *Fac Plast Surg.* 1999;7:347–355.

28. Sykes JM, Rotas N. Orthognathic surgery in the cleft lip and palate patient. In: Larrabee WF, Thomas JR, editors. *Facial plastic surgery clinics of North America*. Philadelphia: WB Saunders; 1996.

29. Ross RB. Treatment variables affecting facial growth in complete unilateral cleft lip and palate. Part 7. An overview of treatment and facial growth. *Cleft Palate J.* 1987;24:71.

30. Herber CS, Lehman JA Jr. Orthognathic surgery in the cleft lip and palate patient. *Clin Plast Surg.* 1993;20(4):755-768.

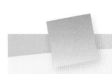

CHAPTER THIRTY-FIVE

Nasal Airway Obstruction

Kimberly Lee • Babak Azizzadeh • Babak Larian

The nasal airway is of paramount importance to the astute rhinoplasty surgeon. Often, great aesthetic results are combined with poor functional outcomes, leading to dissatisfaction and the need for further intervention.[1,2] This problem is curtailed by careful consideration and analysis of the function of the nose as well as its aesthetic value. Even well-experienced surgeons face this problem in a significant number of patients. In the hands of the less-experienced surgeon eager to only please the patient's aesthetic needs, this may be a more common issue. This is complicated by the fact that minor intranasal pathologic conditions that were not clinically significant preoperatively may become distressing and a focal point of complaints in the postoperative setting. As such, surgeons must diagnose both cosmetic and functional issues well in advance so as to ensure a favorable outcome.

NASAL ANATOMY AND FUNCTION

One may assume the anatomy of this area to be simple, but there are some nuances that explain our less than satisfactory outcomes or complications.

SEPTUM

The septum is composed of several components, both bony and cartilaginous. Maxillary, palatine, vomerine, and ethmoid bones contribute to the bony septum. However, the anterior nasal septum is cartilaginous, which allows for the most protruding portion of the nose to be flexible. The cartilaginous septum is attached superiorly to the perpendicular plate of the ethmoid, the bony groove on the undersurface of the nasal bones, and the upper lateral cartilages; these structures are held together by the continuity of the perichondrium and periosteum. Anteriorly fibrous attachments to the medial crura of the lower lateral cartilages determine the integrity of the tip. Inferiorly, the cartilaginous and bony septum lie in the bony groove of the maxillary crest via dense fibrous connective tissue. Embryologically, the cartilaginous septum develops from the perpendicular plate of the ethmoid, yet it remains nonossified. As such, the overlying perichondrium is contiguous with the periosteum of the perpendicular plate. While the vomer has a different embryologic origin and maintains its own periosteum, it is separated at the transition point with the septum of ethmoid bone origin. This seemingly innocuous fact is an important one in that elevation of the mucoperichondrium at the juncture of the perpendicular plate of ethmoid is rarely met with resistance or perforation. The majority of perforations occur at the junction of the cartilage to the vomer due to the noncontinuous covering.

The flow of air in the nasal passage follows the basic tenets of physics and Ohm's law, whereby gases move when there is a pressure gradient, and this flow can be hampered by friction. In laminar flow in a passageway, the fluid in the center has the greatest motion while that which is in contact with the sidewalls is hampered and moves slowly. Turbulent flow results from random, nonlinear motion. In the nasal cavity, laminar flow is of utmost importance because it allows for appropriate humidification and proper mucociliary flow of mucus, while turbulence creates more friction and impairs both functions. The septum helps ensure a laminar flow pattern.

TURBINATES

The three paired turbinates are located on the lateral nasal wall. The superior and middle turbinates arise from the ethmoid bone, whereas the inferior turbinates are made of independent bony structure. Covered by both respiratory and olfactory epithelium, the superior turbinate is located high in the nasal vault and usually arises from the cribriform plate of the ethmoid bone. The middle turbinate has a less consistent site of origin and could arise from the cribriform plate, the lamina papyracea, or the uncinate process in some cases.

The inferior turbinate bone arises on the inferior portion of the lateral nasal walls. The bone itself is penetrated heavily by vascular channels, which supply the overlying respiratory epithelium. The lacrimal duct drains into the nose just lateral to the inferior-anterior portion of the inferior turbinate.

The anterior tip of the turbinates not only directs the air along the passageway to the nasopharynx in a laminar fashion but also acts to deflect some of the air upward towards the olfactory mucosa, thus facilitating olfaction. The *nasal cycle*, a periodic alternating engorgement and enlargement of the inferior turbinates on one side accompanied by contralateral turbinate shrinkage, occurs in about 85% of people. The cycle takes anywhere between 3 to 4 hours to complete, and the total airflow throughout the cycle remain constant. Often, in the postoperative setting, patients complain of alternating nasal obstruction, which is in effect a heightened awareness of the cycle due to surgery and resultant hypersensitivity.

NASAL AIRWAY OBSTRUCTION

There are several components that contribute to nasal airway obstruction. In the pediatric population, congenital anatomic contributions are significant, with adenoid hypertrophy and choanal atresia being the most common. For the adult population, in addition to anatomic considerations, such as septal deviation, septal spurs, and turbinate hypertrophy, the differential diagnoses of tumors and polyps need to be entertained and excluded. A list of nasal airway obstruction components is given in Table 35-1.

PREOPERATIVE ASSESSMENT

Using a headlight, nasal speculum, and an optional endoscope, the surgeon needs to perform diagnostic endoscopy of the nasal vault and nasopharynx. This allows full evaluation of these regions and exclusion of any nonanatomic causes of nasal airway obstruction. Specifically, it allows diagnosis of any visible polyps or malignancies. If purulent discharge or middle meatus obstruction is identified, sinusitis is likely and appropriate treatment with antibiotics is indicated. If an allergic component is considered, nasal steroid sprays, nonsedating antihistamines, and decongestants are first-line treatment. Allergy testing and desensitization should also be considered. Rhinitis medicamentosum must be ruled out and treated in individuals who chronically use oxymetazoline (Afrin), phenylephrine (Neo-Synephrine), and/or xylometazoline (Otrivin or

Inspire). If complete nasal deviation is noted, coexistent pathology needs to be ruled out with computed tomography.

Once adequate examination and workup have been completed and the appropriate diagnosis has been made, attention is then directed to treating the underlying etiology for the patient's nasal airway obstruction. Allergic rhinitis, chronic rhinosinusitis, and turbinate hypertrophy must be initially treated medically. Assuming that all other diagnoses have been ruled out and the patient is diagnosed with only septal deviation as the cause of the nasal aiway obstruction, the decision to perform a septoplasty is entertained. However, the contribution of the nasal turbinates should not be overlooked.

Prior to performing surgery, a thorough history needs to be taken, specifically addressing any coagulopathies, medication allergies, or coexisting medical conditions that can be medically optimized preoperatively. Additionally, patients with nasal polyps may be administered preoperative steroids to facilitate intraoperative bleeding and any associated asthma.

SURGICAL TECHNIQUE

The facial skin is prepared with povidine-iodine or chlorhexidine solution and draped to expose the face. Cotton pledgets soaked with neosynephrine and cocaine are inserted into the nares bilaterally to help achieve vasoconstriction. Using a small syringe and 27-gauge needle, 1% lidocaine with 1 : 100,000 epinephrine is injected to locally anesthetize the region. Local anesthesia is infiltrated externally if the patient is undergoing simultaneous rhinoplasty or internal/external valve reconstruction. The anesthetic is injected into the intercartilaginous region to block the external nasal nerve bilaterally, the edge of the piriform aperture to get the branches of the infrorbital nerve to the nasal ala, and the junction of the caudal septum and columella. Intranasally, it is injected between the perichondrium and the septal cartilage and between the mucoperiosteum and the bone to help achieve anesthesia, hydrodissect the surgical plane, and increase the soft tissue bulk to avoid inadvertent perforation of the mucoperichondrial flap. The inferior turbinates are also anesthetized bilaterally as needed. In the event of a severely deviated septum that precludes injection of the local anesthetic, a long nasal speculum is placed into the narrowed nasal cavity and deflected toward the contralateral side to allow for improved exposure.

In performing a septoplasty, there are two incisions that are typically used—hemitransfixion or Killian—and a decision as to which one to use is made by the surgeon (Figure 35-1). This decision is based on several factors. The hemitransfixion incision allows adequate exposure to address the septal deviation in both anterior and posterior regions. Furthermore, it allows placement of endonasal

Table 35-1 Components of Nasal Airway Obstruction

Septum	Polyps
Maxillary crest	Tumors
Turbinates	Narrowed pyriform aperture
External nasal valve	Stenosis
Internal nasal valve	Choanal atresia
Allergic rhinitis	Adenoid hypertrophy

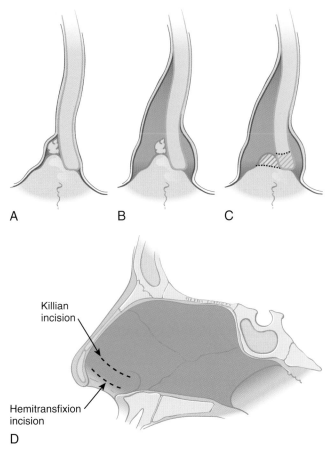

Killian
incision

Hemitransfixion
incision

D

Figure 35-1 A, The septum is deviated off the maxillary crest. **B,** Bilateral mucoperichondrial flaps have been elevated. **C,** Maxillary crest and inferior aspect of septum can be resected to centralize the septum. **D,** In septoplasty, there is a choice of two incisions that are performed: hemitransfixion or Killian. The hemitransfixion incision allows the surgeon adequate exposure to address septal deviation in both anterior and posterior regions. It is placed in the caudal cartilaginous septum extending from the dorsalmost to the caudalmost region. The Killian incision is similar except that it is placed posterior to the location of the hemitransfixion incision. This is often the preferred incision if the septal deviation that needs to be addressed is posterior. In either technique, the surgeon should leave at least a 1-cm strut on the caudal aspect to prevent postoperative loss of tip support.

spreader grafts by having access to the entire length of the upper lateral cartilage. The hemitransfixion incision is placed in the most caudal aspect of the cartilaginous septum.

The Killian incision is placed approximately 1 cm posterior to the location of the hemitransfixion incision. This is often the preferred incision if the septal deviation that needs to be addressed is predominantly posterior as it inherently leaves adequate caudal support. Surgeon preference will play a major role in deciding which incision is performed. In either technique, the surgeon should leave 1 to 2 cm of cartilaginous strut on the caudal and dorsal aspect of the septum to prevent postoperative loss of tip support that can lead to an aesthetically displeasing pollybeak deformity.

Accurate identification of the septal cartilage is the most critical aspect of the septoplasty because it will allow for adequate exposure of the septum and for hemostasis during the procedure. Using a Cottle elevator, the overlying mucoperichondrium is elevated and dissected off of the underlying cartilage. Adequate exposure of the septal cartilage will yield a bluish-grayish color and a gritty texture. Only after accurate identification can the remaining mucoperichondrial layer be elevated posteriorly to the vomer under direct visualization with adequate light and suction.

A septal floor can be encountered inferiorly near the nasal floor during elevation of the mucoperichondrial flaps, and extreme caution is indicated to avoid perforation. The mucosa is usually adhered to the subluxed cartilage, and careful elevation of the mucosa needs to be performed using a Freer or Cottle elevator. The spur should not be removed until there is adequate exposure and detachment from the overlying mucosa (see Figure 35-1A-C).

After adequate elevation of the mucoperichondrium, the septal cartilaginous incision can be made with a D-knife, Cottle elevator, or No. 15 blade scalpel, leaving at least a 1-cm caudal and dorsal strut of cartilage to prevent postoperative loss of tip support. This incision needs to be performed carefully to prevent cutting through the contralateral mucoperichondrium, which would lead to a through-and-through perforation. Once the septal cartilage is incised, the contralateral mucoperichondrium is elevated in a similar fashion in the plane between the cartilage and mucoperichondrium. Upon satisfactory completion of bilateral mucoperichondrial elevation, a nasal speculum is placed to straddle the septal cartilage.

Meticulous analysis of the nasal septum is critical. Only when all of the components contributing to the nasal airway obstruction are addressed will the patient have satisfactory results and clinical relief of the nasal airway obstruction. Several options exist if the mid-portion of the septal cartilage is found to be the culprit of the deviation. The septum can be removed (submucous resection) using a Ballenger swivel knife or D-knife, straightened manually by morselizing or scoring, or removed and replaced between the septal mucosa flaps (Figure 35-2). If a submucous resection is undertaken, a 1- to 2-cm L-strut of cartilage must be preserved in both the dorsal and caudal aspect of the septum to avoid saddle nose deformity as well as loss of tip support. Deviated septal cartilage outside the support structure of the L-strut can be resected in small pieces, preserving as much cartilage in place as possible.

Cartilage-sparing techniques are often preferred to submucous resection, although in many instances, the cartilage will be removed for use during the rhinoplasty portion of the procedure. Although moderately deformed septal cartilage cannot be repositioned without removal of some cartilage in most circumstances, there are some situations where it can be spared. One such situation is septal buckling, which can easily be overlooked without careful attention. Often, despite adequate submucous resection of the septal cartilage, septal buckling remains due to memory, maxillary crest abnormalities, and septal spurs. In these situations, either unilateral or bilateral septal stenting splints can be placed on the side of the septum with horizontal mattresses sutures. This allows support for the septum while straightening it and the septal splints can be removed after 1 to 3 weeks.

In many patients, the septum can be found to be deviated to the side, and on closer examination, the caudal septum is actually subluxed off of the maxillary crest. Two options exist for the surgeon in this situation. The swinging door technique can be used to remove the inferior portion of the septal cartilage followed by suturing the caudal septum in the midline position. Frequently, during the septoplasty, further inspection of the septum reveals that the caudal septum is actually displaced off of the maxillary crest, causing septal deviation and asymmetric nasal airflow. This situation can be easily resolved by excising the redundant and displaced septal cartilage along the nasal floor so that the caudal septum is free. This sufficiently allows positioning of the cartilaginous septum to the midline position.

The other option is to resect the caudal septal cartilage and reconstruct the tip with columellar strut grafts to provide stability and prevent postoperative pollybeak deformity. This can be prevented if the surgeon reserves a 1- to 2-cm L-strut on the caudal and dorsal aspects, which is paramount in resecting septal cartilage and bone.

Using an osteotome or rongeur, the surgeon can resect the bony portion along the maxillary crest. It is important to avoid pulling when removing cartilage or bone. Instead, Takahashi forceps can be used to safely remove tissue. When the forceps have engaged the tissue completely, a twisting motion can free the tissue before gently removing it from the nasal cavity. Pulling on tissue that is not completely detached from the surrounding structures may increase the risk of damage to the cribriform plate, since a large portion of septal tissue is connected to the ethmoid structures.

After correction of the bony deviation, the cartilaginous septum can be replaced on the trough of the maxillary crest and aligned perpendicularly, without deviating into either nasal airway. Sometimes, an anchoring suture, passed through the posterior septal angle and nasal spine, is necessary for stabilization of the cartilaginous septum in the midline.

CARTILAGINOUS INCISIONS OR SCORING OF CARTILAGE

Cartilage-scoring technique weakens the tensile strength of the cartilage and, after postoperative splinting, encourages it to scar into a straighter conformation.

A mucoperichondrial flap can be elevated on the concave side to place full-thickness incisions into the septum. The incisions can be made in either a checkerboard grid or horizontal-line pattern. Alternatively, one can remove small wedges of cartilage from the convex surface of the cartilage.

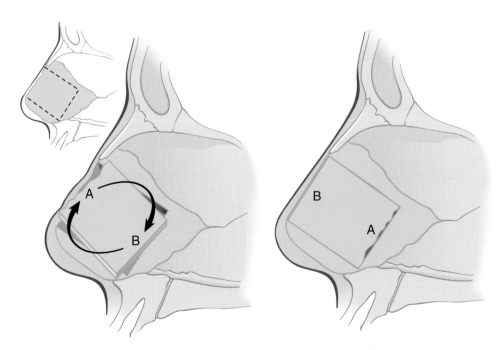

Figure 35-2 In cases where the mid-portion or superior aspect of the septum are severely deviated, the septum can be removed (submucous resection), straightened, rotated, and replaced back in place.

One technique involves incising the septal cartilage and scoring or removing thin wedges of septal cartilage from the convex side of the deviated septum to allow flexibility of the septum to encourage midline repositioning.

Another technique employed is morselization, which involves elevating the mucoperichondrium bilaterally and crushing the cartilage using Adson forceps or specially designed morselization instruments in an effort to destabilize the septal cartilage so that it will be straightened. While theoretically the concept is enticing, unfortunately, the extent of cartilage weakening is unpredictable. Therefore, the results are variable, and consequently, unreliable. The risk of losing dorsal support further contributes to the infrequent use of this particular technique.

Caudal septum: if caused by subluxation off the maxillary crest, use swinging door technique. Otherwise, resect and reconstruct with columellar strut grafts.

If turbinate reduction is not deemed necessary, the operation can conclude with closure of the mucoperichondrium and placement of quilting suture and/or nasal stents. However, if endoscopic sinus surgery, polypectomy, or rhinoplasty is to be performed in the same sitting, the septoplasty is used first and those procedures can be used prior to closing the Killian or hemitransfixion incision for maximum visualization. The septal mucosa is inspected so that any opposing perforations can be closed to prevent any through-and-through defects. This can be accomplished using a 4-0 chromic suture in a purse-string fashion. Isolated perforations limited to only one side do not need to be sutured and can be thought to serve as a drainage route for any potential postoperative hematomas that may accumulate. With a 3-0 chromic suture on a Keith needle, a quilting stitch is placed through both sides of the mucosal flaps to adhere the flaps to the underlying cartilage and prevent postoperative hematoma formation followed by closure of the Killian or hemitransfixion incision. Septal splint placement is optional and depends on the surgeon's preference. Some find it advantageous because it eliminates the need for packing and prevents synechiae or hematoma formation. If splints are used, a stitch is usually loosely placed to secure them to each other in front of the columella and prevent inadvertent displacement posteriorly into the airway. Removal of the splints occurs approximately 1 to 3 weeks postoperatively. Others use antibiotic-impregnated nasal packing combined with oral antibiotics or mattress sutures. Patients with nasal packing must be placed on oral antibiotics to avoid toxic shock syndrome related to staphylococcal infection.

TURBINATE REDUCTION

The subjective sensation of nasal airway obstruction has led surgeons to focus attention to the contributing role of the inferior turbinates. It has been noted that the most common cause of nasal airway obstruction in the 20- to 60-year-old age range is chronic turbinate hypertrophy that can be secondary to anatomy, vasomotor, endocrine, allergic, or environmental rhinitis. Rhinitis medicamentosum must be ruled out and treated in individuals who chronically use Afrin, Neo-Synephrine, and/or Otrivin or Inspire. As medical management is often unsuccessful, surgical turbinate reduction is often used.

Inferior turbinate hypertrophy leading to nasal airway obstruction is often broken down into two categories: (1) enlarged turbinate bone with normal mucosa from either developmental or traumatic causes and (2) thickened turbinate mucosa from inflammation, allergy, endocrine factors, or drug-induced rhinitis. However, the most common etiology is compensatory hypertrophy of the turbinate mucosa secondary to significant septal deviation.

Turbinates form the lateral border of the internal nasal valve, thus exerting most of their obstructive effect anteriorly. Inferior turbinate hypertrophy can cause significant nasal airway obstruction, as it is the most distal region of airflow in the nose. There have been multiple techniques to address turbinate hypertrophy. Submucous resection is the most effective method, especially if bony hypertrophy significantly contributes to the problem. Using this method, the overlying inferior turbinate mucosa is incised and a Cottle elevator is used to free up the underlying bone from the overlying mucosa. Once this is adequately performed, the bony portion is removed and the incision is reapproximated. Other methods include microdebrider submucous resection, radiofrequency ablation (Coblation; ArthroCare, Austin, TX), and cauterization of the inferior turbinate mucosa adjacent to the bony portion. The main goal of achieving improvement in nasal airway obstruction occurs via volume reduction to prevent obstruction of the airflow through the nostrils. Mucosa-sparing techniques lead to faster healing and less crusting, in addition to preventing empty nose syndrome.

INTERNAL NASAL VALVE

The nasal valves are responsible for creating the narrowest region in the nares and, subsequently, the airflow is turbulent in these regions. The external nasal valve is bounded by mobile alar side walls. The internal nasal valve corresponds to the middle nasal vault externally and is situated between the septum, caudal upper lateral cartilages, and inferior turbinates, creating an approximately 10- to 15-degree angle. Despite a successful aesthetic rhinoplasty, if proper attention is not made to nasal functionality, significant problems can arise. Therefore, when performing a rhinoplasty, attention should be directed to avoiding overzealous dorsal reduction and cephalic resection. Patients with short nasal bones, preexisting narrowed internal nasal valves, and/or aggressive dorsal hump reductions are at a high risk of developing postoperative internal nasal valve collapse. Prophylactic nasal valve reconstruction is necessary to avoid significant postoperative functional and aesthetic deformity in the middle nasal vault. Additionally, lateral osteotomies can result in narrowing of the nose resulting in inadequate airflow and clinical awareness of nasal airway obstruction. Furthermore, the location of the intercartilaginous incision should be carefully placed to avoid postoperative cicatrical web formation and stenosis.

The internal nasal valve is the narrowest region of airflow, and it is often necessary to surgically address this region to improve nasal airway obstruction. This can be performed using a variety of techniques (Figure 35-3). A common technique is to use spreader grafts fashioned from septal or rib cartilage. While conchal cartilage can also be used to create spreader grafts, this is less desired as it is likely to have more curvature and less fortitude. Spreader grafts can be placed endonasally or via and external rhinoplasty approach. They are typically placed in between the septum and the upper lateral cartilages. The grafts can be unilateral, bilateral, identical, or asymmetric depending on the problem at hand.

In addition to spreader grafts, flaring sutures can be used to directly improve the internal nasal valve angle. Using the external rhinoplasty approach, the caudal-lateral portion of the upper lateral cartilage is visualized. A 5-0 clear nylon horizontal mattress stitch placed in this region of the upper lateral cartilage across the nasal dorsum is anchored to the contralateral upper lateral cartilage. As the suture is tied, the upper lateral cartilages contract dorsally, and any previously placed spreader grafts and the nasal dorsum serves as a fulcrum. These sutures directly increase the internal valve angle, which can be visualized as the suture is tied. Occasionally, the flaring suture alone can significantly improve nasal airway obstruction caused by internal valve collapse, usually in situations where the middle nasal vault is destabilized.

Other techniques include onlay grafts, autospreader grafts, butterfly grafts, and the orbital suspension suturing method. Butterfly grafts can be used to help improve significant internal nasal valve dysfunction. Using an intercartilaginous incision, previously harvested conchal cartilage grafts fashioned into butterfly grafts are placed in the supratip region and sutured to the caudal edge of the upper lateral cartilages. Although not commonly used for primary surgical intervention, orbital suspension technique can be used in patients who have had unsuccessful middle nasal vault reconstruction. This method suspends a collapsed nasal valve to the orbital rim.

EXTERNAL NASAL VALVES

External nasal valves can also contribute to decreased nasal airflow by collapsing the nasal alae with negative pressure with inspiratory airflow. Multiple factors can also contribute to the lack of support in the external nasal valve, including iatrogenic, traumatic, congenital, and senescent causes. To stabilize the external nasal valve, the most common surgical methods of repair include lateral crural strut or batten grafts (Figure 35-4).

Batten grafts are typically placed on top of existing cartilage in the alar region. Alar batten grafts are used to fortify weakened or absent lower lateral cartilages or nasal sidewalls. Septal, conchal, or rib cartilage serve as excellent sources of graft material. These batten grafts are fashioned and then anchored using 5-0 chromic sutures to the nasal mucosa to reinforce those areas of the side wall or the alar lobule that collapse with inspiration. These grafts do not typically change the resting position of the valve. In thin-skinned patients, it is especially important to thin the grafts and to bevel the edges to prevent external visualization of the graft. Alar batten grafts are sewn in place to act as a reinforcement against dynamic collapse in the area of the lateral crura. Lateral crural strut grafts can also be used to prevent and treat external nasal valve collapse. Lateral crural strut grafts refer to cartilaginous reinforcement that is placed deep to the exisiting alar cartilage.

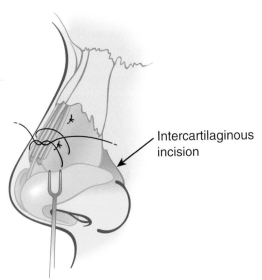

Intercartilaginous incision

Figure 35-3 The internal nasal valve is the narrowest region of airflow, and it is often necessary to surgically address this region to improve nasal airway obstruction. This can be performed using a variety of techniques. A common technique is to use spreader grafts fashioned from septal or costal cartilage. While conchal cartilage can also be used to create spreader grafts, this is less desired as it is more likely to have slight curvature. Two identical thin pieces are fashioned from the cartilage and placed on each side of the remaining septal cartilage strut to widen the region of the internal nasal valve. To maintain their position adjacent to the strut, sutures are placed to anchor the spreader grafts in the location desired for maximal effect. Flaring sutures can also be used to further improve the internal nasal valve.

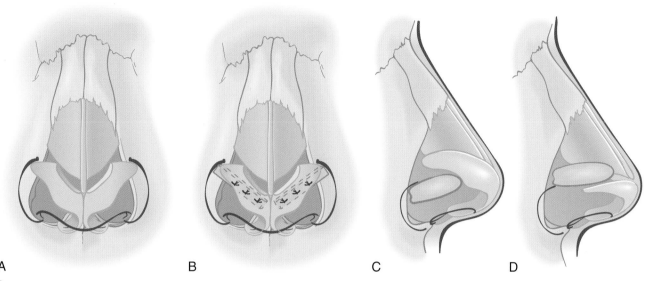

A   B   C   D

Figure 35-4 A, B, Lateral crural strut grafts are placed deep to lateral crura. **C, D,** Alar batten grafts are placed over the lateral crura.

CONCLUSION

Successful treatment of nasal airway obstruction depends largely on careful analysis of the underlying anatomy and structure, while scrutinizing the correct diagnosis preoperatively, intraoperatively, and postoperatively. As many causes for nasal airway obstruction exist, the surgeon needs to properly address all possibilities at the time of surgery and use appropriate surgical planning and intervention.

REFERENCES

1. Goode RL. *Diagnosis and treatment of turbinate dysfunction. A self-instructional package*. Alexandria, CA: American Academy of Otolaryngology–Head and Neck Surgery; 1977.
2. Schlosser RJ, Park SS. Surgery for the dysfunctional nasal valve: cadaveric analysis and clinical outcomes. *Arch Fac Plast Surg*. 1999;1:105–110.

CHAPTER THIRTY-SIX

Nasal Reconstruction

Arnold Lee • Aric Park

The nose occupies a central position both anatomically and aesthetically in determining the overall appearance of the face. Surgery for reconstruction of the nose has a long history, dating back at least to 2000 BC. In India, nasal reconstruction has been performed by specialized castes for millennia. This grew out of necessity as a common punishment for adulterers, thieves, and prisoners was amputation of the tip of the nose to permanently disfigure the offender. Around 600 BC, Sushruta published *Sushruta Samihta*, a detailed text reviewing cheek flaps for reconstruction of the nose. Accounts of the midline forehead flap had been noted since at least 1440 AD by a caste of potters in India known as the Koomas. In 1597, Tagliacozzi published a staged nasal reconstruction using skin from the forearm, the first report in the West. The origins of facial plastic surgery can be found in these early attempts by surgeons to recreate a structure that defines aesthetic appearance.[1]

Centuries of refinement and experience have led to current techniques of nasal reconstruction. Defining the normal appearance and appropriate function of the nose has changed only slightly with passing time and cultural preferences. The importance of understanding the characteristics that create the subtle interplay of light and shadows that are perceived as a nose cannot be understated. Only by understanding the anatomy and topography of the structure to be reconstructed can a comprehensive plan for surgery be created. Once a common groundwork of anatomy and physiometry has been established, the surgeon can begin to explore the art and science of this challenging surgery.

OVERVIEW

When approaching a nasal defect, a systematic method of analyzing the reconstructive options is crucial. Consideration of the location, size, orientation, and depth of the defect are all important. In evaluating the location of the defect, we find it helpful to divide the nose into thirds—upper third, middle third, and lower third, each of which has its own specific reconstructive nuances and pitfalls. The size and orientation of the defect also need to be thoughtfully analyzed when deciding upon a

reconstructive option. The immobile structures surrounding the defect (i.e., hairline, eyelid, melolabial fold, among others) need to be considered. Larger defects may require recruitment of tissue from surrounding areas so as not to cause distortion of adjacent features. Also, the orientation of the defect may allow scars to lie within favorable areas maximally camouflaging resulting scars. Next, the depth of the lesion will determine the extent of repair required. The nose can be broken down to three layers for repair: the skin covering, cartilaginous support, and mucosal lining. All layers that are affected need to be reconstructed. Repairing one or two layers in a full-thickness defect without addressing the remaining layers will result in postoperative scarring and a poor aesthetic outcome as the nose becomes distorted under the cicatricial healing forces of the underlying scar. Finally, the subunits involved should be identified. While this may seem trivial, in wounds that have been allowed to heal by secondary intention, the true magnitude of the defect may be obscured until the initial scar tissue has been excised, allowing a complete, aesthetic repair to be performed. Together, these factors will determine the type of repair used.

There are multiple techniques that are possible for the repair of a given defect, each with their advantages and disadvantages. We will limit our discussion to methods that are commonly used in our practice that have provided acceptable and consistent results—the "workhorse" techniques.

ANATOMY

The basic anatomy of the nose is important to review prior to discussion of surgical techniques. The subunit principle consists of the observation that shadows naturally fall at the junction of the concavities and convexities of the nose. These surface contours divide the nose into nine distinct aesthetic subunits—nasal tip, paired soft tissue triangles, both ala, nasal dorsum, the two lateral nasal walls, and the columella (Figure 36-1). Scars that fall at the junction of the aesthetic subunits tend to be better camouflaged as opposed to scars that cross a subunit. Lesions involving greater than 50% of a subunit are often best repaired with

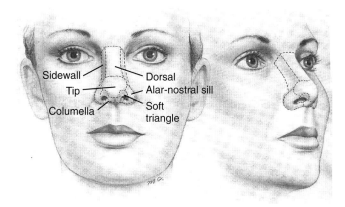

Figure 36-1 Nasal subunits—dorsum, paired lateral sidewalls, nasal tip, nasal alae, columella, soft tissue triangles.

complete excision and reconstruction of the entire subunit. Lesions or defects involving less than 50% of such subunit are often able to be closed without further sacrifice of surrounding unaffected tissue. When the nose and the entire face are viewed in this manner, the surgeon is able to plan the nasal reconstruction by breaking down even a very large defect according to the subunits it encompasses and formulate a plan for repair by approaching each affected subunit as an individual entity. This principle applies mostly to subunits that are convex such as the nasal tip, alae, dorsum, and columella. This concept is critical due to the natural tendency of skin flaps to contract into convex circular mounds of tissue if unopposed by a structural framework to support it. Skin grafts that are supported by a framework of bone or cartilage will resist this contracture and largely keep their form, making them ideal in reconstructing concave areas such as the nasal sidewalls.[2]

The quality of the skin to be repaired is very important in nasal reconstruction. The upper third of the nose, consisting of the nasal dorsum and lateral walls, has a thicker skin with more laxity. The middle third skin is thin and elastic. Skin grafts and local flaps do well in reconstructing this region. The lower third, consisting of the nasal tip, alae, soft tissue triangles, and columella, has thicker, sebaceous, less pliable skin, which poorly matches most skin grafts. The thick, stiff nature of the skin can make local flaps less reliable and may necessitate the use of pedicled flaps, as we will discuss later. The skin of the dorsal nose tapers to the rhinion, where it is the thinnest. In patients with large defects, the opposite side may be used to estimate the quality of the skin to be repaired.

Underlying the skin is loose areolar tissue followed by the musculature of the nose. These are connected by an aponeurotic system of fibrous tissue that is contiguous with the superficial muscular aponeurotic system (SMAS).

The framework of the nose consists of paired quadrangular nasal bones, upper lateral cartilages, lower lateral cartilages, and the septum. The septum acts as the

support for the nose from which the upper and lower lateral cartilages are suspended. An in-depth understanding of the shape, position, and strength of the lower lateral cartilage will prove invaluable in reconstruction of defects involving the nasal alae and tip. Even areas that are not covered by cartilage, such as the soft tissue triangles, must be reconstructed with a supporting framework or risk contraction of the overlying flap or graft.

In evaluating the mucosal lining of the nose, the skin of the vestibule is made up of stratified squamous epithelium. This transitions to the typical pseudostratified ciliated columnar epithelium of the inner lining of the nose just beyond the vibrissae of the vestibule. The thickness of the lining is important to note as reconstruction with thick flaps may lead to obstruction of the external nasal valve. Additionally, use of thinner skin grafts in areas normally covered by mucosa can lead to significant crusting and ozena. Finally, placing mucosa in areas normally covered by stratified squamous epithelium will lead to easy bleeding and irritation due to its proximity to the outside environment and desiccation.

REPAIR OF SURFACE DEFECTS

Repair of superficial cutaneous nasal defects should be based on the size, color, texture, and curvature of the area to be repaired. While many options exist for a given defect, we will approach this issue by dividing the nose into upper two thirds and lower third to simplify the surgical options available. Overall, the goal of surgical reconstruction of unilateral defects should be to replace tissues with those similar in texture and color. The subunit principle should be applied whenever possible. When planning for closure of defects, scars should ideally come to rest in the areas between subunits.

NASAL DEFECTS OF THE UPPER TWO THIRDS OF THE NOSE

The upper two thirds of the nose consists of the nasal dorsum and lateral nasal walls extending from the glabella to the caudal aspect of the nasal bone. The skin tends to be relatively thin, less sebaceous, and more mobile compared to the lower third of the nose. This region is supported by the nasal bones and the upper lateral cartilages. For very small cutaneous lesions primarily over the nasal bones, closure by secondary intention remains an excellent option. Primary closure is possible in this region due to the relative mobility of the soft tissue envelope. Scars that are placed along the relaxed skin tension lines (RSTL) and at the junction of aesthetic subunits tend to camouflage best.[3]

Larger lesions in this region can be reconstructed with full-thickness skin grafts (Figure 36-2). This is ideal for the lateral nasal side walls, which has relatively thin,

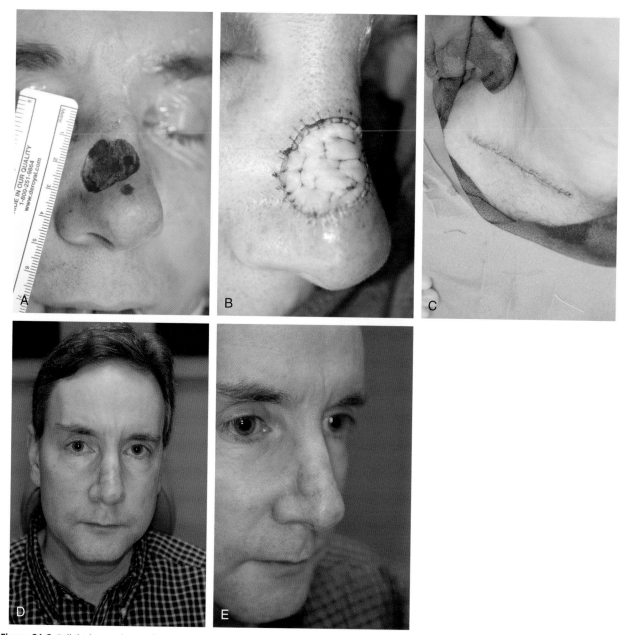

Figure 36-2 Full-thickness skin graft. **A,** Large superficial defect involving the lateral nasal side wall and nasal dorsum. After discussion of treatment options with the patient, he elected for repair with FTSG. **B,** FTSG harvested from excess skin in supraclavicular fossa. Bolstering sutures placed to prevent seroma formation. **C,** Secondary defect in supraclavicular fossa closed. **D,** Repair after 2.5 months. **E,** Close-up of repair at 2.5 months. Some residual hypervascularity is evident around the healing wound.

shiny skin and falls within the natural shadows of the nose. Grafts are most commonly harvested from the preauricular region due to the excellent color and texture match. When additional skin is required, skin from the supraclavicular fossa, nasolabial fold, neck, upper eyelid, or postauricular region can be used (Figure 36-3). A template of the defect is created using the foil from a suture packet, which bends easily to fit the contours of the nose. This is transposed to the proposed donor site. As with all skin grafts, a healthy vascularized wound bed is necessary for graft survival. If the periosteum or perichondrium has been removed with the lesion, a vascularized bed must be in place for successful uptake. Of note, the skin grafts must be supported with either a bony or cartilaginous framework. Without this, the graft will shrink due to contraction of myofibroblasts. During the healing process, the surrounding recipient skin can supply the full-thickness skin graft up to 3 ml away by nutrient and oxygen diffusion. Once the graft is harvested, the surgeon thins the graft by removing the subcutaneous fat until the white portion of the dermis is visible. This increases the likelihood of vascularization and subsequent graft viability. It is worth noting that overaggressive thinning of the graft can lead to loss of the dermal layer,

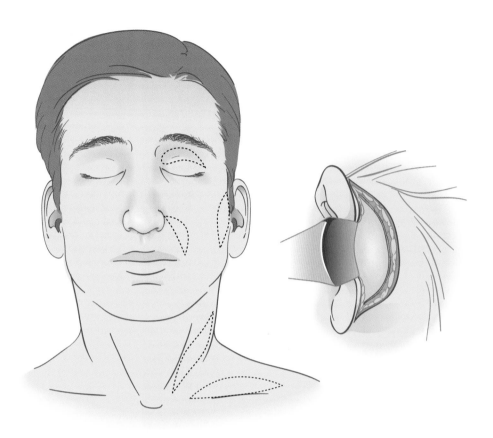

Figure 36-3 Locations for skin graft donor sites on the head and neck.

leaving the patient with a split-thickness skin graft and the potential for postoperative contracture with irregularity of color and texture. The graft is then placed into the defect and any excess skin is gently trimmed. When trimming the edges of the skin graft, we find it helpful to first trim one side of the graft to fit, which is then sutured into place. The second side is then trimmed and inset and so on until the remaining three sides are subsequently cut to fit the defect. Basting sutures are applied between the graft and the vascularized bed with fast absorbing gut suture to prevent seroma or hematoma formation (Figure 36-4). Central basting sutures prevent the graft from lifting off the bed, while peripheral sutures keep the graft aligned in proper position. Those sutures that remain at the first postoperative visit at 5 to 7 days are then removed.

When possible, we try to use local flaps because of the advantage of similar skin color, thickness, and contours as the missing tissue. In the upper two thirds of the nose, transposition flaps such as the bilobed and rhomboid flap may be used with excellent results.

Bilobed flaps are the most commonly used flaps for repair of smaller nasal defects (<1.5 cm) in our practice, our "workhorse" flap (Figure 36-5). They are based on a random blood supply. The initial bilobed flap as described by Esser uses two equal flaps with a 90- and 180-degree rotation. The amount of rotation and large flaps led to excessive tension on the surround tissues, buckling around

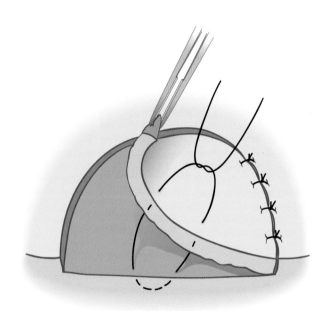

Figure 36-4 Basting sutures applied to prevent seroma formation.

the pivot point, and distal distortion. Multiple modifications have been made on the original design with improved outcomes. We often follow the modifications described by Zitelli in our flap design. The angle of rotation has been decreased to less than 50 degrees per flap, or less than

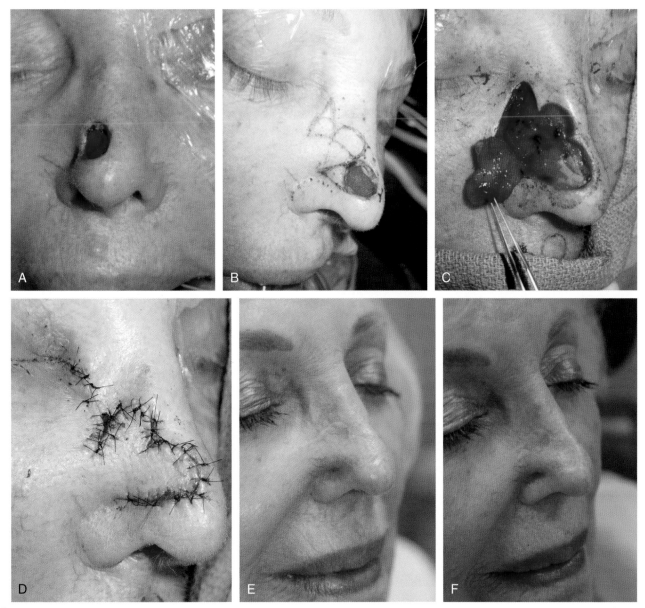

Figure 36-5 Zitelli modification of a bilobed flap. **A,** Superficial defect after MOHS resection of squamous cell cancer involving the lateral nasal side wall, nasal dorsum, and nasal tip about 1.5 cm in diameter. **B,** Bilobed flap designed with laterally based pedicle. The initial flap is equal in size to the defect, while the second flap measures about 80% of the original defect. Burow's triangles have been included in the planning to excise excess tissue and prevent dog ears. **C,** The flap has been mobilized from the SMAS layer. **D,** Inset of the flap with closure of the dog ears. **E,** Repair after 4 months. **F,** Repair after 8 months.

100 degrees for the arc of the entire flap.[4] In general, for the upper two thirds of the nose, a laterally based flap works best. This allows for the majority of the scars to lie within the shadowed lateral nasal wall and can allow for the two relatively linear incisions to lie within junctions of aesthetic subunits.

The initial step in designing the flap is to determine the point of rotation, or the pivot point. This point must be situated sufficiently away from critical adjacent structures such as the lower eyelid, which may cause distortion when the flap is transposed. The pivot point is approximately one radius of the defect away from the edge of a

circular lesion. From the pivot point, a Burow's triangle is marked to account for the standing cone deformity that will occur from the rotation of the flaps. The closure of this limb of the flap will create the first linear scar. We, therefore, attempt to place one side of the Burow's triangle at the junction of aesthetic subunits when possible, such as at the supra-alar crease.

Once the pivot point is determined and the Burow's triangle is marked, we then mark out two arcs: one from the pivot point to the most distal edge of the defect and one from the pivot point to the midpoint of the defect. We use a piece of foil to measure the arc of rotation rather than a straight ruler as the curvature of the nose can add significant extra length to the pivot point. It is between these arcs that our lobes will be marked. The first flap is drawn the same size as the defect. Again, the foil from a suture packet can be used to make a template of the original defect for creation of the primary lobe to ensure adequate size. The second lobe is marked approximately 20% smaller than the original defect to ease in closure. A Burow's triangle is extended from the second lobe to account for the eventual standing cone deformity. The angle between the defect and the secondary flap can be adjusted between 90 degrees and no more than 100 degrees to allow for the closure of the secondary defect to lie at the junction of aesthetic subunits.

Once the markings are complete, wide undermining in the sub-SMAS plane ensues prior to making any releasing incisions. The advantage to undermining in this plane is that it is relatively avascular, the blood supply to the flaps is preserved, and there is less postoperative "pincushioning" of the circular flaps compared to a subcutaneous dissection. Once widely undermined, the flaps are released along the markings, keeping the incisions between the two arcs. The flaps are gently rotated into position and the tension on the flap is assessed. If there is too much tension, the releasing incision along the second lobe is lengthened beyond the lower arc, taking care not to narrow the base of the flap excessively. The incisions are then meticulously closed in layers. This flap is generally limited to defects no larger than 1.5 cm in diameter, as larger flaps will tend to distort surrounding structures when closing the primary and the resulting secondary defects.

In the superior nasal dorsal region, a transposition flap from the glabella works well to repair cutaneous defects. This region has abundant loose skin in comparison to the nasal dorsum and often a unilobed flap such as a banner or rhomboid flap can be used (Figure 36-6). Scars may be oriented vertically to hide in

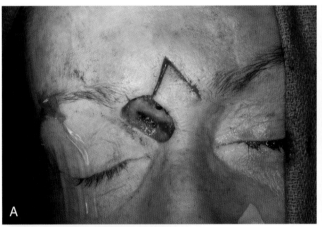

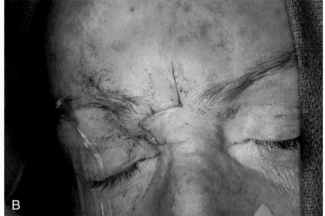

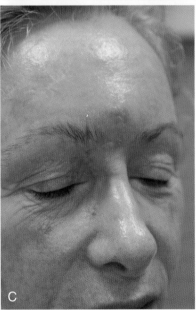

Figure 36-6 Rhomboid flap. **A,** Defect with incision through tissue of the glabella. **B,** Wound after rotation of flap. Note the scars are oriented to hide in the vertical and horizontal rhytids. **C,** One-month postoperative film.

existing glabellar rhytids in the region. Here, undermining is performed in the subcutaneous plane, taking care to avoid injury to the supratrochlear and supraorbital neurovascular bundles.

Defects larger than 1.5 cm in diameter can often be addressed using a superiorly based melolabial flap (Figure 36-7). The skin color and texture can match that of the skin of the nasal dorsum well, but often the flap needs to be thinned of the subcutaneous fat to match the thickness. Generally, defects up to 3 cm can be repaired with these flaps, although the width of the flap is dependent on the inherent laxity of the cheek skin. These random flaps can reach from the lateral nasal sidewall to the nasal tip. The main limitation of the flap occurs when it is carried too far superiorly, at which point distortion of the lower eyelid can occur, leading to ectropion. The flap is marked out along the ipsilateral melolabial crease. The height of the defect is measured and used as the width of the flap. The medial border of the flap is marked out precisely within the existing melolabial crease, and a Burow's triangle is designed to taper distally into the crease as well. The lateral limb is extended no higher than the level of the

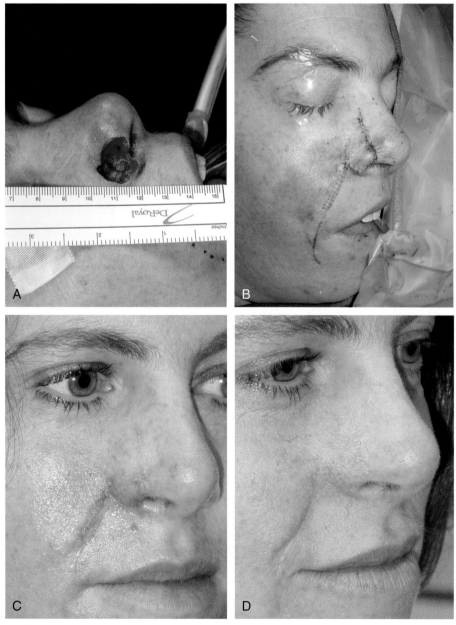

Figure 36-7 Melolabial flap. **A,** Superficial defect involving the nasal ala. A superiorly based melolabial flap was designed to close the wound with minimal tension. **B,** Post flap inset. Note the recreating of the nasolabial sulcus. **C,** Patient after 3 weeks. There is some hyperplasia and edema of the nasolabial sulcal incision. This was treated early with intralesional Kenalog. **D,** At 3 months post surgery, the supra-alar fullness and edema have resolved, leaving a well-camouflaged scar in the nasolabial sulcus.

inferior border of the defect to ensure a sufficiently wide flap base. In men, the border of the bearded and non-bearded skin is marked. If possible, only the non–hair-bearing skin is used for the flap. The nasal defect is undermined in the sub-SMAS plane and releasing incisions are made sharply. The Burow's triangle is elevated along with the flap. This can be very useful if the flap was improperly planned and slightly shorter than anticipated. The cheek skin is undermined in the subcutaneous plane widely and advanced until the donor defect is closed with as little tension as possible. The cheek defect is first closed. This takes tension off of the nasal closure and thus can allow for accurate trimming of the flap to fit the defect. Once transposed and inset, the flap is closed in layers. Disadvantages of this flap include potential blunting of the nasofacial sulcus and asymmetry of the sulcus; however, these problems are easily resolved with minor secondary procedures.[5]

An alternative to the melolabial flap for lesions of the nasal dorsum to nasal tip is the nasal dorsal flap of Reiger. We find this to be an excellent alternative in closure of defects in the middle third. This is a random-based flap that uses loose skin from the glabellar region to assist in closing defects. In performing this procedure, the skin, subcutaneous, and SMAS layers are lifted off the nasal dorsum above the periosteum, the flap is then rotated downward, and the loose skin around the glabella is mobilized to close the subsequent defect in a V-to-Y advancement. A standing cone deformity may develop at the caudal aspect of the flap. The advantages to this flap are that it allows for a single staged repair with excellent color and texture match. This closure, however, does not follow the subunit principle and will leave visible scars in exposed areas. Defects greater than 2.5 cm will lead to significant deformity from closure of the secondary defect. Additionally, it requires the mobilization of a large amount of healthy skin, which may be at risk of necrosis in smokers or those with microvascular disease.[6]

NASAL DEFECTS OF THE LOWER THIRD OF THE NOSE

The lower third of the nose is divided into the nasal tip, ala, columella, soft tissue triangles, and sill. As with small lesions of the upper two thirds, primary closure is a viable alternative for very small defects. The thick skin of the nasal tip does not lend itself well to skin grafting, as the graft will have a noticeable difference in coloration and texture match with the surrounding recipient site. As with lesions of the upper two thirds of the nose, a local flap repair is preferred because of the advantages previously discussed. The technique of choice for lesions up to 1.5 cm in diameter is reconstruction with a bilobed flap. The design is the same as previously discussed but with some specific aspects to consider. When determining a pivot point, the surgeon must be very careful not to orient it

too close to the alar margin. The movement of the flap can distort the margin very easily. Care must be taken in repairing the nasal tip to properly assess the size of the defect using a bendable or pliable template to take into account the convexity of the tip. Because the thicker skin in this region has very poor elasticity, very little margin for error exists in the flap design and a very tight closure can easily result if the convexities are ignored. For defects of the nasal tip, laterally based bilobed flaps work well, whereas medially based flaps can be used with alar defects. The amount of tension that the wound is under can contribute to postoperative alar retraction with dehiscence or scarring, limiting its use in larger defects.

The ala and the alar margin require special attention in planning a reconstruction. These regions are composed of fibrofatty tissue and are devoid of underlying cartilage and therefore are subject to a high rate of distortion due to scar contracture if not properly supported. For smaller lesions, less than 1.5 cm, involving the alar margin, a composite graft offers a simple one-stage solution. A composite graft contains two or more layers of tissue. It is an excellent graft for defects of the alar margin as it can retain the natural thin and delicate quality of the ala without the use of thick, bulky flaps. Due to the lack of a large vascularized bed on which to place the composite graft, it is inherently limited in size by diffusion of nutrients through the wound bed. In practice, we find that defects up to 1.5 cm can be repaired through this technique; attempts at grafting larger defects may result in necrosis of the graft due to the graft's high metabolic demands. Also a limitation of this technique is that the skin eventually takes on the characteristics of the ear and becomes thin and shiny. The composite graft, therefore, may not be ideal for an individual that has a very thick sebaceous alar skin due to the mismatch in skin texture.

Harvesting the graft is relatively uncomplicated. First, a template is created of the defect to be repaired using a piece of foil. This is then transferred onto the skin over the root of the superior helix or posterior concha. In our practice, the most commonly used donor area is the root of the helix (Figure 36-8). We particularly like this area because the helical margin very closely mimics the alar margin. The graft is excised in full thickness, with overlying skin, subcutaneous tissue, cartilage, subcutaneous tissue, and underlying skin en bloc. We will typically harvest a slightly larger graft than the defect and trim the skin to the appropriate size. This leaves a flange of cartilage that can be placed into the undermined defect in a "tongue in groove" method as described by Skouge.[7] This will allow for a greater surface area to be in contact with the vascularized wound bed as compared to a graft that is sutured into position end to end. The skin edges are sutured, and for partial-thickness defects, through-and-though basting sutures are placed to keep the graft well apposed to the wound bed. A light dressing is applied and

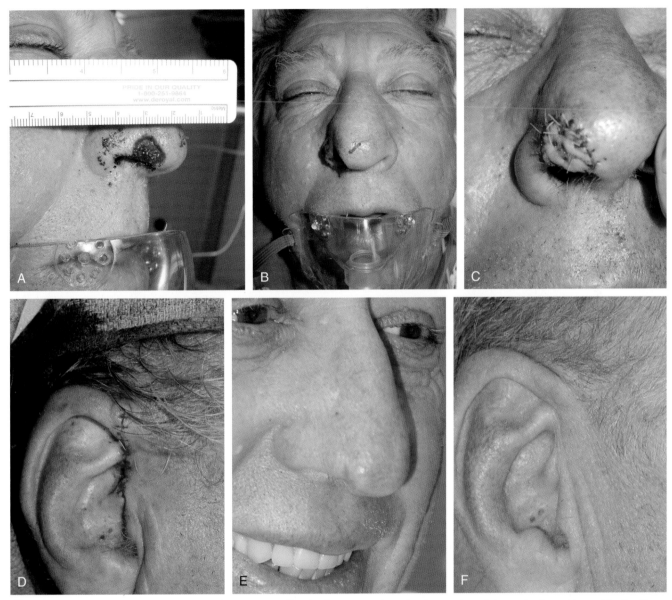

Figure 36-8 Composite grafting. **A,** Defect after resection of basal cell cancer involving the alar margin, soft tissue triangle, and lower lateral cartilage. The defect measures 1 cm in diameter. **B,** On frontal view, there is noticeable collapse of the right ala due to loss of cartilage. **C,** A two-layer composite graft was used to repair the defect. The soft tissues were undermined to allow a flange of cartilage to be inserted in a tongue in groove fashion. **D,** The superior crus after closure of the initial defect. **E,** Repair after 12 months. There is some slight notching of the alar rim on 45-degree view; however, note the excellent color and texture match of the skin. **F,** The auricular defect is almost imperceptible.

the patient is instructed to apply an antibiotic ointment to the graft and donor site incisions three times per day. For lesions between 2 to 3 cm in diameter of the ala and alar margin, a superiorly based melolabial flap can be very effective. These flaps are well vascularized and can therefore support cartilage grafts. The flap is designed as described in the previous section. Disadvantages of this flap for reconstructing the nasal ala is the loss of the superior alar crease as well as possible blunting of the nasofacial sulcus. However, these problems are easily resolved with minor secondary procedures.

PARAMEDIAN FOREHEAD FLAP

For large defects of the nasal surface, the paramedian forehead flap is our reconstructive technique of choice. It is able to provide covering for defects ranging from a single subunit to nearly the entire soft tissue envelope of the nose. Based on the supratrochlear artery running between the corrugator and frontalis muscles, the flap has an excellent blood supply and can support long pedicles, often extending well into the hairline. The vascular supply runs in a vertical direction and can often be identified with a hand-held Doppler.[5] The skin texture and color provide an excellent match to the native skin of the nose (Figure 36-9).

The flap is designed by making a precise template of the defect using a suture foil packet to outline in three dimensions the skin needed. This is then transferred to the forehead and retraced along the distribution of the supratrochlear artery. The flap proceeds in a vertical direction along the path of the artery. It is imperative when tracing the template to ensure that it is oriented correctly for the later transposition. In our experience, the use of the Doppler device enables us to narrow the pedicle. A narrow pedicle (<1.5 cm) allows for an improved arc of rotation. Thicker pedicles increase the tension on the tissue being rotated and may increase the likelihood of flap failure. The flap is then dissected in the subcutaneous plane for 1 to 2 cm distally, unless the patient is a smoker. In nonsmokers, hair follicles can be removed from the distal end of the flap with a sharp pair of iris scissors. At this point, dissection proceeds to just above the periosteum in the subgaleal plane. The dissection continues inferiorly as much as needed until adequate mobility of the flap is achieved. If required, the pedicle can be dissected to the level of the supratrochlear foramen well below the supraorbital rim. The flap is thinned of all galea and frontalis muscle, taking care to visually identify and

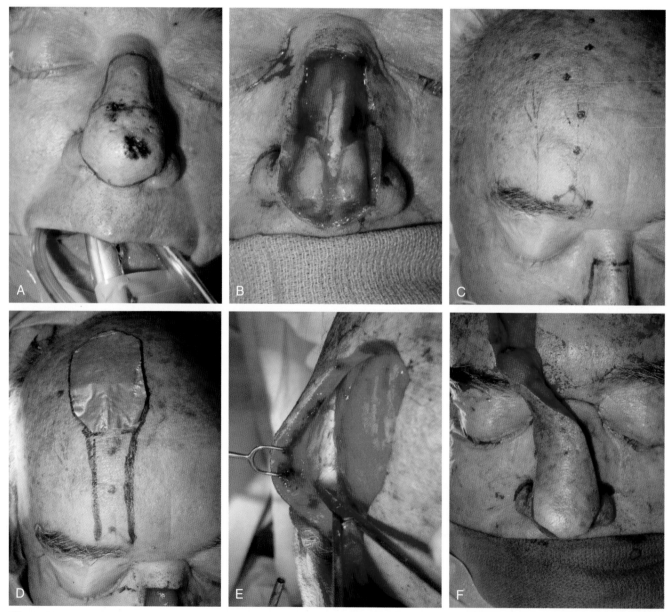

Figure 36-9 Forehead flap cont. **A,** The proposed excision of nasal melanoma along aesthetic subunits. **B,** Defect of the nasal tip and nasal dorsum. **C,** The supratrochlear artery marked out using a hand-held Doppler. **D,** A foil template of the nasal defect transposed over the forehead. **E,** Undermining of the forehead secondary defect. **F,** The transposed flap onto the nasal defect.

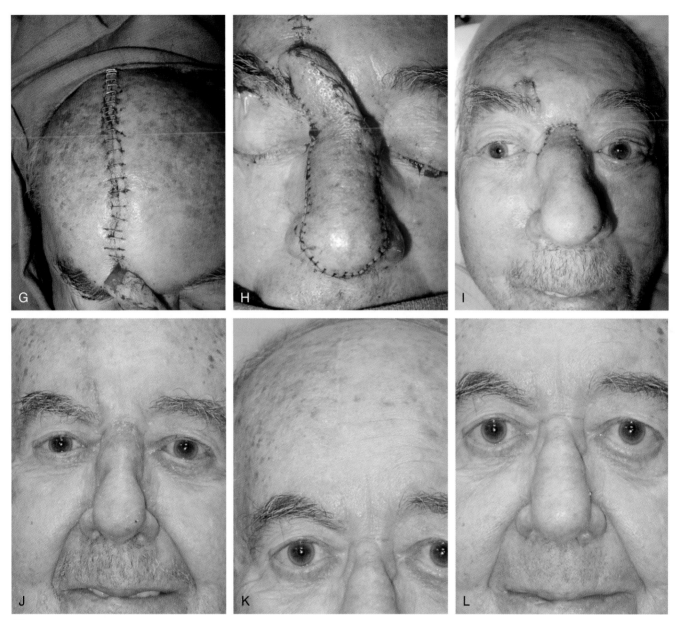

Figure 36-9, cont'd G, Closure of the secondary defect. The surrounding tissues were undermined and underwent intraoperative tissue expansion. This allowed for primary closure of the initial defect. **H,** The exposed surface of the forehead pedicle is covered with an alloderm graft to prevent excessive weeping and improve postoperative comfort. **i,** Flap division occurs after 3 weeks. Note the edema of the tip. **J,** At 1 week after flap division, the swelling has improved. **K,** At 3 months after surgery, the large linear scar over the forehead is barely noticeable. **L,** Some residual fullness of the nasal tip and dorsum is present at 1 year. The patient was offered revision to further thin the flap over his dorsum and side walls; however, he was very happy with his results and deferred further surgery.

preserve the blood vessels coursing though the subcutaneous layer. The flap is rotated 180 degrees away from the eye. Once the defect has been repaired, the exposed raw surface of the pedicle can be covered with a small piece of acellular dermal graft, which can decrease the dripping of transudate during the postoperative period. The donor defect of the forehead is closed primarily with wide undermining of the surrounding forehead skin in the subgaleal plane, taking care to preserve the periosteum. Galeotomies can be used to assist in closure of the forehead donor site by making incisions perpendicular to the vector of tension with a No. 15 blade (i.e., parallel to the incision line).

Each galeotomy can provide approximately 2 to 3 mm of length, and when multiple ones are made in series, up to 5 to 8 mm of extra length can be obtained. In addition, intraoperative tissue expansion with a moist 4 × 8–cm gauze pad placed under the undermined forehead flaps and left in place while the nasal defect is sutured can result in an extra 3 to 4 mm of pliability. If the defect is too large for primary closure, healing by secondary intention is preferable to skin grafting. Potential complications from surgery include flap necrosis and scarring on the forehead. Necrosis is often alleviated by keeping the flap thick distally as the feeding vessels run through the subcutaneous tissue. Scarring of the forehead should be a secondary concern as scars tend to heal well and natural contraction will make a large postoperative defect on the forehead much less apparent.

After approximately 4 weeks, the pedicle is divided and the flap is thinned and inset into the rest of the nasal defect. The eyebrow is replaced into its preoperative position and the pedicle is inset into the forehead as an inverted V. Further refinement of the nasal flap can be performed as needed in subsequent procedures.

REPAIR OF PARTIAL AND FULL THICKNESS DEFECTS

SUBSURFACE FRAMEWORK AND LINING

When repairing partial- and full-thickness defects, the subsurface framework and lining, in addition to the skin covering, may need to be reconstructed. Even those subunits that lack a true cartilaginous framework, such as the soft tissue triangles, must be repaired with a cartilage graft or risk later contraction of the triangle and subsequent deformity. A well-vascularized bed is imperative for the survival of these nonvascularized grafts. Each missing piece of cartilage or bone should be crafted to create a symmetric nose. The other half of the nose can be used as a template to fashion the cartilage grafts. In cases where the lesions extend through the midline, the surgeon's knowledge of the relevant anatomy and local subunits can guide them in the reconstruction.

CARTILAGE GRAFTS

Cartilage support is most easily obtained from septal cartilage. Typically, the septum remains intact after most excisions of skin cancers. Whether or not the mucosa is being harvested for mucosal rotation flaps, a large segment of cartilage may be obtained for use in repairing defects. It is important to ensure that a dorsal and caudal strut of at least 1.5 cm is left intact to prevent potential saddling of the nose in the postoperative period. This strut of cartilage acts as the base for all reconstructive efforts in the repair of larger nasal defects.[9] If the amount of cartilage harvested from the septum is insufficient for the defect, other sources to aid with the repair include conchal cartilage, autogenous rib graft, and cadaveric rib graft. Conchal cartilage has the advantages of ease of harvest without significant morbidity. It is limited in the gross quantity of cartilage available, and its curvature actually can be advantageous when recreating a nasal tip or other curved structure. Autogenous rib graft offers large quantities of cartilage, enough for a total nasal reconstruction in many cases. The cartilage is straight and easy to work with; however, there is usually some moderate donor site discomfort, and the procedure subjects the patient to a small risk of a pneumothorax. Cadaveric cartilage offers similar benefits of autogenous cartilage but has disadvantages, including the potential for late reabsorption and risk of infection from allographic material.

When recreating a nasal subunit, it is imperative to lay down a support even in areas without significant cartilage or risk future contraction of the covering graft or flap. For nasal tip reconstruction, a Peck graft can act to restore proper tip rotation. If further projection is desired, a second graft can be secured to the first. In performing support work with cartilage or bone, it is important that one designs the framework 2 to 3 mm smaller than the actual subunit. This is to ensure that when the cover is applied, the resulting repair will be of the desired size and contour. If a cartilage graft is placed that equals the desired size of the defect, once the layers have been fully reconstructed, the surgeon will find a repair that is too large in comparison to the initial defect.

INTERNAL NASAL LINING

Recreating the lining of the nose is of tremendous importance for its physiologic function as uncontrolled postoperative scarring can lead to vestibular stenosis and nasal airway obstruction. Lining for the nasal cavity can be created with either skin grafts or local mucosal flaps. Skin grafting has several downsides, the first being a need for a well-vascularized bed on which to lay the graft down. Typically with full-thickness defects, this bed is not available as the support graft, be it cartilage or bone, acts as a barrier for osmosis and nutrient supply to a healthy graft. In defects where a vascularized bed of perichondrium is still present, a skin graft has an excellent chance for success. Postoperatively, patients may notice ozena, as the natural mucociliary clearance of the native mucosa has been lost with the grafted skin. This leaves pedicled mucosal flaps from the nasal septum as the optimal choice when approaching full-thickness defects. Often, the septum will be available for lining the defect in most skin cancer excisions. This allows the surgeon to harvest a large flap of mucosa to rotate and to create a lining.

HINGE OVER FLAPS

For alar margin defects, the skin and scar from the healed margins can be mobilized and turned inward to recreate the lining. This leaves a larger cutaneous defect than the original, which can be covered with local or pedicled flaps as the surgeon sees fit. Unfortunately, the blood supply to the turned-in flaps can be variable and does not allow for large defects to be closed in this manner.

CHONDROCUTANEOUS LINING FLAPS

Local flaps designed to harvest vestibular skin can be used for small defects inferior to the nasal valve. The advantages of this technique are that the flaps are well vascularized and can often support immediate placement of cartilage grafts. Additionally, the skin of the vestibule is thin and will not result in a thick, bulky ala with potential for obstruction of the nasal airway.

Intranasal lining flaps offer a one-stage repair for larger defects. Cartilage grafts can be placed at the time of surgery, decreasing the number of potential subsequent procedures. The blood supply to the septal mucosa is important to observe as reconstructing the lining of a full-thickness defect often relies on flaps harvested from the septum. Posteriorly, the septum is supplied from branches of the sphenopalatine artery, and anterosuperiorly, from branches of the ethmoidal artery. Anteroinferiorly, the superior labial arteries contribute to the septal blood supply. Due to its extensive anastomosing network, a septal mucosal flap can be maintained with only one of these blood supplies intact. A pedicle of 1–1.2 cm based over the nasal spine, at the level of the septal perforators from the superior labial artery, will provide adequate nourishment to the flap.

For larger defects of the lining involving the superior, middle, and inferior vaults, a de Quervain flap can be used effectively (Figure 36-10). The lower and middle vaults are relined with a septal mucosal flap from the ipsilateral side. A window of cartilage is removed from the nasal septum, allowing for the contralateral mucosa to be rotated inwards and the upper vault lining to be recreated.[10] This flap may jeopardize dorsal and tip support.

VESTIBULAR ADVANCEMENT

For small defects at the margin of the alae, the vestibular skin can be mobilized and advanced inferiorly 2 to 3 mm (Figure 36-11). As with covering flaps, this flap must be secured in place to a firm support such as cartilage or risk

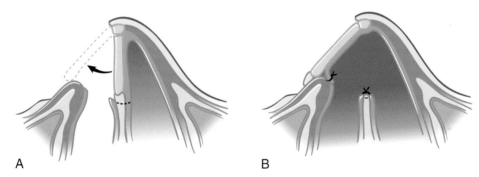

Figure 36-10 De Quervain flap. **A,** Chondromucosal flap, which is useful in cases of large defects of the nasal lining. **B,** The contralateral septal mucosa can be mobilized where it attached cartilage to line the nasal vault.

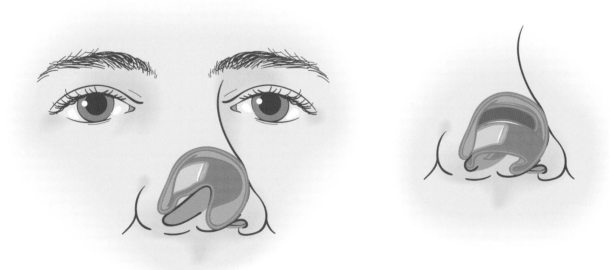

Figure 36-11 Vestibular lining flap. **A,** The vestibular lining is incised and mobilized. **B,** The flap is then freed and mobilized inferiorly. Two small standing cone deformities are left at the pedicles.

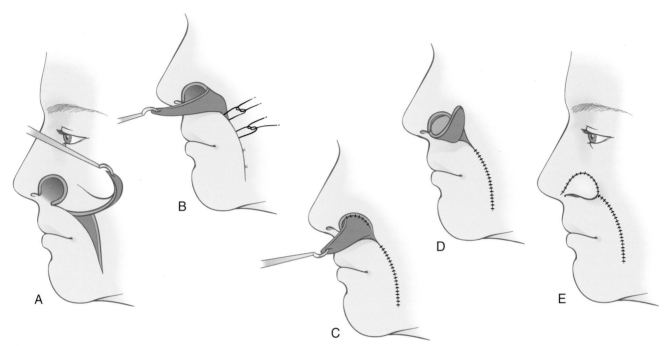

Figure 36-12 Melolabial turn-in flap. **A,** A long melolabial flap is designed with enough excess to rotate a flap over. **B,** The secondary wound is closed. Subcutaneous tissue is left on the flap to preserve the blood supply. **C,** The lining is closed, leading to a rotation of the flap 90 degrees. **D,** The flap is then turned in and used to close the cutaneous defect. **E,** The final resulting flap and closure.

retraction. This technique is limited by the laxity of the vestibular skin and may not be appropriate in patients who have had significant scarring in the region, such as from radiation.

TURN-IN FLAPS

Turn-in flaps require folding a local flap over onto itself to provide both a skin covering and an internal lining (Figure 36-12). Commonly, this technique is used in repairing defects near the alar margin. Due to the inherent thickness of the skin of the flap, however, the flap often becomes bulky, leading to a formless shape with poor match to the delicate surrounding skin of the ala as well as nasal obstruction. These problems can be addressed by using a multistaged reconstruction using a well-vascularized, pedicled flap such as a paramedian forehead flap. A template of both the cutaneous and internal defect is created and transferred to the forehead. The flap is elevated as previously described. Initially, the bulk of the flap will impact both function and aesthetic form of the nasal ala. In 4 to 6 weeks, the flap is divided at the alar margin but left intact at the pedicle. The lining can now be thinned of any excess subcutaneous tissue allowing for a thin, vascularized lining. At this stage, cartilage grafting is performed to support the alar margin as well as the nasal tip and middle vault. The flap, which is still

connected to its blood supply, is thinned as well and replaced. In a third stage 4 to 6 weeks later, the pedicle is divided and the flap is inset. Subsequent revision surgeries are then performed as needed. By proceeding in this manner, a thin well-vascularized lining can be created effectively (Figure 36-13).

CONCLUSION

Repairing nasal defects is a rewarding endeavor, posing new challenges with each case that is encountered. Without treatment, patients would be left disfigured, with the subsequent psychological and social implications that can be associated with severe injuries. While various techniques exist to close and repair these defects, our experience has shown us that perfecting and maximizing several key techniques may be used with consistently excellent results. Determining where and when to use these techniques is based on a thorough knowledge of the regional anatomy and the potential pitfalls associated with each reconstructive technique. While we have touched on our favorite techniques in this chapter, this is by no means intended to be taken as a comprehensive treatise on the subject. We encourage further exploration into the depths of the field to determine the techniques that best suit each individual surgeon.

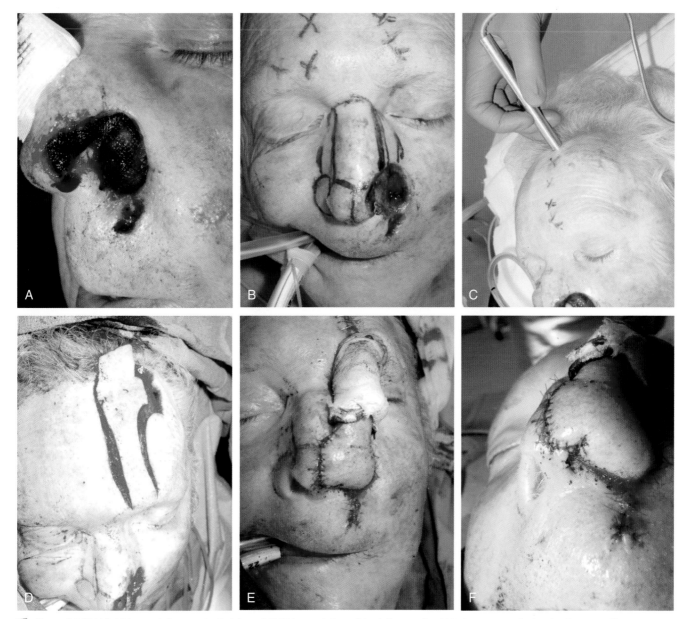

Figure 36-13 Full-thickness defect repair. **A,** A large full-thickness defect of the left nose after MOHS resection of a basal cell cancer. The tumor was deeply invasive, extending to the vestibular skin through the cartilage. **B,** The subunits involved are identified and mapped out for planning of repair. **C,** The course of the supratrochlear artery is identified with Doppler ultrasound. **D,** A forehead flap is designed to cover the defect and resurface the lining of the nasal vestibule as a turn-in flap. The narrow pedicle of the flap prevents strangulation of the supratrochlear artery. **E,** The flap is inset and the forehead defect closed primarily after intraoperative tissue expansion. **F,** Base view of the resulting flap. Note the obstruction of the left nasal passage from the relatively bulky flap.

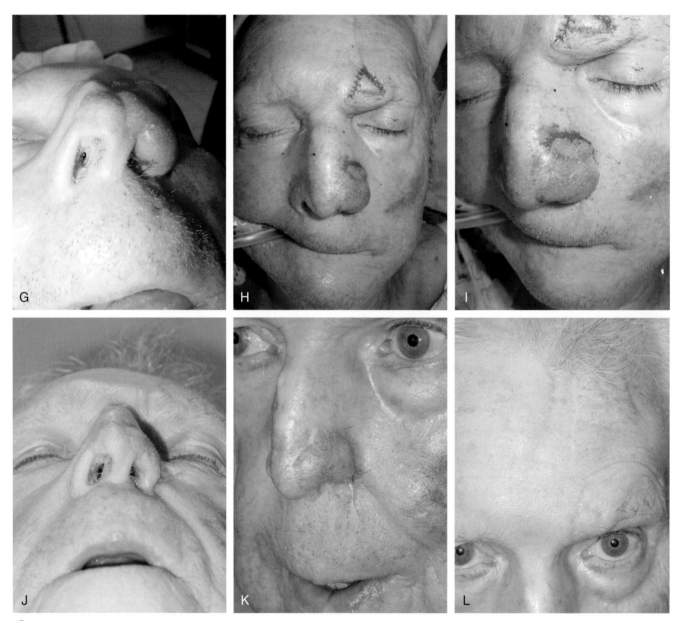

Figure 36-13, cont'd G, Before pedicle division, a secondary procedure was performed through an incision along the alar margin. At this time, a conchal cartilage graft was placed to support the left nasal ala. **H, I,** The flap was inset with further thinning of the nasal ala and recreation of the supra-alar crease. **J,** Base view of the resulting repair shows some vestibular collapse with mild shifting of the nasal pyramid due to the force of scar contraction. Note the patent airway after thinning of the turn-in flap and cartilage grafting. **K,** The supra-alar crease has been recreated with a satisfactory result. **L,** The residual forehead scar is barely noticeable at 3 months.

REFERENCES

1. Yalamachili H, Sclafani AP, Schaefer SD, Presti P. The path of nasal reconstruction: from ancient India to the present. *Fac Plast Surg.* 2008;24(1):3–10.
2. Burget GC, Menick FJ. The subunit principle in nasal reconstruction. *Plast Reconstr Surg.* 1987;76: 239.
3. Gue L, Pribaz JR, Pribaz JJ. Nasal reconstruction with local flaps: a simple algorithm for management of small defects. *PRS.* 2008;122:130–139.
4. Zitelli JA. The bilobed flap for nasal reconstruction. *Arch Dermatol.* 1989;125:957.

5. Carucci JA. Melolabial flap repair in nasal reconstruction. *Dermatol Clin.* 2005;23(1):65–71.
6. Reiger R. A local flap for repair of the nasal tip. *Plast Reconstr Surg.* 1967;40:147.
7. Skouge JW. *Skin grafting.* New York: Churchill Livingstone; 1991.
8. Reece EM, Schaverien M, Rohrich RJ. The paramedian forehead flap: a dynamic anatomical vascular study verifying safety and clinical implications. *Plast Reconstr Surg.* 2008;121(6):1956–1963.
9. Millard DR. Various uses of the septum in rhinoplasty. *Plast Reconstr Surg.* 1988;81:112.
10. Taghinia AH, Pribaz JJ. Complex nasal reconstruction. *Plast Reconstr Surg.* 2008;121(2):15–27.

CHAPTER THIRTY-SEVEN

Nasal Septal Perforation Repair

Marc Cohen • Jeffrey D. Rawnsley

The nasal septum plays a critical role in both the function, as well as the aesthetics, of the human nose. Structurally, the septum forms the foundation of the nasal pyramid and acts as the central support element of the nose, providing support for the cartilaginous and soft-tissue components of the nose and nasal cavity. Functionally, the nasal septum, and its relation with the upper lateral cartilages, forms a critical portion of the internal nasal valve. Disorders of the nasal septum can therefore cause both structural and functional morbidity to the patient.

Nasal septal perforations can be a source of great morbidity to a patient. Structurally, nasal septal perforations may weaken the foundational support of the nasal pyramid so as to cause significant aesthetic deformities. Functionally, septal perforations alter the airflow through the nasal cavity, which in turn may lead to crusting, epistaxis, and pain.

With these morbidities in mind, it is imperative that the rhinoplastic surgeon be thoroughly comfortable with the management of nasal septal perforations. In this chapter, we review the relevant anatomy, etiology, pathophysiology, and management of nasal septal perforations. A review of the different surgical techniques will be discussed as well the appropriate indications for each approach.

RELEVANT ANATOMY

The nasal septum divides the nose into two separate nasal cavities. Each nasal cavity is bounded by the nasal septum, lateral nasal wall, and nasal floor. The nasal septum is composed of a bony and cartilagenous framework covered by a layer of mucoperichondrium and mucoperiosteum. The bony components of the septum include the nasal crest of the palatine bone, the nasal crest of the maxilla and premaxilla, the vomer, the perpendicular plate of the ethmoid, the nasal crest of the frontal bone, and the spine of the paired nasal bones. The anterior septum is composed of the quadrilateral cartilage, with its caudal most projection extending beyond the nasal spine.

The lateral nasal wall is composed of the laminae papyracea of the lacrimal bone, portions of the ethmoid bone, and the inferior and middle nasal conchae or turbinates. The inferior, middle, and superior turbinates are composed of a thin bone for structural support and covered by an adherent mucoperiosteum. Stratified squamous epithelium is found on the anterior tip of the inferior turbinate, whereas pseudostratified ciliated columnar respiratory epithelium covers all other surfaces.

Knowledge of the blood supply to the septum and lateral nasal wall is important for designing mucosal flaps for septal perforation repair. Blood supply and innervation of the nasal septum travel within the mucoperiosteal and mucoperichondrial linings. The arterial blood supply derives from the ophthalmic branch of the internal carotid artery and the maxillary and facial branches of the external carotid artery. The upper nasal septum is supplied by anastomoses of the anterior and posterior ethmoid arteries, which originate from the ophthalmic branch. The external carotid artery contributes via a major branch of the sphenopalatine artery that supplies the posterior and inferior septum. The columella and caudal septum receive blood supply from the septal branch of the superior labial artery. The septal mucosa itself contains complex arteriovenous anastomoses and venous sinusoids that can become engorged or constricted via neural or extrinsic pathways.[1]

The blood supply to the lateral nasal wall is supplied posteroinferiorly by the sphenopalatine artery via the posterior lateral nasal artery and by the anterior and posterior ethmoid arteries superiorly. The posterior lateral nasal artery runs inferiorly on the perpendicular plate of the palatine bone and courses downward at approximately 1 cm anterior to the posterior end of the middle turbinate and approximately 1.5 cm anterior to the posterior end of the superior turbinate. The posterior lateral nasal artery occasionally gives off branches to the superior turbinate and is the predominant supplier of blood to the middle and inferior turbinates.[2]

The arterial supply to the inferior turbinate runs in a direction parallel to the turbinate and nasal floor. Thus, in cases where relaxing incisions are needed to gain length on a mucoperichondrial flap, these incisions should be made immediately below the inferior turbinate bone so as to avoid arterial disruption.[3]

INCIDENCE AND ETIOLOGY

The incidence of nasal septal perforations in adults is 0.9%.[4] In a retrospective review of 74 patients with nasal septal perforations and ulcers, Diamantopoulos and Jones[5] found that 80% of perforations were seen anteriorly, 11% were located posteriorly or superiorly, and 9% were classified as total or subtotal. Although the size of the perforations varied, the majority (39%) had a perforation size of 1 to 2 cm in diameter with an almost equal distribution of perforations less than 1 cm and greater than 2 cm. Crusting, minor bleeding, and erythema were the most common findings on initial presentation.

The etiology of nasal septal perforations is quite varied (Table 37-1). The most common cause of perforation is the result of previous septal surgery. Other causes include nose picking, cocaine use, vasculitis, malignancy, and idiopathic.[6] Proper workup of a patient with a nasal septal perforation should include a thorough history with specific attention to questions that address the wide differential diagnosis.

The history should be followed by a complete nasal endoscopy with documentation of the size and location of the perforation as well as any other findings such as crusting, bleeding, or granulation tissue. The septum should also be inspected to assess the degree of remaining cartilage. This can be assessed by gentle palpation with a cotton swab. In terms of laboratory studies, if the patient does not have a history to suggest a traumatic etiology, then a c-ANCA, antinuclear antibodies, rheumatoid factor, and erythrocyte sedimentation rate tests are sufficient. If any of these are positive, then a rheumatology referral may be warranted.

The previously accepted dogma that all septal perforations should be biopsied has recently come into question. Several studies have shown that septal biopsies have very little diagnostic value.[5,7] Frequently, septal perforation biopsies are nondiagnostic even in the case of known vasculitis or malignant disease. It is therefore suggested that in patients with a clinically unremarkable septal perforation, even in the absence of a diagnostic history, biopsy of the edges does not add to the management of the patient and should not be performed. Biopsy should be reserved for patients in whom a clinical suspicion of malignancy exists and repeated biopsies may be needed to confirm the diagnosis.

MORBIDITY OF NASAL SEPTAL PERFORATION

Patients with nasal septal perforations commonly have a dry and obstructed nose. They also may complain of crusting, bleeding, and a whistling noise during breathing. Pathophysiologically, the airflow jet is directed toward the posterior aspect of the perforation. This leads to an increase in airflow turbulence, which in turn causes desiccation, bleeding, and crusting. These complaints are usually associated with anterior, rather than posterior, perforations. The reason for this finding is that by the time the nasal airflow reaches the posterior nasal cavity, it is sufficiently conditioned at that point. Likewise, smaller perforations are less likely to cause symptoms as would large ones.[8]

Lindemann et al.[9] studied the effects of closure of septal perforations on intranasal humidity and temperature. In a prospective study of 10 patients, surgical closure of the perforation was shown to have a statistically significant increase in nasal airway humidity and temperature. Moreover, clinical symptoms of recurrent epistaxis and nasal dryness were shown to improve after repair. The

Table 37-1 Cause of Nasal Septal Perforation

Traumatic	Inflammatory/Infectious	Neoplastic	Other
Nasal surgery	Sarcoidosis	Carcinoma	Lime dust
Intranasal steroid sprays	Wegener granulomatosis	T-cell Lymphomas	Cryoglobulinemia
Nose ring piercing	Leishmaniasis		Renal failure
Cauterization for epistaxis	Systemic lupus erythematosus		Industrial exposure
Nose picking	Tuberculosis		Nasogastric tube placement
Syphilis	Dermatomyositis		
Nasal cannula oxgen	AIDS		
Nasal foreign body	Diphtheria		
Illicit drugs	Rheumatoid arthritis		
	Crohn disease		

From Lanier (2007).

study provides further evidence to support the proposed mechanism that intranasal dryness secondary to turbulent airflow with septal perforations is responsible for the morbidity of this condition.

MANAGEMENT OF NASAL SEPTAL PERFORATIONS

The first step in the management of nasal septal perforations is to determine whether the perforation needs to be closed. Often, small perforations are asymptomatic and can be left alone. Also, patients with nasal septal perforations may have chronic rhinosinusitis and their symptoms may be attributable to this condition rather than to the perforation.[10] In these circumstances, appropriate medical therapy may provide more benefit than closure of the perforation.

If the patient's symptoms are minor with minimal crusting, then the use of saline sprays or topical petroleum jelly may be sufficient. With more severe crusting, saline irrigation or similar sinus rinses may be needed.

For the patient who does require closure of the septal perforation, two options exist: mechanical obturation and surgical closure.

NONSURGICAL APPROACHES

The mainstay of nonsurgical treatment of septal perforations is the silicone button. Since the 1970s, the use of both prefabricated and custom prostheses has shown some benefit.[11] Recently, Blind et al.[12] studied the impact of custom-made silicone buttons on the quality of life of patients with septal perforations. Their results demonstrated that the use of the silicone obturator led to a decrease in epistaxis, crusting, whistling, dryness, and obstruction in a majority of patients. Moreover, the majority of patients who used the obturator had improved quality of life scores as evidenced with use of a validated questionnaire. The glaring finding in the study was that only 38% of the patients still used their obturator after the follow-up period. The most common reasons given for not using the obturator included difficulty with positioning button, pain, and enlargement of the perforation, rendering the obturator obsolete.

SURGICAL APPROACHES

As Kridel[13] has stated, the goals of septal perforation repair are closure of the perforation and restoration of normal nasal physiology. To achieve these goals, the surgical approach must be tailored for each specific perforation. The size and location of the nasal septal perforation will thus dictate whether to approach repair via a closed or open technique, whether to use an interpositional graft, or which vascular flap to use for repair.

The majority of septal perforations that require surgical closure fall into two main categories: small- to medium-sized anterior perforations and large central perforations. Small posterior perforations are usually asymptomatic and rarely require surgical intervention. The following is a review of several techniques used to repair both types of perforations. The review has been written to provide the reader with an overview of the different approaches and we recommend referring to the original reports for further details on each specific technique.

Small- to Medium-Sized Anterior Perforations

Repair of nasal septal perforations can be achieved by creating well-vascularized transpositions flaps to close the septal defects. Several authors have described their varying techniques and success with these procedures.

De Witt[14] has described the use of a composite flap of mucoperichondrium and a "button" of cartilage at the posterior septum. The flap is created with the base at the flap centered at the posterior edge of the perforation. This composite flap is then rotated into the perforation site as a door hinge. Neighboring mucoperichondrium is then elevated to close the donor site. The author stated success with this method on two patients.

In a similar fashion, Shikowitz[15] describes using a mucoperiosteal flap harvested from the bony septum, which is rotated anteriorly to repair the septal defect. In addition, acellular dermis and occasional autogenous cartilage is used to support the flap. Ninety percent of patients had successful repair of their perforations, with all patients having resolution of their symptoms.

Friedman et al.[16] described their approach and experience with the inferior turbinate flap that was previously described by Vuyk and Versluis.[17] Their indication for use of this flap is for small- to medium-sized perforations. Using nasal endoscopes, the inferior turbinate is incised from a posterior to anterior direction with the pedicle of the flap at the anterior portion of the turbinate. The flap is then rotated anteriorly and sutured to the rimmed perforation. Any exposed bone of the donor site is removed. The pedicle is then taken down 3 weeks later under local anesthesia. Seven of 10 patients had successful closure of their perforation, and one patient required radiofrequency ablation of a bulky flap.

The inferior turbinate flap provides a well-vascularized local flap for repair of small- to medium-sized nasal septal defects. However, disadvantages of this technique are that it requires at least two staged procedures and may lead to nasal obstruction from a bulky flap even after the pedicle is taken down.

Repair of small- to medium-sized anterior perforations can also be achieved by extracting and repositioning the quadrangular cartilage, a technique that was initially described by Sulsenti. In this procedure, the quadrangular cartilage is extracted and then replaced with the perforated end first. This places the perforation in a more posterior location, which no longer matches the perforation in the mucoperichondrium. Local mucoperichondrial flaps are then used to allow a tension-free closure at the perforation site. In a recent series, 87% had successful closure of the perforation at a minimum of 2 years from the time of surgery. However, successful closure was obtained in only 60% of the patients with a greater than 1-cm perforation.[18]

Several authors have described using oral mucosal flaps to repair nasal septal perforations. Both sublabial and buccal flaps have been used with varying degrees of success.[19-22] In general, the flap is harvested and tunneled into the nasal cavity at the gingivolabial sulcus. Meyer[22] describes a three-staged procedure in which a buccal flap is secured to a conchal cartilage graft. The pedicle is then taken down at a later date. Kogan et al.[21] describe their technique of using a medially based sublabial flap without the use of an interpositional graft. The flap is secured into place with absorbable sutures and the donor site is closed, obviating the need for a second procedure to transect the pedicle. They report a 71% success rate based on their experience with seven patients.

Large Perforations

For the repair of large nasal septal perforations, the creation of a large, well-vascularized flap that is not overly bulky is a challenge. Several surgeons have described techniques to accomplish this goal.

Paloma et al.[23] report the use of a pericranial flap to reconstruct large septal perforations. Via a bicoronal incision, a pericranial flap consisting of periosteum and subgaleal fascia is raised and rotated caudally 180 degrees over the supraorbital rim. The flap is tunneled under the glabella inserted into the nasal cavity after detachment of the upper lateral cartilages. The flap is based on the deep branches of the supraorbital and supratrochlear vessels. The advantage of this approach is that it provides a well-vascularized flap of autogenous tissue with an adequate size to repair large septal defects.

Reports of using a free flap for subtotal septal defects have been documented.[24,25] The free flap is anastomosed to the facial artery and vein and tunneled under the upper lip. The flap is inset via an open rhinoplasty approach. This technique is reserved for large perforations in which local tissue for repair is unavailable.

Pedroza et al.[26] reviewed their experience of 100 septal perforation repairs. Their technique shares many of the same principles as several other authors in the literature. The authors use a "postcartilaginous" incision via a closed approach, unless the perforation is greater than 2 cm, in which case the procedure is performed via an open rhinoplasty approach. Bilateral mucoperichondrial flaps are raised at the septum, nasal floors, toward the attachment of the inferior turbinates, and superiorly toward the junction of the upper lateral cartilages and septum. A temporalis fascia graft is harvested and used as an interpositional graft between the mucoperichondrium layers. If tension is found at closure, relaxing longitudinal incisions are made at the floor and superiorly if needed. Their overall success rate of closure was 97%, with 100% closure with perforations less than 2 cm. The follow-up period ranged from 1 to 10 years.

Which Interpositional Graft to Use?

In a study by Mola et al.,[27] New Zealand rabbits had varying materials placed in their nasal septum. Histologic analyses were performed at 3 months. Gore-Tex (Implantech Associates, Ventura, CA) was found to cause the most severe inflammatory reactions, followed by Dacron and acellular dermis (Alloderm; Lifecell, Branchburg, NJ). Autogenic cartilage demonstrated the least immune response.

The use of porcine small intestinal submucosa (SurgiSIS; Cook Biotech Inc., West Lafayette, IN) for the repair of septal perforations has also been shown to be effective. With the use of SurgiSIS positioned between two mucoperichondrial flaps, the authors reported a 100% success rate of closure in 10 patients.[28] In an adjunctive study on rabbits, the placement of SurgiSIS interpositioned between mucoperichondrial flaps demonstrated evidence of cartilage regrowth.[29]

PERSONAL SURGICAL TECHNIQUE

Tissue Graft Selection

Closure of a septal perforation requires the reconstruction of the three layers of the missing septum: bilateral mucosal layers and a connective tissue layer to replace missing cartilage. Interposition grafts have traditionally been composed of either temporalis fascia or pericranium. More recently the use of human acellular dermal grafts (Alloderm) have become increasingly popular due to the fact that they avoid the time and morbidity of harvest as well as the generally thicker nature of the material that eases its use as an interpositional graft.

Graft selection is based on at least two competing concepts. The use of pericranium and temporalis fascia has a theoretically improved success rate over autologous cartilage, due to the rapid neovascularization of these thinner tissues, as well as the lower metabolic activity of these grafts. Alternatively, however, much of the success of closure of the septal perforation relies on complete closure of the perforations. Due to the consistent fact that most closures fail at the point of the suture line, the structural scaffolding of human acellular dermis allows remote mucosalization from the edge of the mucosal flaps. This is important in clinical situations where small, unilateral defects due to incomplete closure or wound breakdown persist after repair. The strength of the acellular dermal graft serves as scaffolding for mucosa to heal upon. In the senior author's experience, these small unilateral and occasionally bilateral defects in the mucosa will fill in from the mucosal wound edge much as remucosalization occurs over exposed bone and cartilage after septoplasty.

When autografts are harvested, the harvest should include a generous amount of temporalis fascia or pericranium that will allow overlay at least 1.5 cm beyond the cartilaginous defect. The harvests of these grafts have been well described and are techniques that most otolaryngologists, facial plastic surgeons, and plastic surgeons are familiar with (i.e., in the harvest of grafts for tympanoplasty).

Operative Approach

While endonasal approaches have been popularized in the past, they are rarely appropriate for most septal perforations except those that are small, low, and anterior, due to the limit of exposure for larger perforations and patients with small nostrils.

The success rate is also affected by size of the perforation, with larger perforations requiring broader undermining of surrounding mucosa to recruit into the defect. This requires extensive exposure necessitating an external approach. Septal perforation repair is one of the most technically difficult procedures to obtain consistent success due to the delicate nature of the tissues, oblique angle of visibility that occurs through most of the surgery, many pitfalls for enlarging the perforation, and production of rents in the mucosal flap as the surgery proceeds. Patient selection is also very important as perforations over 1.5 cm in vertical height, especially in small noses, often do not have sufficient nasal mucosa to allow complete closure. In addition, if the septal perforation is due to cocaine abuse, the vascularity of the tissue involved may be permanently compromised. Preoperative screening may be necessary to ensure the surgeon that the patient has discontinued cocaine, as ongoing use will likely condemn the perforation repair to failure.

At the time of surgery, the patient is placed in the supine position. General endotracheal intubation with a RAE (Ring-Adair-Elwyn) tube is performed and the throat is packed with saline-moistened gauze. The nose is injected with 1% lidocaine with 1:100,000 epinephrine, as is standard in an external rhinoplasty approach, with infiltration of all septal and nasal mucosa. The patient is then prepped and draped in the usual sterile fashion, and careful intranasal examination is performed to confirm the office examination. Any existing synechiae are identified, and the extent of the cartilaginous septal defect, which may be masked by mucosa, is inspected using a 0-degree endoscope and contralateral palpation of the septum.

Marginal incisions are then performed with a No. 15 blade, as well as a transcolumellar incision in an inverted-V fashion using a No. 11 blade. The soft tissue envelope is then undermined and a wide local exposure is begun by sharply disarticulating the intercrural ligaments and

exposing the anterior and caudal septum. Meticulous dissection is required throughout the procedure so as not to perforate the septal flaps. Careful entry into the full submucoperichondrial plane on both sides of the septum is performed sharply with careful attention not to weaken the anterior and caudal septum with multiple knife cuts. A Cottle elevator is then used to create a tunnel underneath the upper lateral cartilages on both sides of the septum. The upper lateral cartilages are then sharply dissected along the dorsum. This may be performed with a No. 15 blade on to the Cottle elevator or with sharp straight Iris scissors. Next, elevation of the mucosal flaps is begun toward the perforation with elevation of the mucoperichondrium surrounding the perforation. The rim of the perforation is incised with a No. 15 blade along its posterior, superior, and inferior edge, and careful blunt dissection is then performed from the remaining septal cartilage toward the perforation to avoid enlargement of the septal defect.

The mucosa of the floor of the nose is then elevated in a submucoperiostial plane. This is performed by first creating a small incision along the ridge of the inferior piriform aperture. Blind dissection is then performed in a subperiostial plane with the Cottle elevator extending up underneath the inferior turbinates and posteriorly. Once this is broadly elevated on both sides, decussation of fibers is performed sharply at the point where the maxillary crest and cartilaginous septal intersection is carefully divided, with careful attention again not to perforate the septal flaps. Backcuts are made underneath the inferior turbinate for the full length of the turbinate with a No. 15 or Beaver blade. Connection of this incision to the subperiosteal plane of the mucuperiosteal flap is then made to increase their mobility and advance them as a bipedicled flap into the defect. Once there has been complete release of the mucoperiosteal flaps, the cartilaginous defect is addressed with the use of either autograft or allograft. The graft is placed with adequate overlap. It is then sutured first anteriorly with two septal mattress sutures using 5-0 chromic suture to anchor the graft. It is then unfurled over the septal cartilaginous defect and sutured posteriorly as well. Septal flaps are then advanced superiorly toward the superior edge of the defect (Figure 37-1). The advancement of the flaps is not strictly in a vertical direction as membranous septum is recruited for its laxity in many cases, such that an anterior-to-posterior direction advancement also occurs (Figure 37-2).

If a tension-free closure is not obtained at this time, further maneuvers are anticipated. The first includes the fortuitous desire of the patient to have a dorsal reduction discussed prior to surgery (Figure 37-3). Resection of bone and cartilage of the dorsum will release the soft tissue attachments and allow lowering of the dorsal septum to relax the superior flap. If dorsal hump reduction is not indicated, an incision can be made in the superior

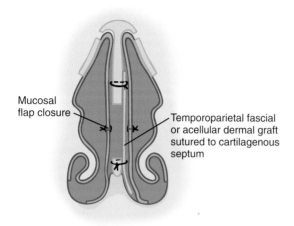

Figure 37-1 Typical three-layer closure of septal perforations.

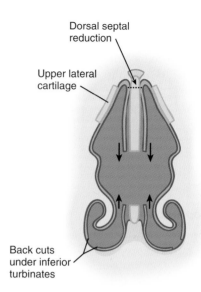

Figure 37-3 Closure of septal perforation with dorsal reduction.

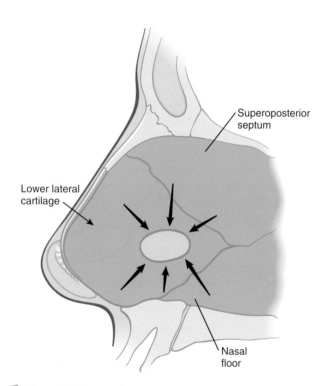

Figure 37-2 Vectors of mucosal recruitment.

flap approximately 5 mm below the upper lateral cartilages (along the length of the upper lateral cartilages) to create a true bipedicled mucosal flap. This should be performed unilaterally to ensure adequate vascularity on closure of the dorsal septum from the contralateral side. Complete closure of one side is a prerequisite of successful long-term closure of the perforation. Although complete bilateral closure is always preferable, incomplete unilateral closure may still allow successful full-thickness closure through postoperative remucosalization. In some

cases, posteriorly based flap of mucosa from the inferior flap is necessary to rotate mucosa into the defect for complete closure (Figure 37-4).

Once the flaps are completely released, reapproximation of the flaps is possible. The flaps are closed with 6-0 chromic suture on a small cutting needle using Castroviejo forceps. Once both septal perforations are closed in this manner, the whole three-layer complex is reapproximated with running 4-0 plain gut suture on a Keith needle to "mattress together" all the elements. This also serves to stabilize the mucosal graft. The upper lateral cartilages are then reapproximated with 5-0 Prolene suture, and the intercrural ligaments are carefully reestablished with tip support if necessary either from a columellar strut or, when appropriate, by suturing the medial crura to the caudal septum in a tongue-in-groove fashion. Under some circumstances, the membranous septum may be pulled with undue tension that will cause tip rotation and columella retraction. This rarely is a long-term problem as this will tend to relax over the course of the first 3 to 6 months. The transcolumellar incision is closed with interrupted 6-0 nylon sutures in a mattress fashion, and the marginal incisions are closed with 4-0 chromic suture. To stabilize the lining and provide a healing moist environment, thin Silastic sheeting is placed over the repaired septum and held in place with 5-0 Prolene sutures through the anterior septum. If gel foam is used as packing, frequent nasal saline spraying in the nostrils at postoperative day 3 will hasten its dissolution.

At 1 week postoperatively, the nasal splint and transcolumellar sutures are removed. At 3 weeks postoperatively, the Silastic sheeting is removed following removal of the anterior retaining sutures. The repaired septum can then be fully examined endoscopically.

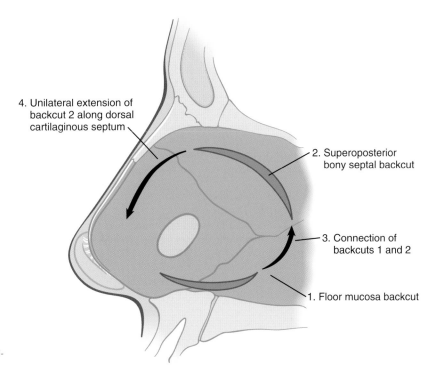

4. Unilateral extension of backcut 2 along dorsal cartilaginous septum

2. Superoposterior bony septal backcut

3. Connection of backcuts 1 and 2

1. Floor mucosa backcut

Figure 37-4 Order of backcuts for progressive mobilization of mucosa.

SURGICAL OUTCOMES

The success of closure is enhanced with proper patient selection; small perforations are more likely to be adequately closed. Complete closure of the septal flaps bilaterally also greatly improves the likelihood of success with complete repair. Meticulous closure and careful preoperative selection of patients will ensure the highest rate of success. Revision septal perforation repair is difficult and usually not recommended; nevertheless, reduction in the size of the perforation can provide significant improvements in nasal physiology and symptoms.

REFERENCES

1. Cummings C, Haughey B, Thomas J, et al. *Cummings Otolaryngology: head and neck surgery.* St Louis: Mosby; 2004.
2. Lee HY, Kim HU, Kim SS, et al. Surgical anatomy of the sphenopalatine artery in lateral nasal wall. *Laryngoscope.* 2002;112:1813–1818.
3. Ribeiro JS, da Silva GS. Technical advances in the correction of septal perforation associated with closed rhinoplasty. *Arch Fac Plast Surg.* 2007;9:321–327.
4. Oberg D, Akerlund A, Johansson L, Bende M. Prevalence of nasal septal perforation: the Skovde population-based study. *Rhinology.* 2003;41:72–75.
5. Diamantopoulos II, Jones NS. The investigation of nasal septal perforations and ulcers. *J Laryngol Otol.* 2001;115:541–544.
6. Dosen LK, Haye R. Nasal septal perforation 1981-2005: changes in etiology, gender and size. *BMC Ear Nose Throat Disord.* 2007;7:1.
7. Murray A, McGarry GW. The clinical value of septal perforation biopsy. *Clin Otolaryngol Allied Sci.* 2000;25:107–109.
8. Grutzenmacher S, Mlynski R, Lang C, et al. The nasal airflow in noses with septal perforation: a model study. *ORL J Otorhinolaryngol Relat Spec.* 2005;67:142–147.
9. Lindemann J, Leiacker R, Stehmer V, et al. Intranasal temperature and humidity profile in patients with nasal septal perforation before and after surgical closure. *Clin Otolaryngol Allied Sci.* 2001;26:433–437.
10. Bhattacharyya N. Clinical symptomatology and paranasal sinus involvement with nasal septal perforation. *Laryngoscope.* 2007;117:691–694.
11. Facer GW, Kern EB. Nasal septal perforations: use of Silastic button in 108 patients. *Rhinology.* 1979;17:115–120.
12. Blind A, Hulterstrom A, Berggren D. Treatment of nasal septal perforations with a custom-made prosthesis. *Eur Arch Otorhinolaryngol.* 2009;266(1):65-69.
13. Kridel RW. Considerations in the etiology, treatment, and repair of septal perforations. *Fac Plast Surg Clin North Am.* 2004;12:435–450, vi.
14. De Witt WS. A new method for closure of small to medium-size nasoseptal perforations. *Ear Nose Throat J.* 2007;86:226–229.
15. Shikowitz MJ. Vascularized mucoperiosteal pull through flap for closure of large septal perforation: a new technique. *Laryngoscope.* 2007;117:750–755.
16. Friedman M, Ibrahim H, Ramakrishnan V. Inferior turbinate flap for repair of nasal septal perforation. *Laryngoscope.* 2003;113:1425–1428.
17. Vuyk HD, Versluis RJ. The inferior turbinate flap for closure of septal perforations. *Clin Otolaryngol Allied Sci.* 1988;13:53–57.

18. Sarandeses-Garcia A, Sulsenti G, Lopez-Amado M, Martinez-Vidal J. Septal perforations closure utilizing the backwards extraction-reposition technique of the quadrangular cartilage. *J Laryngol Otol.* 1999;113:721–724.

19. Tardy ME Jr. "Practical suggestions on facial plastic surgery—how I do it." Sublabial mucosal flap: repair of septal perforations. *Laryngoscope.* 1977;87:275–278.

20. Heller JB, Gabbay JS, Trussler A, et al. Repair of large nasal septal perforations using facial artery musculomucosal (FAMM) flap. *Ann Plast Surg.* 2005;55:456–459.

21. Kogan L, Gilbey P, Samet A, Talmon Y. Nasal septal perforation repair using oral mucosal flaps. *Isr Med Assoc J.* 2007;9:373–375.

22. Meyer R. Nasal septal perforations must and can be closed. *Aesthetic Plast Surg.* 1994;18:345–355.

23. Paloma V, Samper A, Cervera-Paz FJ. Surgical technique for reconstruction of the nasal septum: the pericranial flap. *Head Neck.* 2000;22:90–94.

24. Mobley SR, Boyd JB, Astor FC. Repair of a large septal perforation with a radial forearm free flap: brief report of a case. *Ear Nose Throat J.* 2001;80:512.

25. Murrell GL, Karakla DW, Messa A. Free flap repair of septal perforation. *Plast Reconstr Surg.* 1998;102:818–821.

26. Pedroza F, Patrocinio LG, Arevalo O. A review of 25-year experience of nasal septal perforation repair. *Arch Facial Plast Surg.* 2007;9:12–18.

27. Mola F, Keskin G, Ozturk M, Muezzinoglu B. The comparison of acellular dermal matric (Alloderm), Dacron, Gore-Tex, and autologous cartilage graft materials in an experimental animal model for nasal septal repair surgery. *Am J Rhinol.* 2007;21:330–334.

28. Ambro BT, Zimmerman J, Rosenthal M, Pribitkin EA. Nasal septal perforation repair with porcine small intestinal submucosa. *Arch Facial Plast Surg.* 2003;5:528–529.

29. Pribitkin EA, Ambro BT, Bloeden E, O'Hara BJ. Rabbit ear cartilage regeneration with a small intestinal submucosa graft. *Laryngoscope.* 2004;114:1–19.

CHAPTER THIRTY-EIGHT

Repair of Acute Nasal Fracture

Rami K. Batniji • Kamal A. Batniji

The nasal bones are the most commonly fractured bones in the face. Acute nasal fractures may result in both nasal deformity and nasal airway obstruction. However, some controversy still surrounds the management of acute nasal fractures, in that a review of the literature demonstrates a lack of consensus with respect to the timing of repair of the acute nasal fracture, the anesthesia used during repair, and the type of procedure performed. Furthermore, post-reduction nasal deformities reportedly requiring subsequent rhinoplasty or septorhinoplasty range from 14% to 50%.

A thorough history of the mechanism of injury and a detailed physical examination provide the surgeon with information to adequately decide how to treat the acute nasal fracture, with special attention dedicated to the septum as improper reduction of the injured septum is the usual cause for the high incidence of postreduction nasal deformities. In this chapter, we review the management of the acute nasal fracture.

INCIDENCE

Nasal bones are the most commonly fractured bones in the face. While reports estimate the annual incidence of nasal fractures in the United States as 52,000, the actual number may be higher for a variety of reasons, including the fact that severely traumatized patients with life-threatening injuries may concurrently present with nasal fractures that go unrecognized.[1] The mechanism of injury is usually blunt trauma and can be attributed to assault, motor vehicle accidents, a fall, or a sports-related injury.[2] Previous nasal surgery may have an impact on the incidence of acute nasal fracture[3]; a patient who undergoes rhinoplasty is at an increased risk of nasal fracture, particularly within the first year following the rhinoplasty procedure.[3]

Nasal fractures in the pediatric population may be overlooked. The pediatric nose is mostly cartilaginous and the nasal bones are small; therefore, the pediatric nose is softer and more compliant, therefore being less likely to sustain displacement than the adult nose when fractured. Despite these attributes, pediatric nasal fractures do occur. A review of the pediatric facial fractures in the National

Trauma Data Bank demonstrated a 30.2% incidence of nasal fractures in children and adolescent trauma patients (aged 0 to 18 years).[4] The most common mechanisms of injury are motor vehicle collisions, violence, falls, and sports-related injuries. Another potential cause of nasal fracture in the pediatric population is birth trauma. Birth trauma, from intrauterine forces, breech delivery, or forceps-assisted delivery, may result in congenital deviation of the nasal septum.[5] Although these deviations can be treated easily, expeditiously, and usually without complication in the neonatal period, the identification of a deviated septum can be overlooked. The pediatric nose is very susceptible to septal hematoma following blunt trauma. Unfortunately, childhood nasal trauma is often underappreciated and nasal fracture and/or septal injury is overlooked, resulting in external and internal nasal deformities in adulthood.

MECHANISM OF INJURY

Murray's seminal work in detailing the pathophysiology of nasal bone fractures in fresh cadaver specimens provided valuable insight into the mechanism of injury for nasal trauma.[6] Nasal fractures are most commonly due to a lateral force; this results in two fracture lines running parallel on the ipsilateral thin nasal bone along the dorsum, meeting at the junction of the thick and thin bones (Figure 38-1). In this type of injury, the nose may appear deviated due to the depression of the unilateral bony fragment.

A frontal force must be of greater magnitude to produce a nasal fracture because the nasal bones are buttressed by the frontal process of the maxilla, the nasal spine, and the perpendicular plate of the ethmoid. The resultant injury includes not only a nasal bone fracture (which may be comminuted) but also a C-shaped fracture in the septum extending from just beneath the dorsum of the nose, inferiorly and posteriorly through the perpendicular plate of the ethmoid and curving anteriorly to the inferior cartilaginous septum near the maxillary crest and the angle of the vomer. Frequently, the inferior end of the septum becomes dislodged from its groove and is deflected obliquely into the nasal cavity (Figure 38-2). As a result,

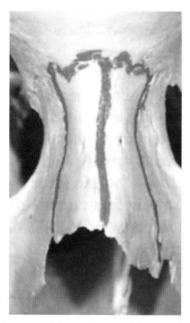

Figure 38-1 The nasal bones. The nasal bony vault is pyramidal in shape and forms the upper third of the nose. The nasal bony vault consists of the paired nasal bones and the ascending frontal process of the maxilla. The nasal bones are thicker and more dense superiorly and are progressively thinner inferiorly. There is a transition zone of relatively thin bone along the frontal processes of the maxilla from the piriform aperture to the radix along the lateral nasal wall.

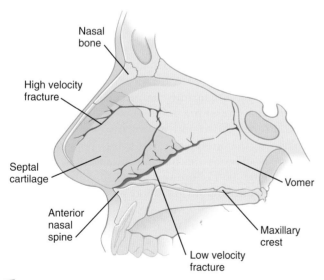

Figure 38-2 The nasal septum and patterns of septal fractures. The septal (aka quadrangular cartilage) articulates with the anterior nasal spine caudally, the perpendicular plate of the ethmoid posteriorly, and the vomer inferiorly; the vomer articulates with the maxillary and palatine crests. The septal cartilage typically rests along a groove at the midline; this is known as the vomerine groove. The most common septal fracture is along this junction between the vomerine groove and quadrangular cartilage. A high-velocity injury or frontal impact can result in a more extensive septal fracture through the thin central region of the septal cartilage and extending to the bony cartilaginous junction.

the ala and nostril on the deflected side can become widened, while the opposite side can become flattened and narrowed.

A high-impact frontal force injury to the nose, such as that sustained during a motor vehicle collision, may produce comminuted or compound nasal fractures. If a patient sustains this type of injury, one must rule out a nasal orbital ethmoid (NOE) complex fracture after the cervical spine, skull, and ophthalmic injuries are cleared. Signs of NOE complex fractures include telecanthus, epiphora, periorbital emphysema, clear rhinorrhea secondary to cerebrospinal fluid leak, and a flattened nasofrontal root. Surgeons should have a low threshold for requesting a noncontrast computed tomography (CT) scan of the facial skeleton if the slightest clinical suspicion for an orbital or facial fracture arises. Further work-up and management of NOE injuries are beyond the scope of this chapter.

DIAGNOSIS

Identification of a nasal fracture is primarily a clinical diagnosis and plain radiographs are rarely, if ever, necessary. Patients may experience epistaxis, edema, ecchymosis, and nasal obstruction. Upon palpation, tenderness, crepitus, and step-off deformities may be appreciated. An obvious deformity may be appreciated, such as a conspicuous concavity or convexity of the nasal bones resulting in a twisted nose appearance. In the acute setting, evidence of nasal deformity may be hidden secondary to the masquerading effects of edema.

Avulsion of the upper lateral cartilage attachments may also result in a concave appearance of the middle third of the nose. The cephalic portion of the upper lateral cartilage is attached to the caudal border of the nasal bone. The medial portion of the upper lateral cartilage is attached to the dorsal cartilaginous septum; this attachment constitutes the internal nasal valve and has been described as a 10- to 15-degree angle on intranasal examination.[7] Placement of a cotton-tipped applicator in the region of the internal nasal valve with subsequent improvement in nasal airway obstruction confirms the diagnosis of internal nasal valve collapse. Closed reduction of the fractured nasal bone may reapproximate the avulsed upper lateral cartilage to the caudal border of the nasal bone. However, avulsion of the upper lateral cartilage from the dorsal cartilaginous septum may require placement of a spreader graft to address the concavity of the middle third of the nose as well as improve nasal function by reconstituting the internal nasal valve.[8]

Intranasal examination should be performed after decongesting the nasal cavities. Topical oxymetazoline is effective and, when mixed with 4% topical lidocaine, can achieve both decongestion and anesthesia. Intranasal examination is performed to evaluate the status of the septum and identify mucosal injuries. If a bulge is appreciated along the septum, this may signify a septal hematoma. If a septal hematoma is suspected, a helpful maneuver is to palpate the intranasal bulge with a cotton-tipped applicator and, if compressible, a fine needle aspiration can be performed. In the pediatric patient, the nose tends to buckle and twist rather than fracture. As such, there is a higher incidence of separation of the perichondrium from the septal cartilage and subsequent potential for hematoma formation. Digital photodocumentation of the resulting nasal deformity can be obtained for the medical record.

TREATMENT

TIMING OF REPAIR

Some controversy surrounds timing of repair for the acute nasal fracture. Edema follows shortly after the initial injury, making it difficult to allow for precise reduction. Therefore, it is best to institute conservative measures to minimize edema and allow for proper analysis of potential deformity 3 to 5 days after injury.[9] These conservative measures include a soft diet, head-of-bed elevation, and the application of an ice compress to the area of injury. Definitive treatment can be carried out 5 to 12 days after the initial injury. During this period, the fractured components of the nasal bone can be easily manipulated. However, if definitive treatment is delayed beyond this time period, fibrosis may result in decreased mobility of the nasal bones, making the closed reduction of the nasal bone fracture more challenging.

ANESTHESIA

Another area of controversy in the management of the acute nasal fracture is the type of anesthesia administered during the surgical repair.[10] Local anesthesia with intravenous sedation, for instance, minimizes the potential risks of general anesthesia, such as nausea. General anesthesia, however, provides the benefit of a controlled airway as well as the opportunity for uncompromised nasal examination, reduction, and manipulation. Typically, a topical vasoconstrictive agent such as oxymetazoline or 4% liquid cocaine is applied to cottonoid pledgets and placed in the nasal passageway to minimize bleeding while a local anesthetic, such as 1% lidocaine with 1 : 100,000 epinephrine, provides more robust anesthesia and vasoconstriction.

Several factors should be weighed when deciding between local or general anesthesia for the management of nasal fractures. The first consideration is the patient's airway. If the surgeon anticipates significant bleeding following reduction of the nasal fracture, then the surgeon should consider the use of a short-acting general anesthetic while the airway is secured and protected.

Another consideration is the severity of the nasal fracture, as well as the presence of an associated septal fracture. Since one of the most common causes for persistent nasal deformity following closed reduction of a nasal fracture includes unrecognized septal fracture or inadequate reduction, the surgeon should consider the use of a short-acting general anesthetic to properly address the causes of the nasal deformity.[11] Pediatric patients should undergo reduction of the nasal fracture under general anesthesia since they are not able to comply with local anesthesia. Finally, patient comfort should also be considered when making this decision. While some patients may tolerate reduction of nasal fracture under local anesthesia, other patients may prefer a short-acting general anesthetic.

CLOSED REDUCTION OF ACUTE NASAL BONE FRACTURE

The authors prefer the use of the Boies elevator to perform closed reduction of acute nasal bone fractures. The Boies elevator is placed intranasally and the impacted nasal bone is reduced, thus restoring the nasal length. The thumb of the contralateral hand is placed over the nasal bone externally to palpate subtle osseous movements (Figure 38-3). If the impacted nasal bone is locked under the ascending process of the maxilla, the Boies elevator is used in an upward and outward motion to reduce the fractured nasal bone; the instrument must not be inserted too deeply, as it may rest under the nasal process of the frontal bone and will be of no value. An external splint is always used. Additionally, in an effort to minimize the possibility of repeat impaction of the recently reduced nasal bone, an internal nasal splint could also be used in the form of nasal packing. A small amount of absorbable packing (Gelfoam; Pfizer) covered with antibiotic ointment strategically positioned intranasally along the medial aspect of the nasal bone usually suffices in maintaining the position of the reduced nasal bone; at the same time, this is well tolerated by the patient and does not require removal given its dissolvable nature. While a variety of dorsal nasal splints are available, the authors prefer the use of PS® Thermoplatic Nasal Splint (Aquaplast Corp., Wyckoff, NJ). First, liquid adhesive (Mastisol®, Ferndale Laboratories, Inc., Ferndale, MI) is applied to the skin. Then, the soft tissues of the nose are taped using ¼-inch paper tape; taping begins at the supratip break to drape the soft tissue in this location intimately to the underlying skeleton. Strips of different lengths are then applied in a transverse fashion over the nose, avoiding excessive pressure. The Aquaplast splint is then applied. The external dorsal splint remains in place for 1 week.

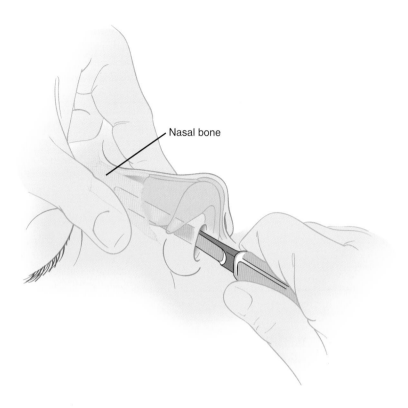

Nasal bone

Figure 38-3 Reduction of nasal fracture. The Boies elevator is placed intranasally. The surgeon's contralateral thumb is used to palpate the nasal bone to ensure adequate reduction.

REPAIR OF SEPTAL FRACTURE

If the septum is deviated, it can be reduced with either an Asch forceps or the Boies elevator to relocate the displaced base to the midline. Following this, the septum should be reevaluated to ensure that proper reduction is achieved. If the septum remains posteriorly displaced or irreducible, then the authors proceed with an open approach to the septum via a hemitransfixion incision. Once bilateral mucoperichondrial flaps are elevated, complete visualization of the septum provides the opportunity to properly identify the extent of the septal injury. In the authors' experience, a small hematoma may be identified at the bony–cartilaginous junction; this is evacuated with suction. If the inferior aspect of the quadrangular cartilage remains dislodged from the vomerine groove, an inferior strip of quandrangular cartilage can be resected, the septum can be repositioned into the vomerine groove in a swinging door fashion, and a figure-of-eight suture with 5-0 Monocryl can be used to keep the posterior caudal septum attached to the anterior septal spine in the midline. Once the hemitransfixion incision is reapproximated using interrupted 5-0 plain gut sutures, internal nasal septal splints are placed. Silicone septal splints are favored to ensure atraumatic placement and removal. Prophylactic gram-positive antibiotic coverage (typically cephalexin) is prescribed following surgical repair and is continued until the silicone splints are removed on postoperative day 7 (Figure 38-4).

IMMEDIATE SEPTORHINOPLASTY

In the literature, some authors advocate an open approach to the nasal pyramid at the time of initial repair using accepted rhinoplasty techniques, including rasping, osteotomies, and cartilaginous resection or augmentation of the dorsum.[12] However, due to the numerous existing variables involved in an acute nasal fracture such as irregularity and/or comminution, the nasal bones may not be easily controlled via the external approach. Also, the healing process and unavoidable fibrosis following surgical repair of the acute nasal fracture may cause shifts in the nasal structures. Ultimately, the absence of a detailed and elective preoperative consultation with the inherent imposition of a time-pressured decision for surgery may generate a series of expectations and obscure the transparency required in the patient's personal decision to go through an elective aesthetic procedure. Therefore, for patients with acute nasal fractures who are interested in cosmetic septorhinoplasty, it behooves both the surgeon and patient to consider delaying treatment for at least a few months for selected cases. However, it is clear that changes will continue to evolve until approximately 1 year after any given traumatic injury.[13]

REPAIR OF THE PEDIATRIC NASAL FRACTURE

While it is unclear whether disruption of the human pediatric septal growth center affects the development of the

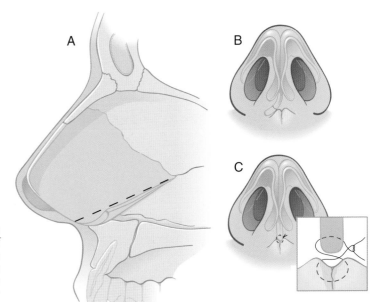

Figure 38-4 Reduction of septal fracture. Adequate exposure to the fractured septum is achieved via a hemitransfixion incision. If the septal fracture is along the junction between the vomerine groove and quadrangular cartilage, a strip of cartilage can be removed (shown in *red*) and the cartilage repositioned within the vomerine groove. A figure-of-eight suture anchors the quadrangular cartilage caudally to the anterior nasal spine at the midline.

nose, there is clear evidence to support the importance of such growth centers in animal models.[14] Therefore, closed reduction is the preferred method of treatment of acute nasal fracture in the pediatric population. To facilitate a thorough examination and complete reduction, general anesthesia is used for the pediatric patient. The technique for closed reduction is similar to that previously described. However, there are a few caveats. For example, internal splinting is typically performed with light absorbable packing such as Gelfoam, thus obviating the need for removal during the postoperative period. Finally, the guardians of the pediatric patient should be properly counseled with respect to the possibility of the child developing delayed nasal deviation and obstruction and may therefore be informed of the possibility of a formal septorhinoplasty in the future.

COMPLICATIONS

Potential complications following repair of the acute nasal fracture include, among other possibilities, epistaxis and septal hematoma. Epistaxis is usually self-limiting; however, if persistent, oxymetazoline nasal spray, head-of-bed elevation, and the application of a cold compress can be used to decrease or stop bleeding. If a septal hematoma is appreciated in the postoperative period, it is dealt with in a manner similar to that described earlier in this chapter. Posttraumatic nasal deformity following reduction efforts is another potential complication. A review of the medical literature demonstrates this

complication ranges from 14% to 50%.[15] Further analysis of these data suggests the possible reason for such a high complication rate is the use of closed techniques to repair the fractured nasal bone, failing to address septal injuries. Indeed, Rohrich and Adams demonstrated a much smaller rate of 9% for posttraumatic nasal deformity following reduction efforts when the septum is properly evaluated and open treatment of the septum is performed when indicated.[16]

CONCLUSION

A detailed history, including the mechanism of injury and a thorough physical examination, provides important information in the treatment of acute nasal fractures. Soft tissue edema, which inevitably accompanies acute nasal fractures, may limit the physical examination; therefore, the decision for definitive therapy should be delayed until the edema has resolved and any underlying acquired nasal deformity can be fully appreciated. It is important to identify and treat septal hematoma early in the process. Definitive treatment should not be delayed beyond 2 weeks as fibrosis will settle in, making mobilization of the fractured nasal bones more difficult. While there are different methods to reduce and treat acute nasal fractures, it is important not to overlook the septum, addressing any existing deviations or fractures at the same time as the fractured nasal bones to minimize the incidence of postreduction nasal deformities requiring subsequent surgical interventions (Figures 38-5 and 38-6).

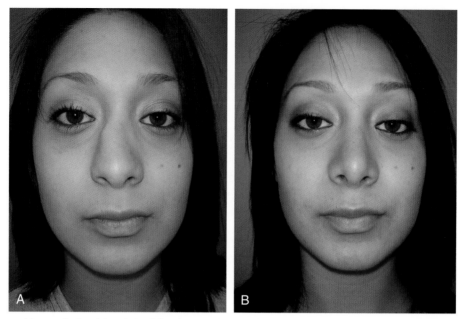

Figure 38-5 Acute nasal fracture before (**A**) and after (**B**) reduction of nasal bone and septal fracture, 1 year postoperatively.

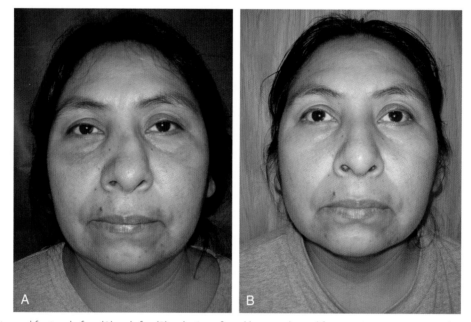

Figure 38-6 Acute nasal fracture before (**A**) and after (**B**) reduction of nasal bone and septal fracture, 1 year postoperatively.

REFERENCES

1. Perkins SW, Dayan SH. Management of nasal trauma. *Aesthet Plast Surg.* 2002;26(Suppl 1):S3.
2. Erdman D, Follmar KE, Debruijin M, et al. A retrospective analysis of facial fracture etiologies. *Ann Plast Surg.* 2008;60(4):398–403.
3. Guyuron B. Does rhinoplasty make the nose more susceptible to fracture? *Plast Reconstr Surg.* 1994;93(2):313–317.
4. Imahara SD, Hopper RA, Wang J, et al. Patterns and outcomes of pediatric facial fractures in the United States:

a survey of the National Trauma Data Bank. *J Am Coll Surg.* 2008;207(5):710–716.
5. Hughes CA, Harley EH, Milmore G, et al. Birth trauma in the head and neck. *Arch Otolaryngol Head Neck Surg.* 1999;125(2):193–199.
6. Murray JA, Maran AG, Busuttil A, et al. A pathological classification of nasal fractures. *Injury.* 1986;17(5):338–344.
7. Howard BK, Rohrich RJ, Landecker A. Nasal physiology. In: Gunter JP, Rohrich RJ, Adams WP, eds. *Dallasrhinoplasty.* St. Louis: Quality Medical Publishing; 2007:29–39.
8. Teichgraeber JF, Wainwright DJ. The treatment of nasal valve obstruction. *Plast Reconstr Surg.* 1994;93:1174–1182.

9. Fischer H, Gubisch W. Nasal valves: importance and surgical procedures. *Fac Plast Surg.* 2006;22:266–280.

10. Ridder GJ, Boedeker CC, Fradis M, et al. Technique and timing for closed reduction of isolated nasal fractures: a retrospective study. *Ear Nose Throat J.* 2002;81(1): 49–54.

11. Khwaja S, Pahade AV, Luff D, et al. Nasal fracture reduction: local versus general anesthesia. *Rhinology.* 2007;45(1):838.

12. Rohrich RJ, Adams WP. Nasal fracture management: minimized secondary nasal deformities. *Plast Reconstr Surg.* 2000;106(2):266–273.

13. Reilly MJ, Davison SP. Open vs closed approach to the nasal pyramid for fracture reduction. *Arch Fac Plast Surg.* 2007;9(2):82–86.

14. Renner GJ. Management of nasal fractures. *Otolaryngol Clin North Am.* 1991;24(1):195–213.

15. Sarnat BG. Normal and abnormal growth at the nasoseptovomeral region. *Ann Otol Rhinol Laryngol.* 1991;100(6):508–515.

16. Rohrich RJ, Adams WP: Acute nasal fracture management: minimizing secondary deformities. In: Gunter JP, Rohrich RJ, Adams WP, editors. *Dallas rhinoplasty.* St Louis: Quality Medical Publishing; 2007:957–971.

Index

The letter t indicates a table, b indicates a box, and f indicates a figure.

Skin–soft tissue envelope *(Continued)*
incisions and elevation of, in secondary rhinoplasty via external approach, 94
in Mestizo patients, 397–398
in Middle Eastern patients, 387–388, 389t
in primary open structure rhinoplasty, 60, 60f, 62, 77
skeletal framework and, 339
stretching of, 339
surgical thinning of, 341
swelling of, 77
tautness of, 339
thickness of, 324–325. *See also* Thick skin
thinness of, 36, 328–329. *See also* Thin skin
tip appearance affected by, 324–325
variations in, 337
Sleep habits, 31–32
Smith, Edward, 1
Social history, 31
Soft tissue fillers, 219
Soft tissue thickening, broadened lobule secondary to, 254–256, 255f–256f
Soft tissue triangles, 22f
Splints, 72–77, 291, 481
Split calvarial bone grafts, 203
Split-thickness skin grafts, 456–458
Spreader grafts, 162–163, 391f–392f
alar, 240, 242f
autospreader grafts, 162f, 163, 164f
bilateral, 401f, 422
creation of, 163
crooked nose corrected with, 291
endonasal approach for placement of, 163, 422
extended, 163, 291, 348, 360–361
external approach for placement of, 163, 163f
flaring sutures and, 163
goals of, 307
horizontal, 162f, 163, 165f, 391f–392f
internal nasal valve narrowing corrected with, 452
inverted-V deformity corrected with, 126
middle nasal vault narrowing corrected with, 422
nasal asymmetry corrected with, 164f
pinched nasal tip deformity correction using, 240, 242f
placement of, 163, 163f
saddle nose deformity corrected with, 294–295, 294f
secondary rhinoplasty use of, 95, 96f
"shim," 289
stabilization uses of, 310
transcartilaginous approach for placement of, 110
types of, 162f
Staff
involvement by, 52
patient dissatisfaction handled by, 52

Stucker, Fred, 16, 17f
Subcognitive perception, 46
Sublabial flaps, 474
Superficial musculoaponeurotic system
anatomy of, 25, 32, 161, 327, 337–338, 350, 374f, 456
debulking technique, 341–343, 342f
Superior turbinates, 447
Supraalar crease, 22f
Supratip
bunching sutures, 252f
debulked, 365f
deficiencies of, 248–249
edema of, 409
fullness of, 174f, 176, 178f
saddle deformity, 311f
Sushruta, 1, 455
Suture techniques
asymmetric lobule corrected with, 256
crooked nose corrected with, 291
double-dome, 256
pinched lobule caused by, 253–254
Suture tiplasty, 183
Suture-based tip modifications, 250–251
algorithm for, 184–186
case examples of, 189, 191f–192f
columella-septal suture, 188–193, 189f–190f
hemitransdomal suture, 184–186, 185f–186f, 193f
history of, 183
improvements in, 183
intercrural suture, 189, 190f, 252f
interdomal suture, 186–187, 187f
intraoperative delayed suture effect, 184
lateral crural mattress suture, 187–188, 188f
in Mestizo patients, 404–406, 406f
models used in, 183, 184f
principles of, 183–184
sutures, 184
transdomal suture, 186–189, 186f, 404–406
"Swinging door" maneuver, 63f, 286–287, 450f, 451

T

Tagliacotian method, 2
Tagliacozzi, Gasparo, 1, 225
Tardy, M. Eugene, 13–14, 13f, 17–18, 18f
Teaching
at Chicago, 12–14
history of, 9–14, 16
at Iowa, 12
Temporalis fascia, 329, 330f, 376–377, 377f, 380–381
"Tension" nose deformity, 36–37, 38f
Thick skin
adverse healing characteristics of, 339–340
anatomy of, 337–338
cartilage framework in, 338–339
description of, 337
disadvantages of, 337

Thick skin *(Continued)*
healing of, 339–340
perioperative management of, 340
physical limitations of, 338–339
skeletal augmentation, 340–341
surgery in patients with
case example of, 344f
compression dressings used after, 343
postoperative steroid treatments, 343
thinning procedures, 341
swelling of, 339–340
thin skin versus, 337–338
Thin skin
adjunctive techniques in, 334–335
aging related, 328
augmentation strategies for, 329–330
bossae in, 331–334, 332f–333f
camouflage strategies for, 329–330
considerations for, 328–329
crooked nose in patients with, 287f
description of, 337
disease-related, 328
lateral crural strut grafts in, 330, 332f
maintenance of, 334–335, 334f
margin of error for, 328
naturally, 327–328
parchment, 328–329
refinements, 334–335, 334f
"shrink wrap" effect, 328, 331
skin–soft tissue envelope elevation and protection, 329
structural correction strategies in, 329–330
technical considerations for, 329–335
thick skin versus, 337–338
types of, 327–328
3:4:5 triangle, 300, 301f
Tip
in African Americans, 369
anatomic determinants of, 169, 245–247, 313, 314f–315f
bifid, 86–87, 88f
blood supply to, 342f
bossae of. *See* Bossae
boxy, 86–87, 88f
broad, 86, 87f, 191f–192f
bulbous, 86–87, 88f, 429f
defining points, 22f–24f, 308, 348–349, 362
dynamics of, 245–247, 246f
foreshortening of, 360
lower lateral cartilage, effects on appearance of, 169
in men, 299
modifications of. *See* Tip modifications
narrowing of, 253–254
palpation of, 39
parenthesis, 241
physical examination of, 282
scarring of, 256f
shape of, 38–39
skin–soft tissue envelope, effect on appearance of, 324–325
support of, 25–27, 27t, 317, 317t